AIDS Vaccine Research and Clinical Trials

AIDS Vaccine Research and Clinical Trials

edited by

Scott D. Putney

Repligen, Inc.
Cambridge, Massachusetts

Dani P. Bolognesi

Duke University Medical Center
Durham, North Carolina

Marcel Dekker, Inc. **New York and Basel**

Library of Congress Cataloging-in-Publication Data

AIDS vaccine research and clinical trials/edited by Scott D. Putney,
   Dani P. Bolognesi.
         p. cm.
   Includes bibliographical references.
   ISBN 0-8247-8221-6 (alk. paper)
   1. AIDS vaccines. 2. Clinical trials. I. Putney, Scott D.
   II. Bolognesi, Dani.
   [DNLM: 1. Acquired Immunodeficiency Syndrome—prevention &
control. 2. Clinical trials. 3. HIV—immunology. 4. Immunity,
Cellular. 5. Vaccines. WD 308 A28876]
   QR189.5.A33A36 1989
   616.97'9205—dc20
   DNLM/DLC
   for Library of Congress   90-2703
                                                                 CIP

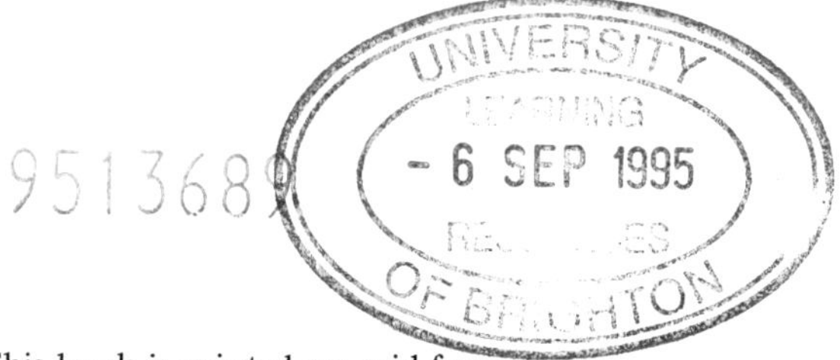

This book is printed on acid-free paper.

Marcel Dekker, Inc.
270 Madison Avenue, New York, New York 10016

Current printing (last digit):
10 9 8 7 6 5 4 3 2 1

Printed in the United States of America

FOREWORD

Vaccination is the only approach that has been successful in arresting or preventing epidemic diseases caused by viruses. From Jenner's discovery that bovine vaccinia virus, a less virulent relative of smallpox virus, could be used to produce lasting immunity against smallpox to the recent advances in vaccination against poliovirus, herpes viruses, hepatitis, and rabies, immunizing preparations have consisted either of attenuated virus strains or of inactivated viruses or their fragments or subunits. The hope of discovering magic bullets such as have been successful in combating bacterial pathogens is likely to be in vain. Bacterial parasites consist themselves of cells; any difference in cellular organization or metabolism is a potential target for some magic bullet, such as the bacterial cell wall synthesis to the penicillins or the requirements for precursors of folic acid that bacteria cannot take up fully formed.

Viruses are not cells; they are parasites at the genetic level, bringing into the cells a genetic apparatus that is directed to producing more virus. Vaccination is the hope for control of the HIV virus, the cause of AIDS. *AIDS Vaccine Research and Clinical Trials* brings together papers on HIV vaccines by leaders in this field of research. The editors are to be congratulated for having produced a useful and complete survey of this important branch of immunology.

Most diseases caused by viruses are epidemic. Clinical finding of persistent immunity to a virus as a result of having successfully overcome an attack of disease has often been the starting point of the search for protective vaccines. No such evidence for acquired immunity is available for HIV viruses. Vaccines consisting of chemically or physically inactivated virions have been tested, but no solid evidence yet exists for immunity to reinoculation in vaccinated human subjects.

Most explored has been the search for vaccines consisting of noninfectious peptides derived from the virus proteins. Some of these peptides retain immunogenic activity and elicit neutralizing antibodies in laboratory animals as well as in macaque monkeys and in chimpanzees.

The search for such immunogenic peptides is guided by the known properties and life course of the HIV viruses. The major protein of the viral envelope, gp160, carries several immunogenic sequences and so does its split product, gp120. Other amino acid sequences serve to bind the virion, still intact, to a protein called CD4 present on the surface of lymphocytes and other infectable cells. More steps follow, which lead to fusion of cell and virus membranes and entry of the virus core. Then other viral gene products are excised from a viral polyprotein and initiate reproduction of the virus. The enzyme reverse transcriptase transcribes the RNA viral genome into a DNA molecule that is then integrated into the cellular genome. Then the DNA is reproduced and also transcribed into RNA for the new virions. The cell surface becomes coated with gp160 protein and can fuse with the membrane of uninfected cells and thereby spread the infection by cell-to-cell contact.

Conceivably, inhibitors of viral enzymes such as reverse transcriptase could be used to arrest the infection. AZT, an analog of thymidine, has limited effects on the course of AIDS, but more powerful inhibitors have not yet been found. The search for vaccines continues to be the most promising approach. Most candidate immunogens are specific fragments of the envelope protein that alone, or with adjuvants, elicit virus-neutralizing antibodies in animals. Such immunogenic activity has been reported for peptides corresponding to different regions of gp160. Especially promising is a sequence of 35 amino acids that form a loop in the viral envelope protein and correspond to one of the hypervariable regions of the virus, that is, a region where field strains of virus exhibit a high degree of different amino acid sequences. The neutralizing antibodies elicited in animals by peptides from this loop are directed specifically to the viral variant from which the peptide is derived. The hypervariability of the viral sequences may be due to selection for mutants resistant to antibodies. It should be possible to construct broad-range peptides that elicit antibodies to a majority of the virus variants present in a population.

Production of neutralizing antibodies is not the only immune response. It occurs when lymphocytes of T4+ cells are stimulated by antigens presented in association with class II histocompatibility proteins. Another class of lymphocytes called T8+ is stimulated by antigen presented with class I MHC proteins and generates a cytolytic response. Both kinds of responses to envelope peptides have been reported.

These and other recent findings reported in *AIDS Vaccine Research and Clinical Trials* raise our hopes that an effective vaccine may become available relatively soon. A major limitation, of course, will remain. The efficacy of vaccines will have to be tested in humans. When an effective vaccine against HIV becomes available, new problems will have to be faced. HIV is not an epidemic virus that spreads like polio or smallpox through entire populations by contact or by excreta. In the United States and in other advanced industrial countries, the virus is spread by unprotected sexual contact or direct blood transfer. Populations within a given society can be roughly, and with significant exceptions, classified as "at risk" or "not at risk." The population at risk will presumably be eager to be vaccinated. Those not at risk may choose to avoid vaccination if it leaves them permanently marked by a seropositive reaction.

In some countries, the AIDS virus is said to be so widespread that a majority of individuals may soon test seropositive. For such situations what is needed is something more than a vaccine. A search for therapeutic intervention by a special class of vaccines should be vigorously pursued. Finding an immunotherapeutic agent is not a priori impossible, but it will require a more intimate understanding of the course of the HIV disease, especially of the events that maintain the seropositive state for years and those that prompt a transition from the asymptomatic to the fully manifested AIDS.

Salvador E. Luria, M.D.
Nobel Laureate in Medicine (1969)
Institute Professor Emeritus
Massachusetts Institute of Technology
Cambridge, Massachusetts

PREFACE

Because vaccination will be the most simple, cost-effective, safe, and efficacious means to prevent and control the spread of AIDS, many laboratories (academic, government, and corporate) are actively engaged in the development and testing of HIV vaccine prototypes. The triumphs of the smallpox and polio vaccines are of landmark proportions, and major advances have also been achieved in the control through vaccination of such diseases as yellow fever, measles, mumps, and rubella. More recently, impressive strides have been made in the development of vaccines against more complex viruses such as hepatitis B. Because HIV is a retrovirus, because it rapidly varies the amino acid sequence of the envelope and other immune targets (discussed in Chapter 5), because readily available animal models for infection and disease do not exist (discussed in Chapters 13–19) and because clinical trials may be difficult, development of an HIV vaccine will be more formidable than for these other viruses. In this book we bring together reports and summaries from the leading researchers involved in this effort. These review progress in understanding the virus and its interactions with host target cells, the identification of target epitopes for humoral and cellular immune responses to the virus, tests that have been conducted on animal models with candidate immunogens, and the initial trials in humans.

Until recently, the science of vaccinology has been largely empirical and based on trial and error using various attenuated or inactivated formulations of the disease-causing organism (this approach for HIV is discussed in Chapter 12). The use of subunit vaccines consisting of selected components of the virus has only recently been pioneered, and their relative efficacy is still being evaluated. The underlying principles of vaccination remain poorly understood in spite of the successes that have been achieved. The morbidity and mortality associated with HIV infection, together with the unique properties of this virus, imply that novel vaccine approaches will have to be developed. Recently, some of the barriers hindering HIV vaccine development have been eroding and these advances come from the identification of important immunological targets on the virus and the infected cell and the recent demonstration of efficacy of inactivated retroviral and lentiviral vaccines.

The latter studies come from Desrosiers, Murphy-Corb, Gardner, Montelaro, and Chesebro. In these studies, immunization with inactivated simian immunodeficiency virus (SIV) (discussed in Chapters 4, 16, 17, and 18), equine infectious anemia virus (EIAV) (Chapter 13), or Friend murine leukemia virus (Chapter 14) was able to delay or prevent onset of disease. In the case of SIV and EIAV, prevention of disease was noted even when infection was not prevented. If this principle applies to HIV, it may not be necessary to completely prevent infection to have an efficacious vaccine as long as the immunity is able to clear viral infection (as is the case with other vaccines).

Although useful during preclinical development, inactivated virus vaccines may not be as attractive as subunit vaccines that consist of protective immune determinants. Numerous advances have been made to define these targets on HIV, and a large part of this book focuses on this work. Advances have been made in the discovery of several neutralizing epitopes (Chapters 1 and 19), T-cell epitopes (some of which are targets for cytotoxic lymphocytes) (Chapters 6 and 8), and regions of the envelope that binds antibodies that mediate antibody-dependent cellular cytotoxicity (ADCC) (Chapter 7).

All this work is crucial because it strongly suggests that a vaccine for HIV can be developed and points to the type of immunity and determinants that will be used to derive effective vaccine prototypes. One must recognize, however, that only human clinical trials can guarantee a successful vaccine. Two vaccines are already being clinically tested after approval of the Food and Drug Administration (Chapters 9, 21, and 22); other candidates are being tested in Europe and Africa. Clearly, HIV vaccine clinical trials will rely on what was learned with the recombinant hepatitis B vaccine (Chapter 20) and additional issues will have to be faced (Chapter 23). Results of these trials have uncovered several key issues that illustrate that it is in this phase of development that HIV vaccines may face the greatest obstacles.

In summary, in spite of the recent progress, the challenges standing before the development of an HIV vaccine are prodigious. Ways to present HIV antigens to the human immune system to evoke and maintain protective humoral and cellular immunity are still being perfected. Much more has to be done to obtain safe and effective adjuvants or innocuous replicating vectors in which critical HIV target epitopes are incorporated. Also, more has to be learned about the role of secretory immunity in a protective response. By far the most formidable barrier, however, will be the evaluation of efficacy of a vaccine candidate in humans because of issues such as the low transmission rate of HIV infection in the population and the long and variable interval between infection and disease. As research produces more compelling vaccine candidates, such obstacles will hopefully be overcome.

Scott D. Putney
Dani P. Bolognesi

CONTENTS

Cellular Immune Response Relevant to Vaccine Development

Development of Vaccine Candidates

Animal Models for Vaccine Development and Efficacy Studies

Contents   xiii

CONTRIBUTORS

Gérard Agius, M.D. Laboratoire de Physiologie Cellulaire, Université P. et M. Curie, Paris, France

Daniel C. Anderson, D.V.M. Associate Research Professor, Yerkes Regional Primate Center, Emory University, Atlanta, Georgia

Noel Barrett, Ph.D. Head, Department of Virology, Biomedical Research Center, Immuno AG, Vienna, Austria

Jay A. Berzofsky, M.D., Ph.D. Chief, Molecular Immunogenetics and Vaccine Research Section, Metabolism Branch, National Cancer Institute, National Institutes of Health, Bethesda, Maryland

Dani P. Bolognesi, M.S., Ph.D. James B. Duke Professor, Department of Surgery, Duke University Medical Center, Durham, North Carolina

Kemp B. Cease, M.D. Assistant Professor, Department of Internal Medicine, University of Michigan Medical School, Ann Arbor, Michigan

Tran C. Chanh Scientist, Department of Virology and Immunology, Southwest Foundation for Biomedical Research, San Antonio, Texas

Bruce Chesebro, M.D. Chief, Laboratory of Persistent Viral Diseases, Rocky Mountain Laboratory, National Institute of Allergy and Infectious Diseases, National Institutes of Health, Hamilton, Montana

Janice E. Clements, Ph.D. Associate Professor, Department of Comparative Medicine, The Johns Hopkins University School of Medicine, Baltimore, Maryland

Sharon E. Crane, Ph.D. candidate Department of Molecular Biology and Genetics, The Johns Hopkins University School of Medicine, Baltimore, Maryland

Muthiah D. Daniel, D.V.M., Ph.D. Senior Research Associate, Division of Microbiology, New England Regional Primate Research Center, Harvard Medical School, Southborough, Massachusetts

Isabelle Desportes, Ph.D. Chargé de recherche au C.N.R.S., Laboratoire de Physiologie Cellulaire, Université P. et M. Curie, Paris, France

Ronald C. Desrosiers, Ph.D. Associate Professor, Microbiology and Molecular Genetics, Harvard Medical School, and Chairman, Division of Microbiology, New England Regional Primate Research Center, Southborough, Massachusetts

Friedrich Dorner, Ph.D. President, Division of Vaccines and Gene Products, Biomedical Research Center, Immuno AG, Vienna, Austria

Jorg W. Eichberg, D.V.M., Ph.D. Scientist, Southwest Foundation for Biomedical Research, San Antonio, Texas

Ronald W. Ellis, Ph.D. Senior Director, Department of Cellular and Molecular Biology, Merck Sharp and Dohme Research Laboratories, West Point, Pennsylvania

Emilio A. Emini, Ph.D. Associate Director, Department of Virus and Cell Biology, Merck Sharp and Dohme Research Laboratories, West Point, Pennsylvania

Max Essex, D.V.M., Ph.D. Professor of Virology and Director, Harvard AIDS Institute, Harvard University, Boston, Massachusetts

Gigliola Flamminio-Zola, M.D. Visiting Scientist, Laboratoire de Physiologie Cellulaire, Université P. et M. Curie, Paris, France

Genoveffa Franchini, M.D. Visiting Scientist, Laboratory of Tumor Cell Biology, National Cancer Institute, National Institutes of Health, Bethesda, Maryland

Patricia N. Fultz, Ph.D. Associate Research Professor, Yerkes Regional Primate Research Center and Department of Pathology, Emory University, Atlanta, Georgia

Robert C. Gallo, M.D. Chief, Laboratory of Tumor Cell Biology, National Cancer Institute, National Institutes of Health, Bethesda, Maryland

Susan L. Gdovin, Ph.D. candidate Department of Immunology and Infectious Diseases, The Johns Hopkins University School of Hygiene and Public Health, Baltimore, Maryland

Merril J. Gersten, M.D.   Senior Research Associate, The Salk Institute for Biological Studies, San Diego, California

Beatrice H. Hahn, M.D.   Associate Professor, Departments of Medicine and Microbiology, University of Alabama at Birmingham, Birmingham, Alabama

William Haseltine, Ph.D.   Professor, Laboratory of Biochemical Pharmacology, Dana-Farber Cancer Institute; Department of Pathology, Harvard Medical School; and Department of Cancer Biology, Harvard School of Public Health, Boston, Massachusetts

Daniel F. Hoth, M.D.   Director, Division of AIDS, National Institute of Allergy and Infectious Diseases, National Institutes of Health, Bethesda, Maryland

Shiu-Lok Hu, Ph.D.   Laboratory Director, Oncogen, Seattle, Washington

Charles J. Issel, D.V.M., Ph.D.   Professor, Department of Veterinary Science and Department of Veterinary Microbiology and Parasitology, Louisiana State University, Baton Rouge, Louisiana

Kashi Javaherian, Ph.D.   Repligen Corporation, Cambridge, Massachusetts

Phyllis J. Kanki, D.V.M., S.D.   Assistant Professor of Pathobiology, Harvard AIDS Institute, Harvard University, Boston, Massachusetts

Ronald C. Kennedy, Ph.D.   Scientist, Department of Virology and Immunology, Southwest Foundation for Biomedical Research, San Antonio, Texas

Wayne C. Koff, Ph.D.   Chief, Vaccine Research and Development Branch, Division of AIDS, National Institute of Allergy and Infectious Diseases, National Institutes of Health, Bethesda, Maryland

Mark Kowalski, M.D., Ph.D.   Instructor, Laboratory of Human Retrovirology, Dana-Farber Cancer Institute, and Department of Pathology, Harvard Medical School, Boston, Massachusetts

Yen Li, Ph.D.   Assistant Professor, Microbiology and Molecular Genetics, Harvard Medical School, and New England Regional Primate Research Center, Southborough, Massachusetts

Z. Lurhuma   Cliniques Universitaires, Kinshasa, Zaire

H. Kim Lyerly, M.D.   Surgical Research Fellow, Department of Surgery, Duke University Medical Center, Durham, North Carolina

Vernon C. Maino, Ph.D.   Senior Scientist, Becton Dickinson Monoclonal Center, Mountain View, California

Thomas Matthews, Ph.D.   Associate Medical Professor of Experimental Surgery, Department of Surgery, Duke University Medical Center, Durham, North Carolina

Harold M. McClure, D.V.M.   Chief, Division of Pathobiology and Immunobiology, Yerkes Regional Primate Research Center, Emory University, Atlanta, Georgia

J. Steven McDougal, M.D.   Chief, Immunology Branch, Division of Host Factors, Center for Infectious Diseases, Centers for Disease Control, and Department of Microbiology/Immunology, Emory University School of Medicine, Atlanta, Georgia

Ronald C. Montelaro, Ph.D.   Professor, Department of Biochemistry, Louisiana State University, Baton Rouge, Louisiana

Bernard Moss, M.D., Ph.D.   Chief, Laboratory of Viral Diseases, National Institute of Allergy and Infectious Diseases, National Institutes of Health, Bethesda, Maryland

Opendra Narayan, D.V.M., Ph.D.   Professor, Department of Comparative Medicine, The Johns Hopkins University School of Medicine, Baltimore, Maryland

Chet L. Nastala, M.D.   Research Investigator, Department of Surgery, Duke University Medical Center, Durham, North Carolina

Gregg M. Orloff, Ph.D. candidate   Immunology Branch, Division of Host Factors, Center for Infectious Diseases, Centers for Disease Control, and Department of Microbiology/Immunology, Emory University School of Medicine, Atlanta, Georgia

Susan L. Payne, Ph.D.   Research Associate, Department of Biochemistry, Louisiana State University, Baton Rouge, Louisiana

Scott D. Putney, Ph.D.   Vice President and Director of Molecular Biology, Repligen Corporation, Cambridge, Massachusetts

Gerald V. Quinnan, Jr., M.D.   Deputy Director, Division of Virology, Center for Biologics Evaluation and Research, Food and Drug Administration, Bethesda, Maryland

James Rusche, Ph.D.   Repligen Corporation, Cambridge, Massachusetts

Keith Rushlow   Cellular and Molecular Biology Section, Battelle Memorial Institute, Columbus, Ohio

J. J. Salaun   Institut National de Recherches Biomédicales, Kinshasa, Zaire

Jonas Salk, M.D.   Distinguished Professor in International Health Sciences, The Salk Institute for Biological Studies, San Diego, California

George M. Shaw, M.D., Ph.D. Associate Professor, Departments of Medicine and Biochemistry, University of Alabama at Birmingham, Birmingham, Alabama

Joseph Sodroski, M.D. Assistant Professor, Laboratory of Human Retrovirology, Dana-Farber Cancer Institute, and Department of Pathology, Harvard Medical School, Boston, Massachusetts

Douglas S. Tyler, M.D. Surgical Research Fellow, Department of Surgery, Duke University Medical Center, Durham, North Carolina

Bruce D. Walker, M.D. Assistant Professor, Department of Medicine, Harvard Medical School and Infectious Disease Unit, Massachusetts General Hospital, Boston, Massachusetts

Noel L. Warner, Ph.D. Vice President, Research, Becton Dickinson Monoclonal Center, Mountain View, California

Kent J. Weinhold, Ph.D. Associate Professor of Experimental Surgery, Department of Surgery, Duke University Medical Center, Durham, North Carolina

Susan L. Wescott Clinical Trials Coordinator, Vaccine Research Development Branch, Division of AIDS, National Institute of Allergy and Infectious Diseases, National Institutes of Health, Bethesda, Maryland

Alec E. Wittek, M.D., C.M. Senior Staff Fellow, Laboratory of Retrovirus Research, Food and Drug Administration, Bethesda, Maryland

Flossie Wong-Staal, Ph.D. Section Chief, Laboratory of Tumor Cell Biology, National Cancer Institute, National Institutes of Health, Bethesda, Maryland

Daniel Zagury, M.D. Professor, Laboratoire de Physiologie Cellulaire, Université P. et M. Curie, Paris, France

PROPERTIES OF HIV RELEVANT TO VACCINE DEVELOPMENT

1

Features of the HIV Envelope and Development of a Subunit Vaccine

Scott D. Putney, Kashi Javaherian, and James Rusche
Repligen Corporation
Cambridge, Massachusetts

Thomas Matthews and Dani P. Bolognesi
Duke University Medical Center
Durham, North Carolina

INTRODUCTION

Since the human immunodeficiency virus (HIV) was identified in 1984 as the causative agent of acquired immunodeficiency syndrome (AIDS), a central effort has been the development of a vaccine. Although effective for other viruses, a vaccine that consists of live attenuated virus particles is considered a poor alternative for HIV. Attenuated HIV may integrate into host cell DNA, and retrovirus infection, which can persist for the life of the host, can cause malignant transformation (1). A vaccine consisting of inactivated virus faces the problem that procedures to inactivate nucleic acid may alter the structure of important epitopes. In addition, the outer envelope protein is readily shed during growth of HIV, resulting in envelope-depleted preparations (2).

For these reasons most efforts are towards development of a subunit vaccine. Because of its surface location and because the envelope is the target for immune protection against other viruses, the HIV envelope is the focus of the majority of studies with regard to vaccine development. The HIV envelope can be produced in eukaryotic or prokaryotic expression systems, and envelope fragments, consisting of critical epitopes, can be chemically synthesized. In addition to purified proteins, attentuated recombinant viruses which undergo limited replication in the host, such as vaccinia (3,4) or adenovirus (5), can be used to deliver the envelope to the immune system. Examples of viruses against which protective immunity is elicited by a surface protein or envelope subunit are herpes simplex 1 and 2 (6-9), rabies (10,11), hepatitis B (12-14), Friend leukemia virus (15-17), feline leukemia virus (18), and the human retrovirus HTLV-I (19,20).

Protective antiviral immune responses can be both antibody mediated, such as virus-neutralizing antibodies, or cell mediated, such as cytotoxic T lymphocytes. A major question in the development of an HIV vaccine is whether the body is capable of mounting an immune response able to prevent initial infection and, if so, which type of immunity is required. In this chapter, we review the structural and functional features of the HIV envelope and the progress that has been made in mapping the determinants on this molecule that are targets for immune responses. We also highlight the ways that these determinants can be used to design vaccine candidates and how knowledge of the role of the envelope in viral infection may lead to strategies for prophylactic and therapeutic intervention.

THE ENVELOPE OF HIV

Structure and Binding to CD4

HIV is surrounded by an envelope that is composed of a lipid bilayer, derived from the infected cell, and a glycosylated protein, encoded by the viral genome (21). The envelope is translated as an 88 kilodalton precursor, and following modification by glucosidase I, the precursor has an apparent molecular weight of 160 kD. gp160 is cleaved by a cellular protease to yield the external envelope, gp120, and the transmembrane glycoprotein, gp41 (21-24). gp120 is anchored to the virion by noncovalent interactions with gp41, and both proteins are present on the surface of both virion particles and virus-infected cells. Electron microscopy and computer image enhancement reveal that the gp120-gp41 complexes are distributed on the surface of the virus particle with the pentagonal and hexagonal positions of T=7 levo symmetry (25-27). The total number of such complexes per virus particle is 72.

Pulse-chase studies show that gp160 is inserted into the rough endoplasmic reticulum where the addition of high mannose N-linked carbohydrate chains takes place (28,29). The glycoprotein is initially produced in a conformation unable to bind CD4, and it attains this conformation with a half-life of about 30 minutes (28). After transport to the Golgi, events leading to glycosylation are completed, the gp160 precursor is cleaved, and the mature envelope proteins are transported to the cell surface (29,30). A majority of the uncleaved gp160 is transferred to the lysozomes and is degraded (29).

The first step in the infection of a cell by HIV is the binding of gp120 to the cell surface protein, CD4 (31–33). HIV tropism for cells of the macrophage/ monocyte and lymphoid lineages is the result of the specific interaction of gp120 and CD4. CD4-specific monoclonal antibodies block HIV infection and prevent binding of CD4 to purified gp120 (31–33). In addition, gp120-CD4 complexes can be immunoprecipitated from virus-infected cells (33). Human cell lines, such as HeLa, become susceptible to HIV infection when transfected with CD4 expression vectors (34). In contrast, murine cell lines transfected with the human CD4 gene express CD4 and bind virus, although virus replication does not ensue. Because HIV replicates in the murine but not human cells when they are transfected with the provirus genome, it is possible that a host factor(s), other than CD4, is necessary for a step after binding and before replication. HIV infection of CD4-bearing cells is blocked by soluble CD4 (see below), but neither soluble CD4 nor anti-CD4 antibodies inhibit infection of glial or muscle cells (35). This suggests that virus entry into CD4 cell types is not CD4 mediated and implicates the existence of another receptor(s).

Using both gp120 purified from virus-infected cells and gp120 produced in Chinese hamster ovary cells using a recombinant expression vector, the gp120-CD4 association constant has been measured to be approximately 10^9 (36,37). Binding is dependent upon the intact conformation of gp120 in that reduced and alkylated or detergent denatured gp120 does not bind with detectable affinity (T. Matthews, unpublished). Studies conducted on intact virions show that reduction and alkalation of cysteines destroy the ability of the virus to bind to CD4-bearing cells but that protein denaturants (SDS, 8M urea, alcohol, or heat) followed by removal of the denaturants do not (38). gp120 contains 18 cysteines (39–42), all of which are specifically joined by disulfide cross-bridges (T. Gregory, personal communication). These cross-bridges appear, therefore, to maintain the conformation necessary for binding. As long as the disulfides are not disrupted, the noncovalent interactions that maintain the native structure appear to be favored.

gp120 has 24 sites for potential *N*-linked glycosylation, and 22 of these are linked to mannose-type carbohydrate chains (T. Gregory, personal communication). *O*-linked glycosylation does not appear to be present (29). Glycosylation of gp120 is required for CD4 binding. Synthesis of envelope in the presence of tunicamycin results in deglycosylated gp120 that is unable to bind CD4 (28). In addition, when gp120 is extensively deglycosylated by treatment with endo-glycosidase F or H, the ability to bind CD4 is lost (28,43). Trimming glycosidase inhibitors that interfere with *N*-linked glycan structure also interfere with infectivity (44–46). Partial deglycosylation of gp120 with endo H, however, does not destroy the CD4-binding ability of gp120 (28,38), and synthesis of the envelope in a mutant cell line, unable to synthesize UDP-galactose and hence unable to synthesize mature N-linked side chains, has no effect on syncytia formation (29). Full glycosylation of gp120 is, therefore, not needed to bind CD4 or to maintain infectivity. Although possible, it is unlikely that there is a direct and specific interaction between carbohydrate moieties on gp120 and CD4. It is more likely that the carbohydrate is needed for gp120 to retain the conformation necessary to bind and that glycosylation of a subset of N-linked sites is critical.

There is one report that proteolytically generated 95 and 25 kD fragments of gp120 bind CD4-bearing cells (47). Other workers (48), however, generated several glycosylated recombinant gp120 fragments and were unable to detect CD4 binding even though these proteins contained these 95 and 25 kD fragments. Because the CD4 binding constants of the 95 and 25 kD fragments were not determined, it is probable that they bind with greatly reduced affinity relative to native gp120. Trypsin digests of HIV destroy the ability of the virus to bind to CD4 lymphocytes (38).

CD4 is composed of both an amino terminal extracellular domain, which contains four tandem immunoglobulin-like domains, and carboxyl-terminal transmembrane and cytoplasmic domains. The region of CD4 that interacts with gp120 has been shown to be the amino-terminal half of the extracellular domain comprised of the first two immunoglobulin-like domains (49–56). Several groups have produced the extracellular domain of CD4 (soluble CD4) (57–61), and this protein is currently being investigated as a therapy for HIV-infected individuals. Soluble CD4 binds gp120 with an affinity equal to that of cell-associated CD4 and, at saturating concentrations, competes with cell-associated CD4 for binding of gp120 and thereby prevents infection. Rhesus monkeys, infected with the simian immunodeficiency virus, treated with soluble CD4, were less viremic than controls, and granulocyte-macrophage and erythrocyte progenitor colonies from the treated monkeys increased to normal levels during treatment (62).

One modification of the soluble CD4 therapeutic approach is to synthesize a hybrid protein with the gp120-binding region of CD4 fused to the Fc portion of a human antibody (63). This protein has a longer half-life than soluble CD4, and the Fc receptor confers properties to the hybrid such as Fc receptor binding, complement fixation, and possibly placental transfer. Another modification of the soluble CD4 approach is to produce a hybrid protein with the gp120-binding portion of CD4 fused to Pseudomonas exotoxin A (64) or to ricin A chain (65). These proteins selectively block protein synthesis of and kill HIV-infected cells.

In addition to infecting as a cell-free virion, HIV can be passed from cell to cell by fusion of an HIV-infected cell with an uninfected CD4-bearing cell. This results in the formation of giant multinucleated cells (termed syncytia). Fusion is initiated by binding of gp120, present on the surface of the infected cell, with

CD4 of the uninfected cell. Direct fusion of the cell membrane following gp120-CD4 binding is believed to be the mechanism of viral entry.

After binding of gp120 to CD4, the steps of virus penetration, virus uncoating, and other molecular steps leading to cellular infection are unknown. Once HIV binds CD4, viral entry can be envisioned as occurring either by direct fusion of the viral envelope with the cell plasma membrane or by internalization of the virus–CD4 complex by CD4-mediated endocytosis. Although CD4 is internalized in response to phorbol-esters or other signals, two findings show that endocytosis of CD4 is not necessary for HIV infection: 1) cells expressing CD4 with mutations in the cytoplasmic domain that impair the ability of CD4 to undergo endocytosis are infected as efficiently as those expressing wild-type CD4 (66,67), and 2) neutralization of the low pH environment of the endosomal compartment does not interfere with viral entry (68,69). This means that the low pH-dependent conformational changes that facilitate direct virus fusion with endosomal membranes are not necessary for entry of HIV. Current thinking holds, therefore, that direct fusion of the virus envelope or the membrane of a virus-infected cell with the membrane of an uninfected CD4-bearing cell occurs. After fusion, the contents of the virus or the infected cell are released into the cytoplasm of the uninfected cell.

The precise role of gp120 or gp41 in the mechanism leading to the direct fusion of either the virus membrane or the infected cell membrane with the membrane of the uninfected CD4-bearing cell has not been established. Further work on understanding the post–CD4 binding molecular steps culminating in virus infection, including the role of any non-CD4 proteins, will assist in understanding how antibodies, such as those elicited by envelope subunits, can interfere with the infectious process.

Variability of Amino Acid Sequence

Early after the molecular cloning of HIV, it was discovered that the sequence of the virus genome varies between HIV isolates. This finding was first made by noting differences in restriction maps of clones of virus isolates from different infected individuals (70). Such variation is expected because variation of other lentiviruses, such as equine infectious anemia virus and visna virus, is well documented (71–73). To date, the nucleotide sequence of the envelope from at least 20 independent HIV-1 isolates has been determined.

Amino acid variability is most prominent in the envelope, which can vary, over gp160, by as much as 15%. The extent of variation is not constant over the whole envelope, and there is a pattern of conserved and hypervariable regions (74–76). This suggests that the protein is divided into regions responsible for different functions and that those regions responsible for functions conserved among all isolates, such as CD4 binding or steps leading to membrane fusion, have conserved structure or sequence. For example, all of the 18 cysteines in gp120 are conserved among all sequenced HIV-1 isolates, and there appears to be strong selective pressure to maintain the tertiary structure conferred by the nine disulfide bonds.

Segments of hypervariable sequence may have no specific function and therefore would be free to mutate as long as the variation does not alter the conformation necessary for proper function of other segments of the envelope. One hypervariable sequence is the target for the two principal types of protective immunity, neutralizing antibodies and cytotoxic T-lymphocytes. One explanation for the hypervariability of this envelope sequence is immunologic selection for mutation in these regions. This leads to the idea that the virus can "outrun" the immune response by mutation and that this results in a population of similar but distinct virus species unaffected by the preexisting immunity. For example, in equine infectious anemia virus infection of horses, which is chronic and life-long, there are periodic cycles of disease outbreaks. Antibodies recovered from an infected animal can effectively neutralize virus isolates recovered during previous outbreaks and do not neutralize virus recovered during subsequent outbreaks (72).

Some evidence for this phenomena in HIV is that variation in the sequence of gp120 is also found between sequential isolates taken from a single infected person (77-79). In this case the amino acid sequence variability of gp120 is on the order of 6%, and the differences appear to be randomly located, primarily in the hypervariable domains. This variation does not occur during in vitro passage of the virus, suggesting that immune selection plays a role in the variability (79). Such variability, particularly in the neutralizing determinants, has important implications for vaccine development. It will be important to understand the mechanism of and the driving force for amino acid sequence variation. To be considered effective, a vaccine would have to protect against infection by a large majority of HIV isolates to which an individual could be exposed.

MECHANISMS OF IMMUNE ATTACK ON HIV

Humoral Immunity

Immune responses to viruses are of two types: humoral, or antibody mediated, and cellular. The most important form of protective immunity against viral particles is neutralizing antibody. Neutralizing antibodies can abrogate any one of several events leading to infection such as receptor attachment, virus penetration, or virus uncoating. Several mechanisms of neutralization have been elucidated for viruses other than HIV.

1. Antibody can cross-link virus particles, which leads to alteration of protein conformation and neutralization (80,81).

2. A monoclonal antibody to the reovirus alpha-1 protein blocks cell attachment (82).
3. Mouse mammary tumor virus is neutralized by steric hindrance by antibody bound to adjacent determinants that function in binding to cell surface receptors (83).
4. Attachment to cell surface occurs without penetration when influenza is neutralized by antibody (84–86).
5. West Nile and rabies viruses are neutralized by antibody that inhibit the intraendosmal acid-catalyzed fusion step that leads to virus uncoating (87,88).

With HIV, neutralization could theoretically occur by antibodies bound to gp120 that prevent attachment to CD4 or that interfere in subsequent steps after attachment but prior to the first replicative event. Monoclonal antibodies that block binding of purified gp120 to CD4 have been isolated but are unable to neutralize virus infectivity (36,48). This is thought to be due to the large binding constant (approximately 10^9) between gp120 and CD4. It is known that the principal mode of antibody neutralization of HIV occurs at a step subsequent to binding.

Antibodies that neutralize HIV are assayed in two ways. The first measures the neutralization of free virus particles and is assayed by incubating serial dilutions of immune antiserum with a known titer of virus particles. This mixture is then incubated with infectable cells such as CD4-bearing lymphocytes. After several days the extent of infectivity is measured by determining the amount of virus produced by the culture by assaying for viral proteins such as reverse transcriptase or the major core protein, p24. The titer of neutralization is the dilution at which a given percentage of the infectivity is reduced. The second assay, termed fusion inhibition, measures the ability of the immune antisera to prevent fusion of an HIV-infected cell with an uninfected CD4-bearing cell. This assay is performed by incubating dilutions of antisera with infected cells and plating the mixture on a lawn of uninfected cells. Cell fusion is assayed by counting syncytia, and the fusion inhibition is the serum dilution that reduces syncytia formation by a given percentage.

Because the mechanism of virus entry, whether as free virus or by fusion of an infected cell with an uninfected cell, is believed to be the same, antisera that inhibit cell fusion also neutralize free virus, and the assay results are often used interchangeably. The sensitivity of the neutralization assay is greater, however, and therefore the reported values of the titer are higher. HIV-neutralizing antibodies are present in the majority of HIV-infected people (89,90). These antibodies appear to bind primarily, if not exclusively, the envelope and are elicited by immunization with gp160, gp120, or fragments thereof (2,91–94).

Most laboratories use the neutralization assay and, unfortunately, there has not been one standard assay adopted. Because the neutralization titer depends on variables such as the sensitivity to neutralization of the virus strain used, the amount of infectious virus and the susceptibility to infection of the cell line used, it is difficult to compare absolute titers from different laboratories even when the same antisera is used (95). In general, however, serum neutralization titers of 100 to 500 using the prototype HTLV-III$_B$ strain are considered moderate to high. Titers of greater than 500 are found in some HIV-infected people and in chimpanzees infected with III$_B$.

Cellular Immunity

Cellular immunity is a broad term describing specific and nonspecific killer, cytotoxic, and helper T cells and other cells that act directly or indirectly to eliminate viral pathogens. The goal of immunization is to induce immunologic memory such that a greatly elevated anamnestic response is generated upon subsequent contact with the invading organism.

T-cell-mediated antiviral responses are considered the most important form of cellular immunity because they are antigen specific and are activated by subsequent viral challenge. T cells recognize foreign antigens only when specific determinants of these antigens are presented on the surface of another cell, termed an antigen-presenting cell (APC). Recognition only occurs in association with proteins encoded by the major histocompatibility complex locus (MHC). Helper T cells recognize antigen in the context of class II MHC molecules and are generally CD4$^+$, whereas CTL recognize antigen on APCs in the presence of class I MHC molecules and can be either CD8$^+$ or CD4$^+$. When activated, helper T cells secrete IL-2, IL-3, gamma interferon, and other lymphokines that lead to B-cell, T-cell, and macrophage activation, whereas cytotoxic T cells lyse cells bearing the foreign antigen in the context of the class I MHC molecule. Helper T cells are found in HIV-infected humans and chimpanzees and are elicited by envelope subunits and other viral proteins (96-100).

Experiments involving adoptive transfer of CTL to unimmunized animals followed by virus challenge suggest that CTL specific for surface or internal viral antigens may serve as a protective host defense. For example, adoptive transfer to mice of either uncloned or cloned CTL specific for influenza A virus results in decreased virus titers and mortality when animals are subsequently challenged with infectious virus (101,102). The effect is seen only when the recipients are of the same MHC I locus as the donor. Similarly, CTL from mice infected with lymphocytic choriomeningitis virus, when transferred to syngenic (but not allogenic) recipients, cause complete clearance of virus from animals previously infected (103). CTL have also been shown to play a protective role in murine leukemia virus infection (104,105). Virus-specific CTL have also been demonstrated in humans for herpesvirus (106), measles (107), cytomegalovirus (108),

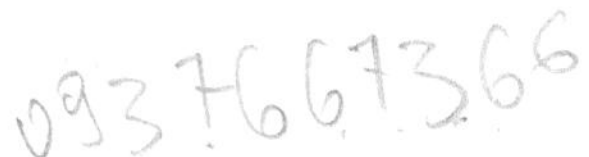

and influenza (109,110). The epitopes recognized by the influenza-specific CTL have been determined (111).

CTL specific for the HIV envelope, core, and reverse transcriptase have been identified in HIV-infected people (112–115), and envelope- and core-specific CTL are elicited by HIV infection of gibbon apes (116). Envelope-specific CTL are elicited by immunization with recombinant vaccinia virus expressing gp160 (99). Because HIV is a chronic infection, the immune system is continually exposed to viral antigen. It is probable that CTL are present, at varying levels, throughout the infection, and one report (117) found CTL and CTL precursor cells with high frequency in HIV-infected individuals. It is possible that CTL reduce the level of free virus or virus-infected cells and CTL thereby serve to lower virus burden. A correlation has been noted (113,117) between the severity of disease symptoms and the level of envelope-specific CTL; Envelope-specific CTL may be an important immune function to elicit by an HIV vaccine because HIV-infected cells present gp120 on their surface and are therefore susceptible to detection and lysis.

An additional type of immune response that involves both antibody and lytic cells is antibody-dependent cellular cytotoxicity (ADCC). This is a process whereby the Fc portion of an antibody that is bound to a viral antigen (such as gp120) presented on the surface of an infected cell is recognized by an Fc receptor on the surface of a natural killer cell, a T cell, or a macrophage. The infected cell is subsequently lysed and the percentage of cells lysed is a function of the antibody titer. HIV-infected people have antibodies that mediate ADCC (118–120) and, theoretically, antibodies able to bind to the exposed portions of surface antigens can direct ADCC. It is not surprising, therefore, that ADCC antibody, resulting from HIV infection, is largely gp120 directed (119,121,122) and not directed to core antigens (122).

MAP OF IMMUNOLOGIC AND FUNCTIONAL DOMAINS ON THE ENVELOPE

Neutralization Epitopes

As we will discuss later, immunization of chimpanzees with envelope has been unable to prevent infection when the animals were challenged with infectious virus. It is now apparent that HIV vaccine development will be more difficult than for other viruses where attenuated or inactivated viruses or envelope subunits confer protection. It is, therefore, important to identify envelope determinants that are the targets of humoral or cellular immune responses because these determinants could be modified to elicit an immune response greater and more focused than that elicited by whole virus or entire envelope preparations or by the infectious virion. For example, it is possible that immunization with a peptide, consisting of only a fraction of gp120, that bears the neutralizing determinant could be appropriately engineered through linking to carrier proteins or peptides with helper T-cell epitopes to elicit a protective antibody response.

To map the neutralization determinants on gp160, we produced recombinant gp160 (r160) in insect cells using a baculovirus expression vector and fragments of gp160, denoted PE3, PB1, and penv9 in *E. coli* (Fig. 1) (92,93). Each of these proteins was expressed from the BH10 molecular clone of the IIIB isolate of HIV-1. r160 comigrates with gp160 isolated from HIV-infected cells and is reduced in molecular weight by *N*-glycanase to about 95 kD, the approximate size of nonglycosylated gp160. This indicates that r160 is glycosylated to about the same extent as native gp160. Each of these proteins were purified under denaturing and reducing conditions and used to generate immune serum in rabbits and goats.

Although immune sera to each of these proteins bind gp120 and gp160 in ELISA and Western blot assays, only sera to r160 and PB1 neutralize the III_B virus isolate. In addition to neutralizing infectivity of cell-free virus, both of these antisera completely inhibit fusion of III_B-infected cells. Cell fusion–inhibiting antibodies elicited by r160 or PB1 can be competitively blocked by PB1 in that antiserum to PB1 or r160 does not inhibit fusion when coincubated with PB1 (123). PB1 competes effectively at concentrations as low as 0.5 μM with a 1:10 dilution of PB1 or r160 antisera in that the same number of syncytia are formed as in the absence of inhibiting antibodies (Fig. 1). These results indicate that all of the neutralizing antibody elicited by gp160 is directed to the PB1 segment of the envelope. In addition, because PB1 is produced in *E. coli*, which does not glycosylate foreign proteins, this indicates that glycosylation is not required to elicit neutralizing antibodies.

To determine the location of the epitope(s) within PB1 recognized by neutralizing antibodies, a number of recombinant polypeptides and synthetic peptides containing regions of PB1 were produced and purified (Fig. 1). Animals were immunized with fragments Sub1, Sub2, Sub6, CNBr1, and CNBr2, and immune sera were assayed for fusion-blocking and virus-neutralizing activities. Antisera to Sub 1, Sub 2, and CNBr1 neutralize virus infectivity and block fusion of III_B-infected cells. Even though Sub6 and CNBr2 elicit high titers of PB1-binding antibody, no neutralization is observed. These purified fragments and sub8 were also tested for their ability to block the fusion-inhibition activity of anti-PB1 and anti-gp160 sera. PB1, Sub1, Sub2, and CNBr1 completely block both sera at approximately equivalent concentrations, whereas the Sub6 and Sub8 fragments have no effect even at 25-fold higher molar concentrations. These results show that the CNBr1 region of PB1 contains the determinant to which fusion-inhibiting and virus-neutralizing antibodies are directed.

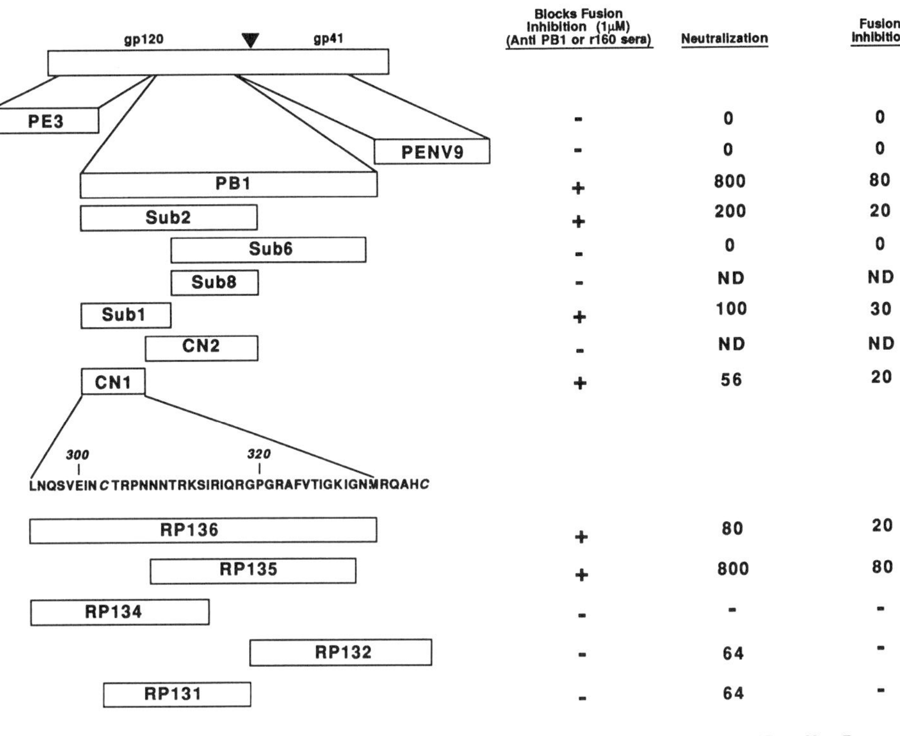

Figure 1   Map of envelope showing location of recombinant and peptide subunit immunogens and activities. On the left are the locations of *E. coli*–produced gp160 fragments and synthetic peptides (RP peptides), and columns on the right indicate the ability of 1 μM concentrations of each to completely absorb antibodies elicited by PB1 or r160 that inhibit fusion of III_B-infected cells with uninfected cells. Also shown are the free virus neutralization titers and fusion inhibition titers (defined in Table 1) elicited by these fragments. CN1 and CN2 are products of a cyanogen bromide digest of Sub2. Synthetic peptide immunogens were covalently coupled to KLH through a C-terminal cysteine.

A series of synthetic peptides from the CNBr1 region were then prepared and assayed for their ability to block fusion inhibition. Peptides RP136 and RP135, a subset of 24 amino acids of RP136, block activity at concentrations equivalent to those of the larger fragments (Fig. 1). Peptides RP131, RP132, and RP134 cover RP136 in an overlapping fashion and do not block fusion inhibition of anti-PB1 or anti-r160 serum. Even though RP131 and RP132 elicit neutralizing antibodies, they are unable to compete for fusion-inhibiting antibodies elicited by the larger PB1 or gp160 immunogens. Because it can compete for all neutralizing antibodies elicited by the entire envelope, RP135 contains the principal neutralization determinant (see Figs. 7b and 8 and Table 3). This determinant has been discovered independently by other laboratories (124-126).

RP135 is from a region of the envelope where the amino acid sequence is highly variable. Figure 2 shows the amino acid sequence of this region from several independent HIV-1 isolates. Whereas the sequence of gp120 differs as much as 20-25% between III_B (BH10) and these isolates, the RP135 region differs as much as 40-50%. There are, however, conserved elements within this region such as the flanking cysteines that are present in all HIV-1 isolates and that are joined to each other by a disulfide cross-bridge (T. Gregory, personal communication). The RP135 determinant is, therefore, contained in a loop in native gp120 (Fig. 3). In addition, the sequences at the base of this loop are relatively conserved. Also relatively conserved is the glycine-proline-glycine in the center of the RP135 determinant, which presumably enables the polypeptide to adopt a β bend structure.

Because of the hypervariability of this domain, antibodies elicited by proteins or peptides comprised of the amino acid sequence from one isolate do not neutralize HIV-1 isolates with different sequences of the RP determinant. For example, antisera to RP135, PB1-III_B, or r160-III_B do not neutralize the divergent isolates HTLV–III_{RF} (RF) or HTLV–III_{MN} (MN), two viruses with different amino acid sequences in this region (Table 1 and Figure 3). In addition to eliciting virus type-specific neutralizing antibodies, blockade of fusion inhibition by the peptides is also virus type-specific. For example, RP135 does not block fusion inhibition of cells infected with RF by antisera to r160-RF (a protein expressed from a baculovirus clone of the HAT-3 molecular clone of RF).

We have synthesized the RP135 analogs from the RF and MN sequences (denoted RP139(RF) and RP142(MN), respectively). RP139 completely competes the fusion-inhibiting antibodies elicited by r160-RF (see below), thus showing that for this variant this domain is also the principal neutralizing determinant. RP139 and RP142 elicit antibodies that neutralize the RF and MN isolates, respectively, but not the heterologous isolates tested (Table 2). Thus, the RP determinant is a neutralization determinant for all three of these isolates.

The principal neutralizing determinant **RP135** spans the region from around position S I R I Q R **G P G** R A F (the boxed Gly‑Pro‑Gly and flanking residues), with the neutralizing epitope shaded.

Isolate	Sequence (C T R P N N N T R K S I R **I Q R G P G R A F** V T I G K · I G N M R Q A H C)	Isolate
III$_B$ (BH10)	C T R P N N N T R K S I R I Q R G P G R A F V T I G K I G N M R Q A H C	III$_B$ (BH10)
RF	C - - - - - - - - - S - T K - - - - V I Y A T - Q I - - D I - K - - C	RF
MN	C - - - - Y - K - - - H I - - - - - - Y - T K N I - - T I - - - - C	MN
SC	C - - - - - - - T R S - H I - - - - - - Y A T - D I - - D I - - - - C	SC
WMJ-2	C - - - Y - - V - R S L S I - - - - - R - R E I - - I I - - - - C	WMJ-2
LAV-MAL	C - - - G - - - - R G - H F - - - Q - L Y - T - I V - D I - R - Y C	LAV-MAL
SF-2	C - - - - - - - - S - Y I - - - - - H - T - R I - - D I - K - - C	SF-2
NY5	C - - - - - - - K - G - A I - - - - T L Y A R E - I - - D I - - - - C	NY5
Z3	C - - - G SDKKI - Q S - R I - - - K V - Y A K - G I T - - - - C	Z3
WMJ1	C - - - - - V - R R H - H I - - - - - Y - G E I R - - I - - - - C	WMJ1
WMJ3	C - - - - D I A - R - - H I - - - - - Y - G K I - - - I - - - - C	WMJ3
Z6	C - - - Y K - - - Q S T P I - L - Q - L Y -TRGRT- I - - - - - - C	Z6
LAVELI	C A - - Y Q - - - Q - T P I - L - Q S L Y - TRSRS I - - - - - - C	LAVELI
CDC451	C - - - - - H - - - - V T L - - - - V W Y - T - E I L - - I - - - - C	CDC451
CDC42	C - - - - - - - - - V T L - - - - V W Y - T - E I L - - I - - - - C	CDC42
BAL	C - - - - - - - - S - H I - - - - - - Y - T - E I - - D I - - - - C	BAL

Figure 2 Amino acid sequences of the principal neutralizing determinant (RP135) from several HIV-1 isolates. The flanking cysteines are conserved in all isolates and are joined by a disulfide cross-bridge (T. Gregory, personal communication), and this region is a loop in the native envelope. The central Gly-Pro-Gly is conserved in the majority of isolates. The relatively conserved amino acids are boxed, and the neutralizing epitope within RP135 is shaded.

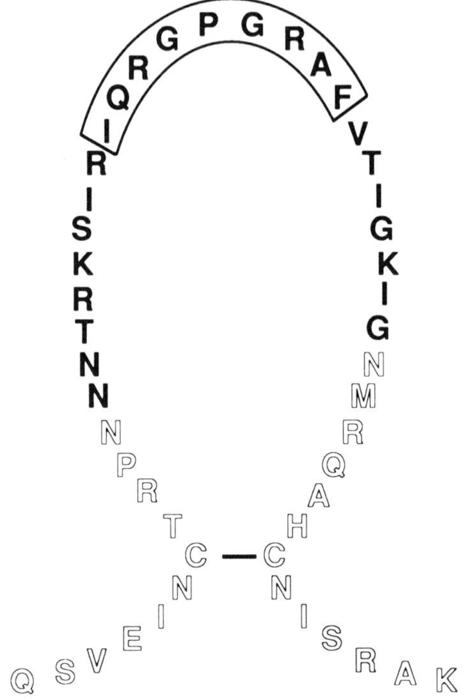

Figure 3 Major neutralizing determinant of HIV-1. The sequences is between amino acids 296–331, and the cysteines are joined by a disulfide cross-bridge. The sequence of RP135 is denoted by bold letters, and the neutralization epitope within RP135 is boxed. The sequence is derived from the BH10 clone of the HTLV-III$_B$ isolate (40).

Several monoclonal antibodies that bind to the RP135 determinant have been characterized (127–131). These antibodies bind to IIIB- or LAV-1–infected cells, and this indicates that the RP135 determinant is positioned on the surface of the infected cells. They also neutralize cell-free III$_B$ and inhibit fusion of cells infected with this virus and do not neutralize the heterologous RF or MN isolates. Our working hypothesis is that an antibody bound to the RP135 determinant, regardless of the HIV-1 isolate, will neutralize that virus.

The function of the RP determinant in virus infectivity, if any, is unknown. It does not appear to act in the binding of gp120 to CD4 because antibodies bound to this determinant do not affect gp120 binding to CD4-bearing cells (37,127) and because insertion mutations in the domain do not disrupt CD4 binding (132). Because antibodies to the RP determinant bind to a different site on gp120 than does CD4, these antibodies do not have to compete for gp120 with CD4, which has a high association constant for the external envelope ($\sim10^9$) (36,37).

The RP determinant domain may act as an "umbrella" to cover more conserved neutralizing epitopes and prevent them from eliciting group-common neutralizing antibodies. The fact that the sequences within the loop may be separated from the remaining gp120 by virtue of the loop structure, and the fact that this loop may have no function, could allow mutational errors without altering important functional or structural features. However, the fact that the Gly-Por-Gly, the sequences of the base of the loop, and the overall length of the loop are generally conserved indicates that there is some constraint on the extent of mutation that can be tolerated. Supporting this is a change of the Gly-Pro-Gly to Gly-Ala-Gly at the tip of the loop in an infectious molecular clone of III_B that greatly reduces viral infectivity (D. Looney and F. Wong-Staal, personal communication).

To further confirm that RP135 is the principal neutralizing determinant, we constructed several versions of r160 (Fig. 4). In addition to r160 of the HTLV-III_B isolate, we constructed two hybrid proteins in which a portion of

Table 1 HIV-1–Neutralizing and Cell Fusion–Inhibiting Antibodies Elicted by Envelope Subunit Immunogens

Antisera	Free virus neutralization[a]			Cell fusion inhibition[b]		
	III_B	RF	MN	III_B	RF	MN
gp160 (III_B)	1000	–	–	60	–	–
gp160 (RF)	–	1200	–	–	90	–
gp160 (III_B + RF) -co-immunization	145	66	–	40	40	–
PB1 (III_B)	1000	–	–	120	–	–
PB1 (RF)	–	500	–	–	80	–
PB1 (III_B + RF) -co-immunization	620	80	–	10	10	–
Seropositive human	300	250	300	20	20	20

[a]Neutralization titer is the reciprocal serum dilution that reduces infectivity, as measured by reverse transcriptase activity, by 50% compared to nonimmune serum.
[b]Fusion inhibition titers are the reciprocal serum dilution that reduces the number of syncytia to zero.
– indicates that titers are less than 10.

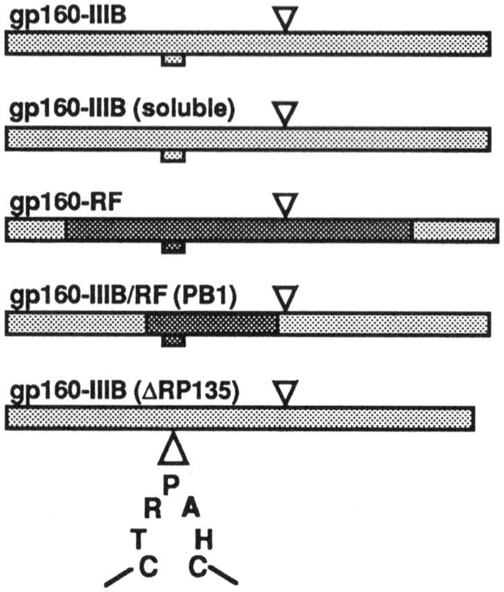

	Free-Virus Neutralization Titers		Fusion Inhibition Titers	
	IIIB	RF	IIIB	RF
gp160-IIIB	1200	0	80	0
gp160-IIIB (soluble)	2560	0	160	0
gp160-RF	0	1200	0	90
gp160-IIIB/RF (PB1)	0	320	0	90
gp160-IIIB (ΔRP135)	0	0	0	0

Figure 4 Recombinant r160 proteins. These proteins were produced in recombinant baculovirus-infected insect cells. Proteins (a) and (c)-(e) were purified using denaturing and reducing conditions, and soluble r160 (b) was purified under nondenaturing/nonreducing conditions. Each was used to immunize goats with Freund's complete/incomplete adjuvant. Titers are defined in Table 1. ▒ and ▓ denote III_B- and RF-specific sequences, respectively.

the protein was derived from the HTLV-III RF isolate (75). One of these, r160-RF, contains approximately 85% of the amino acids from the RF isolate, whereas r160-III_B/RF (PB1) contains essentially the BP1 region from the RF isolate and the remainder of the envelope from the III_B isolate. These purified proteins elicit antibodies that neutralize only the RF isolate, and this indicates that the neutralization activity is directed to the PB1 region. In addition to the hybrid envelope proteins, we also constructed, using oligonucleotide mutagensis, r160 in which the RP135 region is deleted. When this protein is purified and used as an immunogen, even though it elicits antibodies that bind gp160, gp120, and gp41 on a Western blot, these antibodies do not neutralize either the III_B or the RF isolates. Thus, by deleting the RP135 region we abrogate the ability of the envelope to elicit neutralizing antibodies.

To more precisely localize the amino acids of the RP135 determinants that elicits neutralizing and fusion-inhibiting antibodies, we synthesized a series of hybrid peptides (containing sequences from both the III_B and RF isolates) and a series of RP135 fragments (Fig. 5). Peptide RP138 is a hybrid that has the same number of amino acids as RP135 but has the amino acid sequence of III_B on the left and of RF on the right side of the Gly-Pro-Gly, repectively. RP138 completely abrogates the fusion-inhibiting antibodies elicited by both PB1-III_B and PB1-RF (Table 2) although at different concentrations. The concentration of RP138 required to block PB1-IIIB sera is the same as that required for RP135 to block the same sera (0.1 μM), and this indicates that the neutralizing determinant in RP138 is the same as that presented in RP135. On the other hand, the blockade of PB1-RF sera by RP138 is achieved only at a concentration 100 times greater than with RP139 (0.01 μM for RP139 and 1 μM for RP138). RP138 is therefore less efficient in binding the fusion-inhibiting antibodies, and thus some of the RF specific amino acids composing the neutralizing determinant of PB1-RF are not present in RP138. The result with RP339 (see below) shows that these amino acids are those immediately to the left of the Gly-Pro-Gly. Hybrid peptide RP140 with the RF sequence on the left and the III_B sequence on the right of Gly-Pro-Gly is unable to block either PB1-III_B or PB1-RF antisera.

These data indicate that the neutralizing epitope in PB1-III_B is composed of the Gly-Pro-Gly and amino acids on the left and the neutralizing epitope in PB1-RF is the Gly-Pro-Gly and amino acids on the right. A shorter hybrid peptide, RP73 (14 amino acids), with a sequence arrangement similar to RP138 (III_B sequence on the left and RF sequence on the right) blocks both PB1-III_B and PB1-RF sera demonstrating the sequence at the tip of the loop defines neutralizing epitopes for both of these isolates. (As with RP138, micromolar concentrations of RP73 are required to block the PB1-RF sera.)

The neutralization determinants for III_B and RF were further defined by competition experiments using RP335 and RP339, peptides with 9 or 10 amino acids from the tip of the loop. RP339 contains a C-terminal sequence identical to RP73 and three additional RF-specific amino acids on the left of Gly-Pro-Gly. RP339 completely blocks PB1-RF at the same concentration as RP139 (0.01 μM), indicating that the neutralization determinant presented in RP139 is identical to that in RP339. This demonstrates that the amino acids Ile-Thr-Lys on the amino terminus of RP339 contribute to the RF neutralizing epitope in PB1-RF. RP335, a similar peptide of nine amino acids with a III_B-specific amino acid sequence, is not able to block PB1-III_B sera even at a 40 μM concentration. Additional amino acids N-terminal to the Ile-Gln-Arg in RP73 or RP135 are therefore part of the neutralizing epitope of PB1-III_B.

The ability of these peptides to elicit neutralizing antibody was also studied. Both peptides, RP335 and RP339, excluding the C-terminal cysteine used to

Peptide	Viral Isolate	Sequence
	IIIB	I N C T R P N N N T R K S I R I Q R G P G R A F V T I G K I G N M R Q A H C N I S
RP135	IIIB	N N T R K S I R I Q R G P G R A F V T I G K I G(C)
RP139	RF	- - - - - - - T K - - - - V I Y A T - Q I - -(C)
RP142	MN	Y - K - - R - H - - - - - - - Y - T K N I - -(C)
RP335	IIIB	- - - - - - - -(C)
RP79	IIIB	- - - - - - - -(C)
RP339	RF	- T K - - - - V I Y(C)
RP138	IIIB-RF	- - - - - - - - - - - - - V I Y A T - - - -(C)
RP140	RF-IIIB	- - - - - - - T K - - - - - - - - - - - -(C)
RP73	IIIB-RF	- - - - - - - - - - - V I Y(C)
RP55	IIIB,RF,MN	A H C N I S
RP57	IIIB,RF,MN	I N C T R P A H C N I S
RP59	IIIB,RF,MN	I G D I R Q A H C N I S
RP60	IIIB,RF,MN	I N C T R P N N N T R K S I

Figure 5 Synthetic peptides used to map the neutralization epitope within RP135. The sequence of the III_B (BH10) isolate is shown at the top. Cysteines (in parentheses) were added to the C-terminus of most of the peptides and were used to link the peptide to KLH. Peptide 57 has amino acids surrounding the cysteines that flank RP135 peptide.

Table 2 Neutralization and Fusion-Inhibition Titers of Antisera Elicited by Peptides from the RP135 Determinant

Peptide	Fusion inhibition[a] titer			Neutralization[a] titer			Complete Blockade[b] of fusion inhibition (μM)	
	III$_B$	RF	MN	III$_B$	RF	MN	PB1-III$_B$	PB1-RF
RP135	40	—	—	1500	—	—	0.1	—
RP139	—	320	—	—	2560	—	—	0.01
RP142	—	—	20	—	—	280	—	—
RP335	160	—	—	2560	—	ND	—	—
RP79	10	—	—	190	—	—	—	—
RP339	—	90	—	—	1300	—	—	0.01
RP138	40	40	—	340	1250	—	0.1	1
RP140	—	—	—	—	—	ND	—	—
RP73	20	40	—	1600	1300	ND	0.5	5
RP55	—	—	—	—	—	—	—	—
RP57	—	—	—	—	—	—	—	—
RP59	—	—	—	—	—	—	—	—
RP60	—	—	—	—	—	—	—	—

[a]Titers are defined in Table 1.
[b]Indicates the minimum concentration of peptide that completely blocks fusion inhibition of the indicated PB1 antisera.
ND = not determined.

link the peptides to KLH carrier, elicit high titer-neutralizing and cell fusion-inhibiting antibody to the homologous isolate (Table 2). RP79, which is one amino acid shorter than RP335, also elicits neutralizing antibody albeit at approximately a 10-fold lower titer. It is probable, therefore, that the isoleucine on the N-terminus of RP335, not present in RP79, is required to elicit higher titer·neutralizing antibody.

The amino acid sequences flanking the cysteines at the base of the loop (Figs. 2 and 3) are generally conserved among HIV-1 isolates and in light of the ability of epitope at the tip of the loop to elicit only type-specific neutralizing antibodies, we investigated the ability of peptides from these conserved regions to elicit neutralizing antibodies (Fig 4 and Table 2). Although these peptides elicit antibodies that bind the immunogen, the sera do not bind PB1-IIIB or r160-IIIB on Western blots. No fusion-inhibiting antibodies to either the IIIB or RF isolates is observed. This is consistent with the data showing that peptides containing only the tip of the loop are sufficient to block the PB1 antisera. It is possible that, whereas the tip of the loop is exposed and accessible to neutralizing antibody, the base is buried within the gp120 structure and inaccessible to antibody. It is not known whether antibodies that bind the base of the loop bind virus-infected cells. A similar result has been observed by others (126).

Hybrid peptides RP138 and RP73 elicit antibodies that neutralize both the IIIB and the RF isolates, whereas antisera elicited by RP140 do not neutralize either isolate (Table 2). This further supports the finding of the competition experiments that the neutralizing epitope of IIIB consists of the Gly-Pro-Gly and amino acids to the left and that the neutralizing epitope of RF is Gly-Pro-Gly and the amino acids to the right. These results show that hybrid peptides can be designed to elicit antibodies that neutralize more than one virus isolate.

In contrast to the virus type–specific antibodies elicited by these and other recombinant or synthetic peptide immunogens (125,133–136), immune sera generated by infectious virus neutralizes a number of different isolates. Antisera from chimpanzees (137) or a laboratory worker infected with the IIIB virus isolate (138) taken within a year after seroconverson neutralize only IIIB, and this neutralization can be competitively blocked with RP135 (Fig. 6). After the first year the peptide can no longer effectively compete for these antibodies. Antisera taken 18 months after seroconversion neutralize RF and several other isolates. After this transition from type-specific to group-common neutralization, these antisera behave as do many immune sera from seropositive individuals, which neutralize multiple isolates.

This data suggests that after one year the nature of the neutralizing antibody response changes. Because these antibodies cannot be competitively blocked by a peptide consisting of the principal neutralizing domain of the test virus, these neutralizing antibodies do not bind this domain. These antibodies probably bind

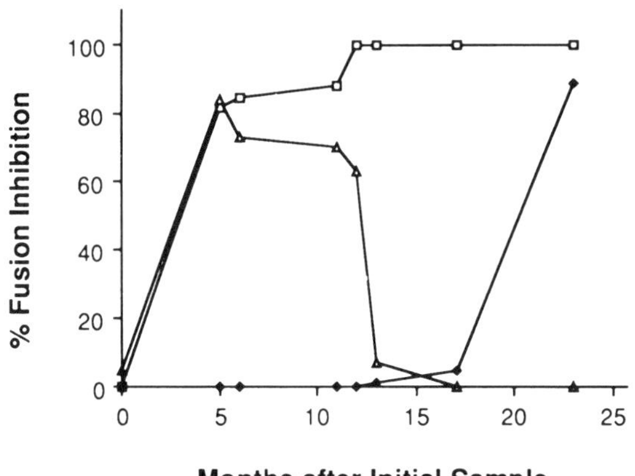

Figure 6 Time course of fusion-inhibition antibody response in a HTLV–III$_B$-infected human. □ and ◆ indicate the ability of a 1:10 dilution of serum to inhibit fusion of cells infected both III$_B$ and RF, respectively. △ indicates the ability of RP135 to block the fusion inhibition of III$_B$-infected cells by the antisera. After 13 months the peptide can no longer block the activity.

more conserved regions of the envelope, and because gp120 and r160 are unable to elicit measurable titers of these group-common neutralizing antibodies, it is possible that this epitope(s) is formed by a particular conformation the envelope adopts in virus or in virus-infected cells which is not present or not readily accessible in purified gp120 or r160. One possibility is that antibodies that block binding of gp120 to CD4 and that are found in a majority of HIV positive human sera (37,139) can neutralize virus infectivity. However, there is no correlation between binding inhibition titer and HIV neutralizing activity in such sera (139). Another possibility is that antibodies to determinants on the p17 core antigen neutralize in a group-common fashion (140,141).

We thought it possible that the denaturing and reducing conditions used to purify the r160 immunogens may destroy noncontinuous neutralizing determinants. This purification procedure uses high concentrations of urea and β-mercaptoethanol to solubilize the r160-containing insect cells. This is followed by lentil-lectin Sepharose chromatography and gel filtration chromatography using buffers containing reducing agent, urea, and, in the final step, SDS. To purify the protein using gentler conditions, we devised another procedure using the same solubilization and chromatographic steps in which the urea, SDS, and β-mercaptoethanol was substituted by the nonionic detergent deoxycholate. This resulted in a protein, denoted soluble r160, which presumably contains intact disulfide cross-bridges. When soluble r160 is used an an immunogen (Fig. 4), only type-specific neutralizing antibodies are observed. Thus, at least when purified under these conditions, r160 is unable to elicit antibodies to any additional conserved neutralizing determinants.

In contrast to our and others' (134,136) inability to elicit cross-neutralizing antibodies with a single envelope subunit, group-common neutralizing antibodies have been elicited by immunization of a human volunteer with recombinant vaccinia virus expressing gp160 followed by boosting with formalin-fixed autologous cells infected with this recombinant vaccinia virus (97). Group-common neutralization was observed only after the boost and immunization with only the gp160-expressing vaccinia virus was unable to elicit group-common neutralizing antibodies. It is possible that the vaccinia virus in combination with the boost of the infected cells more readily present conformationally dependent neutralizing epitopes to the immune system, and it therefore may be possible to design a subunit immunogen to do the same. Some conserved segments of the envelope have been reported to elicit low titers of neutralizing antibodies (Figs. 7b and 8 and Table 3) (131,142–145), and it is possible that one or more of these regions contribute to this conserved epitope.

In an experiment designed to study the effect of mutations on the neutralizing antibody susceptibility of a molecular clone of III$_B$, a mutant virus resistant to neutralization by human seropositive antisera was selected (146). The envelope was sequenced and the only change, which was confirmed to confer the neutralization resistant phenotype, was an Ala to Thr replacement in the amino-terminal half of gp41 (Figs. 7b and 8 and Table 3) (147). Synthetic peptides or envelope fragments containing this region of gp41 are unable to elicit or bind neutralizing antibodies, and this mutant virus is neutralized by antibodies to the neutralizing loop. It is likely that the neutralization resistance is due to a conformational change in gp120, induced by the mutation, that affects distant neutralization epitopes. It is also possible that this region contributes to part of a neutralization determinant formed by one or more gp120 domains, distant in the linear sequence, that are proximal in the three-dimensional structure.

T–Cell Epitopes

Antigen recognition by T cells differs from that of antibodies in two major respects. First, T cells recognize the specific sequence only when it is presented on the surface of the APC in association with products of the MHC. Second, T-cell recognition is limited to a small number of immunodominant sites, whereas antibodies recognize a larger number of sites. The properties of a peptide or epitope that make it a T-cell site are not fully understood, and algorithms have been developed to predict the location of these determinants (148,149).

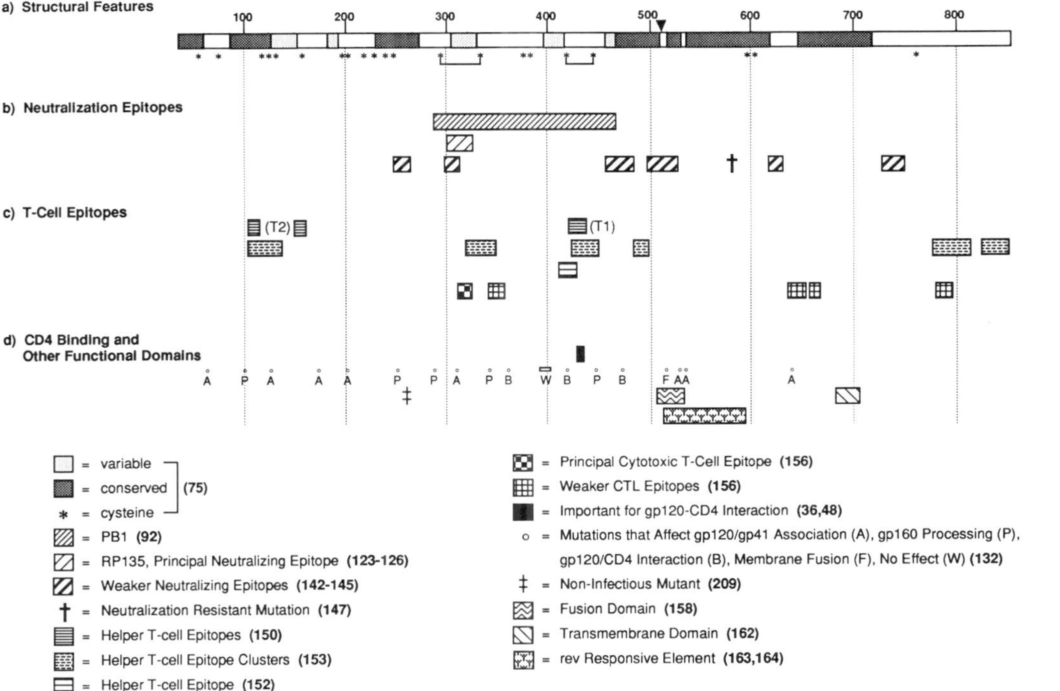

Figure 7 (a) Map of HIV-1 envelope showing the external envelope, gp120, and the transmembrane envelope, gp41. The cysteines, conserved in gp120 in all HIV-1 isolates, are shown by asterisks (*). Cysteines joined by disulfide bonds (T. Gregory, personal communication) are also shown. Shown are location of (b) neutralizing epitopes, (c) T-cell epitopes, and (d) regions involved in CD4 binding and other functions. Shown are the locations of mutations affecting CD4 binding (B), gp120–gp41 association (A), gp160 processing (P) and membrane fusion (F). Also shown in (d) is the location of a mutation that renders virus noninfectious but that does not interfere with envelope synthesis or processing, the stability of gp41 or the binding of gp120 to CD4 (209).

One study used an algorithm to predict amphipathicity of gp160 to locate two immunodominant helper T-cell epitopes (150). These peptides, denoted T1 and T2, stimulate proliferation and lymphokine release from lymphocytes of mice immunized with native or recombinant gp120 (Figs. 7c and 8 and Table 3). Conversely, the T2 peptide induces T-cell immunity to native gp120 in that mice immunized with T2 are primed for a response to gp120. T2 is recognized by 8 of 14 and T1 by 4 of 14 humans immunized with vaccinia virus expressing gp160 and boosted with recombinant envelope (151). This indicates that T1 and T2 function as T-cell epitopes in humans. Both T1 and T2 are in relatively conserved regions of gp120, and T2 overlaps a segment of gp120 required for interaction with CD4. In addition to T1 and T2, six additional regions of gp160, mapped using overlapping peptides, have been found to contain clusters of T-helper-cell epitopes (Figs 7c and 8 and Table 3) (152). Four of the six regions are conserved, and all six are recognized by mice of either three or four MHC types.

In other experiments, CD4$^+$,CD8$^-$ T-cell clones responding to gp120 were isolated from HIV-seronegative human donors (153). The T-cell epitope on the linear gp120 sequence recognized by one of these clones was mapped using synthetic peptides and fragments from an acetic acid digest of gp120. The sequence recognized by this clone overlaps with, but is not identical to, T2 (Figs. 7c and 8). Although this region has a relatively conserved polypeptide sequence among different HIV-1 isolates, a single amino acid substitution abolishes recognition by this clone.

The same gp120-specific CD4$^+$,CD8$^-$ clones from the same donor are cytolytic in that either autologous CD4 peripheral blood lymphocytes or an autologous CD4$^+$ lymphocyte clone, when incubated with gp120, are targets for lysis. The uptake of gp120 by CD4$^+$ clones and hence their lysis is prevented by soluble CD4 and monoclonal antibodies that block binding of gp120 to CD4. This and similar studies (154,155) provide evidence for a mechanism of CD4$^+$ cell depletion in HIV infection in which gp120 shed from the virus is picked up by uninfected CD4$^+$ cells and presented as antigen in association with class II MHC. These cells would then be targets for class II-restricted killing by CD4$^+$ cytotoxic cells specific for gp120. CD4$^+$ cells with gp120 bound to CD4 are also targets for lysis by ADCC (155).

A target within gp120 for MHC class I-restricted CTL has been mapped (156), and this epitope is within the RP135 principal neutralizing determinant discussed earlier (Fig. 7c). H-2^d mice immunized with vaccinia virus expressing

---

Figure 8 The envelope amino acid sequence encoded by the BH10 molecular clone of the HTLV-III$_B$ isolate (40). The functional and structural features are shown and are described and referenced in Figure 7 and Table 3. (Figure continues over following five pages.)

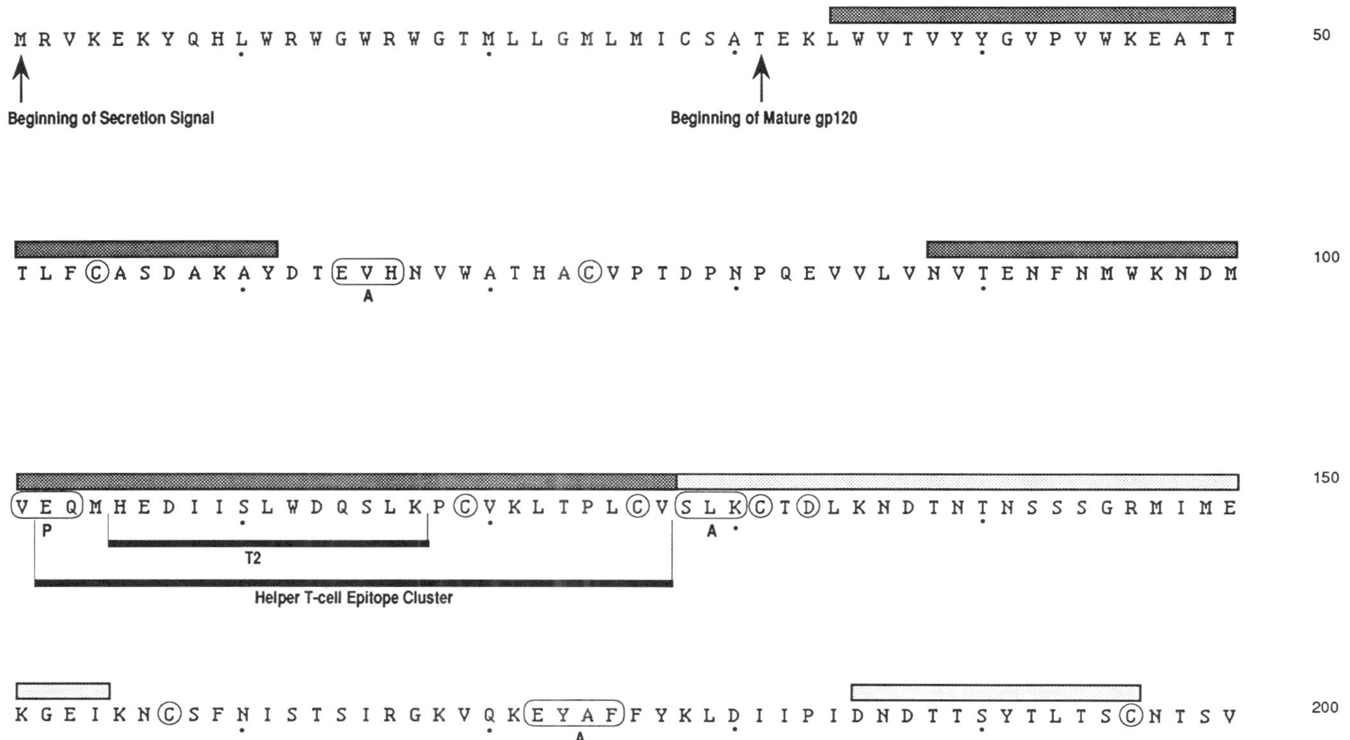

M R V K E K Y Q H L W R W G W R W G T M L L G M L M I C S A T E K L W V T V Y Y G V P V W K E A T T   50
Beginning of Secretion Signal
Beginning of Mature gp120
T L F C A S D A K A Y D T E V H N V W A T H A C V P T D P N P Q E V V L V N V T E N F N M W K N D M   100
A
V E Q M H E D I I S L W D Q S L K P C V K L T P L C V S L K C T D L K N D T N T N S S S G R M I M E   150
P
A
T2
Helper T-cell Epitope Cluster
K G E I K N C S F N I S T S I R G K V Q K E Y A F F Y K L D I I P I D N D T T S Y T L T S C N T S V   200
A

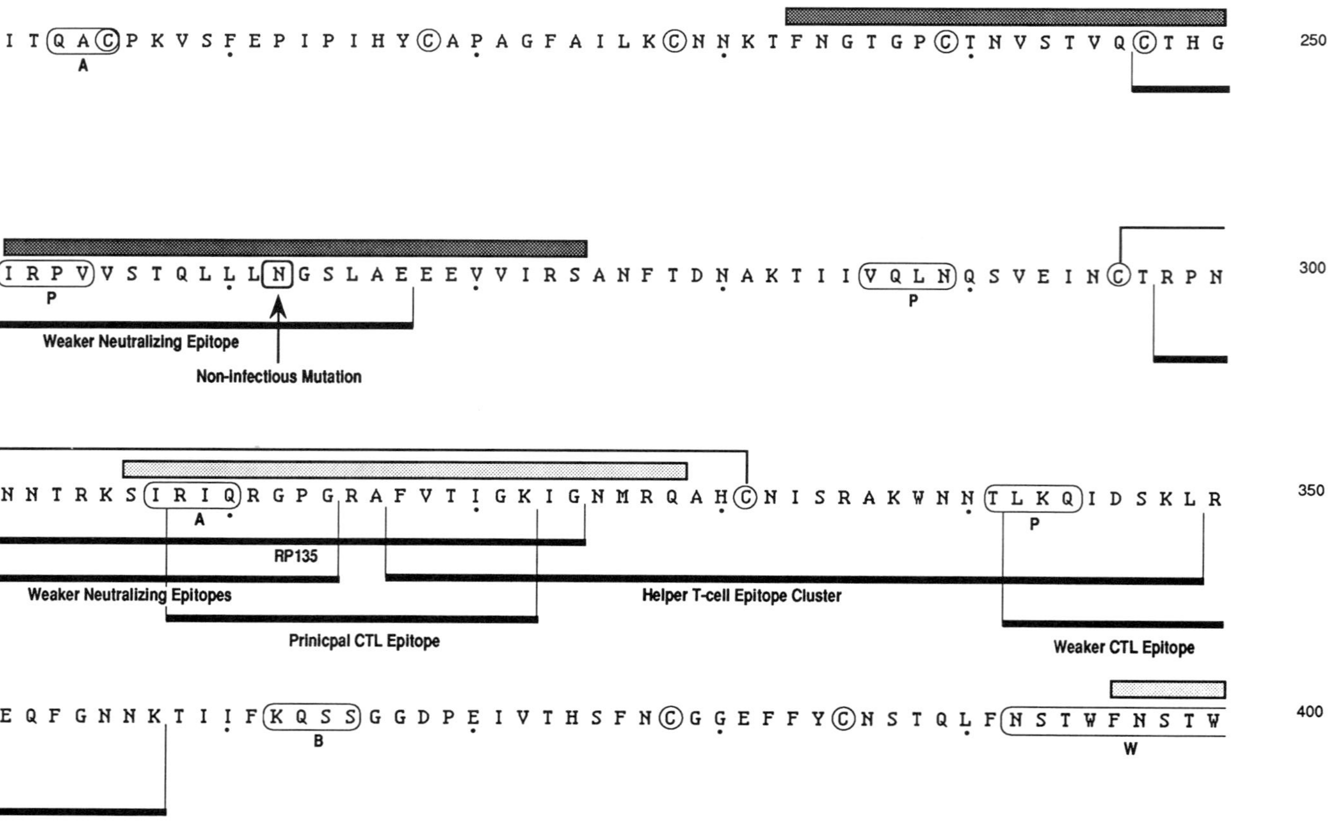
I T Q A C P K V S F E P I P I H Y C A P A G F A I L K C N N K T F N G T G P C T N V S T V Q C T H G
A
250

I R P V V S T Q L L L N G S L A E E E V V I R S A N F T D N A K T I I V Q L N Q S V E I N C T R P N
P
Weaker Neutralizing Epitope
Non-Infectious Mutation
300

N N T R K S I R I Q R G P G R A F V T I G K I G N M R Q A H C N I S R A K W N N T L K Q I D S K L R
A
P
RP135
Weaker Neutralizing Epitopes
Helper T-cell Epitope Cluster
Prinicpal CTL Epitope
Weaker CTL Epitope
350

E Q F G N N K T I I F K Q S S G G D P E I V T H S F N C G G E F F Y C N S T Q L F N S T W F N S T W
B
W
400

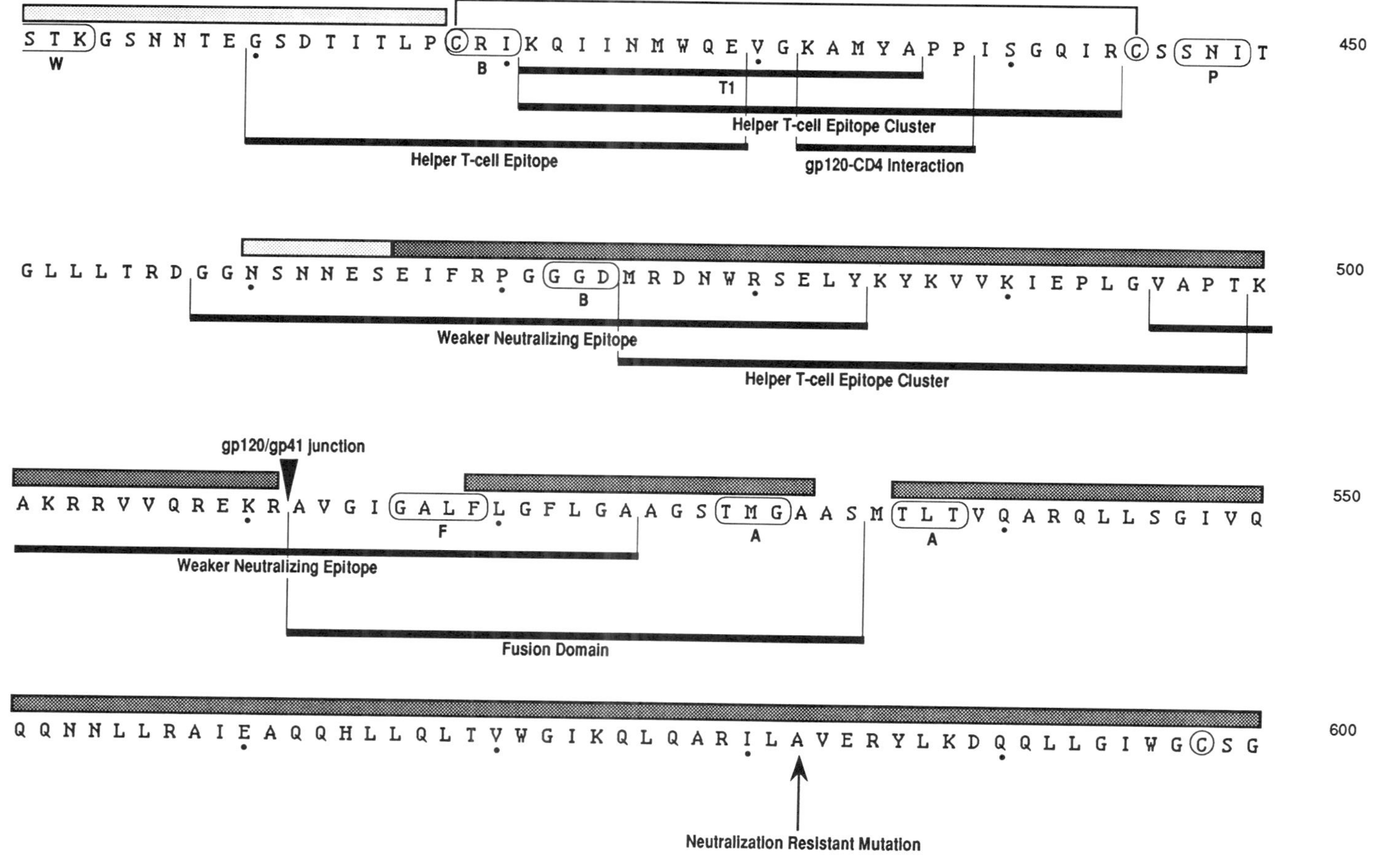

Figure 8   (Continued)

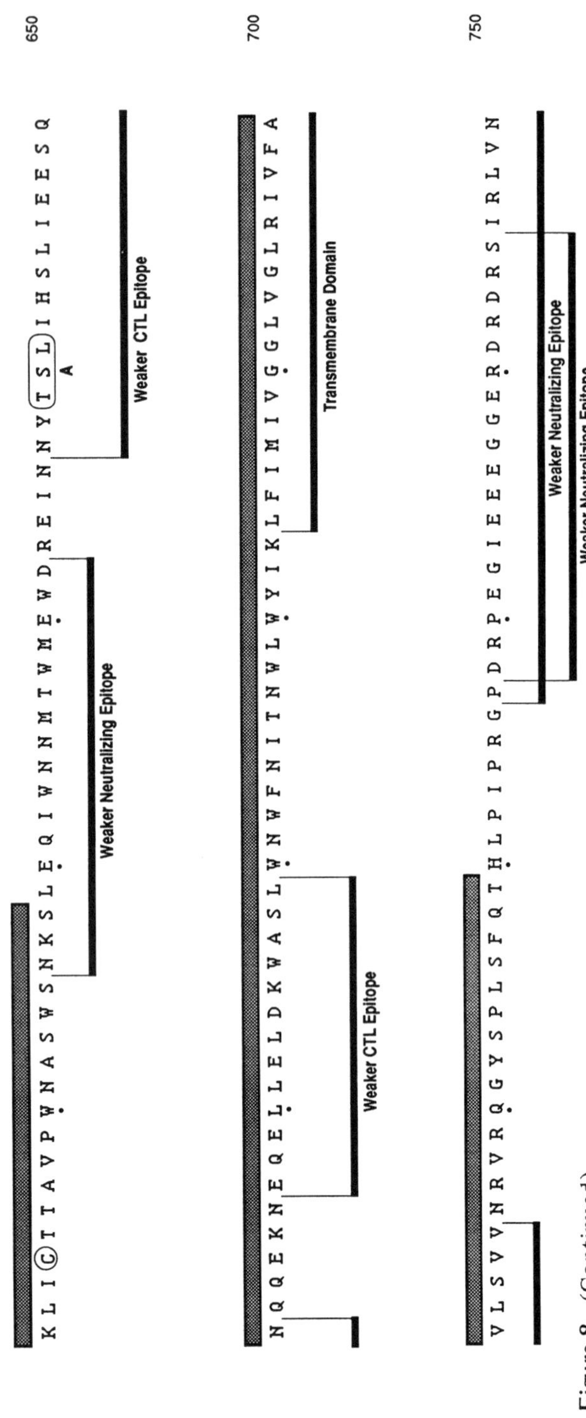

Figure 8 (Continued)

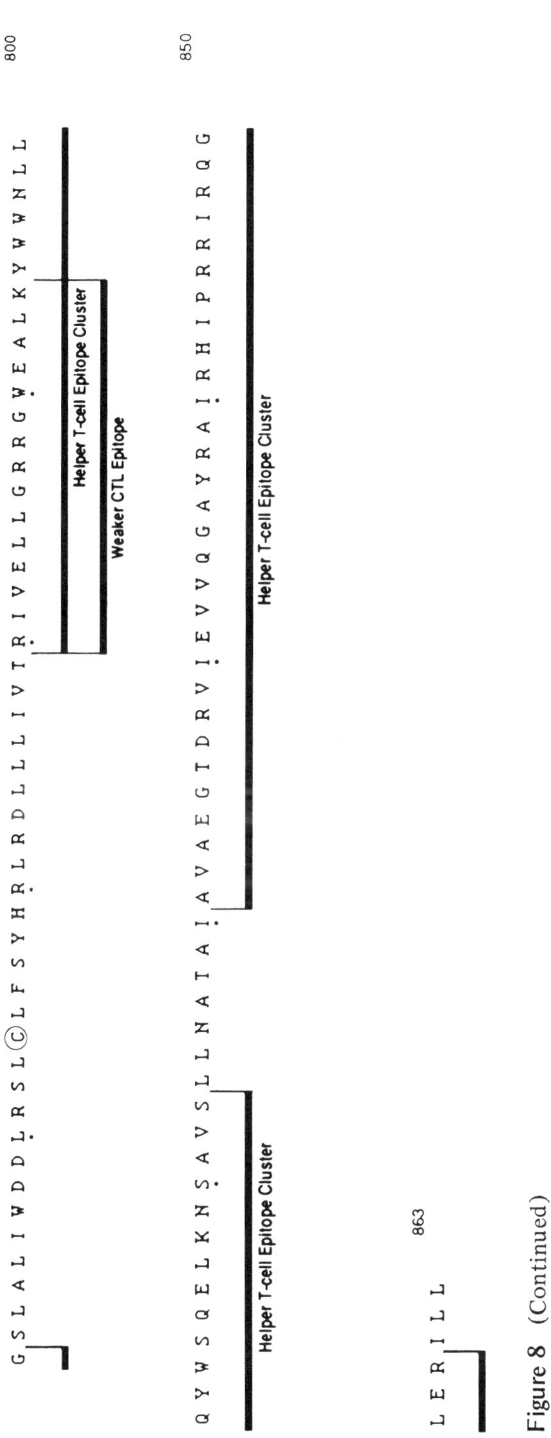

Figure 8 (Continued)

Table 3 Location of Important Regions of gp160 (HTLV-III$_B$; BH10)

	Amino acid positions[a]	References
a. Envelope structure		
Beginning of secretion signal	1	40
Beginning of mature gp120	31	
End of gp120	511	
Beginning of gp41	512	
End of gp41	856	
Cysteines in gp120[b]	54,74,119,126, 131,157,196,205, 218,228,239,247 296,331,378,385, 418,445	
Cysteines in gp41	598,604,764	
Conserved regions	34-61,88-127 233-274,466-511, 519-532,536-618, 647-719	75
Variable regions	128-154,185-196, 306-328,396-417, 460-465	
b. Neutralization epitopes		
PB1	289-466	92
Principal neutralizing domain (RP135)	301-324	123-126
Weaker neutralizing epitopes	247-267, 298-314, 458-484,616-632, 727-751, 496-525,728-745	144,145 142,143
Neutralization-resistant-mutation	582	147
c. T-cell epitopes		
Helper T-cell epitopes	105-117(T2),421- 436(T1) 410-429	150 153
Helper T-cell epitope clusters	102-127,317-349, 421-444, 475-499,780-813, 821-853	152
Principal CTL epitope	308-322	156
Weaker CTL epitopes	342-357,637-651, 657-669,780-794	156

Table 3   (Continued)

	Amino acid positions[a]	References
d. CD4 binding and other functional domains		
gp120-CD4 Interaction	432–437	36,48
Noninfectious mutation	262	208
Fusion domain	512–534	158
Transmembrane domain	684–705	162
Mutations that affect gp120/gp41 association	64,129 173,204,308 530,537,640	132
Mutations that affect gp160 processing	102,252,287 342,448	132
Mutations that affect gp120/CD4 interaction	363,419,473	132
Mutation that affects membrane fusion	517	132
Deletion that has no apparent effect	392–403	132
Location of *rev*-responsive element	516–593	163,164

[a]Numbered with position 1 as the beginning of the secretion signal.
[b]In mature envelope (excluding secretion signal).

gp160 generate CD8$^+$, CD4$^-$ lymphocytes that recognize principally an epitope within the neutralizing determinant. These CTL responses were detected in only one of four MHC class I murine molecules tested and this suggests that the CTL repertoire elicited by the envelope is limited. Because of the variability of the sequence in this epitope, this CTL response is virus isolate-specific in that a CTL clone specific for the loop of IIIB does not lyse target cells presenting peptide antigen from four other isolates (J. Berzofsky, personal communication). Other regions of the envelope act as CTL targets, although they are not recognized as efficiently as that within the RP135 determinant (156). These are denoted as weaker CTL epitopes in Figures 7c and 8.

Although the epitopes recognized by human class I- or II-restricted CTL have not yet been determined, envelope-specific CTL clones isolated from seropositive donors are both virus type-specific or group-common in their target selection (117,157). This suggests that these epitopes are from both variable and conserved regions of the envelope. The response of T cells to the envelope, therefore, appears to be broader than that of neutralizing antibody, which recognizes principally one epitope.

CD4 Binding

Several experiments have delineated regions of gp120 that interact with CD4. One study (36,48) generated three monoclonal antibodies to gp120 that block binding to CD4. These antibodies bind to gp120 with an association constant of about 10^8 and, because this is more than an order of magnitude lower than the gp120-CD4 association constant, they are unable to block HIV infection of CD4-bearing cells. A peptide of gp120 that binds to one of these antibodies was isolated and sequenced. Although this peptide cannot bind to CD4, several mutations introduced into this domain (Figs. 7d and 8 and Table 3) in a clone expressing the envelope result in purified gp120 unable to bind CD4. The gp160-binding region of all three blocking antibodies were mapped using proteolytic fragments of gp120 and gp120 fragments expressed using the λgt11 expression system (48). All blocking antibodies bind to this domain.

In separate experiments in vitro mutagenesis was used to insert linkers and delete sequences randomly throughout the envelope (132). The mutants were introduced into a vector that expressed envelope after transfection into $CD4^+$ cells, and the ability of gp120 to bind CD4 was measured. Mutations in three locations at the carboxyl-terminal half of gp120 interfere with binding (Figs. 17d and 8 and Table 3). These positions are separated by approximately 50 amino acids, and the CD4-binding determinant identified by mapping blocking monoclonal antibodies falls midway between the second and third of these positions.

The regions of gp120 associated with CD4 binding are relatively conserved in amino acid sequence between HIV-1, HIV-2, and SIV isolates. This is understandable considering that each of these molecules binds CD4. The regions of gp120 defined by these mutations have an overall hydrophobic composition suggesting that they are buried within the envelope. This is consistent with the fact that no monoclonal antibodies that neutralize viral infectivity by preventing binding of gp120 to CD4 have been identified.

Fusion Peptide, Mechanism of Membrane Fusion, and other Domains

The amino terminus of gp41 (Figs. 7d and 8 and Table 3) has homology with the amino terminus of the F_1 glycoprotein of paramyxoviruses (158). The F_1 protein is generated by cleavage of a precursor, Fc, by a trypsin-like enzyme to expose the amino terminus of F_1, which is hydrophobic and contains the peptide Phe-X-Gly. This amino terminus of F_1 is responsible for both envelope-cell fusion and cell–cell fusion induced by these viruses. The amino terminus of

HIV gp41, which is generated after cleavage of gp160, is also hydrophobic and contains Phe-Leu-Gly. Mutations that affect the ability of the envelope to induce syncytia formation map to this region (132).

Endoproteolytic cleavage of gp160 is required to generate infectious virus (159). If the trypsin-like cleavage site is replaced with a chymotrypsin-like site, the mutant virus is phenotypically wild type with respect to proviral replication, RNA processing, protein expression, and viral assembly. The virus mutant is noninfectious unless it is exposed to chymotrypsin. The ability of the envelope to induce syncitia is also inhibited when gp160 cleavage is inhibited by monensin (160).

A model for the role of gp41 in initiating membrane fusion, reflecting this data, has been proposed (132). Binding of gp120 to CD4 leads to a conformational change in gp120 that allows the amino terminus of gp41 to penetrate the membrane of the CD4-bearing cell. Whether there is a protein that acts as a receptor for gp41 has not been determined. Once gp41 spans the gap between the membranes, direct membrane fusion occurs and the contents of the virus particle or infected cell are released into the uninfected cell. Similar models for the role of the envelope glycoproteins in fusion have been proposed for the paramyxoviruses (161).

This model suggests that antibodies that bind the amino terminus of gp41 may neutralize viral infectivity. Antibodies elicited by a peptide consisting of the C-terminus of gp120 and the N-terminus of gp41 have been reported to have a weak neutralizing effect (142). It is possible that this segment of gp41 is buried in the envelope structure and therefore inaccessible to antibodies. The amino terminus of gp41 appears to directly associate with the amino terminal half of gp120 because mutations in either of these two regions disrupt this association (132). gp120 produced by these mutations is in the supernatant rather than associated with the cell. It is possible that antibodies bound to the RP135-neutralizing determinant either interfere with the gp120 conformational change resulting in membrane insertion of gp41 or directly interfere with gp41 insertion.

The carboxyl-terminal half of gp41 contains a hydrophobic stretch of amino acids that spans the membrane once (Figs. 7d and 8 and Table 3). This was shown by studying the effect of translation termination mutations inserted in the envelope on the secretion of gp160 (162). In addition, translation termination insertions, mutations that introduce hydrophilic amino acids, or deletions of amino acids in this region result in quantitative release of the envelope into the supernatant (132). These mutations also eliminate syncytia formation.

The *rev* gene product augments the production of viral structural gene products (core, *pol*, and envelope) by increasing the concentration of the messenger RNAs specific for these proteins. It is currently thought that *rev* acts to export the incompletely spliced mRNA from the cell nucleus to the cytoplasm. The action of *rev* requires a 200-nucleotide-long sequence within the mRNA encoding gp41 (163,164) that presumably adopts a stable secondary structure, and *rev* may act by directly binding to this *rev*-responsive element (Figs. 7d and 8 and Table 3). Because *rev* is required for the virus life cycle, there is strong selective pressure to preserve the sequence of the *rev*-responsive element, and this may be the reason the amino acid sequence of the envelope is conserved in this region. The second exons of *tat* and *rev* are also located in regions encoding the carboxyl-terminal half of gp41, and this presumably places constraints on the amount of variability that can be tolerated in this region.

HIV VACCINE DEVELOPMENT AND TESTING EFFICACY

Can HIV or Subunits Elicit Protective Immunity?

Central unanswered questions in HIV vaccine development are "Does HIV elicit protective immunity? If so, can this immunity be elicited by a subunit and sustained for a period long enough to make a vaccine practical?" These are difficult questions because, although HIV-infected individuals develop immune responses such as neutralizing and ADCC antibodies and helper and cytotoxic T lymphocytes, virus infection persists and disease progression continues in the face of this immunity. Although the answers remain unclear, several things suggest that infected persons do develop a protective immune response.

Figure 9 shows a generalized model of the progression of an HIV infection, and this model is supported by the following correlative evidence. Once the virus infects an individual, there is a rapid burst of virus replication, and p24 core antigen can be found in the blood or cerebral spinal fluid prior to development of virus-specific antibodies in some infected persons (165,166). In addition, some individuals experience flu-like symptoms or swollen lymph nodes during this period (167). As antibody to p24 approaches detectable levels, p24 antigen becomes undetectable and remains low until ARC or AIDS clinical symptoms develop (165,166). During this asymptomatic period, virus isolation is difficult. As clinical symptoms become more severe and as immune dysfunction increases, as measured by CD4/CD8 cell ratios and other parameters, HIV viremia increases and viral antigen levels increase to detectable levels (168,169).

One interpretation of these observations is that an immune response generated early in infection, such as neutralizing antibodies, eliminates cell-free virus and only cell-associated virus sustains the infection during the asymptomatic period. During the asymptomatic period, virus replication proceeds and, as explained earlier, there is hypervariability in the sequence of the envelope suggesting that selection of nonneutralized viral mutants is occurring. As these mutants are generated, neutralizing antibodies specific for the new variants are

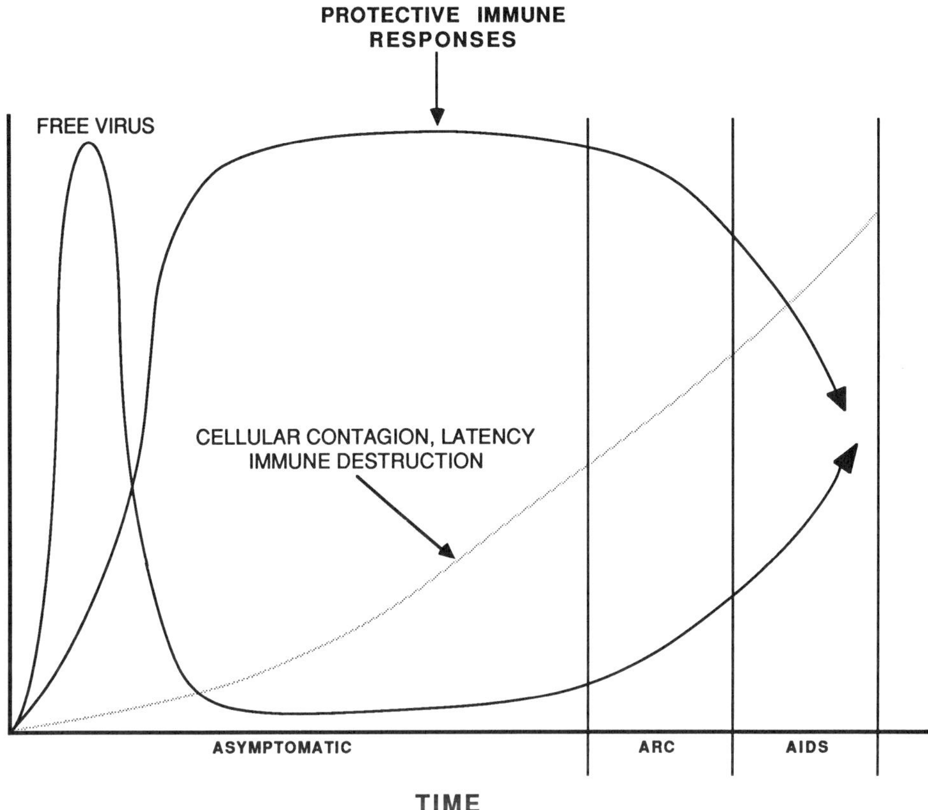

Figure 9   Generalized model of an HIV-1 infection.

generated. The infection is held in check until enough CD4 cells are destroyed or more cytopathic forms of the virus are generated and the infection is no longer contained. Antigenemia and viremia then increase resulting in further CD4-cell depletion and disease progression. An effective vaccine would have to, therefore, establish this protective immunity prior to or, via an anamnestic response, during the early stages of infection. It may also be possible that a vaccine could be effective, even if it does not prevent infection, by reducing virus burden early in infection and prolonging or extending indefinitely the asymptomatic period.

There is some evidence that HIV isolates obtained from individuals more advanced in disease progression are more cytopathic and infect a wider range of human cell types (170-172). One interpretation of this is that, in the face of protective immunity, intercellular virus transmission is limited until more cytopathic variants with a larger host range are generated. These variants, with a selective advantage, are then able to deplete the CD4 population before an immune response to those variants can be generated.

The only method that can be used to test the efficacy of an experimental vaccine immunogen is to immunize an animal able to sustain viral infection and then to experimentally challenge the animal with titered, infectious virus. Such a challenge experiment is successful when unimmunized but not immunized animals become infected or when only the immunized animals can rapidly clear the infection without progression to disease. Although several animaals are being investigated for the ability to sustain HIV infection, the only ones found to do so reliably are the chimpanzee (173) and the gibbon ape (116).

Six immunization/challenge experiments designed to test the ability of immunogens to protect chimpanzees from HIV infection have been performed (Table 4). Four of these were active immunizations using in two cases gp120 (174-176), in one case a synthetic peptide of gp41 (177), and in one case vaccinia virus expressing gp160 (178). Two additional experiments were done by immunizing with HIV-specific antibodies (179,180). The basic design of the active immunization experiments was to immunize the animals and assay for envelope antibody titer, neutralizing antibodies, and in some cases cellular immunity as measured by a proliferative T-cell response to intact virus or envelope antigen. The animals are then challenged by an intravenous injection of infectious HIV. Following challenge, infection in the experimental and control animals is monitored by seroconversion to nonenvelope antigens and the ability to culture virus from peripheral blood lymphocytes.

One experiment used a recombinant vaccinia virus expressing gp160 of the LAV-1 strain of HIV-1 (178). After the initial immunization and one boost, low gp120-specific antibody titers and no neutralizing antibodies were detected. The immunized animals did have helper and cytotoxic T lymphocytes specific for LAV-1-infected cells. The animals were challenged with, in one experiment, 3×10^5 tissue culture infectious doses ($TCID_{50}$) of LAV-1 and, in a subsequent experiment, 3×10^2 $TCID_{50}$.

Two of the active immunization experiments used as immunogen gp120 purified from either HTLV-IIIB (III_B)-infected cells (174) (native gp120) or purified from a CHO cell line producing recombinant gp120 expressed from a molecular clone of the III_B isolate (recombinant gp120) (175). Both proteins were formulated with aluminum hydroxide, which is the only adjuvant approved for human use. Five 50 μg immunizations of native gp120 and four 1 mg doses of recombinant gp120 elicited antibodies that both bound gp120 as assayed by radioimmunoprecipitation and Western blotting and neutralized the III_B virus. Although detectable, the neutralization titers, which were approximately 10-20, were approximately a factor of 10 lower than those elicited using Freund's

Table 4 Vaccine Efficacy Experiments

	Immunogen						
	gp120 native	gp120 recombinant	gp160 vaccinia	gp41 peptide	IgG-infected human	IgG-IIIB-infected chimpanzee	0.5β monoclonal
Immunogen strain	III$_B$	III$_B$	LAV-1	III$_B$	NA	III$_B$	III$_B$
Number of animals	2	2	2,2[a]	2	2,2[b]	1	1
Dose	$5 \times 50\ \mu g$	5×1 mg	$2\times (2 \times 10^8\ \text{pfu})$	$4 \times 200\ \mu g$	1 ml/kg, 10 ml/kg	NA	NA
Adjuvant	Alum	Alum	NA	CFA/IFA	NA	NA	NA
Binding antibody	αgp120	αgp120	αgp120,gp41	αgp120	αenv, core RT	αenv, core RT	αgp120
Neutralizing antibody	+	+	−	+/−	+	+	+
ADCC	+	ND	ND	ND	+	ND	ND
T-helper response	+	+	+	ND	NA	NA	NA
CTL response	ND	ND	+	ND	NA	NA	NA
Challenge strain	III$_B$	III$_B$	LAV-1	NY-5	III$_B$	III$_B$	III$_B$
Challenge dose (TCID$_{50}$)	10^2	10^2	$3.2 \times 10^5, 10^2$	10^3	10^2	10^2	10^2
Reference	176	175	178	177	179	180	180

[a]Two animals were challenged with 3.2×10^5 TCID$_{50}$ and two with 10^2 TCID$_{50}$
[b]Two animals received 1 ml/kg and two received 10 mg/kg.
ND = not determined.
NA = not applicable.

adjuvant with the same immunogen. Both forms of the gp120 immunogen elicit T cells that proliferate in response to both III_B and gp120. Immunized and control animals were challenged with 100 $TCID_{50}$ of $HTLV-III_B$ virus. This infectious dose had been determined from an in vivo infection titration experiment to be the minimum dose of virus that ensures infection.

In one early experiment (177), two chimpanzees were immunized with four 200 μg doses of a synthetic peptide consisting of amino acids 735-752 of the III_B (BH10) sequence. Complete Freund's followed by incomplete Freund's adjuvant was used, and the animals developed gp41-binding antibody but a very lower titer of neutralizing antibody to the NY-5 strain of HIV-1. The animals were challenged with 10^3 $TCID_{50}$ of NY-5.

For the passive immunization experiment (179), plasma from seropositive donors was screened for neutralizing antibody to $HTLV-III_B$, and samples from approximately 20 people that had relatively high neutralizing titer (>128) were pooled. After treatment to inactivate infectious virions, IgG was isolated and concentrated to about 50 mg/ml. This IgG has a neutralization titer 5- to 10-fold higher than that in the unfractionated plasma, but subsequent experiments (see below) showed that there was no antibody present to the RP135 determinant. In two separate experiments IgG was administered intravenously at doses of 1 ml/kg and 10 ml/kg body weight to immunized animals. Control animals received similar doses of immunoglobulin devoid of HIV antibodies. The dilution factors were roughly 1:100 and 1:10 with the low and high doses, respectively. One day after receiving immunoglobulin, the animals were challenged with 100 $TCID_{50}$ of $HTLV-III_B$.

When animals immunized with any of these preparations were challenged, they seroconverted as rapidly as the unimmunized controls, and there were no statistically significant differences from controls in the ability to isolate virus. No analysis has yet been done to determine whether there are any differences, particularly in the ability to be neutralized by the immune antisera, between the virus recovered from the infected animals and the virus used for the challenge. One explanation for the disappointing results, therefore, is that the animals were protected from infection by a subset of the viruses in the challenee inoculation and were infected by variants within the population that were resistant to neutralization. This is of particular concern because the virus challenge inoculum was isolated from a seropositive individual, and such viruses consist of a population of similar but sequence heterogenous viruses. This is particularly true for the III_B virus isolate, from which four independent molecular clones have been sequenced and differ in amino acid sequence of the envelope by 1 or 2 percent (40). For this reason, challenge inoculums to be used in subsequent experiments should consist of infectious virus generated from an infectious proviral molecular clone.

Another possible reason for the infection is that the binding and neutralizing antibody titers at the time of challenge were too low so that only a fraction of the challenge virus was neutralized. This is of concern particularly in the active immunization experiments where the neutralization titers were relatively low. It will be important in subsequent experiments to use an adjuvant or modified immunogens able to elicit higher titers.

The results of these experiments leave doubt as to whether neutralizing antibody, which can prevent infection in vitro, can prevent infection in vivo. An experiment was therefore performed (180) to assess the ability of neutralizing antibodies, when complexed with infectious virion, to prevent infection following inoculation of the virion-antibody complexes (Table 4). The experiment consisted of incubating HTLV-III$_B$ virus with antibody for 90 minutes, inoculating uninfected chimpanzees with the antibody-virus complex, and monitoring for subsequent seroconversion to viral antigens. (In previous experiments it was shown that, with the antibody used, the 90-minute incubation ensured complete in vitro neutralization of the challenge virus for 8 weeks.) Antibodies used in this experiment include an IgG fraction isolated from polyclonal antisera from an uninfected chimpanzee, a mouse monoclonal antibody (0.5β), which neutralizes the III$_B$ isolate and binds to the RP135 determinant (128), and an IgG fraction isolated from polyclonal antisera from a chimpanzee which had been infected with the III$_B$ isolate for approximately 1 year. This IgG fraction had a III$_B$-neutralizing titer of 640.

The chimpanzee inoculated with the IgG fraction taken from the uninfected chimpanzee seroconverted in 6 weeks, which is consistent with other animals challenged with the III$_B$ virus. The animal inoculated with the virus preincubated with the 0.5β monoclonal, however, did not seroconvert until 12 weeks and showed a significantly lower antibody titer than the control animal. The chimpanzee receiving the IgG fraction taken from the III$_B$-infected chimpanzee has shown no signs of seroconversion even after 50 weeks. All of the neutralizing antibody in the IgG fraction which was protective can be absorbed with the RP135 peptide, thus indicating that all of the III$_B$-neutralizing antibody in this fraction binds the RP135 determinant.

These results show that the RP135-directed monoclonal antibody delays infection and strongly suggests that the RP135-directed neutralizing antibodies in the polyclonal antisera protected against infection. Although encouraging, these experiments do not prove rigorously that RP135-directed antibodies can protect against infection and this must await an immunization/challenge experiment with an RP135 immunogen. The experiment does, however, show that antibody immunity is sufficient to prevent infection and also shows that, at least in the presence of high neutralizing antibody concentration, antibody-dependent enhancement of infection does not occur. These results offer an explanation of

why the human immunoglobin with high neutralizing antibody titer administered passively before challenge (179) did not prevent infection. As described
earlier, there are at least two types of neutralizing antibody. One binds to the
RP135 determinant and is induced by immunization with envelope subunits, and
the other binds elsewhere and is induced only by infectious virion. Because the
immunoglobulin used in the passive immunization experiment did not contain
antibody to RP135 but did contain neutralizing antibody directed elsewhere,
this suggests that neutralizing antibody not directed to RP135 is unable to
prevent infection.

Design of Vaccine Candidates

How can the information learned about the HIV envelope be used to design an
effective subunit vaccine? Although the in vitro neutralization/challenge experiment (180) showed that antibody can prevent infection, CTL reduce virus
burden and could prevent infection if the levels were high enough at the time of
exposure. Vaccine candidates should, therefore, be designed to elicit both
humoral and cellular immunity and epitopes for neutralizing, and ADCC antibody as well as helper and cytotoxic T-cell epitopes should be included in
current vaccine candidates.

One advantage to a subunit vaccine is that it can be engineered to contain
epitopes representing immune targets while eliminating unimportant or potentially detrimental epitopes. Another advantage is that epitopes could be engineered to elicit a response higher than that elicited by the infection virus. This
may be particularly important for an HIV vaccine because HIV may not elicit,
or elicit only in some cases, protective immunity.

One possible approach to vaccine design is to construct a hybrid immunogen
consisting of a B-cell epitope, such as the neutralizing domain, and a T-helper-
cell epitope. The T-cell epitope could be chosen to elicit high titers and a
potent anamnestic response to the attached neutralizing epitope. Because the
response to T-helper-cell epitopes is MHC restricted, not all of the population
will generate a good immune response to a vaccine with one particular T-helper
epitope. This nonresponsiveness could be overcome by using a cocktail of
T-helper epitopes which will elicit a universal response. For example, H-2^d mice
are nonresponders to the neutralizing epitope of the foot-and-mouth disease
virus. When a 20-amino-acid-long peptide containing this epitope is coupled to
T-helper-cell epitopes derived from either ovalbumin or sperm whale myoglobin,
this nonresponsiveness is overcome (181). In addition, H-2 congenic mouse
strains, which are unable to mount an antibody response to a peptide containing
the major B-cell site on the malaria circumsporozoite protein, respond to this
sequence when it is coupled to a helper-T-cell site from the same protein (182).
These data suggest that by incorporating a series of T-helper-cell sites in the

vaccine subunit, MHC restriction could be overcome and a large percentage of the population may respond to the immunogen.

Another problem that must be overcome is the amino acid sequence variability of the envelope. A vaccine must protect against a diverse array of HIV isolates. One possible solution is to devise a subunit immunogen to elicit a protective immune response targeted towards the conserved envelope segments. This strategy may work with helper and cytotoxic T-cell responses that recognize relatively conserved sequences, but the major neutralizing epitope is highly variable. Another approach is to use a "cocktail" immunogen consisting of neutralizing epitopes from more than one HIV isolate. This assumes that the variability of HIV is limited and that a limited number of serotype classes can be defined. This will allow induction of protective immunity by the envelope of one member of the class that will protect against infection by other members in than class.

In preliminary cocktail studies, we have shown that immunization of a single animal with PB1 or gp160 from both the III$_B$ and RF viral isolates elicits antibodies that neutralize both isolates, whereas immunization with a single immunogen elicits only a type-specific response (Table 1). In addition, a trivalent cocktail of three peptides of the RP135 determinant from the III$_B$, RF, and MN isolates elicits antisera that neutralize all three isolates (183). Another approach is to construct hybrid proteins or peptides containing epitopes from several serotype classes. This approach was used to generate hybrid polioviruses containing neutralization determinants from both the type 1 and type 3 serotypes (184,185). Immune sera to either type 1 and type 3 virus neutralized the hybrid virus, and the hybrid virus elicits neutralizing antibodies to both serotypes. As discussed earlier, with hybrid peptides containing both III$_B$ and RF sequences, we have designed peptides that elicit antibodies that neutralize more than one virus isolate (Table 2). To develop a cocktail or hybrid polypeptide vaccine based on the RP135 determinant, HIV-1 strains must be grouped into serotypes based on the sequence of the RP135 determinant. Because the Gly-Pro-Gly is highly conserved, it may serve as an anchor around which to design such hybrid peptides. For example, hybrid peptides could be constructed with the amino acid sequence of serotype A on the left of the Gly-Pro-Gly and with serotype B on the right. Such a peptide would elicit antibodies able to neutralize members of both serotype classes. Obviously, deciphering such serotype classes will be an important part of vaccine development.

There are also epitopes in the envelope that may be detrimental to the recipient and, therefore, should not be included in a subunit vaccine. For example, peptides consisting of amino acid sequence of the transmembrane envelope protein suppress the proliferative response to mitogens of normal human lymphocytes (186). Peptides and recombinant proteins, also from the transmembrane protein, cause a proliferative response of peripheral blood mono-nuclear cells and of both CD3[+] and CD3[−] lymphocyte subpopulations (187). These effects, if functional in vivo, could have a detrimental effect on the immune function of vaccines. No such activities, however, have been ascribed to regions of the external envelope.

Another example of potentially harmful epitopes are those that participate in antibody-dependent enhancement (ADE) of HIV infection. It has been found that antibodies from some sera from HIV-infected individuals enhance infection of Fc receptor–bearing cells (188-190). One mechanism for this is Fc receptor-mediated uptake of an antibody bound to a viral particle. ADE would imply that the presence of HIV-specific antibody may make vaccinees more susceptible to infection. Although it may be that any virus-specific antibody could partici-pate in ADE, it may also be that antibody bound to particular epitopes are more efficient in ADE. These sites, if they do not overlap with protective epitopes, could be eliminated in the subunit immunogen. The results of the in vitro neutralization–virus challenge experiment described earlier (180), however, showed that ADE did not occur in that case.

Another advantage unique to the subunit approach is that detrimental effects of inactivated virus or native viral proteins can be eliminated in the subunit immunogen. For example, there are several immunosuppressive activities that are mediated by gp120 binding to CD4 lymphocytes. Native gp120 activates resting CD4 lymphocytes as measured by an increase in intracellular levels of inositol triphosphate and calcium and elevates interleukin-2 receptor levels (191). gp120 also inhibits antigen-specific CD4 lymphocyte responses of cells from normal donors (192,193), and native and recombinant gp120 suppresses PHA-induced lymphocyte blastogenesis and has other effects on functions of immune cells from uninfected donors (194,195). In addition to these effects, which could potentially be seen in uninfected vaccinees, gp120, either bound or processed and presented on an APC, could target for destruction uninfected CD4 lympho-cytes in HIV-infected vaccinees (119,155).

Because binding to CD4 is necessary for gp120 to exert these effects, immu-nization with an envelope subunit unable to bind CD4 would be a preferable immunogen to the native envelope. This could consist of mutant gp120 with amino acid substitutions that eliminate CD4 binding but that preserve native overall conformation of the protein. This would allow the presentation of epitopes, possibly those that elicit group-common neutralizing antibodies, that depend on the native conformation.

Efficacy Testing of Vaccine Candidates

Efficacy testing of vaccine candidates has been a severe bottleneck for vaccine development because HIV infects only chimpanzees (173) and gibbon apes

(116), and these species are in limited supply. It is estimated that there are less than 1000 chimpanzees currently available for AIDS research (196). Another drawback to using chimpanzees is that infected animals have not yet shown AIDS-like symptoms so that vaccine candidates could only be tested for the ability to prevent infection or to reduce viremia if infection occurs. An important advance in vaccine development will be in an in vivo model system in which the animals are plentiful, inexpensive, easy to manage, able to support HIV infection and manifest disease syndromes.

Recently, rabbits have been shown to be susceptible to HIV infection (197). Rabbit T-cell and macrophage cell lines, transformed with oncogenic viruses, can be infected with HIV-1 (198). Animals inoculated with HIV or virus-producing cells develop persistent infection and seroconvert. Virus can be isolated months after infection by co-cultivating rabbit lymphocytes with CD4 human cells. Infected animals may experience some disease symptoms (199).

Another approach to animal model development is to generate mice that can be infected with HIV. Mice with severe combined immune deficiency (SCID), harboring a human thymus or lymph nodes, have been inoculated intrathymically or intranodally with a cloned HIV-1 isolate and become infected (200). Virus spread within the lymphoid organs and infection was shown by immuno-histochemistry and by in vitro hybridization of RNA transcripts, and some cells express both viral-specific RNA and protein. Another approach (201) is to generate transgenic mice to incorporating infectious HIV genomic clones. Founder mice with incorporated provirus do not express HIV, but some offspring contain infectious virus, show disease symptoms, and die.

Even if such preliminary work does develop into a reliable model that can be used to develop viable vaccine candidates able to confer protection, subsequent efficacy studies should be done in chimpanzees before progressing to human clinical trials. Human trials have already begun with some vaccine candidates (202,203; J. Zarling, personal communication). Phase I clinical trials should be performed with low-risk volunteers and assess only safety and not efficacy. Human efficacy of vaccines has traditionally been tested only with a large number of uninfected high-risk volunteers (Phase III clinical trials). The expense and duration of such a study with an HIV vaccine will depend on the clinical endpoint. If the endpoint is prevention of seroconversion (i.e., prevention of infection), efficacy studies could potentially be completed in 1–2 years because seroconversion occurs relatively soon after infection. If, however, the endpoint is prevention of disease, the study could last several years because of the long asymptomatic period (204-207). Clearly, thorough efficacy data should be gathered in animal models before large-scale human efficacy experiments are begun.

Once the safety of a vaccine candidate is established, it may be reasonable to use a serologic endpoint to determine potential efficacy. For example, if vaccinated humans develop an immune response (e.g., neutralizing antibody) identical to that which was previously shown to protect chimpanzees from infection, it could be argued that because chimpanzees and humans are immunologically similar such an immune response will also protect humans. This approach would considerably reduce the length and expanse of clinical trials. Considering the urgency to develop and obtain approval for widespread human use for an HIV vaccine, a serologic endpoint for efficacy seems attractive.

ACKNOWLEDGMENTS

The authors thank colleagues at Repligen, Duke, and the National Cancer Institue who have contributed to the work described herein. These include Walter Herlihy, Karen Ross, All Profy, Larry Eckler, Paul Salinas, Ray Grimaila, Joan Petro, Cindy Jellis, Tom Mueller, Charlene McDanal, Marjorie Robert-Guroff, Kent Weinhold, Flossie Wong-Staal, and Robert Gallo. We thank Stephanie Palms and Elizabeth Bothwell for preparation of the manuscript.

REFERENCES

1. Varmus H. Retroviruses. Science 1988; 333:504.
2. Robey WG, Arthur LO, Matthews TJ, Langlois A, Copeland TD, Lerche NW, Oroszlan S, Bolognesi DP, Gilden RV, Fischinger PJ. Prospect for prevention of human immunodeficiency virus infection: purified 120-kDa envelope glycoprotein induces neutralizing antibody. Proc Natl Acad Sci USA 1986; 83:7023-7.
3. Chakrabarti S, Robert-Guroff M, Wong-Staal F, Gallo RC, Moss B. Expression of the HTLV-III envelope gene by a recombinant vaccinia virus. Nature 1986; 320:535-40.
4. Hu SL, Kosowski SG, Dalrymple JM. Expression of AIDS virus envelope gene in recombinant vaccinia viruses. Nature 1986; 320:537-40.
5. Dewar RL, Natarajan V, Vasudevachari MB, Salzman NP. Synthesis and processing of human immunodeficiency virus type 1 envelope proteins encoded by a recombinant human adenovirus. J Virol 1989; 63:129-36.
6. Berman PW, Gregory T, Crase D, Lasky LA. Protection from genital herpes simplex virus type 2 infection by vaccination with cloned type 1 glycoprotein D. Science 1985; 227:1490-2.
7. Cantin EM, Eberle R, Baldwick JL, Moss B, Willey DE, Notkins AL, Openshaw H. Expression of herpes simplex virus 1 glycoprotein B by a recombinant vaccinia virus and protection of mice against lethal herpes simples virus 1 infection. Proc Natl Acad Sci USA 1987; 84:5908-12.
8. Lasky LA, Dowbenko D, Simonsen CC, Berman PW. Protection of mice from lethal herpes simplex virus infection by vaccination with a secreted form of cloned glycoprotein D. Biotechnology 1984; 2:527-32.

9. Torseth JW, Cohen GH, Eisenberg RJ, Berman PW, Lasky LA, Cerini CP, Heilman CJ, Kerwar S, Merigan TC. Native and recombinant herpes simplex virus type 1 envelope proteins induce human immune T-lymphocyte responses. J Virol 1987; 61:1532-9.

10. Blancou J, Kieny MP, Lathe R, Lecocq JP, Pastore PP, Soulebot JP, Desmettre P. Oral vaccination of the fox against rabies using a live recombinant vaccinia virus. Nature 1986; 322:373-5.

11. Rupprecht CE, Wiktor TJ, Johnston DH, Hamir AN, Dietzschold B, Wunner WH, Glickman LT, Koprowski H. Oral immunization and protection of raccoons (Procyon lotor) with a vaccinia-rabies glycoprotein recombinant virus vaccine. Proc Natl Acad Sci USA 1987; 83:7947-50.

12. Morin JE, Lubeck MD, Barton JE, Conley AJ, Davis AR, Hung PP. Recombinant adenovirus induces antibody response to hepatitis B virus surface antigen in hamsters. Proc Natl Acad Sci USA 1987; 84:4626-30.

13. Scolnick EM, McLean AA, West DJ, McAleer WJ, Miller WJ, Buynak EB. Clinical evaluation in healthy adults of a hepatitis B vaccine made by recombinant DNA. J Amer Med Assoc 1984; 251:2812-5.

14. Valenzuela P, Medina A, Rutter WJ, Ammerer G, Hall BD. Nature 1982; 298:347-50.

15. Hunsmann G, Schneider J, Schulz A. Immunoprevention of Friend virus-induced erythroleukemia by vaccination with viral envelope glycoprotein complexes. Virology 1981; 113:602-12.

16. Earl PL, B. M, Morrison RP, Wehrly K, Nishio J, Chesebro B. T-lymphocyte priming and protection against Friend leukemia by vaccinia-retrovirus env gene recombinant. Science 1986; 234:728-31.

17. Kleiser C, Schneider J, Bayer H, Hunsmann G. Immunosuppression of Friend Leukemia virus-induced erythroleukemia by vaccination with aggregated gp70. J Gen Virol 1986; 67:1901-94.

18. Lewis MG, Mathes LE, Olson RG. Protection against feline leukemia by vaccination with a subunit vaccine. Infection and Immunity 1981; 34:888-94.

19. Nakamura H, Hayami M, Ohta Y, Ishikawa K, Tsujimoto H, Kiyokawa T, Yoshida M, Sasagawa A, Honjo S. Protection of cynomolgus monkeys against infected by human T-cell leukemia virus type 1 by immunization with viral env gene products produced by Escherichia coli. Internat'l J Cancer 1987; 40:403-7.

20. Shida H, Tochikura T, Sato T, Konno T, Hirayoshi K, Seki M, Ito Y, Hatanka M, Hinuma Y, Sugimoto M, Takahashi-Nishimaki F, Maruyama T, Miki K, Suzuki K, Morita M, Sashiyama H, Hayami M. Effect of the recombinant vaccinia viruses that express HTLV-I envelope gene on HTLV-I infection. European Mol Biol J 1987; 6:3379-84.

21. Allan JS, Coligan JE, Barin F, McLane MF, Sodroski JG, Rosen JA, Haseltine WA, Lee TH, Essex M. Major glycoprotein antigens that induce antibodies in AIDS patients are encoded by HTLV-III. Science 1985; 228:1091-4.

22. Barin F, McLane MF, Allan JS, Lee TH, Groopman JE, Essex M. Virus envelope protein of HTLV–III represents major target antigen for antibodies in AIDS patients. Science 1985; 228:1094-6.

23. Robey WG, Safai B, Oroszlan S, Arthur LO, Gonda MA, Gallo RC, Fischinger PJ. Characterization of envelope and core structure gene products of HTLV–III with sera from AIDS patients. Science 1985; 228:593-5.

24. Veronese FD, DeVico AL, Copeland TD, Oroszlan S, Gallo RC, Sarngadharan MG. Characterization of gp41 as the transmembrane protein coded by the HTLV–III/LAV envelope gene. Science 1985; 229:1402-5.

25. Gelderblom HR, Ozel M, Hausmann EHS, Winkel T, Pauli G, Koch MA. Fine structure of human immunodeficiency virus (HIV), immunocalization of structural proteins and virus-cell relation. Micron Microscopia 1988; 19: 41-60.

26. Ozel M, Pauli G, Gelderblom HR. The organization of the envelope projections on the surface of HIV. Arch Virology 1988; 100:255-66.

27. Takahashi I, Takama M, Ladhoff A, Scholz D. Envelope structure model of human immunodeficiency virus type I. J AIDS 1989; 2:136-40.

28. Fennie C, Lasky LA. Model for intracellular folding of the human immunodeficiency virus type 1 gp120. J Virol 1989; 63:639-46.

29. Kozarsky K, Penman M, Basiripour L, Haseltine W, Sodroski J, Krieger M. Glycosylation and processing of the human immunodeficiency virus type I envelope protein. J AIDS 1989; 2:163-9.

30. Willey RL, Bonifacino JS, Potts BJ, Martin MA, Klausner RD. Biosynthesis, cleavage, and degradation of the human immunodeficiency virus 1 envelope glycoprotein gp160. Proc Natl Acad Sci USA 1988; 85:9580-4.

31. Dalgleish AG, Beverley PCL, Clapham PR, Crawford DH, Greaves MF, Weiss R. The CD4 (T4) antigen is an essential component of the receptor for the AIDS retrovirus. Nature 1984; 312:763-8.

32. Klatzmann D, Champagne E, Chamaret S, Gruest J, Guetard D, Hercend T, Gluckman JC, Montagnier L. T-lymphocyte T4 molecule behaves as the receptor for human retrovirus LAV. Nature 1984; 312:767-8.

33. McDougal JS, Kennedy MS, Sligh JM, Cort SP, Mawle A, Nicholson JKA. Binding of HTLV–III/LAV to T4$^+$ T cells by a complex of the 110K viral protein and the T4 molecule. Science 1986; 231:382-5.

34. Maddon PJ, Dalgleish AG, McDougal JS, Clapham RP, Weiss RA, Axel R. The T-4 gene encodes the acquired immune deficiency syndrome virus receptor and is expressed in the immune system and the brain. Cell 1986; 42:333-48.

35. Clapham PR, Weber JN, Whitby D, McIntosh K, Dalgleish AG, Maddon PJ, Deen KC, Sweet RW, Weiss RA. Soluble CD4 blocks the infectivity of diverse strains of HIV and SIV for T cells and monocytes but not for brain and muscle cells. Nature 1989; 337:368-70.

36. Lasky LA, Nakamura G, Smith DH, Fennie C, Shimasaki C, Patzer E, Berman P, Gregory T, Capon DJ. Delineation of a region of the human immunodeficiency virus type 1 gp120 glycoprotein critical for interaction with the CD4 receptor. Cell 1987; 50:975-85.

37. Skinner MA, Langlois AJ, McDanal CB, McDougal JS, Bolognesi DP, Matthews TJ. Neutralizing antibodies to an immunodominant envelope sequence do not prevent gp120 binding to CD4. J Virol 1988; 62:4195–200.

38. McDougal JS, Nicholson KA, Cross GD, Cort SA, Kennedy MS, Mawle AC. Binding of the human retrovirus HTLV–III/LAV/ARV/HIV to the CD4 (T4) molecule: conformation dependence, epitope mapping, antibody inhibition, and potential for idiotypic mimicry. J Immunol 1986; 137: 2937–44.

39. Muesing MA, Smith DH, Cabradilla CD, Benton CV, Lasky LA, Capon DJ. Nucleic acid structure and expression of the human AIDS/lymphadeno-pathy retrovirus. Nature 1985; 313:450–8.

40. Ratner L, Haseltine W, Patarca R, Livak KJ, Starcich B, Josephs SF, Doran ER, Rafalski AN, Whitehorn EA, Baumeister K, Ivanoff L, Petteway SR, Pearson ML, Lautenberger JA, Papas TS, Ghrayeb J, Chang NT, Gallo RC, Wong-Staal F. Complete nucleotide sequence of the AIDS virus, HTLV-III. Nature 1985; 313:277–84.

41. Sanchez-Pescador R, Power MD. Barr PJ, Steimer KS, Stempien MM, Brown-Shimer SL, Gee WW, Renard A, Randolph A, Levy JA, Dina D, Luciw PA. Nucleotide sequence and expression of an AIDS-associated retrovirus (ARV-2). Nature 1985; 227:484–503.

42. Wain-Hobson S, Sonigo P, Danos O, Cole S, Alizon M. Nucleotide sequence of the AIDS virus, LAV. Cell 1985; 40:9–17.

43. Matthews TJ, Weinhold KJ, Lyerly HK, Langlois AJ, Wigzell H, Bolognesi DP. Interaction between the human T-cell lymphotropic virus type IIIB envelope glycoprotein gp120 and the surface antigen CD4: role of carbo-hydrate in binding and cell fusion. Proc Natl Acad Sci USA 1987; 84:5424–8.

44. Gruters RA, Neefjes JJ, Tersmette M, de Goede REY, Tulp A, Huisman HG, Miedema F, Ploegh HL. Interference with HIV-induced syncytium formation and viral infectivity by inhibitors of trimming glucosidase. Nature 1987; 330:74–7.

45. Walker BD, Kowalski M, Goh WC, Kozarsky K, Krieger M, Rosen C, Rohschneider L, Haseltine WA, Sodroski J. Inhibition of human immuno-deficiency virus syncytium formation and virus replication by castanosper-mine. Proc Natl Acad Sci USA 1987; 84:8120–214.

46. Montefiori DC, Robinson WE, Mitchell WM. Role of protein N-glycosyla-tion in pathogenesis of human immunodeficiency virus type 1. Proc Natl Acad Sci USA 1988; 85:9248–52.

47. Nygren A, Bergman T, Matthews T, Jornvall H, Wigzell H. 95- and 25-kDa fragments of the human immunodeficiency virus envelope glycoprotein gp120 bind to the CD4 receptor. Proc Natl Acad Sci USA 1988; 85:6543–6.

48. Dowbenko D, Nakamura G, Fennie C, Shimasaki C, Riddle L, Harris R, Gregory T, Lasky L. Epitope mapping of the human immunodeficiency virus type 1 gp120 with monoclonal antibodies. J Virol 1988; 62:4703–11.

49. Berger EA, Fuerst TR, Moss B. A soluble recombinant polypeptide comprising the amino-terminal half of the extracellular region of the CD4 molecule contains an active binding site of human immunodeficiency virus. Proc Natl Acad Sci USA 1988; 85:2357–61.

50. Clayton LK, Hussey RE, Steinbrich R, Ramachandran H, Husain Y, Reinherz EL. Substitution of murine for human CD4 residues identifies amino acids critical for HIV-gp120 binding. Nature 1988; 335:363–6.

51. Jameson BA, Rao PE, Kong LI, Hahn BH, Shaw GM, Hood LE, Kent SBH. Location and chemical synthesis of a binding site for HIV-1 on the CD4 protein. Science 1988; 240:1335–9.

52. Landau NR, Warton M, Littman DR. The envelope glycoprotein of the human immunodeficiency virus binds to the immunoglobulin-like domain of CD4. Nature 1988; 334:159–62.

53. Peterson A, Seed B. Genetic analysis of monoclonal antibody and HIV binding sites on the human lymphocyte antigen CD4. Cell 1988; 54: 65–72.

54. Richardson NE, Brown NR, Hussey RE, Vaid A, Matthews TJ, Bolognesi DP, Reinherz EL. Binding site for human immunodeficiency birus coat protein gp120 is located in the NH2-terminal region of T4 (CD4) and requires the intact variable-region-like domain. Proc Natl Acad Sci USA 1988; 85:6102–6106.

55. Mizukami T, Fuerst TR, Berger EA, Moss B. Binding region for human immunodeficiency virus (HIV) and epitopes for HIV-blocking monoclonal antibodies of the CD4 molecule defined by site-directed mutagenesis. Proc Natl Acad Sci USA 1988; 85:9273–7.

56. Sattenau QJ. Dalgleish AG, Weiss RA, Beverly PC. Epitopes of the CD4 antigens and HIV infection. Science 1986; 234:1120–3.

57. Deen KC, McDougal S, Inacker R, Folena-Wasserman G, Arthos J, Rosenberg J, Maddon PJ, Axel R, Sweet RW. A soluble form of CD4 (T4) protein inhibits AIDS virus infection. Nature 1988; 331:82–4.

58. Fisher RA, Bertonis JM, Meier W, Johnson VA, Costopoulos DS, Liu T, Tizard R, Walker BD, Hirsch MS, Schooley RT, Flavell RA. HIV infection is blocked in vitro by recombinant soluble CD4. Nature 1988; 331:76–8.

59. Hussey RE, Richardson NE, Kowalski M, Brown NR, Chang HC, Siliciano RF, Dorfman R, Walker B, Sodroski J, Reinherz EL. A soluble CD4 protein selectively inhibits HIV replication and syncytium formation. Nature 1988; 331:78–81.

60. Smith DH, Byrn RA, Marsters SA, Gregory T, Groopman JE, Capon DJ. Blocking of HIV-1 infectivity by a soluble, secreted form of the CD4 antigen. Science 1987; 238:1704–7.

61. Traunecker A, Luke W, Karjalainen K. Soluble CD4 molecules neutralize human immunodeficiency virus type I. Nature 1988; 331:84–6.

62. Watanabe M, Reimann KA, DeLong PA, Liu T, Risher RA, Letvin NL. Effect of recombinant soluble CD4 in rhesus monkeys infected with simian immunodeficiency virus of macaques. Nature 1989; 337:267–70.

63. Capon DJ, Chamow SM, Mordenti, Marsters SA, Gregory T, Mitsuya H, Byrn RA, Lucas C, Wurm FM, Groopman JE, Broder S, Smith DH. Designing CD4 immunoadhesions for AIDS therapy. Nature 1989; 337:525-531.

64. Chaudhary VK, Mizukami T, Fuerst TR, Fitzgerald DJ, Moss B, Pastan I, Berger EA. Selective killing of HIV-infected cells by recombinant CD4-Pseudomonas exotoxin hybrid protein. Nature 1988; 335:369-72.

65. Till MA, Ghettie V, Gregory T, Patzer EJ, Porter JP, Uhr JW, Capon DJ, Vitetta ES. HIV-infected cells are killed by rCD4-ricin A chain. Science 1988; 242:1166-8.

66. Bedinger P, Moriarty A, von Borstel RC II, Donovan NJ, Steimer KS, Littman DR. Internalization of the human immunodeficiency virus does not require the cytoplasmic domain of CD4. Nature 1988; 334:162-5.

67. Maddon PJ, McDougal JS, Clapham PR, Dalgleish AG, Jamal S, Weiss RA, Axel R. HIV infection does not require endocytosis of its receptor, CD4. Cell 1988; 54:865-74.

68. McClure MO, Marsh M, Weiss RA. Human immunodeficiency virus infection of CD4-bearing cells occurs by a pH-independent mechanism. European Mol Bio J 1988; 7:513-8.

69. Stein BS, Gowda SD, Lifson JD, Penhallow RC, Bensch KG, Engleman EG. pH-independent HIV entry into CD4-positive T cells via virus envelope fusion to the plasma membrane. Cell 1987; 49:659-68.

70. Wong-Staal F, Shaw GM, Hahn BH, Salahuddin SZ, Popovic M, Markham P, Redfield R, Gallo RC. Genomic diversity of human T-lymphotropic virus type III (HTLV-III). Science 1985; 229:759-62.

71. Braun DA, Clements JE, Gonda MA. The Visna virus genome: evidence for a hypervariable site in the env gene and sequence homology among lentivirus envelope proteins. J Virol 1987; 61:4046-54.

72. Payne SL, Salinovich O, Montelaro RC, Issel CJ, Nauman SM. Course and extent of variation of equine infectious anemia virus during parallel persistent infections. J Virol 1987; 61:1266-70.

73. Payne SL, Fang FD, Lui CP, Dhruva B, Rwambo P, Issel CJ, Montelaro RC. Antigenic variation and lentivirus persistence: variations in envelope gene sequences during EIAV infection resemble changes reported for sequential isolates of HIV. Virology 1987; 161:321-31.

74. Alizon M, Wain-Hobson S, Montagnier L, Sonigo P. Genetic variability of the AIDS virus: nucleotide sequence analysis of two isolates from African patients. Cell 1986; 46:63-74.

75. Starcich DH, Hahn BH, Shaw GM, McNeely PD, Modrow S, Wolf H, Parks ES, Parks WP, Josephs SF, Gallo RC, Wong-Staal F. Identification and characterization of conserved and variable regions in the envelope gene of HTLV-III/LAV, the retrovirus of AIDS. Cell 1986; 45:637-48.

76. Willey RL, Rutledge RA, Dias S, Folks T, Theodore T, Buckler CE, Martin MA. Identification of conserved and divergent domains within the envelope gene of the acquired immunodeficiency syndrome retrovirus. Proc Natl Acad Sci USA 1986; 83:5038-42.

77. Fisher AG, Ensoli B, Looney D, Rose A, Gallo RC, Saag MS, Shaw GM, Hahn BH, Wong-Staal F. Biologically diverse molecular variants within a single HIV-1 isolate. Nature 1988; 334:444-7.
78. Hahn BH, Shaw GM, Taylor ME, Redfield RR, Markham PD, Salahuddin SZ, Wong-Staal F, Gallo RC, Parks ES, Parks WP. Genetic variation in HTLV-III/LAV over time in patients with AIDS or at risk for AIDS. Science 1986; 232:1548-53.
79. Saag MS, Hahn BH, Gibbons J, Li Y, Parks ES, Parks WP, Shaw GM. Extensive variation of human immunodeficiency virus type-1 in vivo. Nature 1988; 334:440-4.
80. Emini EA, Ostapchuk P, Wimmer E. Bivalent attachment of antibody and polio virus leads to conformational alteration and neutralization. J Virol 1983; 48:547-50.
81. Icenogle J, Schiwen J, Duke G, Gilbert S, Rueckert R, Anderegg J. Neutralization of poliovirus by a monoclonal antibody: kinetics and stoichiometry. Virology 1983; 127:412-25.
82. Lee PWK, Hayes EC, Joklik WK. Characterization of anti retrovirus immunoglobins secreted by cloned hydridoma cell lines. Virology 1981; 108: 134-46.
83. Massey RJ, Schochetman G. Tropographical analysis of viral epitopes using monoclonal antibodies: mechanism of virus neutralization. Virology 1981; 115:20-32.
84. Possee RD, Schild GC, Dimmock NJ. Studies on the mechanism of influenza virus by antibody: evidence that neutralizing antibody (anti-haemagglutinen) inactivates influenza virus in vitro by inhibiting virion transcriptase activity. J Gen Virol 1982; 58:373-86.
85. Taylor HP, Dimmock NJ. Mechanism of neutralization of influenza virus by secretory immunoglobulin A is different from that of monomeric immunoglobulin A or immunoglobulin G. J Exp Med 1985; 161:198-209.
86. Taylor HP, Dimmock NJ. Mechanisms of neutralization of influenza virus by immunoglobulin. J Gen Vir 1985; 66:903-8.
87. Dietzschold B, Tollis M, Lafon M, Wunner WH, Koprowski H. Mechanisms of rabies virus neutralization by glycoprotein-specific monoclonal antibodies. Virology 1987; 161:29-36.
88. Gollins SW, Porterfield JS. A new mechanism for the neutralization of enveloped viruses by antiviral antibody. Nature 1986; 321:244-6.
89. Robert-Guroff M, Brown M, Gallo RC. HTLV-III-neutralizing antibodies in patients with AIDS and AIDS-related complex. Nature 1985; 316: 72-4.
90. Weiss RA, Clapham PR, Cheingsong-Popov R, Dalgleish AG, Carne CA, Weller IVD, Tedder RS. Neutralization of human T-lymphotropic virus type III by sera of AIDS and AIDS-risk patients. Nature 1985; 316:69-71.
91. Lasky LA, Groopman JE, Fennie CW, Benz PM, Capon DJ, Dowbenko DJ, Nakamura GR, Nunes WM, Renz ME, Berman PW. Neutralization of the AIDS retrovirus by antibodies to a recombinant envelope glycoprotein. Science 1986; 233:209-12.

92. Putney SD, Matthews TJ, Robey WG, Lynn DL, Robert-Guroff M, Mueller WT, Langlois AJ, Ghrayeb J, Petteway SR Jr., Wienhold KJ, Fischinger PJ, Wong-Staal F, Gallo RC, Bolognesi DP. HTLV–III/LAV-neutralizing antibodies to an E. coli produced fragment of the virus envelope. Science 1986;234:1392–5.

93. Rusche JR, Lynn DL, Robert-Guroff M, Langlois AJ, Lyerly HK, Carson H, Krohn K, Ranki A, Gallo RC, Bolognesi DP, Putney SD, Matthews TK. Humoral immune response to the entire human immunodeficiency virus envelope glycoprotein made in insect cells. Proc Natl Acad Sci USA 1987; 84:6924–8.

94. Steimer KS, Van Nest G, Dina D, Barr P, Luciw PA, Miller ET. Genetically engineered human immunodeficiency envelope glycoprotein gp120 produced in yeast is the target of neutralizing antibodies. In Vaccines 87. Chanock RM, Lerner RA, Brown F, Ginsberg H, eds. 1987 Cold Spring Harbor Laboratory. Cold Spring Harbor.

95. Martin MA, Quinnan G. Personal communication.

96. Eichberg JW, Zarling JM, Alter HJ, Levy JA, Berman PW, Gregory T, Lasky LA, McClure J, Cobb KE, Moran PA, Hu SL, Kennedy RC, Chanh TC, Dreesman GR. T-cell responses to human immunodeficiency virus (HIV) and its recombinant antigens in HIV-infected chimpanzees. J Virol 1987;61:3804–8.

97. Zagury D, Bernard J, Sheynier R, Desportes I, Leonard R, Fouchard M, Reveil B, Ittele D, Lurhuma Z, Mbayo K, Wane J, Salaun JJ, Goussars B, Dechazal L, Burney A, Nara P, Gallo RC. A group specific anamnestic immune reaction against HIV-1 induced by a candidate vaccine against AIDS. Nature 1988;332:728–31.

98. Zarling JM, Morton W, Moran PA, McClure J, Kosowski SG, Hu SL. T-cell responses to human AIDS virus in macaques immunized with recombinant vaccinia viruses. Nature 1986;323:344–6.

99. Zarling JM, Eichberg JW, Moran PA, Mcclure J, Sridhar P, Hu SL. Proliferation and cytotoxic T-cells to AIDS virus glycoproteins in chimpanzees immunized with a recombinant vaccinia virus expressing AIDS virus envelope glycoproteins. J Immunol 1987;139:988–90.

100. Walker CM, Steimer KS, Rosenthal KL, Levy JA, Identification of human immunodeficiency virus (HIV) envelope type-specific T helper cells in an HIV-infected individual. J Clin Invest 1988;82:2172–5.

101. Lin YL, Askinos BA. Biological properties of an influenza A virus-specific killer T cell clone. J Exp Med 1981;154:225–34.

102. Yap KL, Ada GL, McKenzie IFC. Transfer of specific cytotoxic T lymphocytes protects mice inoculated with influenza virus. Nature 1978;273: 238.

103. Byrne JA, Oldstone MBA. Biology of clones cytotoxic T lymphocytes specific for lymphocytic choriomenengitis virus: clearance of virus in vivo. J Virol 1984;51:682–6.

104. Chesebro B, Wehrly K. Studies on the role of the host immune response in recovery from frined virus leukemia II. J Exp Med 1976;143:85–99.

105. Plata F, Langlade-Demoyen P, Abastado JP, Berbar T, Kourlisky P. Retrovirus antigens recognized by cytolytic T lymphocytes activate tumor rejection in vivo. Cell 1987; 48:231.

106. Schmidt DS. The human MHC-restricted cellular response to herpes simplex virus Type I is mediated by CD4+, CD8– T cells and is restricted to the DR region of the MHC complex. J Immunol 1988; 140:3610–6.

107. Jacobson S, Rose JW, Flerlage ML, McFarlin DE, McFarland MF. Induction of measles virus-specific human cytotoxic T cells by purified measles virus nucleocapsid and hemagglutinin polypeptides. Viral Immunol 1988; 1:153–62.

108. Rook AH, Manischewitz JF, Frederick WR, Epstein JS, Jackson L, Gelmann E, Steis R, Masur H, Quinnan G. Deficient HLA-restricted, cytomegalovirus-specific cytotoxic T cells and natural killer cells in patients with the acquired immunodeficiency syndrome. J Infect Dis 1985; 152:627–30.

109. McMichael AJ, Gotch FM, Noble GZ, Beare PAS. Cytotoxic T-cell immunity to influenza. N Eng J Med 1983; 309:13–17.

110. Townsend ARM, McMichael AJ. HLA class-I restriction of T cell mediated cytotoxicity. Prog Allergy 1985; 36:10–43.

111. Townsend ARM, Rothbard J, Gotch FM, Bahadur G, Wraith D, McMichael AJ. The epitopes of influenza nucleoprotein recognized by cytotoxic T lymphocytes can be defined with short synthetic peptide. Cell 1986; 44:959–68.

112. Plata F, Autran B, Martins LP, Wain-Hobson S, Raphael M, Mayaud C, Denis M, Guillon JM, Debre P. AIDS virus-specific cytotoxic T lymphocytes in lung disorders. Nature 1987; 328:348–51.

113. Walker BD, Chakrabarti S, Moss B, Paradis TJ, Flynn T, Durno AG, Blumberg RS, Kaplan JC, Hirsch MS, Schooley RT. HIV-specific cytotoxic T lymphocytes in seropositive individuals. Nature 1987; 328:345–8.

114. Walker BD, Flexner C, Paradis TJ, Fuller TC, Hirsch MS, Schooley RT, Moss B. HIV-1 reverse trancriptase is a target for cytotoxic T lymphocytes in infected individuals. Science 1988; 240:64–6.

115. Sethi KK, Naher H, Stroehmann I. Phenotypic heterogeneity of cerebrospinal fluid-derived HIV-specific and HLA-restricted cytotoxic T-cell clones. Nature 1988; 335:178–81.

116. Lusso P, Markham PD, Ranki A, Earl P, Moss B, Dorner F, Gallo RC, Krohn K. Cell-mediated immune response toward viral envelope and core antigens in gibbon apes (Hylobates lar) chronically infected with human immunodeficiency virus-1. J Immunol 1988; 141:2467–73.

117. Hoffenbach A, Langlade-Demoyen P, Dadaglio G, Vilmer E, Michel F, Mayaud C, Autran B, Plata F. Unusually high frequencies of HIV-specific cytotoxic T lymphocytes in humans. J Immunol 1989; 142:452–62.

118. Ljunggren K, Bottiger B, Biberfeld G, Karlson A, Fenyo EM, Jondal M. Antibody-dependent cellular cytotoxicity-inducing antibodies against human immunodeficiency virus. J Immunol 1987; 139:2263–7.

119. Lyerly HK, Reed DL, Matthews TJ, Langlois AJ, Ahearne PA, Petteway SR Jr, Weinhold KJ. Anti-GP120 antibodies from HIV seropositive individuals mediate broadly reactive anti-HIV ADCC. AIDS Research and Human Retroviruses 1987; 3:409-22.

120. Rook AH, Lane HC, Folks T, McCoy S, Alter H, Fauci AS. Sera from HTLV-III/LAV antibody-positive individuals mediate antibody-dependent cellular cytotoxicity against HTLV-III/LAV-infected T cells J Immunol 1987; 138:1064-7.

121. Ljunggren K, Chiodi F, Beberfeld G, Norrby E, Jondal M, Fenyo EM. Lack of cross-reaction in antibody-dependent cellular cytotoxicity between human immunodeficiency virus (HIV) and HIV-related West African strains. J Immunol 1988; 140:602-5.

122. Koup RA, Sullivan JL, Levine PH, Brewster F, Mark A, Mazzara G, McKenzie S, Panicali D. Antigenic specificity of antibody-dependent cell-mediated cytotoxicity directed against human immunodeficiency virus in antibody-positive sera. J Virol 1989; 63:584-90.

123. Rusche JR, Javaherian K, McDanal C, Petro J, Lynn DL, Grimaila R, Langlois A, Gallo RC, Arthur LO, Fischinger PJ, Bolognesi DP, Putney SD, Matthews TJ. Antibodies that inhibit fusion of human immunodeficiency virus-infected cells bind a 24-amino acid sequence of the viral envelope, gp120. Proc Natl Acad Sci USA 1988; 85:3198-202.

124. Goudsmit J, Debouck C, Meloen RH, Smit L, Bakker M, Asher DM, Wolff AV, Gibbs CJ Jr., Gajdusek DC. Human immunodeficiency virus type 1 neutralization epitope with conserved architecture elicits early type-specific antibodies in experimentally infected chimpanzees. Proc Natl Acad Sci USA 1988; 85:4478-82.

125. Palker TJ, Clark ME, Langlois AJ, Matthews TJ, Weinhold KJ, Randall RR, Bolognesi DP, Haynes BF. Type-specific neutralization of the human immunodeficiency virus with antibodies to env-coded sythetic peptides. Proc Natl Acad Sci USA 1988; 85:1932-6.

126. Kenealy WR, Matthews TJ, Ganfield M, Langlois AJ, Waselefsky DM, Petteway SR. Antibodies from human immunodeficiency virus-infected individuals bind to a short amino acid sequence that elicits neutralizing antibodies in animals. AIDS Research and Human Retroviruses 1989; 5:173-82.

127. Linsley PS, Ledbetter JA, Kinney-Thomas E, Hu SL. Effects of anti-gp120 monoclonal antibodies on CD4 receptor binding by the env protein of human immunodeficiency virys type 1. J Virol 1988; 62:3695-702.

128. Matsushita S, Robert-Guroff M, Rusche J, Koito A, Hattori T, Hoshino H, Javaherian K, Takatsuki K, Putney S. Characterization of a human immunodeficiency virus neutralization monoclonal antibody and mapping of the neutralizing epitope. J Virol 1988; 62:2107-14.

129. Skinner MA, Ting R, Langlois AK, Weinhold KJ, Lyerly HK, Javaherian K, Matthews TJ. Characteristics of a neutralizing monoclonal antibody to

HTLV-IIIB envelope glycoprotein. AIDS Research and Human Retroviruses 1988; 4:187-97.

130. Kinney-Thomas E, Weber JN, McClure J, Clapham PR, Singhal MC, Sriver MK, Weiss R. Neutralizing monoclonal antibodies to the AIDS virus. AIDS 1988; 2:25-9.

131. Fung MSC, Sun C, Sun N, Chang NT, Chang TW. Monoclonal antibodies that neutralize HIV-1 virions and inhibit syncytium formation by infected cells. Bio/Technology 1987; 5:940.

132. Kowalski M, Potz J, Basiripour L, Dorfman T, Goh WC, Terwilliger E, Dayton A, Rosen C, Haseltine W, Sodroski. Functional regions of the envelope glycoprotein of human immunodeficiency virus type 1. Science 1987; 237:1351-5.

133. Looney DJ, Fisher AG, Putney SD, Rusche JR, Redfield RR, Burke DS, Gallo RC, Wong-Staal F. Type-restricted neutralization of molecular clones of human immunodeficiency virus. Science 1988; 241:357-9.

134. Matthews TJ, Langlois AJ, Robey WG, Chang NT, Gallo RC, Fischinger PJ, Bolognesi DP. Restricted neutralization of divergent human T-lymphotropic virus type III isolates by antibodies to the major envelope glycoprotein. Proc Natl Acad Sci USA 1986; 83:9709-13.

135. Weiss RA, Clapham PR, Weber JN, Dalgleish AG, Lasky LS, Berman PW. Variable and conserved neutralization antigens of human immunodeficiency virus. Nature 1986; 324:572-5.

136. Nara PL, Robey WG, Pyle SW, Hatch WC, Dunlop NM, Bess JW, Kelliher JC, Arthur LO, Fischinger PJ. Purified envelope glycoproteins from human immunideficiency virus type 1 variants induce individual, type-specific neutralizing antibodies. J Virol 1988; 62:2622-8.

137. Goudsmit J, Thiriart C, Smit L, Bruck C, Gibbs CJ. Temporal development of cross-neutralization between HTLV-IIIB and HTLV-III RF in experimentally infected chimpanzees. Vaccine 1988; 6:229-32.

138. Weiss SH, Goedert JJ, Gartner S, Popovid M, Waters D, Markham P, diMarzo G, Gail MH, Barkley WE, Gibbons J, Gill FA, Leuther M, Shae GM, Gallo RC, Blattner WA. Risk of human immunodeficiency virus (HIV-1) infection among laboratory workers. Science 1988; 239: 68-71.

139. Schnittman SM, Lane HC, Roth J, Burrows A, Folks TM, Kehrl JH, Koenig S, Berman P, Fauci AS. Characterization of gp120 binding to CD4 and an assay that measures ability of sera to inhibit this binding. J Immunol 1988; 141:4181-6.

140. Naylor PH, Naylor CW, Badamchian M, Wada S, Goldstein AL, Wang S, Sun DK, Thornton AH, Sarin PS. Human immunodeficiency virus contains an epitope immunoreactive with thymosin α_1 and the 30-amino acid synthetic p17 group-specific antigen peptide HGP-30. Proc Natl Acad Sci USA 1987; 84:2951-5.

141. Papsidero LD, Sheu M, Ruscetti FW. Human immunodeficiency virus type 2-neutralizing monoclonal antibodies which react with p17 core protein: characterization and epitope mapping. J Virol 1989; 63:267-72.

142. Chanh TC, Dreesman GR, Kanda P, Linette GP, Sparrow JT, Ho DD, Kennedy RC. Induction of anti-HIV neutralizing antibodies by synthetic peptides. European Mol Bio J 1986; 5:11:3065–71.

143. Dalgleish AG, Chanh TC, Kennedy RC, Kanda P, Clapham PR, Weiss R. Neutralization of diverse HIV-1 strains by monoclonal antibodies raised against a gp41 synthetic peptide. Virology 1988; 165:209–15.

144. Ho DD, Sarngadharan MG, Hirsch MS, Schooley RT, Rota TR, Kennedy RC, Chahn TC, Sato VL. Human immunodeficiency virus neutralizing antibodies recognize several conserved domains on the envelope glycoproteins. J Virol 1987; 61:2024–8.

145. Ho DD, Kaplan JC, Rackauskas IE, Gurney ME. Second conserved domain of gp120 is important for HIV infectivity and antibody neutralization. Science 1988; 239:1021–3.

146. Robert-Guroff M, Reitz MSJ, Robey WG, Gallo RC. In vitro generation of an HTLV-III variant by neutralizing antibody. J Immunol 1986; 137:3306–9.

147. Reitz MS Jr., Wilson C, Naugle C, Gallo RC, Robert-Guroff M. Generation of a neutralization-resistant variant of HIV-1 due to selection for a point mutation in the envelope gene. Cell 1988; 54:57–63.

148. Berzofsky JA, Cease KB, Cornette JL, Souge JL, Margalit H, Berkower IJ, Good MF, Miller LH, Delisi C. Protein antigenic structures recognized by T cells: Potential applications to vaccine design. Immunol Rev 1987; 98:9–52.

149. Rothbard J. Peptides and the cellular immune response. Annual Int Pasteur 1986; 137E:518–26.

150. Cease KB, Margalit H, Cornette JL, Putney SD, Robey WG, Ouyang C, Streicher HZ, Fischinger PJ, Gallo RC, DeLisi C, Berzofsky JA. Helper T-cell antigenic site identification in the acquired immunodeficiency syndrome virus gp120 envelope protein and induction of immunity in mice to the native protein using a 16-residue synthetic peptide. Proc Natl Acad Sci USA 1987; 84:4249–53.

151. Berzofsky JA, Bensussan A, Cease KB, Bourge JF, Cheynier R, Lurhuma Z, Salaun JJ, Gallo R, Shearer GM, Zagury D. Antigenic peptides recognized by T-lymphocytes from AIDS viral envelope-immune humans. Nature 1988; 334:706–8.

152. Hale PM, Cease KB, Hougton RA, Ouyang C, Putney SD, Javaherian K, Margalit H, Cornette JL, Spouge JL, DeLisi C, Berzofsky JA. T-cell epitope clusters in the HIV envelope: towards overcoming the problem of MHC restriction. Int Immunol 1989; 1:409–415.

153. Siliciano RF, Lawton T, Knall C, Karr RW, Berman P, Gregory T, Reinherz EL. Analysis of host-virus interaction in AIDS with anti-gp120 T cell clones: effect of HIV sequence variation and a mechanism for CD4$^+$ cell depletion. Cell 1988; 54:561–75.

154. Lanzavecchia A, Roosnek E, Gregory T, Berman P, Abrignani S. T cells can present antigens such as HIV gp120 targeted to their own surface molecules. Nature 1988; 530–2.

155. Lyerly HK, Matthews TJ, Langlois AJ, Bolognesi DP, Weinhold KJ. Human T-cell lymphotropic virus IIIB glycoprotein (gp120) bound to CD4 determinants on normal lymphocytes and expressed by infected cell serves as target for immune attack. Proc Natl Acad Sci USA 1987; 84: 4601–5.

156. Takahashi H, Cohen J, Hosmalin A, Cease KB, Houghton R, Cornette JL, DeLisi C, Moss B, Germain RN, Berzofsky JA. An immunodominant epitope of the human immunodeficiency virus envelope glycoprotein gp160 recognized by class I major histocompatability complex molecule-restricted murine cytotoxic T lymphocytes. Proc Natl Acad Sci USA 1988; 85: 3105–9.

157. Koenig S, Earl P, Powell D, Pantaleo G, Merli S, Moss B, Fauci AS. Group-specific, major histocompatibility complex class I-restricted cytotoxic responses to human immunodeficiency virus (HIV-1) envelope proteins by cloned peripheral blood T cells from an HIV-1-infected individual. Proc Natl Acad Sci USA 1988; 85:8638–42.

158. Gallaher WR. Detection of a fusion peptide sequence in the transmembrane protein of human immunodeficiency virus. Cell 1987; 50:327–8.

159. McCune JM, Rabin LB, Feinberg MB, Lieberman M, Kosek JC, Reyes GR, Weissman IL. Endoproteolytic cleavage of gp160 is required for the activation of human immunodeficiency virus. Cell 1988; 53:55–67.

160. Pal R, Gallo RC, Sarngadharan MG. Processing of the structural proteins of human immunodeficiency virus type 1 in the presence of monensin and cerulenin. Proc Natl Acad Sci USA 1988; 85:9283–6.

161. White J, Kielian M, Helenius A. Membrane fusion proteins of enveloped viruses. Q Rev Biophys 1983; 16:151–95.

162. Berman PW, Nunes WM, Haffar OK. Expression of membrane-associated and secreted variants of gp160 of human immunodeficiency virus type 1 in vitro and in continuous cell lines. J Virol 1988; 62:3135–42.

163. Malim MH, Hauber J, Le S, Maizel JV, Cullen BR. The HIV-1 rev trans-activator acts through a structured target sequence to activate nuclear export of unspliced mRNA. Nature 1989; 338:254–6.

164. Dayton AL, Terwilliger EF, Potz J, Kowalski M, Sodroski JG, Haseltine WA. Cis-acting sequences responsive to the rev gene product of the human immunodeficiency virus. J AIDS 1988; 1:441–52.

165. Allain JP, Laurian Y, Paul DA, Senn D. Serological markers in early stages of human immunodeficiency virus infection in haemophiliacs. Lancet 1986; 2:1233–6.

166. Goudsmit J, Paul DA, Lange JMA, Speelman H, Van Der Noordaa J, Van Der Helm HJ, DeWolf F, Epstein LG, Krone WJA, Wolters EC, Oleske JM, Coutinho RA. Expression of human immunideficiency virus antigen (HIV–Ag) in serum and cerebrospinal fluid during acute and chronic infection. Lancet 1986; 2:177–80.

167. Redfield RR, Wright DC, Tramont EC. The Walter Reed staging classification of HTLV–III/LAV infection. J Med 1986; 314:131–2.

168. Pederson C, Nielsen CM, Vestergaard BF, Gerstoft J, Krogsgaard K, Nielsen JO. Temporal relation of antigenaemia and loss of antibodies to core antigens to development of clinical disease in HIV infection. British Med J 1987; 295:567-9.

169. deWolf F, Goudsmit DA, Lange JMA, Hooijkaas C, Schellekens P, Coutinho RA, van der Noordaa J. Risk of AIDS related complex and AIDS in homosexual men with perisistent HIV antigenemia. British Med J 1987; 295:569-72.

170. Cheng-Mayer C, Seto D, Tateno M, Levy M. Biologic features of HIV-1 that correlate with virulence in the host. Science 1988; 240:80-2.

171. Fenyo EV, Morfeldt-Manson L, Chiodi F, Lind B, von Gegerfelt A, Albert J, Olausson E, Asjo B. Distinct replicative and cytopathic characteristics of human immunodeficiency virus isolates. J Virol 1988; 62: 4414-9.

172. Sakai K, Dewhurst S, Ma X, Volsky DJ. Differences in cytopathogenecity and host cell range among infectious molecular clones of human immunodeficiency virus type 1 simultaneously isolated from an individual. J Virol 1988; 62:4087-95.

173. Alter JS, Eichberg JW, Masur H, Saxinger WC, Gallo R, Macher AM, Lane HC, Fauci AS. Transmission of HTLV-III infection from human plasma to chimpanzees: an animal model for AIDS. Science 1984; 226:549-52.

174. Arthur LO, Pyle SW, Nara PL, Jr., Bess JW, Jr., Gonda MA, Kelliher JC, Gilden RV, Robey WG, Bolognesi DP, Gallo RC, Fischinger PJ. Serological responses in chimpanzees inoculated with human immunodeficiency virus glycoprotein (gp120) subunit vaccine. Proc Natl Acad Sci USA 1987; 84: 8583-7.

175. Berman PW, Groopman JE, Gregory T, Clapham PR, Weiss RA, Ferriani R, Riddle L, Shimasaski C, Lucas C, Lasky LA, Eichberg JW. Human immunodeficiency virus type 1 challenge of chimpanzees immunized with recombinant envelope glycoprotein gp120. Proc Natl Acad Sci USA 1988; 85:5200-4.

176. Arthur L, Nara P, Fischinger P. Personal communication. 1987.

177. Kennedy RC, Kanda P, Dressman GR, Eichberg JW, Chanh TC. Properties of synthetic peptides that identify meturalizing epitopes on the HIV envelope glycoprotein. In Vaccines '87. Chanock, Lerner, Brown, and Ginsberg ed. Cold Spring Harbor Laboratory, Cold Spring Harbor, 1987.

178. Hu SL, Fultz PN, McClure HM, Eichberg JW, Thomas EK, Zarling J, Singhal MC, Kosowski SG, Swenson RB, Anderson DC, Todaro G. Effect of immunization with a vaccinia-HIV env recombinant on HIV infection of chimpanzees. Nature 1987; 328:721-3.

179. Prince AM, Horowitz B, Baker L, Shulman RW, Ralph H, Valinsky J, Cundell A, Brotman B, Boehle W, Rey F, Piet M, Reesink H, Lelie N, Tersmette M, Miedema F, Barbosa L, Nemo G, Nastala CL, Allan JS, Lee DR, Eichberg JW. Failure of a human immunodeficiency virus (HIV)

immune globulin to protect chimpanzees against experimental challenge with HIV. Proc Natl Acad Sci USA 1988; 85:6944–8.

180. Emini E. et al. in preparation. 1989.

181. Francis MJ, Hastings GZ, Syred AD, McGinn B, Brown F, Rowlands DJ. Non-responsiveness to a foot-and-mouth disease virus peptide overcome by addition of foreign helper T-cell determinants. Nature 1987; 330:168–70.

182. Good MF, Maloy WL, Lunde MN, Margalit H, Cornette JL, Smith GL, Moss B, Miller LH, Berzofsky JA. Construction of synthetic immunogen: use of new T-helper epitope on malaria circumsporozoite protein. Science 1987; 235:1059–62.

183. Palker TJ, Matthews TJ, Langlois A, Tanner ME, Martin ME, Scearce RM, Kim JE, Bersofsky JA, Bolognesi DP, Haynes BF. Polyvalent human immunodeficiency virus synthetic immogen comprised of envelope gp120 T helper cell sites and B cell neutralization epitopes. J Immunol 1989; 142:3612–9.

184. Burke KL, Dunn G, Ferguson M, Minor PD, Almond JW. Antigen chimaeras of poliovirus as potential new vaccines. Nature 1988; 332:81–2.

185. Murray MG, Kuhn RJ, Arita M, Kawamura N, Nomoto A, Wimmer E. Poliovirus type 1/type 3 antigenic hybrid virus constructed in vitro elicits type 1 and type 3 neutralizing antibodies in rabbits and monkeys. Proc Natl Acad Sci USA 1988; 85:3203–7.

186. Chanh TC, Kennedy RC, Kanda P. Synthetic peptides homologous to HIV transmembrane glycoprotein suppress normal human lymphocyte blastogenic response. Cellular Immunol 1988; 111:77–86.

187. Nair MPN, Pottathil R, Heimer EP, Schwartz SA. Immunoregulatory activities of human immunodeficiency virus (HIV) proteins: effect of HIV recombinant and synthetic peptides on immunoglobulin synthesis and proliferative responses by normal lymphocytes. Proc Natl Acad Sci USA 1988; 85:6498–502.

188. Homsy J, Tateno M, Levy JA. Antibody-dependent enhancement of HIV infection. Lancet 1988; 1285–6.

189. Robinson WEJ, Montefiori DC, Mitchell WM. Antibody-dependent enhancement of human immunodeficiency virus type 1 infection. Lance 1988; 790–4.

190. Takeda A, Tuazon CU, Ennis FA. Antibody-enhanced infection by HIV-1 via Fc receptor-mediated entry. Science 1988; 242:580–3.

191. Kornfeld H, Cruikshank WH, Pyle SW, Berman JS, Center DM. Lymphocyte activation by HIV-1 envelope glycoprotein. Nature 1988; 335:445–8.

192. Diamond DC, Sleckman BP, Gregory T, Lasky LA, Greenstein JL, Burakoff SJ. Inhibition of $CD4^+$ T cell function by the HIV envelope protein gp120. J Immunol 1988; 141:3715–7.

193. Chirmule N, Kalyanaraman V, Oyaizu N, Pahwa S. Inhibitory influences of envelope glycoproteins of HIV-1 on normal immune responses J AIDS 1988; 1:425–30.

194. Mann DL, Lasane F, Popovic M, Arthur LO, Robey WG, Blattner WA, Newman MJ. HTLV-III large envelope protein (gp120) suppresses PHA-induced lymphocyte blastogenesis. J Immunol 1987; 138:2640.

195. Shalaby MR, Krowka JF, Gregory TJ, Hirabayashi SE, McCabe SM, Kaufman DS, Stites DP, Ammann AJ. The effects of human immunodeficiency virus recombinant envelope glycoprotein on immuno cell functions in vitro. Cell 1987; 110:140.

196. Prince AM, Moor-Jankowski J, Eichberg JW, Schellekens H, Mauler RF, Girard M, Goodall J. Chimpanzees and AIDS research. Nature 1988; 333: 513.

197. Filice G, Cereda PM, Varnier OE. Infection of rabbits with human immunodeficiency virus. Nature 1988; 335:366-9.

198. Kulaga H, Folks TM, Rutledge R, Kindt TJ. Infection of rabbit T-cell and macrophage lines with human immunodeficiency virus. Proc Natl Acad Sci USA 1988; 85:4455-9.

199. Kulaga H, Folks TM, D. H, Rutledge R, Kindt TJ. HIV-1 infection of a rabbit macrophage cell line: absence of RT activity in infected cell supernatants. IV International Conference on AIDS. Book 1 1988, 179.

200. Namikawa R, Kaneshima H, Lieverman M, Weissman IL, McCune JM. Infection of the SCID-hu mouse by HIV-1. Science 1988; 242:1684-6.

201. Leonard JM, Abramczuk JW, Pezen DS, Rutledge R, Belcher JH, Hakim F, Shearer G, Lamperth L, Travis W, Frederickson T, Notkins AL, Martin MA. Development of disease and virus recovery in transgenic mice containing HIV proviral DNA. Science 1988; 242:1665-70.

202. Megil ME, Deyton L, Metcalf JA, Salzman N, Vasudevachari M, Baseler M, Martin M, Folks TM, Smith G, Cochran M, Volvovitz F, Masur H, Fauci AS, Lane HC. Phase I trial of a recombinant gp160 candidate AIDS vaccine. IV International Conference on AIDS. Book 2, 1987, 289.

203. Zagury D, Leonard R, Fouchard M, Reveil B, Bernard J, Ittele D, Cattan A, Zirimwabagabo L, Kalumbu M, Justin W, Salaun J, Goussard B. Immunization against AIDS in humans. Nature 1987; 326:249-50.

204. Costagliola D, Mary JY, Brouard N, Laporte A, Valleron AJ. Incubation time for AIDS from French transfusion-associated cases. Nature 1989; 338:768-9.

205. Kalbfleisch JD, Lawless JF. Estimating the incubation period for AIDS patients. Nature 1988; 333:504-5.

206. Medley GF, Anderson RM. Estimating the incubation period for AIDS patients. Nature 1988; 333:505.

207. Auger I, Thomas P, De Gruttola V, Morse D, Moore D, Williams R, Truman B, Lawrence CE. Incubation periods for paediatric AIDS patients. Nature 1988; 336:575-7.

208. Willey RL, Smith DH, Lasky LA, Theodore TS, Earl PL, Moss B, Capon DJ, Martin MA. In vitro mutagenesis identifies a region within the envelope gene of the human immunodeficiency virus that is critical for infectivity. J Virol 1988; 62:139-47.

2

Interaction of HIV with
Its Cellular Receptor, CD4
Prospects for Immunologic Intervention

Gregg M. Orloff and J. Steven McDougal
Center for Infectious Diseases
Centers for Disease Control
and Emory University School of Medicine
Atlanta, Georgia

INTRODUCTION

The identification of immune specificities or epitopes of the human immunodeficiency virus (HIV) that, as immunogens, elicit cellular or humoral responses
that limit or prevent HIV infectivity is critical for vaccine development. Because
the initial interaction between virus and host cells involves binding of the HIV
outer envelope glycoprotein gp120 to the CD4 molecule, much attention has
been focused on the envelope and its binding site. The focus on the CD4 binding
site of gp120 is attractive because the site is likely to be conserved between
strains. An immune intervention targeted to the site should be a universal inhibitor of HIV infection. However, lacking complete definition of the site, it is not
clear whether the site is immunogenic in humans or even accessible to antibody.
In fact there is some reason for pessimism. For instance, serum samples from
patients infected with HIV do not react with (or rarely react with) the envelope
of LAV-2 or HTLV–IV (now called HIV-2) (1,2). If the two viruses have identical CD4-binding sites, one must conclude that the precise site is not immunogenic in humans. Moreover, the affinity of gp120 for CD4 is relatively high (3)
giving virus somewhat of a thermodynamic advantage over potentially inhibitory
antibodies. Other functional domains of virus proteins should not be overlooked

and also need to be defined. It is likely that regions involved in cell penetration, fusion, or intermolecular adhesion of envelope to the rest of the virus particle are immunogenic and that immune responses directed against these regions would disrupt or interfere with virus spread. Nevertheless, definition of the molecular nature of the CD4 receptor-HIV envelope interaction is not only a key to understanding virus tropism, but, along with other functional domains of HIV proteins, will be required to understand mechanisms of immune interference or escape. It will be essential to define the functional relevance of antigenic epitopes that are immunogenic or nonimmunogenic, immunodominant or silent, accessible or not accessible, strain-specific or group-common, and protective or nonprotective. In this chapter, we focus on the CD4 receptor-HIV interaction by reviewing the CD4 molecule, its receptor function, and the nature of the interaction. Relevant immune responses would seem to us to indicate the potential for defining immunogens that elicit responses that may be universal inhibitors of HIV-CD4 interaction.

THE CD4 MOLECULE

In 1979, Kung and coworkers and, independently, Ledbetter and coworkers described antilymphocyte monoclonal antibodies (mAb) (now called OKT4 and Leu3a, respectively) that reacted with the cell surface of a subset of human lymphocytes (4,5). Subsequently designated CD4 T cells, this T cell subset recognizes antigen and subsequently helps or induces other cell populations to perform their respective immunologic functions. It is thus a pivotal cell in the inductive and effector stages of immune responses. A reciprocal population of T cells, CD8 T cells, perform suppressor and cytotoxic cell functions and, together with CD4 T cells, comprise the majority of the mature T-cell pool. The predominant association of the CD4 phenotype is with helper/inducer function, but this is not absolute. CD4 T cells with suppressor and cytotoxic function have been described (6,7). A more stringent association of the CD4 phenotype with function is in the mode of antigen recognition rather than with the resultant cellular function. CD4 T cells recognize antigen in the context of class II major histocompatibility (MHC) structures, whereas CD8 T cells recognize antigen in the context of class I MHC (6-10). The association of these and other cell surface phenotypes with specific immune functions has become a central theme in investigations dissecting cellular interactions in the normal immune system and perturbations associated with disease states.

The gene encoding human CD4 was first cloned and sequenced by Maddon et al. (11). The gene encodes a leader sequence of 23 amino acids and a processed protein of 435 amino acids. The processed protein consists of a carboxy-terminal cytoplasmic segment, a hydrophobic transmembrane region, and an extracellular region having four domain-like structures formed by (potential but uncon-firmed) intrachain disulfide loops reminiscent of immunoglobulin and MHC molecules. The penultimate domain shares some sequence homology with immunoglobulin, T-cell receptor, and MHC sequences (11). The molecule is glycosylated but is not covalently bound to other proteins and migrates in gels as a single 55–62 kD species (5,11,12). CD4 is constitutively produced by T cells although cell surface expression is subject to down-modulation (presumably via endocytic cycling) following T-cell activation. The regulatory mechanism in-volves phosphokinase C activity and phosphorylation of the cytoplasmic seg-ment of CD4 (13-15). Direct perturbation of the molecule with mAb may transmit a negative regulatory signal—one that prevents the increased flux of intracellular calcium that occurs with T-cell activation (16-19).

Although expression of CD4 is a useful marker for a subset of T cells whose T-cell antigen receptor recognizes antigen in the context of class II MHC struc-tures, the precise role of the CD4 molecule itself in this recognition event and the resultant response remains unclear. There is evidence indicating that CD4 functions in associative recognition of nonpolymorphic regions of class II MHC structures. The activity of MHC class-II restricted, antigen-specific T-cell clones can often be dampened or abrogated by blocking CD4 with CD4 mAb, especially clones that are weakly responsive or of an apparently low affinity (9,10,18-23). In a zenogeneic system, the response of a murine T-cell hybridoma subclone that had lost the CD4 homologue (L3T4) was greatly enhanced by transfection of human CD4 into the subclone and human MHC class II into the antigen-present-ing cell (24). These experiments indicate that a functional interaction occurs between CD4 and MHC class II and between CD4 and the T-cell receptor complex and indirectly imply that physical (binding) interactions occur. How-ever, only recently has any direct evidence been obtained for a physical interac-tion between CD4 on one cell and MHC class II on another (25).

CD4 AS A RECEPTOR FOR HIV

Whatever its role in T-cell physiology and immune responses, CD4 is also the target or receptor for HIV. HIV has evolved an envelope with affinity for CD4, and cellular expression of CD4 is the prime determinant of the tropism of this virus in man. Compelling justification for those conclusions comes from six types of experimental investigations. First, the tropism in vitro and in vivo of HIV for CD4 T cells does not constitute proof but is a consistent and expected finding if CD4 functions as a relevant receptor. HIV infection in vivo results in a numerical and functional deficiency of CD4 T cells. In vitro, HIV infection and replication has only been consistently and reliably detected in cells that express CD4, such as T cells. Cells with lesser density of CD4 expression (monocytes and some B-cell lines) are also susceptible (26–37). Second, Popovic, Klatzmann, Dalgleish, and their respective coworkers demonstrated that certain CD4 mAb prevented or substantially reduced the infectivity of HIV for T cells (30,37,39). Furthermore, CD4 mAb were shown to block penetration of a pseudotype virus formed between HIV and vesicular stomatitis virus and to block fusion (syncytia) of HIV-infected cells with uninfected CD4 cells, providing more direct evidence that CD4 mAb act early in infection and at the cell membrane (30). Third, by indirect immunofluorescence, HIV was shown to bind to the surface of CD4 cells but not to CD4-negative cells (34) (Fig. 1). Binding is saturable, specifically inhibited by certain CD4 mAb (but not by a fairly comprehensive panel of mAb to other cell surface molecules), and reciprocal in that HIV and CD4 mAb inhibit binding of each other to CD4 cells (34). Fourth, radioimmuno-precipitation experiments wherein virus is reacted with CD4 cells followed by lysis and immunoprecipitation have demonstrated bimolecular complexes of the CD4 molecule and the gp120 envelope glycoprotein (40). Further evidence that gp120 is the principal viral protein that binds CD4 has been provided by Matthews and colleagues and Lasky and colleagues using highly purified native gp120 and recombinant gp120, respectively (3,41). The latter group measured the affinity of interaction by Scatchard analysis and found an extraordinarily high association constant on the order of 10^9 (3). Fifth, transfection of the CD4 gene into CD4-negative and noninfectable human cell lines renders them CD4-positive, HIV binding, and infectable (42). Murine cell lines transfected with the CD4 gene, like human cell lines, express CD4 and bind virus but, unlike human cell lines, HIV replication does not ensue (42). Since murine cells will replicate HIV when HIV is transfected as proviral DNA (43–45), the block in murine CD4-transfectants must be in a step after binding and before replication, most likely a penetration step, but the precise basis has yet to be elucidated. Finally, several groups using recombinant DNA technology have produced a soluble form of CD4 containing the extracellular domains of CD4. This material, purified to apparent homogeneity, dramatically blocks HIV binding and infectivity for CD4 cells (46–51).

Taken together, these experiments indicate that: 1) the CD4 molecule specifically binds the HIV envelope glycoprotein gp120 with characteristics of a receptor-ligand interaction: binding has measurable affinity, is saturable, and is specifically and reversibly inhibited, 2) CD4 expression is both sufficient and necessary for binding and infectivity of HIV for human cells, 3) virtually all the affinity of binding is provided by the gp120:CD4 interaction, as attested to by the fact that soluble purified CD4 completely inhibits binding to CD4 cells. If another viral or cellular protein is involved, it must be of exceedingly low affinity or require prior CD4:gp120 binding.

As a receptor with high affinity, CD4 functions to focus HIV on susceptible cells by overcoming the natural repulsive forces that occur between membranes.

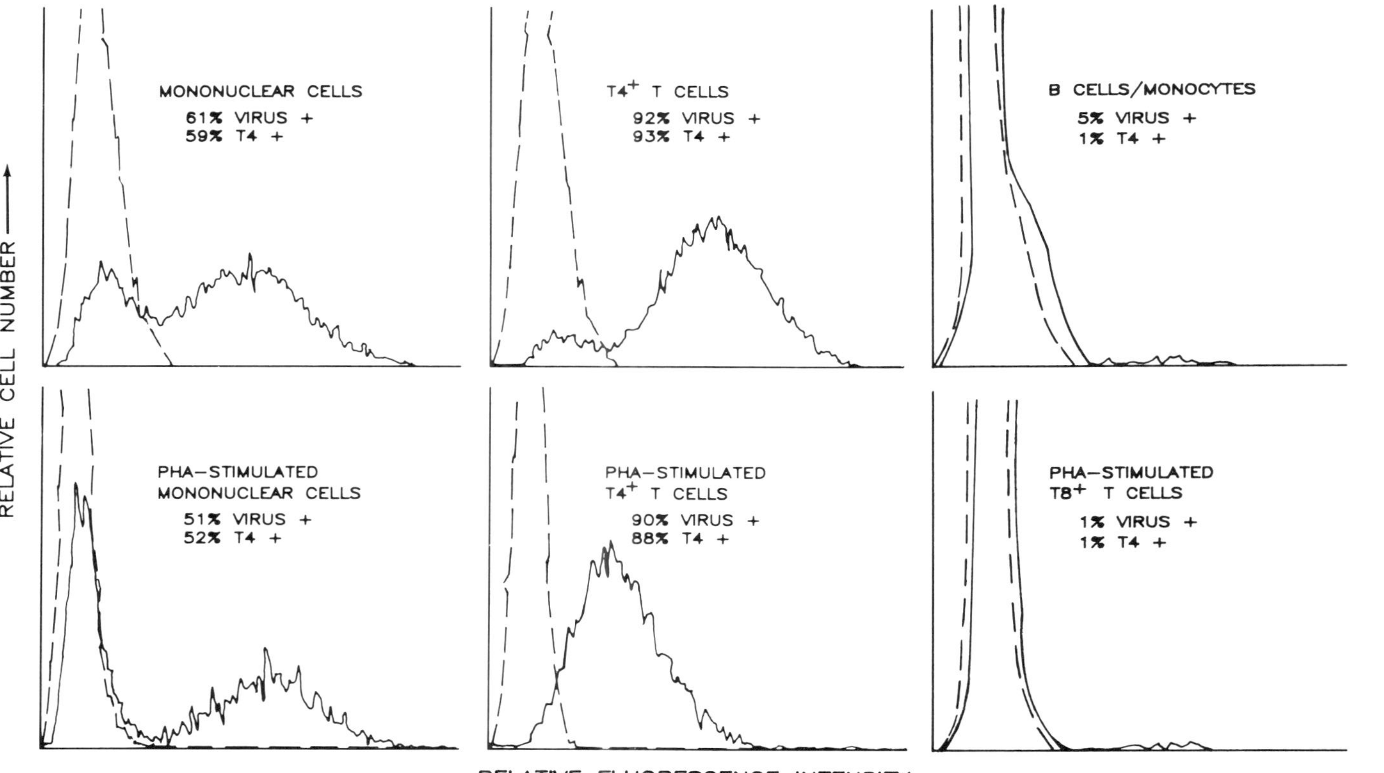

Figure 1 HIV binding to human lymphocytes. Ficoll-Hypaque–separated peripheral blood mononuclear cells, negatively selected CD4+ T cells or CD8+ T cells, and a B-cell/monocyte population were incubated with HIV (———) or buffer (– – – –) followed by fluorescein-conjugated anti-HIV. (From Ref. 34, with permission, American Association of Immunologists.)

Both infectivity by cell-free virus and syncytia formation between HIV-infected cells and uninfected CD4 cells involve the HIV envelope–CD4 interaction, and both are inhibited by soluble CD4 or CD4 mAb (51). By virtue of the potential for multipoint attachment, the syncytia phenomenon probably has a much higher net avidity than does attachment by cell-free virus, and this may explain why inhibition of syncytia formation by HIV antibody has been more difficult to demonstrate than neutralization of cell-free HIV infectivity.

Beyond the focusing function, it is not clear what role CD4 or other viral and cellular structures play in virus penetration. CD4 can be internalized through an endocytic pathway by stimulation with phorbol esters, a pathway involving phosphokinase C (PKC) activation and phosphorylation of the CD4 molecule (13–15). However, HIV attachment and initial infectivity does not result in CD4 phosphorylation (16), is not affected by PKC inhibition (J. S. McDougal and P. J. Maddon, unpublished), and is not associated with an initial loss of CD4 from the membrane (34,52). Although T-cell activation substantially influences the amount of virus replication and rate of cell death, T-cell activation is not a requirement for HIV binding and infectivity (34,53). Stein et al. (54) have shown convincingly that the integrity of the low pH-dependent endocytic pathway is not essential for HIV penetration of T cells, nor is it required for infection of monocytes (36), although an acidic compartment (possibly trans-Golgi transport) is required for later stages of virus replication (42). The transmembrane protein of HIV has a short sequence that is homologous with the fusion domains of influenza and paramyxoviruses (55), and it may be that penetration is a function of this protein, with CD4 playing no role in penetration (other than bringing HIV into proximity with the cell membrane).

CD4 may function later in the life cycle of HIV as well. Infected CD4 T cells eventually lose cell surface expression of CD4 (34,52), and intracellular CD4 protein is found complexed to gp120 (52). Several recent investigations suggest that CD4 expression is a necessary requisite for cell death. One of the earliest experiments was that of DeRossi et al. (56), who "forced" HIV into CD4-negative CD8 T cells and found that HIV replication was equivalent to that of CD4 cells, but the cells did not die. Asjo et al. (57) have shown a correlation between the degree of CD4 expression before infection and the cytopathic effect. Numerous studies of deletion and site-directed mutants of HIV regulatory genes or transfection studies using cloned HIV genes have failed to implicate any of the HIV regulatory genes in the cytopathic effect. However, Fisher et al. (58) produced a mutant of HIV with a deletion in the *env* gene that was replication competent but not cytopathic. Sodroski et al. (59) and Lifson et al. (60) found that transfection of the *env* gene into CD4-positive cells results in syncytia formation and cell death. Transfection of the *env* gene into CD4-negative cells does not result in syncytia, although these cells will form syncytia with CD4-positive cells (59,60). Thus it seems quite likely that CD4 expression is both a determinant of tropism and a requisite for cell death.

LOCATION AND CONFORMATIONAL REQUIREMENTS OF THE CD4-BINDING SITE OF THE HIV OUTER ENVELOPE GP120

Kowalski et al. (61) generated a series of envelope mutations and have defined regions of the molecule critical for envelope binding to CD4. Mutations affecting amino acids in the carboxy-end of the molecule at positions 363, 419, and 473 abolished CD4-binding capacity. In an alternate but complementary approach, Lasky et al. (3) defined a region of gp120 that reacted with an anti-gp120 mAb. This mAb inhibits gp120:CD4 binding and reacts within a region of gp120 spanning amino acids 397 to 439. They then performed site-directed mutagenesis in this region to confirm that its integrity was essential for binding.

For reasons outlined below, the binding site on gp120 requires a proper three-dimensional orientation or conformation formed by approximating discontiguous amino acid sequences. We treated HIV with the physical, chemical, and enzymatic regimens listed in Table 1 and assessed their effect on HIV binding capacity. Specific details of the manipulations and controls to assure or deny authentic binding to CD4 are given elsewhere (62). Reduction of disulfide bonds with dithiothreitol and alkylation with iodoacetamide followed by dialysis

Table 1 Physical, Enzymatic, and Chemical Treatments of HIV: Effect on HIV Binding to CD4 T Cells

Treatments that abolished HIV binding capacity:
$100°C \times 10$ min
reduction and alkylation
trypsin

Treatments that did not affect HIV binding capacity:
$65°C \times 30$ min
$56°C \times 30$ min
8 M Urea
1% SDS
95% alcohol
alkylation
periodate oxidation and borohydrate reduction
endoglycosidase F
endoglycosidase H
neuraminidase

Source: Ref. 62, with permission, American Association of Immunologists.

abolished the capacity of HIV to bind. The effect is likely on intramolecular disulfide bonds since there is no evidence that gp120 is covalently bound to other gp120 molecules or other viral proteins. If the tertiary structure conferred by covalent disulfide bonding is not disrupted, the proper secondary structure required for binding appears to be thermodynamically favored because treatment with heat or denaturants followed by their removal did not affect binding. Proteolysis with trypsin destroyed binding, but derivatization of carbohydrate by periodate oxidation and borohydride reduction or glycolytic digestion did not. Our carbohydrate digestions were not complete as assessed by reduction in apparent molecular weight, and this may explain differences in results from other groups who have found that deglycosylation or carbohydrate-binding lectins interfere with HIV:CD4 interactions (41,63). Carbohydrate may function to maintain conformation or protect the molecule from degradation, but it seems unlikely (or at least unappealing) that the binding site is composed only of carbohydrate because it would require that HIV (which has no glycosylation enzymes of its own) acquire its highly specific CD4-binding capacity from the host cell glycosylation system.

RELEVANCE OF ANTI-GP120 ANTIBODIES: CLUES FROM NATURAL HISTORY STUDIES

In theory, if natural infection induces an immune response favorable to the host, one should be able to identify such responses in clinical studies. All one needs is a measure of the response and analysis of its association with the course of infection. The concept is simple; the process is not. With respect to antibody, the measurement of HIV-specific responses has been relatively straightforward, and most HIV-infected individuals mount and sustain a vigorous humoral response. Detection of antibody has become a clinically useful marker for past exposure and probable current infection; however, distinguishing whether these responses are clinically important, effective in controlling infection, or potentially protective has been difficult.

Although complicated, we feel that natural history studies do provide a useful and objective framework against which the importance and relevance of a particular immune response can be measured. Generally, such studies are designed by dividing HIV-infected subjects into two groups—one with a favorable clinical outcome and one with an unfavorable outcome—and comparing the particular immune response between the groups. The simplest study design is a comparison of HIV-infected subjects with and without AIDS. Such studies provide a description of changes that occur with clinical AIDS but provide little insight as to whether the changes are a consequence or determinant of the severe immunodeficiency of AIDS. Longitudinal studies, initiated at seroconversion, are more appropriate for detecting determinants of progressive disease. Unfortunately, collecting subjects with a known seroconversion date is difficult. A more common design is the study of HIV-infected subjects at a time when they are relatively asymptomatic and in whom the subsequent clinical course is known. Numerous studies of this sort (most appropriately termed cross-sectional with longitudinal followup) have been conducted seeking to identify features that predict progression to AIDS. Only two features have consistently and reproducibly emerged as predictors: longer duration of infection (seropositivity) (64–70) and lower levels of CD4 T cells (67–76). For any cumulative event or endpoint (clinical AIDS in this case), a relation to duration or seropositivity would be expected regardless of whether the event was random in time, occurred at homogeneous rates, or occurred in subgroups with markedly different rates. Although it remains unclear whether some, most, or all HIV-infected persons will eventually develop clinical manifestations of AIDS, it is quite clear that there is marked heterogeneity in the rates at which different people progress to severe immunodeficiency. Indeed, the distinction between "progressors" and "nonprogressors" may be one of relative rates of progression rather than an absolute characteristic. The second, lower CD4 T-cell levels, increases the probability of clinical manifestations and thus is a determinant of progression when AIDS is the endpoint. In the context of progressive disease, it is better interpreted as a marker (rather than determinant) for more severe infection and immunodeficiency, which, in turn, increases the likelihood of developing clinical complications that meet criteria for AIDS. The hallmark of HIV infection is a numerical and functional depletion of CD4 T cells, a notion supported by the strong association of CD4 T-cell levels with disease manifestation, prognosis, and progression (64–76). Other candidates for determinants of progression fall into three general categories: relative differences in virulence or cytopathicity of different HIV strains; so-called environmental or infectious cofactors that presumably act through T-cell stimulation to increase virus replication; and host factors (most notably the immune response) that may govern or regulate virus replication and spread. In vitro observations support cogent arguments that any of the three possibilities may contribute, but clinical and epidemiologic verification has been difficult to obtain. Thus, natural history studies provide ample justification for the use of CD4 cell levels as an objective measure of severity of infection, and the heterogeneity in rates of progression should provide clinical subgroups for assessing the importance of specific immune responses and/or cofactors.

There are differences in the pattern of antibody reactivity with specific HIV proteins for patients with AIDS and infected persons without AIDS and for infected persons destined to develop AIDS and those with a relatively stable clinical course. Progressive disease has been associated with lower levels of

Table 2 Antibody Titers and IgG Levels in Homosexual Men

Group[a]		HIV p17	HIV p24	HIV p31
AIDS	Geometric mean[b]	778	3,676	800
(n = 25)	SD	X/÷12.1	X/÷8.6	X/÷4.4
	Median	400	1,600	1,600
PGL	Geometric mean	11,143	67,559	6,850
(n = 20)	SD	X/÷10.1	X/÷9.1	X/÷13.5
	Median	6,400	102,400	6,400
Asymptomatic	Geometric mean	7,003	48,100	5,930
(n = 37)	SD	X/÷11.8	X/÷11.4	X/÷6.3
	Median	6,400	25,600	6,400
Progressor	Geometric mean	4,106	7,558	3,478
(n = 25)	SD	X/÷7.0	X/÷6.9	X/÷9.3
	Median	1,600	6,400	6,400
Nonprogressor	Geometric mean	8,214	54,119	6,225
(n = 57)	SD	X/÷11.0	X/÷10.4	X/÷8.3
	Median	6,400	102,400	6,400
Statistics[c] (p value)				
AIDS vs. PGL		0.0002	0.0002	0.0036
AIDS vs. asymptomatic		0.0010	0.0001	0.0001
PGL vs. asymptomatic		ns	ns	ns
Progressor vs. nonprogressor		ns	0.0004	ns

[a]PGL and asymptomatic groups have had a stable clinical course, and their data were pooled (nonprogressors) for comparison with PGL and asymptomatic persons who subsequent to testing developed AIDS (progressors).
[b]Anti-log$_2$ of the average of log$_2$-transformed titers.
[c]Wilcoxon rank sum test.
Source: Ref. 76.

antibody to most viral proteins with the notable exception of the transmembrane protein gp41 (76–83). Loss or absence of antibody that inhibits reverse transcriptase activity (84) and loss of antibody reactive with denatured as opposed to native outer envelope protein gp120 (reduced verses nonreduced protein) (85) have both been associated with progression.

We determined the titers and isotypes of HIV antibody to specific HIV proteins by Western blot and performed lymphocyte studies on 82 HIV-infected homosexual men who were asymptomatic or had persistent generalized lymphadenopathy (PGL) at the time of specimen collection (76). Twenty-five (30%) of

HIV gp41	HIV p51	HIV p65	HIV gp120	Tetanus toxoid	IgG
					mg/dl
3,112	1,600	2,111	894	1,364	1,677
X/÷3.3	X/÷13.6	X/÷12.5	X/÷7.9	X/÷1.5	X/÷1.5
1,600	1,600	1,600	1,600	1,600	1,547
4,850	33,779	54,875	2,425	2,216	1,865
X/÷4.3	X/÷8.5	X/÷8.5	X/÷4.2	X/÷1.7	X/÷1.6
6,400	25,600	25,600	6,400	1,600	1,853
10,043	24,728	56,028	3,027	1,392	1,442
X/÷6.7	X/÷12.4	X/÷5.2	X/÷7.8	X/÷1.2	X/÷1.5
6,400	25,600	102,400	6,400	1,600	1,505
6,400	3,478	6,225	217	1,255	1,713
X/÷4.2	X/÷12.5	X/÷12.0	X/÷7.2	X/÷1.9	X/÷1.4
6,400	1,600	6,400	<100	1,600	1,862
7,771	27,628	55,641	2,805	1,634	1,581
X/÷6.0	X/÷10.8	X/÷6.1	X/÷6.4	X/÷1.4	X/÷1.7
6,400	25,600	102,400	6,400	1,600	1,547
ns	0.0003	0.0001	0.048	ns	ns
ns	0.0002	X0.0001	0.0310	ns	ns
ns	ns	ns	ns	ns	ns
ns	0.0007	0.0002	<0.0001	ns	ns

the men subsequently progressed to AIDS. The other 57 (70%) have been followed for an equal or greater period of time (17–46 months) and have had a stable clinical course. In 59 men for whom it could be ascertained, progressors did not differ from nonprogressors in duration of seropositivity or duration of lymphadenopathy at the time of study. Twenty-five patients with AIDS were also studied. Antibody titers were generally lower in sera from patients with AIDS and in sera from men whose condition subsequently progressed to AIDS than in sera from men who did not progress to AIDS. Specifically, antibody titers to the envelope protein gp120, the core protein p24, and the reverse transcriptase enzyme p51/65 were lower (Table 2). Antibody titers to the transmembrane protein gp41 are an exception in that they are well preserved and similar in AIDS patients and HIV-exposed persons who do and do not eventually develop AIDS. We found no evidence for isotypic restriction or prominence in the HIV response. The frequency of isotypic responses generally parallels the anticipated concentration of the different isotypes in serum, and all isotypes may participate in the response, which is characteristic of a mature, ongoing response to complex T-dependent antigens.

Lymphocyte and titer data were entered into a multivariate analysis as independent variables with progression/nonprogression to AIDS as the dependent variable (Table 3). Lower levels of CD4 T cells were most highly associated with progression to AIDS in seropositive asymptomatic men or men with PGL. Other lymphocyte enumerations of which CD4 is a component were significantly associated with progression but did not retain the association when the analysis was corrected for CD4 T-cell levels. Several clinical studies have shown that CD4 T-cell levels are lower in persons with severe clinical manifestations of HIV infection (65-67), that levels decline with increasing duration of infection (64-67), and that a low CD4 cell level is a poor prognostic sign in HIV-infected persons (67-74). Other immunologic abnormalities are observed in HIV-infected persons, but these are highly correlated with CD4 T-cell levels (65-67,75), and their association with HIV infection is not independent of their relationship to CD4 T-cell levels (75). Thus, this and other clinical studies indicate that CD4 T-cell levels are the best immunologic marker for severity of HIV infection, a concept supported by the known tropism and cytopathic effect of HIV for CD4 T cells in vitro (26-39).

Lower antibody titers to gp120, p51/65, and p24 did correlate with lower CD4 T-cell levels and are thus, in part, a reflection (consequence) of immunodeficiency. However, they were also predictive of progression to AIDS independent of their association with CD4 T-cell levels. Furthermore, titers to gp120 were associated with progression independent of titers to p51/65 and p24 (Table 3). The finding of several independent associations with progression makes it unlikely that a single underlying factor is responsible. For instance, if the data associated with progression were all surrogate markers for a single factor (such as duration of infection), which in turn was the major determinant of progression, one would not expect these "surrogates" to retain an independent association with progression when the multivariate model was adjusted for any one of them. Finally, it is difficult to explain lower titers to most proteins as a general consequence of progressive immunodeficiency when titers to gp41 remain stable and when titers to an irrelevant antigen (tetanus toxoid) do not show a similar relationship.

Lee et al. (85) also detected a qualitative loss of antibody to gp120 in those who progress. The loss was apparent when denatured (reduced) HIV was used as antigen but not when native (nonreduced) HIV was used (our data was generated using reduced antigen). They suggest that antibodies reactive with conformation-dependent epitopes of gp120 are relatively better preserved. Because gp120 is a likely target for antibody-mediated interruption of virus spread, the association

Table 3 Logistic Stepwise Regression

Independent variables significantly associated with progression	Step 0		Step 1 (adjust analysis for CD4 cells)		Step 2 (adjust analysis for CD4 cells and gp120 titer)		Step 3 (adjust analysis for CD4 cells, gp120 titer, and p65 titer)	
	F	p	F	p	F	p	F	p
Lower CD4 cells	27.8	<0.0001	adjusted		adjusted		adjusted	
Lower α-gp120 titer	27.5	<0.0001	19.7	<0.0001	adjusted		adjusted	
Lower α-p65 titer	19.3	<0.0001	10.4	0.0019	6.7	0.0116	adjusted	
Lower CD4/CD8 ratio	17.6	0.0001		ns		ns		ns
Lower α-p24 titer	13.3	0.0005	7.0	0.0100	5.7	0.0192		ns
Lower α-p51 titer	12.1	0.0008	8.7	0.0042	6.5	0.0131		ns
Lower CD3 cells	12.0	0.0009		ns		ns		ns
Lower lymphocytes	9.4	0.0030		ns		ns		ns

Dependent variable: progression/nonprogression to AIDS. Independent variables: lymphocyte and titer data.

of lower anti-gp120 titers with progression makes sense. Changes in titers to *gag*- and *pol*-encoded proteins are more difficult to explain by any postulated effect on virus infection. Laurence et al. (84) have reported loss of antibody that inhibits reverse transcriptase activity in progressive disease. It is possible that *gag* and *pol* responses as well as the gp120 response are not important for their functin as antigen-binding effector molecules; rather, their levels may be a marker for some other process that is important in the control of infection. For instance, *env, gag*, and, recently, *pol* gene products have been shown to be expressed on the cell surface and serve as targets for cytotoxic T cells (86–88). Because of the nature of the study, we do not know if the serologic differences we found are an inherent feature of the initial response to HIV or whether they represent a decline over time from previously higher levels; however, the decline does ante-date immune deterioration and is not simply another concomitant of the general immune deterioration. The fact that HIV-infected people progress to AIDS despite the presence of antibody does not rule out a role for antibody, either as a direct effector or as a marker for some other immunologic process, that limits the pace at which virus replication, CD4 T-cell depletion, and clinical AIDS occur.

ANTIBODY IDIOTOPES AS MOLECULAR MIMICS OF HIV GP120

One tenet of the idiotype network theory can be stated as follows: Given that antibodies combine with antigen by approximation of complementary molecular structures and that the immune system responds to the universe of antigenic structures, it follows that the antigen-combining site of antibody (the idiotope) itself can be antigenic and that within the antibody repertoire there exist anti-idiotypic antibodies that are structural homologues of antigenic epitopes found in nature. In the case of HIV, if an anti-CD4 antibody and gp120 bound to precisely the same region of CD4, the two may share some structural homology in their binding sites. If so, antisera raised to one should react with the other. The anti-CD4 antibody itself might be a potent vaccine inducing antibodies targeted against the critical site of gp120 required for the initial HIV–CD4 cell interaction. Aside from its theoretical appeal, the anti-idiotype approach has practical advantages. The surrogate vaccine would not be a viral product, and, to the extent to which conformational epitopes are critical for induction of potent antibodies, these epitopes may be relatively better preserved in an idiotype vaccine than in a viral subunit vaccine. However, this approach assumes that the dimensions of the CD4 binding site of gp120 and the CD4 antibody are similar, that such a CD4 antibody can be identified, and that it reliably induces an anti-idiotypic response in humans that reacts with gp120. It is also essential that protective effects in vivo and in vitro be reproducibly observed, and that the idiotype not induce an idiotype–anti-idiotype cascade deleterious to the host.

We and others have screened a relatively large panel of CD4 mAb for their effect on the HIV gp120:CD4 interaction (62,89). We found that OKT4A, OKT4D, OKT4F, and Leu3a mAb were potent inhibitors of HIV binding, whereas binding was not inhibited by OKT4 and OKT4C mAb and only partially inhibited by OKT4B and OKT4E (62). Similar results were reported by Sattentau et al. (89) for inhibition of syncytia. The CD4 epitopes detected by these mAb map as clusters on the molecule (90), and the pattern of inhibition indicates that HIV binds to a restricted portion of CD4, most probably in the distal amino-end of the molecule. The CD4 epitope recognized by Leu3A is highly conserved in primates and highly concordant with the infectivity of HIV for primate cells (91), making Leu3a, in a sense, the best candidate compared to other CD4 mAb.

Anti-idiotypic sera were prepared in rabbits to each of the four CD4 mAb that inhibited HIV binding. The sera were anti-idiotypic by the criteria that they reacted uniquely with the respective CD4 mAb used as the immunogen in ELISA and Western blot under nonreducing conditions, and they inhibited binding of the respective CD4 mAb to CD4. They did not react with HIV in ELISA or Western blot under nonreducing conditions, nor did they inhibit HIV binding to CD4 cells (Table 4).

One other group, using Leu3a, has generated a murine monoclonal anti-idiotypic antibody that reacts with Leu3a and with gp120 and inhibits Leu3a binding to CD4 as well as HIV syncytia formation and infectivity (92,93). This anti-idiotypic mAb also reacts with OKT4A, a cross-specificity that was not present in or was adsorbed from our rabbit anti-Leu3a (or anti-OKT4A) reagent. We examined serum samples from the Leu3a-immunized rabbit that had not been adsorbed to render them idiotype-specific and found no anti-HIV activity. If Leu3a contains a partial or whole "internal image" of the CD4 binding site of HIV, Leu3a becomes a candidate vaccine. It remains to be determined if Leu3a, as an immunogen in humans, reliably induces an anti-HIV response. It doesn't do so in rabbits, and the isolation of a murine monoclonal antibody with anti-Leu3a and anti-HIV activity does not mean that such an antibody is a major component of the polyclonal anti-Leu3a response in mice (93). Further search or different approaches may yet yield an antibody whose idiotope is an internal image of HIV and reliably induces an anti-HIV response. One such approach is to generate monoclonal antibodies to polyclonal anti-CD4 antibodies hoping to isolate an internal image of CD4 which in turn could be used to generate an anti-idiotypic antibody with an internal image of HIV (94). Another approach that we have tried without success is to immunize mice with conformation-dependent human anti-gp120 antibodies purified by affinity chromatography hoping to induce anti-idiotypic antibodies that also react with CD4. The mice produce potent antihuman Ig responses but no detectable anti-CD4 response and three fusions have thus far failed to select for an anti-CD4 mAb that mimics HIV.

Table 4 Summary of α-HIV and α-(α-CD4) Idiotypic Sera

Reagent	Direct reaction with[a]				
	gp120	OKT4A	OKT4D	OKT4F	Leu-3a
Rabbit α-OKT4A idiotype	−	+ (3,200)	−	−	−
Rabbit α-OKT4D idiotype	−	−	+ 3,200)	−	−
Rabbit α-OKT4F idiotype	−	−	−	+ 3,200	−
Rabbit α-Leu-3a idiotype	−	−	−	−	+ (1,600)
Rabbit α-HIV	+ (800)	−	−	−	−
Human α-HIV serum 1	+ (12,800)	−	−	−	−
Human α-HIV serum 2	+ (25,600)	−	−	−	−
Human α-HIV serum 3	+ (25,600)	−	−	−	−
Human α-HIV serum 4	+ (6,400)	−	−	−	−
Human α-HIV serum 5	+ (3,200)	−	−	−	−
Murine α-gp120 mAb	+ (10,000)				

[a]Reactions with gp120 were tested by immunoblot. Reactions with CD4 mAb were tested by ELISA. Lowest dilution tested was 1/10. Titers are indicated in parentheses.
[b]Lowest dilution tested was 1/10. End-point titers resulting in 50% inhibition of binding are indicated in parentheses.
Source: Ref. 62, with permission, American Association of Immunologists.

	Inhibition of[b]			
Virus binding	OKT4A binding	OKT4D binding	OKT4F binding	Leu-3a binding
−	+ (800)	−	−	−
−	−	+ (800)	−	−
−	−	−	+ (400)	−
−	−	−	−	+ (400)
+ (200)	−	−	−	−
+ (6,400)	−	−	−	−
+ (6,400)	−	−	−	−
+ (6,400)	−	−	−	−
+ (6,400)	−	−	−	−
+ (1,600)	−	−	−	−
+ (10,000)	−	−	−	−

PROSPECTS FOR A LIGAND OR IMMUNOGEN ELICITING ANTIBODY THAT BLOCKS THE CD4:GP120 INTERACTION

There are four possibilities: ligands that react with the binding sites of CD4 or gp120 and immunogens that induce antibodies reactive with these sites. Clearly it is possible to construct a ligand that binds to the CD4-binding site of gp120 and is a universal inhibitor of HIV infectivity. Soluble CD4 fulfills these criteria. Furthermore, antibodies to CD4 block HIV binding and infectivity. Mimics of gp120 as ligands or immunogens are more of a problem. Nothing short of full-length and conformationally intact gp120 has been shown (reliably and reproducibly) to bind to CD4 or interfere with HIV:CD4 interaction (3,40,41,61,62,95, 96). The fact that binding of gp120 is sensitive to cleavage of disulfide bonds as noted above indicates that the binding site requires a proper protein conformation and not simply the proper primary amino acid sequence. Thus it is unlikely that synthetic peptides matching portions of the gp120 molecule would bind to CD4 or inhibit virus binding unless, of course, they were formulated in the proper tertiary structure. Nevertheless, it is possible that a receptor that apparently binds to a ligand formed by approximating discontiguous amino acid sequences might have some affinity for contiguous sequences that form part of the bond. We tested a panel of 22 peptides corresponding to gp120 sequences spanning most portions of the molecule (97) (Table 5). They were tested for inhibition of HIV binding at $\geqslant$10:1 ratio by weight of peptide to HIV, which is conservatively estimated to be at least a 1000:1 molar ratio. We also tested peptide preparations that were covalently coupled to bovine serum albumin on the premise that the relative avidity of a low affinity interaction between putative peptide inhibitor and CD4 cells would be enhanced by virtue of the potential for multipoint attachment. None of the peptides inhibited HIV binding (not shown). This panel was by no means comprehensive, and perhaps some peptide could bind to CD4 as a mimic of gp120. However, in view of the conformation requirements noted above, it seems unlikely that such a peptide would be constructed solely from a single primary sequence. On the other hand, antiserum to the peptides may be sufficiently reactive with native gp120 to be useful for mapping the portion(s) of gp120 involved in binding. Accordingly, we prepared immunogens by covalently conjugating the peptides to keyhole limpet hemocyanin. The resultant antisera were strongly reactive in ELISA with the respective peptide coupled to a heterologous protein (BSA) using a heterologous coupling agent. However, most of the antipeptide sera did not react with native HIV in a sensitive radioimmunoprecipitation assay suggesting that most of the sequences are relatively inaccessible perhaps because they are buried or surrounded by a carbohydrate shell (Table 5). Only two of the antipeptide sera inhibited binding, and the inhibition was not as complete as that obtained with antiserum raised to the whole molecule, nor was inhibition increased by pooling

Table 5 Anti-*env* Peptide Sera

Peptide	gp120[a] residue numbers	Reactivity with peptide (ELISA)	Reactivity with HIV (ELISA)	Reactivity with gp120 (RIP)	Inhibition of HIV binding
24	54– 83	+++	++	++	–
25	89–108	+++	–	–	–
26	113–134	+++	+	++	–
27	166–190	+++	++	–	–
28	268–280	++	–	–	–
29	308–328	+++	–	–	–
30	323–336	+++	++	++	–
31	345–360	++	++	–	–
32	362–382	++	–	–	–
33	398–423	+	++	–	–
34	424–450	++	–	++	++
35	469–493	+++	++	–	–
36	494–517	+++	++	++	++
37	488–499	++	+	+	+
41	252–266	++	–	–	–
42	224–233	+	–	–	–
43	210–222	++	–	++	–
44	192–201	++	–	–	–
45	147–162	+++	–	–	–

[a]Residue numbers from Ref. 101.

the antipeptide sera. The partial inhibition was not due to inadequate amounts or affinity of antibody because the partial inhibition was sustained with dilution of the antisera—suggesting that they inhibit sterically or interfere with only a portion of the site.

The epitope mapping approach using antipeptide sera could potentially complement the site-directed or deletion mutation approach for localizing the CD4-binding site of gp120 if, for instance, the pool of anti-peptide sera completely inhibited binding and one dissected which serum components, alone or in combination, were responsible for inhibition. Both approaches have problems in interpretation related to the distinction of direct effects from steric effects or effects at a distance. Nevertheless, similar localization by dissimilar techniques would be complementary and overcome some of these difficulties. Our results with antipeptide sera were disappointing but not unusual. Most reported antipeptide sera or monoclonal antibodies reactive with conserved sequences of gp120 have been only partially inhibitory or neutralizing (3,95–99). More potent antibodies tend to be strain-specific and are unlikely to be reactive with the CD4-binding site, which is conserved and thus likely to be composed of conserved sequences.

For instance, Matthews and Putney and coworkers (95,96) reported that gp120 or a recombinant peptide derived from the HTLV-III$_B$ strain of HIV induced antibodies that neutralized the HTLV-III$_B$ strain but not the HTLV-IIIRF strain (which differ by about 20% in envelope amino acid sequence). They also demonstrated that human antibodies adsorbed to and eluted from immobilized gp120 of HTLV-III$_B$ preferentially neutralized HTLV-III$_B$. However, antibodies from the same serum samples that did not adsorb to the gp120 column were broadly neutralizing. We have also found that serum samples from humans infected with HIV inevitably contain binding-inhibition activity which, like soluble CD4 and anti-CD4 mAb, is complete and present in high titer. The effect is due to reaction with HIV rather than reaction wtih test cells or due to interference with the fluorescence reagent used to detect bound virus (Fig. 2, Table 6). Clearly, natural infection induces a population of antibodies that neutralize or inhibit binding of other (presumably diverse) strains and, by definition, are

Table 6 All Anti–HIV-Seropositive Human Sera Tested Inhibit HIV Binding

Serum source	No.	Anti-HIV	HIV binding inhibition median titer[a] (range)
Homosexual men with AIDS	25	+	1:800 (1:100–1:3200)
Homosexual men with lymphadenopathy	38	+	1:1600 (1:200–1:6400)
Asymptomatic seropositive homosexual men	44	+	1:1600 (1:400–1:6400)
Asymptomatic seronegative homosexual men	14	−	<1:100 (<1:100)
Heterosexual seronegative persons	15	−	<1:100 (<1:100)

[a]Titer equals highest serum dilution resulting in ⩾50% inhibition of binding.

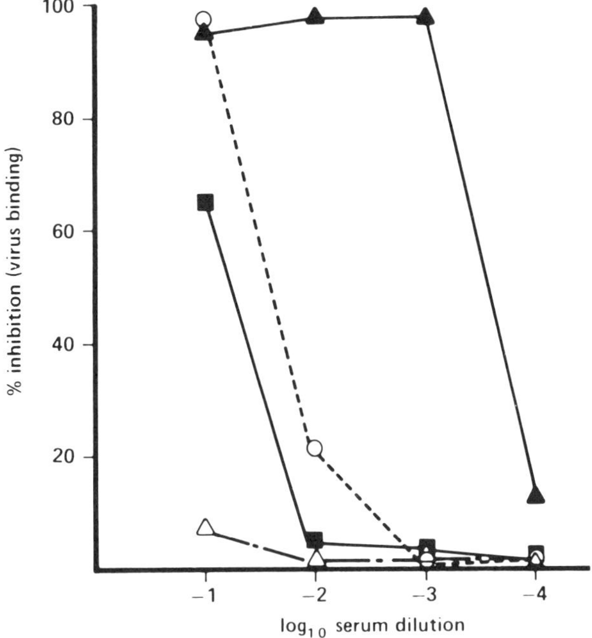

Figure 2   Inhibition of HIV binding to CD4 T cells by human anti-HIV serum. HIV was preincubated with a human anti-HIV serum (▲—▲) or a nonimmune serum (△—△) in the dilutions indicated. The mixtures were added to CD4 cells, and HIV binding was detected with fluorescein anti-HIV. As controls to rule out reaction with cells or interference with detection of bound HIV, CD4 cells were pretreated with human anti-HIV serum and washed once before addition of HIV (O—O), or CD4 cells that had bound HIV were incubated with human anti-HIV serum and washed once before addition of fluorescein anti-HIV (■—■). (From Ref. 62, with permission, American Association of Immunologists.)

not strain specific. Yet immunization with peptides or absorption to peptides has failed to identify the responsible epitope(s). Some of this data might be reconciled by postulating the existence of antibodies that detect conformational determinants on gp120. Such antibodies would not be induced or detected by denatured immunogens or absorbants. Two sets of data indicate to us that such antibodies exist in human sera. First, in a set of 30 human anti-HIV sera, binding inhibition titers correlate better with antibody titers to unreduced gp120 (by Western blot) than with antibody titers to reduced gp120 (100). Second, HIV immunoadsorbants were prepared containing Sepharose-amine linked to HIV through its carbohydrate groups which were oxidized to aldehydes (a procedure that does not destroy CD4 binding activity) (Table 1). Antibody adsorbed to and eluted from native HIV, on a weight basis, was a much more potent inhibitor of virus binding compared to antibody adsorbed to and eluted from reduced and alkylated HIV (100). Although the nature of the conformational determinants recognized by these sera have yet to be identified, they are likely to be conserved, and antibody to them interferes with HIV binding. It remains to be determined, once these determinants are defined, whether they will elicit protective anti-HIV responses.

CONCLUSION

The fact that disease progresses despite the presence of an immune response in HIV-infected people does not mean that such responses are totally ineffective. If induced before infection, it is conceivable that protection from initial infection would be observed when virus inoculum and load is less than in established infection. Clearly, serum and cells from HIV-infected people have substantial antiviral effects in vitro that have yet to be reproduced by artificial immunization. Regardless of whether the precise CD4 binding site of gp120 is immunogenic or accessible to antibody, further research on the structure of this site or other functional domains of HIV may define immunogens that elicit protective anti-HIV responses, perhaps even superior to those obtained during natural infection.

REFERENCES

1. Clavel F, Guetard F, Brun-Venzinet F, Chamaret S, Rey M, Santos-Feureira MO, Laurent AG, Dauguet C, Katlama C, Rouzioux C, Klatzman D, Champalimaud JL, Montagnier L. Isolation of a new human retrovirus from West African patients with AIDS. Science 1986; 233:343–6.
2. Kanki PJ, Barin F, M'Boup S, Allan JS, Romet-Lemonne JC, Marlink R, McLane MF, Lee T, Arbeille B, Denis F, Essex M. New human T-lymphotropic retrovirus related to simian-T-lymphotropic virus type III (STLV–III/AGM). Science 1986; 232:238–43.
3. Lasky LA, Nakamura G, Smith DH, Fennie C, Shimaski C, Patzer E, Berman P, Gregory T, Capon DJ. Delineation of a region of the human immunodeficiency virus type 1 gp120 glycoprotein critical for interaction with the CD4 receptor. Cell 1987; 50:975–85.
4. Kung PC, Goldstein G, Reinherz EL, Schlossman SF. Monoclonal antibodies defining distinctive human T cell surface antigens. Science 1979; 206:347–9.
5. Ledbetter J, Evans RL, Lipinski M, Cunningham-Rundles C, Good RA, Herzenberg LA. Evolutionary conservation of surface molecules that distinguish T lymphocyte helper/inducer and cytotoxic/suppressor subpopulations in mouse and man. J Exp Med 1981; 153:310–23.

6. Thomas Y, Rogozinski L, Irigoyen O, Friedman SM, Kung PC, Goldstein G, Chess L. Functional analysis of human T cell subsets defined by monoclonal antibodies. IV. Induction of suppressor cells within the OKT4[+] population. J Exp Med 1981; 154:459–67.

7. Meur SC, Schlossman SF, Reinherz EL. Clonal analysis of human cytotoxic T lymphocytes. T4[+] and T8[+] effector cells recognize products of different histocompatibility complex regions. Proc Natl Acad Sci USA 1982; 79: 4395–9.

8. Reinherz EL, Kung PC, Goldstein G, Schlossman SF. Separation of functional subsets of human T cells by a monoclonal antibody. Proc Natl Acad Sci USA 1979; 76:4061–3.

9. Engleman EG, Benike C, Grumet C, Evans RL. Activation of human T lymphocyte subsets: helper and suppressor/cytotoxic T cells recognize and respond to distinct histocompatibility antigens. J Immunol 1981; 127: 2124–9.

10. Swain SL. T cell subsets and the recognition of MHC class. Immunol Rev 1983;   74:129–42.

11. Maddon PJ, Littman DR, Godfrey M, Maddon DE, Chess L, and Axel R. The isolation and nucleotide sequence of a cDNA encoding the T cell surface protein T4: a new member of the immunoglobulin gene family. Cell 1985; 42:93–104.

12. Terhorst C, Van Agthhoven A, Reinherz EL, Schlossman S. Biochemical analysis of human T lymphocyte differentiation antigens T4 and T5. Science 1980; 209:520–1.

13. Acres RB, Conion PJ, Mochizuki DY, Gallis B. Rapid phosphorylation and modulation of the T4 antigen on cloned helper T cells induced by phorbol myristate acetate or antigen. J Biol Chem 1986; 261:16210–4.

14. Hoxie JA, Matthews DM, Callahan KD, Cassel DL, Cooper RA. Transient modulation and internalization of T4 antigens induced by phorbol esters. J Immunol 1986; 137:1194–7.

15. Hoxie JA, Rackowski JL, Haggarty BS, Gaulton GN. T4 endocytosis and phosphorylation induced by phorbol esters but not by mitogen or HIV HIV infection. J Immunol 1988; 140:786–95.

16. Wassmer P, Chan C, Lodgberg L, Shevach E. Role of L3T4 antigen in T cell activation. II. Inhibition of T cell activation by monoclonal anti-L3T4 antibodies in the absence of accessory cells. J Immunol 1985; 135: 2237–41.

17. Bank I, Chess L. Perturbation of the T4 molecule transmits a negative signal to T cells. J Exp Med 1985; 162:1294–1303.

18. Tite JP, Sloan A, Janeway CA. The role of L3T4 in T cell activation: L3T4 may be both an Ia-binding protein and a receptor that transduces a negative signal. J Mol Cell Immunol 1986; 2:179–83.

19. Rosoff PM, Burakoff SJ, Greenstein JL. The role of L3T4 molecule in mitogen and antigen-activated signal transduction. Cell 1987; 49:845–53.

20. Biddison WE, Rao PE, Talle MA, Goldstein G, Shaw S. Possible involvement of the OKT4 molecule in T cell recognition of class II HLA antigens. J Exp Med 1982; 156:1065–76.

21. Marrack P, Endres R, Schimon-Kevitz R, Ziotnik A, Dialynas D, Fitch F, Kappler J. The major histocompatibility complex-restricted antigen receptor on T cells. II. Role of the L3T4 product. J Exp Med 1983; 158:1077–91.

22. Rogozinski L, Bass A, Glickman E, Tulle MA, Goldstein G, Wang J, Chess L, Thomas Y. The T4 surface antigen is involved in the induction of helper function. J Immunol 1984; 132:735–9.

23. Saizawa K, Rojo J, Janeway CA. Evidence for a physical association of CD4 and the CD3:α:β T-cell receptor. Nature 1987; 328:260–3.

24. Gay D, Maddon, P, Sekaly R, Talle MA, Godfrey M, Long E, Goldstein G, Chess L, Axel R, Kappler J, Marrack P. Functional interaction between human T-cell protein CD4 and the major histocompatibility complex HLA–DR antigen. Nature 1987; 328:626–9.

25. Doyle C, Strominger JL. Interaction between CD4 and class II MHC molecules mediates cells adhesion. Nature 1987; 330:256–257.

26. Gallo RC, Salahuddin SZ, Popovic M, Shearer AM, Kaplan M, Haynes BF, Palker PJ, Redfield R, Oleske J, Safai B, White G, Foster P, Markham PD. Frequent detection and isolation of cytopathic retroviruses (HTLV-III) from patients with AIDS and at risk for AIDS. Science 1984; 224: 500–2.

27. Klatzmann D, Barre Sinoussi F, Nugeyre MT, Dauguet C, Vilmer E, Griscelli C, Brun-Venzinet F, Rouzioux C, Gluckman JC, Chermann JC, Montagnier L. Selective tropism of lymphadenopathy associated virus (LAV) for helper-inducer T lymphocytes. Science 1984; 225:59–62.

28. Montagnier L, Gruest J, Chamaret S, Dauguet C, Axler C, Guetard D, Nugeyre MT, Barre-Sinoussi F, Chermann JC, Brunet JB, Klatzmann D, Gluckman JC. Adaptation of lymphadenopathy associated virus (LAV) to replication in EBV-transformed B-lymphoblastoid cell lines. Science 1984; 225:63–7.

29. Popovic M, Read-Connole E, Gallo RC. T4 positive human neoplastic cell lines susceptible to and permissive for HTLV-III. Lancet 1984; 2:1472.

30. Dalgleish AG, Beverley PCL, Clapham PR, Crawford DH, Greaves MF, Weiss RA. The CD4 (T4) antigen is an essential component of the receptor for the AIDS retrovirus. Nature 1985; 312:763–7.

31. Fauci AS, Masur H, Gelmann EP, Markham, PD, Hahn BH, Lane HC. The acquired immunodeficiency syndrome: an update. Ann Intern Med 1985; 102:800–13.

32. Dalgleish AG, Clapham P. B cells in the pathogenesis of AIDS. Immunol Today 1985; 6:71.

33. Levy JA, Shimabukuro J, McHugh T, Casavant C, Stites DP, Oschiro LS. AIDS-associated retroviruses (ARV) can productively infect other cells besides human T helper cells. Virology 1985; 147:441–8.

34. McDougal JS, Mawle A, Cort SP, Nicholson JKA, Cross GD, Scheppler-Campbell JA, Hicks D, Sligh J. Cellular tropism of the human retrovirus HTLV–III/LAV. I. Role of T cell activation and expression of the T4 molecule. J Immunol 1985; 135:3151-62.

35. Ho DD, Rota TR, Hirsch MS. Infection of monocyte/macrophages by human T lymphotropic virus type III. J Clin Invest 1986; 77:1712-5.

36. Nicholson JKA, Cross GD, Calloway CS, McDougal JS. In vitro infection of human monocytes with HTLV–III/LAV. J Immunol 1986 137:232-9.

37. Gartner S, Markovits P, Markovitz CM, Kaplan MH, Gallo RC, Popovic M. The role of mononuclear phagocytes in HTLV–III/LAV infection. Science 1986; 233:215-9.

38. Popovic M, Gallo RC, Mann DL. OKT4 bearing molecule is a receptor for the human retrovirus HTLV–III. Clin Res 1984; 33:560A.

39. Klatzmann D, Champagne E, Chamaret S, Gruest J, Guetard D, Hercend T, Gluckman JC, Montagnier L. T-lymphocyte T4 molecule behaves as the receptor for human retrovirus LAV. Nature 1985; 312:767-8.

40. McDougal JS, Kennedy MS, Sligh JM, Cort SP, Mawle A, Nicholson JKA. Binding of HTLV–III/LAV to T4$^+$ cells by a complex of the 110k viral protein and the T4 molecule. Science 1986; 231:382-5.

41. Matthews TJ, Weinhold KJ, Lyerly HK, Langlois AJ, Wigzell H, Bolognesi DP. Interaction between the human T-cell lymphotropic virus type III B envelope glycoprotein gp120 and the surface antigen CD4: Role of carbohydrate in binding and cell fusion. Proc Natl Acad Sci USA 1987; 84: 5424-8.

42. Maddon PJ, Dalgleish AG, McDougal JS, Clapham PR, Weiss RA, Axel R. The T4 gene encodes the AIDS virus receptor and is expressed in the immune system and the brain. Cell 1986; 47:333-8.

43. Rosen CA, Sodroski JG, Haseltine WA. The location of cis-acting regulatory sequences in the human T cell lymphotropic virus type III (HTLV–III/ LAV) long terminal repeat. Cell 1985; 41:813-23.

44. Fisher AG, Collalti E, Ratner L, Gallo RC, Wong-Staal F. A molecular clone of HTLV–III with biological activity. Nature 1985; 316:262-5.

45. Levy JA, Cheng-Mayer C, Dina D, Luciw PA. AIDS retrovirus (ARV-2) clone replicates in transfected human and animal fibroblasts. Science 1986; 232:998-1000.

46. Smith DH, Byrn RA, Marsters SA, Gregory T, Groopman JE, Capon DJ. Blocking of HIV-1 infectivity by a soluble, secreted form of the CD4 antigen. Science 1987; 238:1704-7.

47. Fisher RA, Bertonis JM, Meier W, Johnson VA, Costapoulos DS, Liu T, Tizard R, Walker BD, Hirsh MS, Schooley RT, Flavell RA. HIV infection is blocked in vitro by recombinant soluble CD4. Nature 1988; 331:76-8.

48. Hussey RE, Richardson NE, Kowalski M, Brown NR, Chang H, Silicano RF, Dorfman T, Walker B, Sodroski J, Reinherz EL. A soluble CD4 protein selectively inhibits HIV replication and syncytium formation. Nature 1988; 331:78-81.

49. Deen KC, McDougal, JS, Inacker R, Folena-Wasserman G, Arthos J, Rosenberg J, Maddon PJ, Axel R, Sweet RW. A soluble form of CD4 (T4) protein inhibits AIDS virus infection. Nature 1988;331:82-4.

50. Traunecker A, Luke W, Karjalainen K. Soluble CD4 molecules neutralize human immunodeficiency virus type 1. Nature 1988;331:84-6.

51. Weiss RA. Receptor molecule blocks HIV. Nature 1988;331:15.

52. Hoxie JA, Alpers JD, Rackowski J, Huebner K, Haggarty BS, Cedarbaum AJ, Reed JC. Alterations in T4 (CD4) protein and mRNA synthesis in cells infected with HIV. Science 1986;234:1123-7.

53. Zagury D, Bernard J, Leonard R, Cheynier R, Feldman M, Sarin PS, Gallo RC. Long term cultures of HTLV-III infected T cells: a model of cytopathology of T cell depleiton in AIDS. Science 1986;231:850-3.

54. Stein BS, Gowda SD, Lifson JD, Penhallow RC, Bensch KG, Engleman EG. pH-independent HIV entry into CD4-positive T cells via virus envelope fusion to the plasma membrane. Cell 1987;49:659-68.

55. Gallaher WR. Detection of a fusion peptide sequence in the transmembrane protein of human immunodeficiency virus. Cell 1987;50:327-8.

56. DeRossi A, Franchini G, Aldovini A, Del Mistro A, Chieco-Bianchi L, Gallo RC, Wong-Staal F. Differential response to the cytopathic effects of human T-cell lymphotropic virus type III (HTLV-III) superinfection in T4$^+$ (helper) and T8$^+$ (suppressor) T cell clones transformed by HTLV-1. Proc Natl Acad Sci USA 1986;83:4297-301.

57. Asjo B, Irhed I, Gridlund M, Fuerstenberg S, Feuyo EM, Nilsson K, Wigzell H. Susceptibility to infection by the human immunodeficiency virus (HIV) correlates with T4 expression in a parental monocytoid cell line and its subclones. Virology 1987;157:359-65.

58. Fisher AG, Ratner L, Mitsuya H, Marselle LM, Harper ME, Broder S, Gallo RC, Wong-staal F. Infectious mutants of HTLV-III with changes in the 3^1 region and markedly reduced cytopathic effects. Science 1986;233:655-9.

59. Sodroski J, Goh WC, Rosen C, Campbell K, Haseltine W. Role of the HTLV-III/LAV envelope in syncytium formation and cytopathicity. Nature 1986;470-4.

60. Lifson JD, Feinberg MD, Reyes GR, Rabin L, Banapour B, Chakrabarti S, Moss B, Wong-Staal F, Steimer KS, Engleman EG. Induction of CD4-dependent cell fusion by the HTLV-III/LAV envelope glycoprotein. Nature 1986;323:725-8.

61. Kowalski M, Potz J, Basiripour L, Dorfman T, Goh WC, Terwilliger E, Dayton A, Rosen C, Haseltine W, Sodroski J. Functional regions of the envelope glycoprotein of human immunodeficiency virus type 1. Science 1987;237:1351-55.

62. McDougal JS, Nicholson JKA, Cross GD, Cort SP, Kennedy MS, Mawle AC. Binding of the human retrovirus HTLV-III/LAV/ARV/HIV to the CD4 (T4) molecule: conformation dependence, epitope mapping, antibody inhibition, and potential for idiotypic mimicry. J Immunol 1986; 137:2937-44.

63. Lifson J, Coutre S, Huang E, Engleman E. Role of envelope glycoprotein carbohydrate in human immunodeficiency virus (HIV) infectivity and virus-induced cell fusion. J Exp Med 1986; 164:2101–6.

64. Jaffe HW, Feorino PM, Darrow WW, O'Malley PM, Getchell JP, Warfield DT, Jones BM, Echenberg DF, Francis DP, Curran JW. Persistent infection with HTLV–III/LAV in apparently healthy homosexual men. Ann Intern Med 1985; 102:627–8.

65. Ammann AJ, Abrams D, Conant M, Chudwin D, Cowan M, Volberding P, Lewis B, Casavant C. Acquired immune dysfunction in homosexual men: immunologic profiles. Clin Immunol Immunopathol 1983; 27:315–25.

66. Schroff RW, Gottlieb MS, Prince HE, Chai U, Fahey JL. Immunological studies of homosexual men with immunodeficiency and Kaposi's sarcoma. Clin Immunol Immunopathol 1983; 27:300–14.

67. Lane HC, Masur H, Gelmann EP, Longo DL, Steiss RG, Chused T, Whalen G, Edgar L, Fauci AS. Correlation between immunologic function and clinical subpopulations of patients with the acquired immunodeficiency syndrome. Am J Med 1985; 78:417–22.

68. Eyster ME, Goerdert JJ, Sarngadharan MG, Weiss SH, Gallo RC, Blattner WA. Development and early natural history of HTLV–III an antibodies in persons with hemophilia. JAMA 1985; 253:2219–23.

69. Schwartz K, Visscher BR, Detels R, Taylor J, Nishanian P, Fahey JL. Immunologic changes in lymphadenopathy virus positive and negative symptomless male homosexuals: two years of observation. Lancet 1985; 2:831–2.

70. Melbye M, Biggar RJ, Ebbesen P, Neuland C, Goerdert JJ, Faber V, Lovenzen I, Skinhog P, Gallo RC, Blattner WA. Long-term seropositivity for human T-lymphotropic virus type III in homosexual men without the acquired immunodeficiency syndrome: development of immunologic and clinical abnormalities. Ann Intern Med 1986; 104:496–500.

71. Metroka CD, Cunningham-Rundles S, Pollack MS, Sonnabend JA, Davis JM, Gordon B, Fernandez RD, Mouradian J. Generalized lymphadenopathy in homosexual men. Ann Intern Med 1983; 99:585–91.

72. Goerdert JJ, Sarngadharan MG, Biggar TJ, Weiss SH, Winn D, Grossman RJ, Greene MH, Bodner A, Mann DL, Strong DM, Gallo RC, Blattner WA. Determinants of retrovirus (HTLV–III) antibodies and immunodeficiency in homosexual men. Lancet 1984; 2:711–6.

73. Mathur-Wagh W, Enlow RE, Spigland L, Winchester RJ, Sacks HS, Rorat E, Yancovitz SR, Klein MJ, Williams DC, Mildvan D. Longitudinal study of persistent generalized lymphadenopathy in homosexual men: relation to AIDS. Lancet 1984; 1:1033–7.

74. Fishbein DB, Kaplan JE, Spira TJ, Miller B, Schonberger LB, Pinsky PF, Getchell JP, Kalyanaraman VS, Braude JS. Unexplained lymphadenopathy in homosexual men: a longitudinal study. JAMA 1985; 254:930–5.

75. Nicholson, JKA, McDougal JS, Jaffe HW, Spira TJ, Kennedy MS, Jones BM, Darrow WW, Morgan M, Hubbard M. Exposure to human T-lymphotropic

virus type III/lymphadenopathy associated virus and immunologic abnormalities in asymptomatic homosexual men. Ann Intern Med 1985; 103;37–42.

76. McDougal JS, Kennedy MS, Nicholson JKA, Spira TJ, Jaffe HW, Kaplan JE, Fishbein DB, O'Malley P, Aloisio CH, Black CM, Hubbard M, Reimer CB. Antibody response to human immunodeficiency virus in homosexual men. Relation of antibody specificity, titer, and isotype to clinical status, severity of immunodeficiency, and disease progression. J Clin Invest 1987; 80:316–24.

77. Safai B, Groopman JE, Popovic M, Schupbach J, Sarngadharan MG, Arnett K, Sliski A, Gallo RC. Seroepidemiological studies of human T-lymphotropic retrovirus type III in acquired immunodeficiency syndrome. Lancet 1984; 1:1438–40.

78. Schupbach J, Haller O, Vogt M, Luthy R, Joller H, Oelz O, Popovic M, Sarngadharan MG, Gallo RC. Antibodies to HTLV–III in Swiss patients with AIDS and pre-AIDS and in groups at risk for AIDS. N Engl J Med 1985; 312:265–70.

79. Sarngadharan MG, di Marzo Veronese F, Lee S, Gallo RC. Immunological properties of HTLV–III antigens recognized by sera of patients with AIDS and AIDS-related complex and of asymptomatic carriers of HTLV–III infection. Cancer Res 1985; 45:4574s–7s.

80. Biggar TJ, Melbye M, Ebbesen P, Alexander S, Nielson JO, Sarin P, Faber F. Variation in human T lymphotropic virustype III (HTLV–III) antibodies in homosexual men: decline before onset of illness related to acquired immune deficiency syndrome (AIDS). Br Med J 1985; 291:997–8.

81. Kaminsky LS, McHugh T, Stites D, Volberding P, Henle G, Levy JA. High prevalence of antibodies to acquired immune deficiency syndrome (AIDS)-associated retrovirus (ARV) in AIDS and related conditions but not in other disease states. Proc Natl Acad Sci USA 1985; 82:5535–9.

82. Steimer K, Puma JP, Power MD, Powers MA, Nacimento CG, Stephans JC, Levy JA, Sanchez-Pescador R, Luciw PA, Barr PJ, Hallewell RA. Differential antibody responses of individuals infected with AIDS-associated retroviruses surveyed using the viral core p25 gag expressed in bacteria. Virology 1986; 150:283–90.

83. Lange JMA, Coutinho RA, Krone WJA, Verdonck LF, Danner SA, Van der Noordaa J, Goudsmit J. Distinct IgG recognition patterns during progression of subclinical and clinical infection with lymphadenopathy associated virus/human T lymphotropic virus. Br Med J 1986; 292:228–30.

84. Laurence J, Saunders A, Kulkowsky J. Characterization and clinical association of antibody inhibitory to HIV reverse transcriptase activity. Science 1987; 235:1501–4.

85. Lee T, Redfield, R, Chou MJ, Allan J, Burke D, Essex M. Differential recognition of HTLV–III/HIV envelope antigens is correlated with clinical outcome. III International Conference on AIDS. Washington, D.C. 1987; abstract WP17:p113.

86. Walker BD, Chakrabarti S, Moss B, Paradis TJ, Flynn T, Durno AG, Blumberg RS, Kaplan JC, Hirsch MS, Schooley RT. HIV-specific cytotoxic T lymphocytes in seropositive individuals. Nature 1987; 328:345–8.

87. Plata F, Autran B, Martins LP, Wain-Hobson S, Raphael M, Mayaud C, Denis M, Guillon JM, Debre P. AIDS virus-specific cytotoxic T lymphocytes in lung disorders. Nature 1987; 328:348–51.

88. Walker BD, Flexner C, Pardis TJ, Fuller TC, Hirsch MS, Schooley RT, Moss B. HIV-1 reverse transcriptase is a target for cytotoxic T lymphocytes in infected individuals. Science 1988; 240:64–6.

89. Sattentau QJ, Dalgleish AG, Weiss RA, Beverley PCL. Epitopes of the CD4 antigen and HIV infection. Science 1986; 234:1120–3.

90. Fuller TC, Trvithick JE, Fuller AA, Colvin RB, Cosimi AB, Kung PC. Antigenic polymorphism of the T4 differentiation antigen expressed on human T helper/inducer lymphocytes. Hum Immunol 1984; 9:89–102.

91. McClure MO, Sattentau QJ, Beverley PC, Hearn JP, Fitzgerald AK, Zuckerman AJ, Weiss RA. HIV infection of primate lymphocytes and conservation of the CD4 receptor. Nature 1987; 330:487–9.

92. Chanh TC, Dreeman GR, Kennedy RC. Monoclonal anti-idiotypic antibody mimics the CD4 receptor and binds human immunodeficiency virus. Proc Natl Acad Sci USA 1987; 84:3891–5.

93. Dalgleish AG, Thomson BJ, Chanh TC, Malkovsky M, Kennedy RC. Neutralisation of HIV isolates by anti-idiotypic antibodies which mimic the T4 (CD4) epitope: a potential AIDS vaccine. Lancet 1987; 2:1047–9.

94. Ludwig DS, Schoolnik GK. Anti-receptor antibodies designed to elicit "internal image"-bearing anti anti-idiotypes: a possible AIDS vaccine. Med Hypoth 1987; 23:303–7.

95. Putney SD, Matthews TJ, Robey WG, Lynn DL, Robert-Guroff M, Mueller WT, Langlois AJ, Ghrayeb J, Petteway SR, Weinhold KJ, Fischinger PJ, Wong-Staal F, Gallo RC, Bolognesi DP. HTLV–III/LAV-neutralizing antibodies to an E. coli-produced fragment of the virus envelope. Science 1986; 234:1392–95.

96. Matthews TJ, Langlois AJ, Robey WG, Chang NT, Gallo RC, Fischinger PJ, Bolognesi DP. Restricted neutralization of divergent human T-lymphotropic virus type III isolates by antibodies to the major envelope glycoprotein. Proc Natl Acad Sci USA 1986; 83:9709–14.

97. McDougal JS, Nicholson JKA, Cosand WL, Cross GD, Cort SP, Kennedy MS, Mawle AC. HIV binding to the CD4 molecule: conformation dependence and binding inhibition studies. In Human Retroviruses, Cancer, and AIDS. D Bolognesi ed. New York: Alan R. Liss, Inc., 1988: 269–81.

98. Palker PJ, Matthews TJ, Clark ME, Cinaciolo EJ, Randall RR, Langlois AJ, White GC, Safai B, Snyderman R, Bolognesi DP, Haynes BF. A conserved region of the COOH terminus of human immunodeficiency virus gp120 envelope protein contains an immunodominant epitope. Proc Natl Acad Sci 1987; 2479–2483.

99. Ho DD, Sarngadharan MG, Hirsch MS, Schooley RT, Rota TR, Kennedy
     RC, Chanh TC, Sato VL. Human immunodeficiency virus neutralizing
     antibodies recognize several conserved omains on the envelope glycopro-
     teins. J Virol 1987; 61:2024–8.
100. McDougal JS, Nicholson JKA, Cross GD, Cort SP, Kennedy MS, Mawle A.
     HIV binding to the CD4 molecule: conformation dependence and anti-
     body inhibition. III International Conference on AIDS. Washington, D.C.
     1987; abstract TP108:p80.
101. Wain-Hobson S, Sonigo P, Danos O, Coles S, Alizon M. Nucleotide
     sequence of the AIDS virus, LAV. Cell 1985; 40:9–17.

3

Structure and Function of the HIV Envelope
Implications for Vaccine Development

Joseph Sodroski, Mark Kowalski, and William Haseltine
Dana-Farber Cancer Institute
Harvard Medical School
Boston, Massachusetts

Human immunodeficiency virus (HIV), the etiologic agent of acquired immuno-deficiency syndrome (AIDS) (1-3), is surrounded by an envelope composed of a lipid bilayer and envelope glycoproteins. The lipid bilayer is derived from the host cell as the virus buds, while the envelope glycoproteins are encoded by the virus.

The HIV envelope is synthesized as an 88 kilodalton (kD) precursor (4,5). High mannose-type sugar chains are added to the envelope precursor and, following modification by glucosidase I, the glycosylated precursor migrates as a 160 kD glycoprotein (gp160) (4-6). The gp160 glycoprotein is not expressed appreciably on the surface of infected cells nor is it incorporated into the virion (6).

Cleavage of the gp160 glycoprotein by a cellular protease yields the exterior glycoprotein, gp120, and the transmembrane glycoprotein, gp41. Both proteins are expressed on the surface of the infected cell and are incorporated into the virion. Close in time to the cleavage of gp160, some of the high-mannose sugar chains are converted to the complex type of carbohydrate, so that the mature gp120 glycoprotein contains both complex and high-mannose sugar residues (7). The gp41 transmembrane glycoprotein contains complex sugar side chains. Following these modifications in the golgi complex, the mature gp120 and gp41 proteins are either incorporated into virion particles or are channeled to the surface of the infected cell.

HIV ENTRY INTO THE HOST CELL

The gp120 and gp41 envelope glycoproteins play central roles in the process of virus entry into the target cell. The major determinant of the tropism of HIV for cells of the macrophage/monocyte and lymphoid lineages appears to be a specific binding that occurs between the gp120 exterior glycoprotein and the virus receptor, the CD4 or T4 glycoprotein (8-10). Cells infectible by HIV express the CD4 protein on their surface. Following gp120–CD4 binding, other events, including fusion of the virion and target cell membranes and entry of the viral core containing the virion RNA, are probably necessary for initiation of infection (11). Host cell factors other than CD4 are likely to be involved in the fusion process, since animal cells transfected with and expressing the human CD4 gene are not infectible by HIV (12). These cells also are resistant to the formation of syncytia when cultivated with cells expressing the HIV envelope (see below). Thus, CD4 would appear to be necessary but not sufficient for infectivity by HIV.

The necessity of the membrane fusion event for virus entry is based primarily upon analogy with other enveloped viruses (for review, see Ref. 13). While the fusion of viral and host cell membranes has been observed by electron microscopy to occur at the plasma membrane and within endosomes, it is not yet clear which of these modes of entry is most efficient. Based on studies of syncytium formation (see below) and studies involving inhibitors of endosomal acidification, it is unlikely that a decrease in pH is a necessary step in HIV envelope-mediated fusion (11). In this respect, HIV resembles the paramyxoviruses rather than members of the orthomyxoviruses, rhabdoviruses, or togaviruses, all of which depend upon endocytosis and endosomal acidification for the fusion process involved in virus entry to occur.

HIV CYTOPATHICITY

The envelope glycoproteins of HIV have also been implicated in the cytopathic effect of the virus, which is specific for cells bearing high levels of virus receptor (14). In tissue culture, the cytopathic effects of HIV consist of multinucleated giant cell (syncytium) formation and the lysis of single cells (2,15). Syncytium formation is mediated solely by the HIV envelope expressed on the infected cell surface (16,17). The envelope binds to the CD4 receptor present on adjacent cells and then, via a fusion reaction analogous to that involved in virus entry, the apposed cell membranes are fused so that heterokaryons are formed. The lifespan of a syncytium formed between lymphocytes in tissue culture is limited to several days, at which time cell membrane lysis and nuclear pyknosis occur (16). Syncytium formation probably involves the interaction of multiple envelope glycoproteins and receptor molecules, so that it is prominent early in the course of HIV infection in vitro. At this time, when multiplicities of infection are lower, higher levels of free receptor are available for syncytium formation.

At higher multiplicities of infection or in cell lines where less receptor is available, single cell killing is the predominant cytopathic effect observed (15). The HIV envelope, probably via similar receptor-binding and membrane fusion events as those involved in syncytium formation, has been implicated in single cell killing. First, involvement of the novel retroviral genes possessed by HIV in the killing process has been ruled out. Deletion of the R, *sor*, or 3' *orf* genes results in viruses that are still capable of killing CD4-positive lymphocytes, both by syncytium formation and by single cell killing (18,19). Expression of particular viral genes such as *tat, art,* or *sor* at high levels in cells susceptible to HIV killing is not sufficient for induction of cytopathic effect (20). Second, the HIV cytopathic effect is specific for cells that have higher levels of receptor, independent of the level of viral protein expression or viral DNA in the infected cell (14). Implication of the viral receptor in the cytopathic process in turn implicates the viral protein that interacts with that receptor, the gp120 envelope glycoprotein. Third, the HIV envelope has been shown to be capable alone of initiating cell damage during syncytium formation (16,17). It is reasonable to suggest that similar events might damage the membranes of single infected cells. Finally, mutations in the envelope gene generate viruses that are compromised in their ability to kill single cells (21).

HIV CELL–TO–CELL TRANSMISSION

In tissue culture, HIV infection has been demonstrated to spread via cell-free virions as well as via contact of uninfected and infected cells (22,23). This latter mode of cell-to-cell transmission is the predominant means of spread of HIV viruses compromised in their ability to encode the 23 kD *sor* gene product. Cell-to-cell transmission has been observed for other fusogenic viruses and probably involves the fusion of elements of the infected cell with the uninfected cell. Cell-to-cell transmission is likely to be dependent upon many of the same parameters important for the process of syncytium formation.

THE NEUTRALIZING ANTIBODY PARADOX

High titers of antienvelope antibodies are found in most infected people (24-26). However, these antibodies do not completely prevent virus infection or syncytium formation even at low dilution of the patient sera (15,27). The absence of complete inhibition is all the more surprising as HIV-1–infected patient sera generally contains high titers of antibodies that recognize the envelope proteins as judged both by immunoprecipitation reactions and immunofluorescence reactions with the virus-infected cells (2,24,28). Often, the titers of antibodies directed to the envelope in patients exceeds 1 to 10,000 (29). At best, patient antibodies may slow down the process of syncytium formation or virus infectivity without completely blocking these reactions (16, 27). This observation suggests that the surface of the virus is constructed to evade the immune response. The failure of the natural immune response to prevent these reactions may account for both the progressive nature of AIDS virus infection in the face of a vigorous immune response and the failure of antibodies to protect chimpanzees from de novo infections. This observation suggests that regions of the envelope protein that are recognized by antibodies in infected patients may not correspond to those regions important for the functioning of the envelope glycoprotein.

MUTATIONAL ANALYSIS OF ENVELOPE FUNCTIONS

The development of effective HIV vaccines will require the elicitation of humoral and cellular immune responses against the regions of the HIV envelope critical for its function in virus entry, cell-to-cell transmission, syncytium formation, and cytopathic effect. We have attempted to determine the regions of the envelope protein that encode functions required for receptor-binding and membrane fusion reactions.

Our approach to localization of functions necessary for the receptor binding and membrane fusion reactions has been to introduce mutations into the envelope glycoprotein gene by linker scanning mutagenesis and deletion mutagenesis (30). The mutants were introduced into a clone of the envelope glycoprotein gene that was expressed at high concentrations upon transfection into uninfected cells. The envelope glycoprotein gene was functional as judged by the ability of the gene to induce syncytia upon transfection into CD4$^+$ cells and also by the ability of the gene to complement infectivity of an HIV-1 provirus defective in the envelope gene.

Measurement of properties of the mutants included:

1. Determination of the size and amount of protein produced.
2. Determination of partitioning of the envelope protein between the transfected cells and the cell supernatant.
3. Determination of the ability of the transfected envelope glycoprotein gene to induce syncytia when transfected into CD4$^+$ cells in culture.
4. Determination of the ability of gp120 produced by the mutants to bind to the CD4 receptor.
5. Determination of the ability of the mutant envelope envelope gene to complement *env*-deleted viruses for replication.

The effects of the introduced mutations could be divided into five different groups depending on phenotype (Figure 1).

MUTATIONS THAT AFFECT gp120–CD4 BINDING

Envelope mutations that affect the ablity of the virus to bind to the CD4 receptor were found to be located in the 3′ region of gp120. These mutant envelope genes synthesize normal amounts of gp120 and gp41 on the cell surface and excrete normal amounts of gp120 into the supernatant fluid. However, the gp120 was not able to bind to the CD4 receptor.

CD4 binding mutants were located in three noncontiguous regions corresponding to amino acid sequences that have been shown to be well conserved among HIV-1, HIV-2, and simian immunodeficiency virus (SIV) isolates, all of which utilize the CD4 molecule as a receptor. All three conserved regions are located near the carboxyl terminus of gp120. These three conserved regions are separated by regions of amino acids that vary from isolate to isolate. Mutations in the variable regions were not found to affect CD4 binding.

Based on these observations, it is likely that the binding site for CD4 is

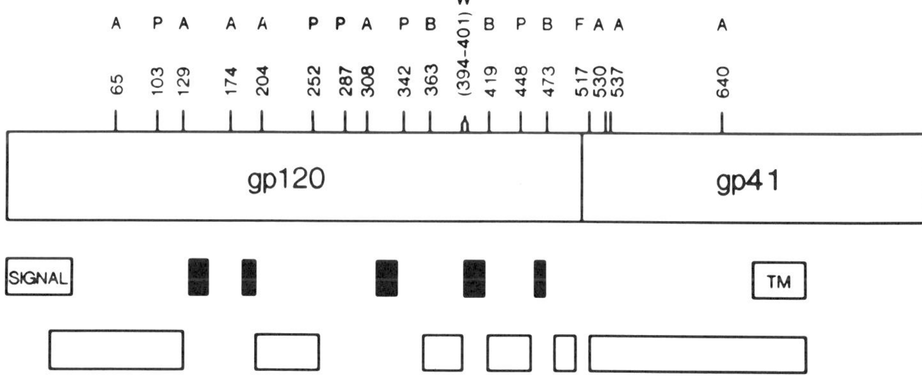

Figure 1 Phenotype of mutations in the HIV envelope. A linear diagram of the HIV envelope is shown, with the location of the signal sequences (SIGNAL) and membrane-spanning region (TM) labeled. The relatively conserved regions between HIV-1, HIV-2, and SIV are depicted by open boxes, while the variable regions are depicted as black boxes. At each of the designated positions, mutations consisting of four or five amino acid insertions were introduced. The phenotype of each mutation is shown (W = wild type, A - gp120–gp41 association, P = processing, B = gp120–CD4 binding, F = membrane fusion).

located near the carboxyl terminus of gp120. The three defined regions of conserved amino acids within the carboxyl terminus of the gp120 protein might comprise three faces of the CD4-binding pocket, brought into juxtaposition by the formation of disulfydryl bonds between two pairs of cysteine residues that are also shown to be conserved in this region. The three regions of the gp120 molecule defined by mutagenesis to be important for CD4 receptor binding contain relatively hydrophobic amino acids, while the more variable regions separating them contain more hydrophilic amino acids or sites for potential glycosylation. Thus, it is possible that the CD4-binding pocket is deeply recessed within the envelope glycoprotein and that the conserved regions important for receptor recognition are not readily available to the surface. By contrast, the hypervariable regions that flank the binding region may be exposed to the surface.

Other evidence supports the localization of the CD4 binding region to the 3' half of gp120. Several polyclonal and monoclonal antisera raised to peptides corresponding to gp120 sequences interfere with gp120 binding of CD4. Lasky and coworkers find that monoclonal antibodies that are raised to amino acid sequences corresponding to the middle of the three conserved regions defined by our mutagenesis also block CD4 binding (31). McDougal and coworkers find that antibodies to the carboxy terminal conserved regions of gp120 inhibit CD4 binding (McDougal, personal communication). Antisera to other oligopeptides corresponding in sequence to a hypervariable region of gp120 immediately amino terminal to the conserved regions defined in our studies were found to inhibit CD4 binding. Mutations in other regions of gp120 and gp41 were not found not to inhibit gp120-CD4 interaction, and antipeptide antibodies raised against the amino terminal half of gp120 do not inhibit CD4 binding (31,32).

MUTATIONS THAT AFFECT MEMBRANE FUSION

Mutations that affect membrane fusion are located in the extreme amino terminus of the gp41 protein. The amount and size of the envelope protein produced by these mutants is normal. The gp120 encoded by such mutants binds CD4 normally. However, the envelope mutants in this region are markedly attenuated in their ability to induce syncytia.

The region affected by these mutations is a hydrophobic region. The hydrophobic character of this region as well as its location immediately adjacent to a site of proteolytic cleavage is reminiscent of fusion domains of the paramyxoviruses and orthomyxoviruses (13).

Based on these results, we propose that the membrane fusion reaction is mediated by the hydrophobic amino terminus of gp41 and occurs when the virus and cellular membranes are brought into juxtaposition by the binding of gp120 to the CD4 receptor.

MEMBRANE ANCHORAGE

Mutations resulting in a loss of the HIV envelope glycoprotein from the cell surface affect a hydrophobic region of the gp41 located at the center of the protein. Deletion of the hydrophobic region or a change in the sequence of this region such that it specifies hydrophilic rather than hydrophobic amino acids results in quantitative release of the envelope glycoprotein from the cell into the supernatant.

Based on these results, it appears there is a *single* membrane anchorage sequence, and that this sequence is comprised of hydrophobic amino acids located near the center of the gp41 protein. Membrane anchorage of the HIV envelope is necessary for syncytium induction.

gp120-gp41 ASSOCIATION

Two classes of envelope mutations affected the association of the gp120 and gp41 envelope glycoproteins. These mutations were found to be located within the amino-terminal region of gp120 or the amino-terminal region of gp41. The amount and size of the envelope protein produced by these mutants were the same as those of the wild type. Moreover, the gp120 protein produced by these mutants was capable of binding to CD4. However, the gp120 produced by such mutants was not found to be associated with the surface of the transfected cells but rather was found to be located predominantly in the supernatant. No syncytia were induced by mutants of this phenotype, and such mutants were found to be defective for complementation of viruses defective for *env* gene function.

The simplest explanation for these observations is that the amino termini of the gp120 and gp41 proteins are in contact, and that the binding of gp120 to gp41 is specified by multiple noncovalent contacts. Analysis of envelope glycoprotein migration on reducing or nonreducing SDS-polyacrylamide gels indicates that no covalent disulfide bonds link the gp120 and gp41 glycoprotein (29,30). Alteration of these contacts or changes in the structure in these regions of the protein disrupts the gp120-gp41 association. Since the noncovalent association of gp120 and gp41 is dependent upon the structure of the amino-terminal halves of both gp120 and gp41, mutations in either of these regions leads to a similar phenotype.

These results also suggest that the regions of gp120 that specify CD4 binding are distinct from the regions that specify gp41 binding. Functionally, the gp120 protein appears to be comprised of at least *two independent domains*, the amino terminal domain which binds to the gp41 and the carboxy terminal domain that binds to CD4. Mutants in either one of these domains do not necessarily affect the function of the other domain.

PROTEOLYTIC CLEAVAGE OF THE ENVELOPE PRECURSOR

A series of mutations scattered throughout the gp120 coding sequences affect the processing of the protein precursor. The phenotype of such mutations is that normal amounts of envelope protein are produced but the product accumulates as a gp160 precursor. Gp120 and gp41 are not found in such cells. The surface labeling of cells transfected with envelope glycoprotein genes that contain such mutations demonstrate little or no envelope on the surface. We suggest that these mutants affect the folding of the gp160 protein and that proper folding is required both for proteolytic cleavage of the envelope precursor and for transport to the cell surface.

MUTANTS AT THE CARBOXYL TERMINUS OF THE gp41

The HIV gp41 protein is unusual among retroviral transmembrane proteins in the presence of approximately 150 amino acid residues carboxy terminal to the membrane-spanning region. Mutants in the carboxyl terminus of gp41 do not affect the ability of the transfected envelope glycoprotein gene to induce syncytia in CD4$^+$ cells in culture. However, mutants that delete substantial portions of the carboxyl terminus of gp41 are attenuated in their ability to support viral replication (19). We conclude that whereas the carboxy terminal region of the gp41 envelope glycoprotein is not required for the binding and fusion reactions, it is required for virion infectivity.

A MODEL FOR BINDING AND FUSION

These experiments permit us to construct a model for the functions of the HIV envelope involved in syncytium formation. Such a model is likely to be relevant to the processes of virus entry, cell-to-cell transmission, and single cell cytolysis as well. Following the translation, glycosylation, processing, and association of the gp120 and gp41 proteins, the envelope glycoproteins move to the cell surface or onto the virion. The initial step in the HIV envelope function is the recognition and high affinity binding of CD4 by the carboxy terminal region of gp120 (Figure 2). This reaction brings the two membranes—one bearing the integral membrane protein CD4 and the second bearing the gp120-gp41 complex—into close juxtaposition. The reaction depends upon the noncovalent association of the amino terminal region of gp120 with gp41 as well as upon the anchorage of gp41 to the membrane of the virus or infected cell. Upon juxtaposition of the membranes by this "molecular bridge," conformational changes resulting from gp120-CD4 interaction might allow the hydrophobic amino terminus of gp41 to interact with the membrane of the uninfected target cell.

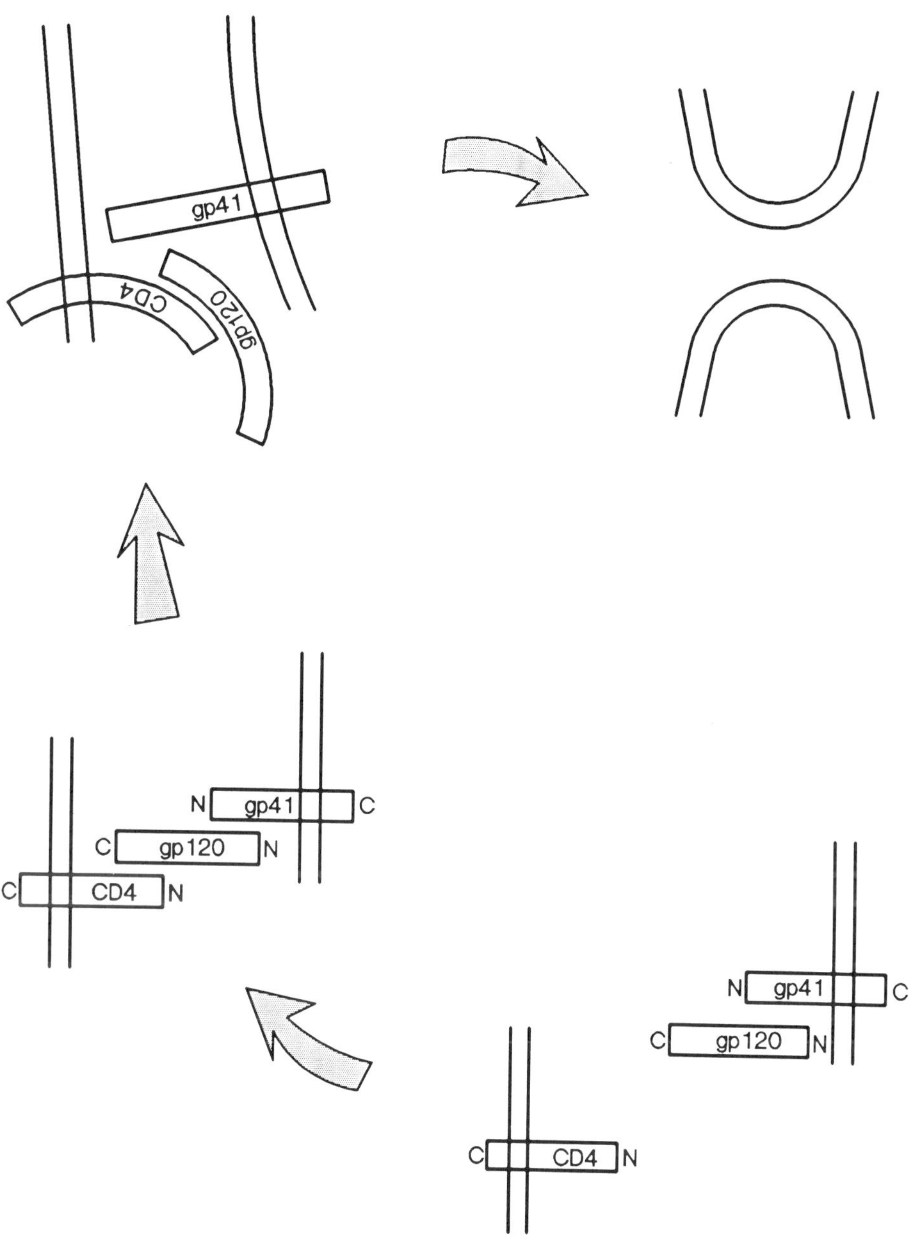

Figure 2 A functional model of the HIV envelope. The initial event in virus entry or cell membrane fusion is the binding of gp120, via carboxy-terminal sequences, to the CD4 receptor (N = amino terminus, C = carboxyl terminus). The amino-terminal half of gp120 is involved in a noncovalent association with the exterior amino-terminal half of the gp41 transmembrane protein. Following binding of gp120 to the CD4 receptor, conformational changes might allow the hydrophobic fusion region located at the amino terminus of gp41 to insert into the target cell membrane. Finally, the gp41 glycoprotein mediates the fusion of the two apposed membranes to allow either virus entry or cell membrane fusion.

Insertion of the hydrophobic amino terminus of gp41 into the apposed membrane disrupts the membrane of the uninfected cell and leads to a membrane-to-membrane fusion event. Similar models have been proposed for the envelope glycoproteins of the ortho- and paramyxoviruses (13).

THE NEUTRALIZATION PARADOX RESOLVED

How might this model for the envelope glycoprotein resolve the paradox that the high titer immune response to the envelope glycoprotein in infected people inhibits the function of the envelope only weakly?

Individuals infected with HIV-1 raise a humoral immune response that recognizes both conformation-dependent and linear determinants on the HIV envelope glycoproteins. One of the immunodominant epitopes on the gp120 glycoprotein is conformation dependent since it is not recognized once the gp120 protein is reduced and denatured (T. H. Lee, personal communication). The majority of the conformation-dependent reactivity to the gp120 glycoprotein is ineffectual at inhibiting the binding of gp120 to CD4; however, a fraction of this conformation-dependent antibody is capable of a group-specific inhibition of gp120–CD4 binding. This conclusion follows from the observation that all infected individuals examined generate a weak group-specific anti-gp120 binding response, despite the inability of some of these patient sera to recognize denatured gp120 on Western blots (Kowalski, Lee, and Sodroski, unpublished data). These latter patient sera contain relatively high titers of antibodies that recognize the native gp120 glycoprotein, either by radioimmunoprecipitation or by nondenaturing Western blotting. Thus, only a small fraction of the total conformation-dependent antibody response in infected individuals is directed at conserved regions of gp120 involved in receptor binding.

Experiments with fragments of unglycosylated peptides corresponding in sequence to the envelope protein demonstrate that most of the human antienvelope antibodies that recognize *linear* polypeptide determinants recognize two regions of the envelope protein (33,34). These two regions are highly conserved among all HIV-1 strains. One of these sequences is located at the extreme carboxyl terminus of gp120, and the second is located within the exterior portion of gp41. According to our proposed model of gp120–gp41 structure and function, the immunodominant region of gp41 is located at the interface between gp120 and gp41. We suggest that in the functional configuration of envelope, where gp120 and gp41 are associated, this region of gp41 is not accessible to antibodies. For that reason this subset of the humoral response does not inhibit virus infection or syncytium formation. However, this region of the gp41 may be exposed on the surface of virions or infected cells as about half of the gp120 is rapidly shed into the supernatant, leaving an excess of uncomplexed exposed gp41 on the surface of the virus and infected cell. This may account for the ability of human sera to recognize such cells in immunofluorescence reactions.

The extreme carboxyl terminus of gp120, which constitutes the second immunodominant *linear* envelope deterinant, is near one of the proposed CD4-binding regions. Antibodies to this region have been reported to weakly inhibit gp120-CD4 binding, perhaps because they recognize an outer edge of the binding region.

A second class of antibodies to gp120 is reported to neutralize HIV. These antibodies are directed against a hypervariable region that is located just amino terminal to the CD4 binding region (35). Antibodies to this region inhibit virus infectivity in a type-specific manner. Such antibodies do not inhibit the binding of gp120 to CD4 and therefore may inhibit postreceptor binding steps involved in virus entry. That gp120-gp41 interaction may be involved in these steps is suggested by the observation that a linker-insertion mutation in this region disrupts gp120–gp41 association (30). This region is presumably exposed at the surface of the envelope protein. The region is not required for receptor binding and therefore may vary among HIV isolates without affecting CD4 binding.

The fusion region of the gp41 envelope protein is highly hydrophobic and is probably exposed only for limited time periods during the fusion process. Antibodies to this region have not been demonstrated in sera from HIV-infected individuals.

IMPLICATIONS FOR VACCINE DEVELOPMENT

The natural response to HIV infection includes both humoral and cellular arms. Neutralizing antibodies, antibody-dependent cytotoxic responses, and generation of cytotoxic T cells all directed against the HIV gp120 exterior glycoprotein have been documented (27,33,36). These responses, in some cases, have been shown to be directed against regions of gp120 that are conserved among isolates from different geographic areas. Despite these immune responses, virus replication and CD4 lymphocyte depletion in most cases is not completely eliminated. Eventually, perhaps due to progressive weakening of the immune system by persistent virus infection and perhaps due to as yet unidentified factors, virus replication achieves high levels. The high level of p24 antigenemia and CD4 lymphocyte depletion that signals this high level of virus replication is a harbinger of imminent clinical deterioration (37,38). Thus, for the majority of infected individuals, the natural immune response appears to delay but not to prevent disease.

Other studies with chimpanzees indicate that humoral and cellular immune responses already in place prior to HIV exposure may not be capable of preventing initiation of infection (39 and Fischinger, Lasky, and Desrosiers, personal communication). These observations suggest that elicitation of immune responses either qualitatively or quantitatively better than those induced by natural HIV exposure must be achieved if protection against HIV infection is to be attained.

Is it reasonable to believe that protective immune responses against HIV infection can be achieved based on our analysis of the functional regions of the envelope glycoproteins? The present data allow for both optimistic and pessimistic replies to this question. On the positive side, the same regions of the HIV envelope important for cell-free virus entry appear to be critical for cell-to-cell transmission of the virus. With the exception of the gp41 carboxyl terminus, the same regions defined to be important for viral replicative processes are likely to be essential for syncytium formation, single cell killing and CD4-positive lymphocyte depletion. Thus, it would be reasonable to focus our efforts on several critical regions and their respective function: 1) the carboxy-terminal half of gp120 (CD4 binding), 2) the amino terminus of gp41 (membrane fusion), and 3) the amino terminal regions of gp120 and gp41 (gp120-gp41 association). These regions are well conserved among HIV-1 isolates and are conserved to a reasonable extent between HIV-1, HIV-2, and SIV. Thus, novel members of the family of CD4-tropic, immunodepletive retroviruses that the human population is likely to encounter in the near future may utilize common schemes for replication and pathogenesis.

On a more pessimistic note, the ability of the human immune system to raise a virogous humoral or cellular response to the regions of gp120 and gp41 important for function is presently unknown. Several potential problems can be envisioned. The CD4-binding region of gp120 is likely to be recessed, surrounded by glycosylated hypervariable regions that are functionally unimportant. The affinity of antibodies that recognize conserved regions within the CD4-binding pocket may be far less than the affinity of the CD4 receptor for gp120, thus making long-term blockade of infection or membrane fusion events unlikely. The hydrophobicity of the gp41 fusion domain will make elicitation of antibodies to this region difficult, and lessens the likelihood that such antibodies will have access to the region at the appropriate point in virus entry or cell membrane fusion.The sequences that specify the interaction of gp120 and gp41 are juxtaposed when the envelope is in a functional configuration and thus may not be accessible to antibody at the desired times. Recent evidence, however, indicates that some sequences in the amino-terminal half of gp120 not recognized by patient antisera can elicit neutralizing antibodies in animals (32). The carboxyl terminus of gp41 may be located on the inner surface of the viral or infected cell membrane and not be available to antibody recognition for that reason.

In summary, the same features of the envelope glycoproteins that mask important functional regions from the natural immune response following HIV infection render elicitation of the desired responses a formidable task.

ACKNOWLEDGMENTS

We thank Drs. Robert Gallo, Flossie Wong-Staal, Peter Nara, Peter Fischinger, Mary Fran McLane, Myron Essex, and Tun Hou Lee for gifts of reagents and plasmids. We acknowledge the assistance of Joseph Potz, Ladan Basiripour, Tatyana Dorfman, Ernest Terwilliger, Wei Chun Goh, and Andrew Dayton in this work. Support for this work was received from the State of Massachusetts, the National Institutes of Health, the American Foundation for AIDS Research, the Leukemia Society of America, and the Department of the Army.

REFERENCES

1. Barre-Sinoussi F et al. Science 1983; 220:868.
2. Popovic M et al. Science 1984; 224:497–500.
3. Gallo RC et al. Science 1984; 224:500.
4. Allen JS et al. Science 1985; 228:1091.
5. Robey WG et al. Science 1985; 228:593.
6. Walker B et al. Proc Natl Acad Sci USA 1987; 84:8120.
7. Kozarsky K et al. J AIDS 1989; 2:163.
8. Dalgleish AG et al. Nature 1985; 312:763.
9. Klatzman DE et al. Nature 1985; 312:767.
10. McDougal JS et al. Science 1986; 231(4736):382-5.
11. Stein BS et al. Cell 1987; 49:659.
12. Maddon PJ et al. Cell 1986; 47(3):333–48.
13. White J, Kielian M, Helenius A. Q Rev Biophys 1983; 16(2):151.
14. De Rossi A et al. Proc Natl Acad Sci USA 1986; 83:4297.
15. Somsundarin M, Robinson HL. J Virol 1987; 61(10):3114-9.
16. Sodroski J et al. Nature 1986; 322(6078):470-4.
17. Lifson JD et al. Nature 1986; 323(6090):725-8.
18. Sodroski J et al. Science 1986; 231:1549.
19. Terwilliger E et al. J Virol 1986; 60:754-60.
20. Dayton A et al. Cell 1986; 44:941.
21. Fisher A et al. Science 1986; 233:655.
22. Fisher A et al. Science 1987; 237:888.
23. Strebel K et al. Nature 1987; 328:728.
24. Barin F et al. Science 1985; 228:1094.
25. Sarngadharan MG et al. Science 1984; 224:506.
26. Kitchen LW et al. Nature 2984; 312:367.
27. Weiss RA et al. Nature 1985; 316:69.
28. Schupbach J et al. Science 1984; 224:503.
29. McDougal JS et al. J Immunol 1986; 137(9):2937.
30. Kowalski M et al. Science 1987; 237:1351.
31. Lasky L et al. Cell 1987; 50:975.
32. Ho D et al. Science 1988; 239:1021.
33. Matthews T J et al. Proc Natl Acad Sci 1986; 83:9709.

                                    Sodroski et al.

34. Palker TJ et al. Proc Natl Acad Sci 1987; 84:2479.
35. Putney S et al. Science 1986; 234:1392.
36. Walker B et al. Nature 1987; 328:345.
37. Goudsmit J et al. J Inf Dis 1987; 156:558.
38. Goudsmit J et al. Lancet 1986; 2:177.

4

Conserved and Divergent Features of Human and Simian Immunodeficiency Viruses

Genoveffa Franchini and Flossie Wong-Staal
National Cancer Institute
National Institutes of Health
Bethesda, Maryland

INTRODUCTION

The discovery of the human T-cell leukemia virus (HTLV–I) as the etiologic agent of adult T-cell leukemia (ATL) has provided the impetus for investigation of retroviruses as possible etiologic agents of other human diseases (1). Within a decade, retroviruses have been shown to be etiologic agents of neurologic and immunologic disorders of man and subhuman primates (2–12). The human immunodeficiency virus type-1 (HIV-1) has been associated with the majority of acquired immunodeficiency syndrome (AIDS) cases worldwide, while the type-2 virus (HIV-2) is associated with infection prevalent in West Africa (6–7). Interesting parallels can be drawn between HTLV–I and HIVs (HIV-1 and HIV-2); among these are 1) a common major target cell ($CD4^+$ T-lymphocyte), 2) association with diseases of the immune system and central nervous system, 3) presence of highly related viruses that naturally infect Old World primates, and 4) common regulatory pathways for viral gene expression. The simian immunodeficiency virus (SIV_{mac}) has been isolated from captive rhesus macaques with clinical signs of immunodeficiency, as well as chronic degenerative brain disorders, resembling the manifestations of human AIDS. Experimental inoculation of SIV in macaques induces immunodeficiency at high frequency (11–12), providing an excellent animal model to study pathogenesis, prevention, and treatment of human AIDS. Although macaques in the wild are not known to be infected with SIV_{mac}, several other captive Old World monkey species (pig-tailed macaques, sooty mangabey, macaque nemestzina) appear to be naturally infected with viruses related to, but distinct from SIV$_{mac}$. SIV$_{mac}$ is quite divergent from the simian virus isolated from wild African green monkeys (SIV$_{agm}$) (13), but ironically is closely related to a second human immunodeficiency virus (HIV-2) (14-18). HIV-2 infection in humans appears to induce a lower morbidity rate than HIV-1 infection (19), although the biological behavior in vitro of different strains of HIV-2 and HIV-1 appear to be comparable (18). However, several HIV-2 isolates have been obtained from patients with AIDS (6,7) or immunodeficiency. HIV-1, HIV-2, and SIV share common biological features: 1) their host range appears to be restricted to cells expressing the CD4 antigen, which is probably an essential component of the virus receptor, and 2) they exert a cytopathic effect on some cell types, not necessarily the same for each virus, either by inducing fusion of the infected cells or by direct killing of the cells through an unknown mechanism. The biological similarity among these primate viruses suggests evolutionary conservation of their functionally active genes. We will try to summarize their genetic similarities and differences which could be relevant to their biological effects in vitro and in vivo, with particular references to the isolates analyzed in our own laboratory.

ACCESSORY GENES OF HUMAN AND MONKEY IMMUNODEFICIENCY VIRUSES

The HIV-1 genome has been extensively studied in the last few years and found to be far more complex than that of most known retroviruses (20). Several accessory genes, in addition to the structural genes for the core proteins (*gag*), the viral enzymes (*pol*), and the envelope proteins (*env*), have been identified either serologically or functionally. Several of these accessory genes are regulatory in function (Table 1). Sequential expression of the regulatory genes induces modulation of viral expression, which appears to be the key event in determining viral replication and latency. Two gene products (*tat* and *rev*) have been shown to directly modulate viral expression vira transcriptional (*tat*) and posttranscriptional (*tat* and *rev*) mechanisms. The *rev* gene in particular positively regulates the expression of structural proteins but negatively regulates the regulatory proteins including itself (21-23). In turn, the *nef* gene product is a negative regulator of viral expression (Ratner et al., personal communication).

The *vif* gene product is critical for the capability of the extracellular virus to propagate efficiently in target human cells in vitro (24-25). The *vpr* gene product has not been identified yet, and the gene appears to be nonessential for viral replication in vitro. *Vpu* (26) encodes a kD protein, and its expression, like *vpr*, is not required for viral replication since a replication-competent molecular clone of HIV-1 has a termination codon after the initiating AUG and efficiently produces virus in vitro.

Table 1 Regulatory Accessory Genes

New gene name	Previous name	Molecular weight of protein	Known function
HIV			
tat proteins	*tat*-3, TA	p14	transactivator of all viral
rev (transregulator of expression of virion proteins)	*art, trs*	p19	regulates expression of virion proteins
vif (virion infectivity protein)	*sor*, A, P′, Q	p23	determines virus infectivity
vpr (R)	R	?	unknown
nef (retrovirus inhibitory factor)	3′ *orf*, B, E′, F	p27	reduces virus expression, GTP-binding
vpx (X) (in HIV-2 and SIV)	X	p16 p14	unknown

In the HIV-2 and SIV genomes characterized thus far, we and others (14–18) could identify the equivalent open reading frames corresponding to most HIV-1 genes, but some differences could also be observed (Fig. 1). It is noteworthy that an additional gene (X) can be found in HIV-2, SIV_{mac}, and SIV_{agm} which does not have an obvious counterpart in HIV-1. This gene encodes for a 16 kD protein associated with mature HIV-2 virion (27–29). On the other hand, the *vpu* gene is apparently present only in HIV-1. The SIV_{agm} that has been characterized (13) appears to lack the *vpr* gene (Fig. 1), but it is not clear whether such a finding has any meaning for the biology of this virus.

The high degree of conservation in the amino acids sequence of the putative functional domains of these genes and the biological similarities among HIV-1/ SIV and HIV-1 can lead to the assumption that what we have learned about HIV-1 may apply to HIV-2 and SIV as well.

The overall amino acid similarity among the HIV-2s (rod, NIH–Z, SBL6669), the HIV-1s, SIV_{mac}, and SIV_{agm} regulatory proteins is not very high compared to the overall conservation of the amino acid sequence of the *gag* and *pol* protein genes. However, there are some structural features or short regions that are conserved. For example, the cysteine- and arginine-rich regions in the first exon of the *tat* gene and the arginine-rich region in the second exon of the *rev* gene are highly conserved among all these viral isolates.

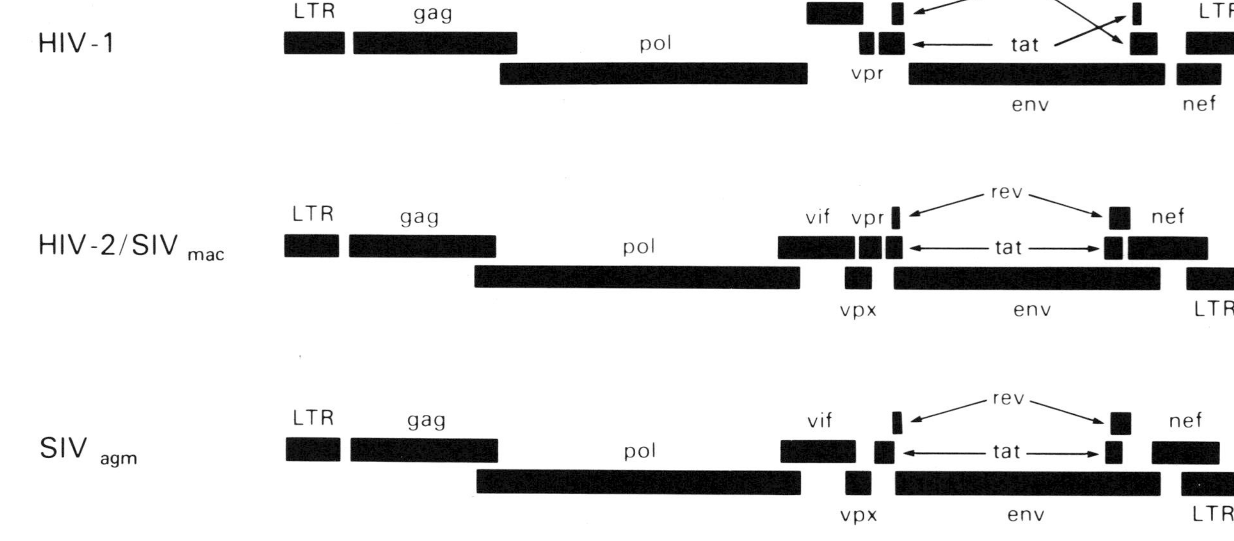

Figure 1 The proviral genome of HIV-1, HIV-2/SIV$_{mac}$, and SIV$_{agm}$. The bars represent, with the exception of the LTRs, open reading frames corresponding to the various genes. For the names and functions of the various genes, refer to Table 1.

MAPPING THE FUNCTIONAL SITES IN THE ENVELOPE GENES OF HIV AND SIV

The envelope gene of HIV-1, especially the region encoding the extracellular glycoprotein (gp120), has been shown to be the most variable among different isolates (30). Interstrain variations occur consistently in the same areas of the envelope gene. The same regions that vary in the envelope of HIV-1 are also poorly conserved among the HIV-2 and SIV isolates characterized. A highly immunogenic region of the HIV-1 envelope which elicits a type-specific immune response in the infected individuals (31,34) resides in one of these variable regions (V3) flanked by two cysteine residues (Fig. 2). A current hypothesis is that such an epitope could assume the form of a loop in the native envelope protein. In the middle of the putative loop is the amino acid sequence GlyProGly, which is identical in all the HIV-1 isolates sequenced so far, with the exception of HIV-1$_{eli}$, HIV1$_{z6}$, and HIV-1$_{jyl}$, in which the proline is substituted by a leucine (Fig. 2). Such a change leaves a nonpolar amino acid between the two glycines. In the HIV-2 isolates and both SIV$_{mac}$ and SIV$_{agm}$, the amino acid sequence of this epitope is also not conserved, but the two cysteines flanking this region are (Fig. 2). Interestingly, the GlyProGly motif is not retained in the HIV-2 and SIV, but analysis of the amino acid sequence of the HIV-2 putative loops suggest that their secondary structure could be very similar to the HIV-1 loops.

HIV-1, HIV-2, SIV$_{mac}$, and SIV$_{agm}$ bind to and infect cells bearing the CD4 molecule, which is thought to be their cellular receptor (35,36). A binding site of the viral envelope to the receptor has been identified in the extracellular portion of the envelope of HIV-1 (37). The binding region, also included between two cysteines, is conserved among the HIV-1 isolates and among HIV-2 isolates and SIVs (Fig. 3).

The existence of a region responsible for the induction of cell fusion was hypothesized based on the amino acid similarity at the amino terminus of the transmembrane portion of the envelope of HIV-1, HIV-2, SIV, and ortho- and paramyxoviruses (38) (Fig. 4).

Mutagenesis by insertion at the N-terminus of the transmembrane glycoprotein (gp41) of HIV-1 showed abolishment of the capability of HIV-1 to induce syncytia in CD4$^+$ cells (39). Point mutations in the putative fusogenic domain of SIV, expressed in a heterologous system, induced either increase or abolishment of syncytia in CD4$^+$ cells (40). These studies confirm the localization of a fusion domain of the N-terminus of gp41. Although the mechanism of T cells killing probably involves more than one pathway, one important in vitro parameter is syncytia formation. Accumulating evidence, in the study of the simian model for disease induced by SIV, indicates that syncytia formation occurs in vivo as well. Therefore, recombinant viruses with modified fusion domains may

```
HIV-1  HXB2   276   C T R P N N N · T R K R · · · I R I Q R G P G R A F V T I G K · · · · I G N M R Q A H C   329
       BRU    299   - - - - - - - - - - - S - - - - - - - - - - - - - - - - - - - - - - - - - - - - - -   330
       MN     299   - - - - - Y - - K - - - - - - - H - · - - - - - - - Y - T K N - - - I - - T I         329
       SC     277   - - - - - - - - T R S - - - - H - · - - - - - - Y A T - D - - - I - - D I - -          324
       SF2    297   - - - - - - - - - - S - - - - Y - · - - - - - - H - T - R - - - I - - D I - K          337
       NY5    289   - - - - - - - - K - G - - - - A - · - - - - - T L Y A R E - - - - I - - D I - - -       315
       CDC4   303   - - - - - - H - - - - - V T L · · · - · - - - - V W Y - T - E - - - I L - - I - - -      333
       WMJ2   291   - - - - Y - - - V - R S - - - L S - · - · - - - - - R - R · E - - I - - I I - - -       320
       RF     307   - - - - - - - - - - S - - - - T K - · - - - - V L Y A T - Q - - - I - - D I - K ·       337
       MAL    299   - - - - G - - - - - R G - - - H F · · - - - Q - L Y - T - · - - - I V - D I - R  Y       326
       ELI    295   - A - - Y Q - - - - Q - - - - T P - · · - L - Q S L Y - T R S R - S I - - - · · · -      324
       Z6     294   - - - - Y K - - - - Q S - - - T P - · · - L - Q - L Y - T R G R T K I - - · · - -        326
       Z3     291   - - - - G S D - K K I - - - - Q S - R I - - - K V - Y A K - G - - - I T - · · · - -      320
       Z321   295   - M - - - - - - - - - S - - - - S - · · - - - - - - F A T - D - - - I - - D I - - -      325
       JY1    307   - - - - D - K I - - Q S - - - T P - · · - L - Q - L Y - T R · - - - I K - D I - - - Y -   336


HIV-2  ROD    304   C K R P G N K I V K Q I M L M S G H V F H S H Y Q P · I N K R P R Q A W C   339
       NIHZ   294   - - - - - - - T - L P - T F - - - F K - - - · · - - V - - - K - - - - -       328
       SBL/ISY 296  - R - - E - - T - V P - T - - - - R R - - - - · · - K I - - - K - - - - -      330
SIV    MM142  313   - R - - - - - T - L P V T I - - A L - - - - - · · - - V · - E - - K - - - -    346
       K6W    312   - R - - - - - T - L P V T I - - - L - - - - - · · - - L · T D - - K - - - -    345
       AGM    —     - R - - - - - T - L P V T I - A - L - - - - - · · - K Y N M - L - - - - - -    —
```

Figure 2 Amino acid sequences of the hypervariable (V3) region of various HIV isolates (upper part) and HIV-2 and SIV (lower part). The amino acids are represented with the single letter code. The dashes represent identity, whereas dots indicate the lack of an amino acid in the specific viral sequence.

```
HIV-1  BRU    I T L P C R I K Q F I N M W Q E V G K A M Y A P P I S G Q I R C S S N I T G L L L T R D G G
       MN     - - - - - K - - - I - - - - - - - - - - - - - - - - - - E - - - - - - - - - - - - - - - - -
       SC     - - - - - - - - E I - - - - - - - - - - - - - - - - - - K - - V K - - - - - - - - - - - - -
       SF2    - I - - - - - - - I - - - - - - - - - - - - - - - - - - G - Q - S - - - - - - - - - - - - -
       CDC4   - - - - - - - - - I - - R - - V - - - - - - - - - - - - L - - K - L - - - - - - - - - - - -
       WMJ2   - - - - - - - - - I - - - G - - - - - - - - - - - - - - Q - - - - - - - - - - - - - - - - -
       RF     - - - - - - - - - I V - - - - - - - - - - - - - - - - - - - - K - I - - - - - - - - - - - -
       ELI    - - - Q - - - - - I - - - V A G · R - - I - - - - - - E R N - L - - - - - - - - - - - - - -
       MAL    - - - - - - - - - I - - - - - K T - - - - - - - - - - - - A - V - N - L - - - - - I - - - - -
       Z6     - - Q - - - - - - I - - - G - - - - - - - - - - - - - - E - - N - - - - - - - - - - - - - -
       Z3     - - - - - - - - - V V R T - - G - - Q - - - - - - - - - E - T - - - - - - - - - - - - - - - -
       Z321   - I - - - - - - - I V - - - - - R - - Q - - - - - - - - K - V - K - V - - - - - I - - - - V
       JY1    - K - - - - - - - I - - - - - G - - - - - - - - - - - - E - L - K - T - - - - - - - - - - -

HIV-2  ROD    N Y A P C H I K Q I I N T W H K V G R N V Y L P P R E G E L S C N S T V T S I I A N I D W Q
       NIHZ   - - - - - R - R - - - - - - - - R - - K - L - - - - - - - - - T - - - - - - - - - - - - A G
       SBL/ISY - - V - - - - E - - - - - - - - - - - K - - - - - - - - - - - - - - E - - - - - - - - - V D
SIV    K6W    - - V - - - - R - - - - - - - - - - - K - - - - - - - - - - - D - T - - - - - - L - - - - T
       MM142  - - V - - - - R - - - - - - - - - - - K - - - - - - - - - - - D - T - - - - - - L - - - N - T
       AGM    T - V A Y - - R S V - - D S Y T L S K K T - A - - - - - H - Q - R - - - - G M T V E L N Y N
```

Figure 3 Amino acid sequences of one of the putative envelope regions binding to the receptor CD4 molecule. Symbols as in Figure 2.

Cleavage Site
▼
HIV-1 HXB2   E K R A V G · I G A L F L G F L G A A G S T
           BRU   –
           MN   – – – – A · – – – – – – – – – – – – – – – – –
           SC   – – – – – – T – – – M – – – – – – – – – – –
           SF2   – – – – – – I V – – M – – – – – – – – – – –
           NY5
           CDC4   – – – – – – M L – – M – – – – – – – – – – –
           WMJ2   – – – – – – T – – – M – – – – – – – – – – –
           RF   – – – – – – T – – – M – – – – – – – – – – –
           MAL   – – – – I – – L – – M – – – – – – – – – – –
           ELI   – – – – I – – L – – M – – – – – – – – – – –
           Z6   – – – – I – – L – – M – – – – – – – – – – –
           Z3
           Z321   – – – – I – M · – – F – – – – – – – – – – –
           JY1   – – – – I – – L – – V – – – – – – – – – – –

Cleavage Site
▽
HIV-2 ROD   H T R G V F V L G · · F L G F L A T A G S A
           NIHZ   –
           SBL/ISY – K – – – L – – – – · · – – – – – T – – – A –
SIV   MM142   N K – – – – – – – · · – – – – – – – – –
           K6W   N K – – – – – – · · – – – – – – – – –
           AGM   Q K – V P – – – – · · – – – – – G A – – T –

Figure 4 Comparison of the amino-terminus region of the human and simian immunodeficiency virus transmembrane proteins. The triangle denotes the cleavage site in the envelope precursor protein gp160.

show increased or decreased virulence in vivo and would be valuable in developing animal models for studying pathogenesis by this group of viruses. Furthermore, the conservation of the amino acid sequence of the fusogenic domain make it a suitable candidate for the development of specific reagents that could not only elicit a protective immune response in at-risk individuals but also be potentially therapeutic in already infected individuals. In this regard, it is very encouraging that peptides obtained from this region elicit in the immunized animal neutralizing antibodies that appear to be group specific (D. Ho, personal communications).

SIV AND HIV-2 INFECTION OF RHESUS MACAQUE AS AN ANIMAL MODEL FOR VACCINE STUDIES

The restricted host range of HIV-1 has greatly limited animal studies that are crucial for vaccine development and evaluation. Other than man, HIV-1 appears to infect efficiently only chimpanzees (41,44) and gibbons (P. Markham, personnel communication), two great ape species that are very expensive and scarcely available for experimental studies. In contrast, the SIVs and HIV-2 readily infect the lower primates. SIV_{mac} and other related simian retroviruses (SIV_{mne} and SIV_{delta}) induce immunodeficiency in the infected animals with high efficiency (10,11). Since inoculation of monkeys with HIV-2 has been performed only recently, the available data are not enough to evaluate the in vivo pathogenicity of this virus in animals. Since the biological behavior, the genomic complexity and the target cell specificity of HIV-1 and HIV-2 strains are similar, in vivo studies with HIV-2 may shed some light on the host virus interaction as well as on the role of different genes in maintaining HIV-I infection in man.

Studies on the genetic variability of HIV-1 in a single infected human did not evaluate precisely the extent of variability within a single provirus since viral strains do contain intrastrain variants which prevail at different times during the infection. Infecting animals with a single viral genotype will provide more precise information in this regard and allow a better understanding of the biological meaning and the immunologic consequences of the rate of variability of viral RNA in vivo.

REFERENCES

1. Gallo RC. The first human retrovirus. Sci Am 1986; 255:88–98.
2. Gallo RC, Salahuddin SZ, Popovic M, Shearer GM, Kaplan M, Haynes BF, Palker TJ, Redfield R, Oleske J, Safai B, Whitte G, Foster P, Markham PD. Frequent detection and isolation of cytopathic retroviruses (HTLV–III) from patients with AIDS and at risk for AIDS. Science 1984; 224:550–553.

3. Popovic M, Sarngadharan MG, Read E, Gallo RC. Detection, isolation, and continuous production of cytopathic human T-lymphotropic retroviruses (HTLV–III) from patients with AIDS and pre-AIDS. Science 1984; 224: 497–500.

4. Barre-Sinoussi F, Chermann JC, Rey F, Nugeybe MT, Chamaret S, Gruest J, Dauguet C, Axler-Blin C, Brun-Vezinet F, Rouzioux C, Rozenbaum W, Montagnier L. Isolation of a T-lymphotropic retrovirus from a patient at risk for acquired immune deficiency syndrome (AIDS). Science 1983; 220: 868–870.

5. Gottlieb MS, Schroff R, Schanler HM, Weisman JD, Fan PT, Wold RA Saxon A. Pneumocystis carinii pneumonia and mucosal candidiasis in previously healthy homosexual men. Evidence of a new acquired cellular immunodeficiency. 1981; 305:1426–1431.

6. Clavel F, Guetard D, Brun-Vezinet F, Charmaret S, Rey MA, Santos-Ferreira MO, Laurent AG, Dauguet C, Katlama C, Rouzioux C, Klatzmann D, Champalimaud JL, Montagnier L. Isolation of a new human retrovirus from West African patients with AIDS. Science 1986; 223:343–3466.

7. Albert J, Bredberg U, Chiodi F, Bottiger B, Fenyo EM, Norrby E, Biberfeld G. A new pathogenic human retrovirus of West African origin (SBL-6669) and its relationship to HTLV–IV, LAV–II and HTLV–IIB. AIDS Res Hum Retroviruses 1987; 3:3–10.

8. Daniel MD, Letvin NL, King NW, Kannagi M, Sehgal PK, Hunt RD, Kanki PJ, Essex M, Desrosiers RC. Isolation of T-cell tropic HTLV–III-like retrovirus from macaques. Science 1985; 228:1201–1204.

9. Fultz PM, McClure HM, Anderson DC, Brent-Swenson R, Anand R, Srinivasan A. Isolation of a T-lymphotropic retrovirus from naturally infected sooty mangabey monkeys (Cerecebus atys). Proc Natl Acad Sci USA 1986; 83:5286–5290.

10. Murphey-Corb M, Martin LN, Rangan SRS, Bashin GB, Gormus BJ, Wolf RH, Andes WA, West M, Montelaro RC. Isolation of an HTLV–III-related retrovirus from macaques with simian AIDS and its possible origin in asymptomatic mangabeys. Nature 1986; 321:435–437.

11. Benveniste, R. E, Morton WR, Clark EA, Tsai C-C, Ochs HD, Ward JM, Kuller L, Knott WB, Hill RW, Gale MJ, Thouless ME. Inoculation of baboons and macaques with simian immunodeficiency virus/Mne, a primate lentivirus closely related to human immunodeficiency virus Type 2. J Virol 1988; 62:2091–101.

12. Letvin NL, Daniel MD, Sehgal PK, Derosiers RC, Hunt L, Waldrom LM, Mackey JJ, Schmidt DK, Chalifoux LV, King NW. Induction of AIDS-like disease in macaque monkeys with T-cell tropic retrovirus STLV–III. Science 1985; 230:71–73.

13. Fukasawa M, Miura T, Hasegawa A, Morikawa S, Tsujimoto H, Miki K, Kitamura T, Hayami M. Sequence of simian immunodeficiency virus from African green monkey, a new member of the HIV/SIV Group. Nature 1988; 333:457–4661.

14. Franchini G, Gallo RC, Gurgo C, Guo H-G, Collalti E, Fargnoli KA, Hall LF, Wong-Staal, F. Reitz MS Jr. Sequence of simian immunodeficiency virus and its relationship to the human immunodeficiency viruses. Nature 1987; 328:539–543.

15. Hirsh MS, Riedel M, Mullins J. The genome organization of STLV-3 is similar to that of the AIDS virus except for a truncated transmembrane protein. Cell 1987; 49:307–319.

16. Chakrabarti L, Guyader M, Alizon M, Daniel MD, Desrosiers RC, Tiollais P, Sonigo P. Sequence of simian immunodeficiency virus from macaque and its relationship to other human and simian retrovirus. Nature 1987; 328: 543–547.

17. Zagury JF, Franchini G, Reitz MS Jr, Collalti E, Starcich B, Hall L, Fargnoli KA, Jagodzinski L, Guo H-G, Laure F, Zagury JF, Arya SK, Josephs SF, Wong-Staal F, Gallo RC. The genetic variability between HIV-2 isolates is comparable to the variability among HIV-1. Proc Natl Acad Sci USA 1988; 85:5941–5945.

18. Franchini G, Fargnoli KA, Giombini F, Jagodzinsky L, De Rossi A, Bosch M, Biberfeld G, Fenyo EM, Alberts J, Gallo RC, Wong-Staal F. Molecular and biological characterization of a replication compentent human immunodeficiency type 2 (HIV-2) proviral clone. Proc Natl Acad Sci USA 1989; 86:2433–2437.

19. Marlink RG, Ricard D, M'Boup S, Kanki PJ, Romet-Lemonne J-L, N'Doye I, Diop K, Simpson MA, Greco F, Chou M-J, Degruttola V, Hsieh C-C, Boye C, Barin F, Denis F, McLane MF, Essex M. AIDS Res Hum Retroviruses 1988; 4:137–147.

20. Haseltine WA, Wong-Staal F. The molecular biology of the AIDS virus. Sci Am 1988; 259:52–62.

21. Feinberg MB, Jarrett RF, Aldovini A, Gallo RC, Wong-Staal F. HTLV–III expression and production involve complex regulation at the levels of splicing and translation of viral RNA. Cell 1986; 46:807–817.

22. Rosen CA, Terwilliger E, Dayton A, Sodroski JG, Haseltine WA. Intragenic cis-acting *art* gene-responsive sequences of the human immunodeficiency virus. Proc Natl Acad Sci USA 1988; 85:2071–2075.

23. Malim MH, Hauber J, Fenrick R, Cullen BR. Immunodeficiency virus *rev* *trans*-activator modulates the expression of the viral regulatory genes. Nature 1988; 335:181–183.

24. Fisher AG, Ensoli B, Ivanoff L, Chamberlain M, Petteway S, Ratner L, Gallo RC, Wong-Staal F. The *sor* gene of HIV-1 is required for efficient virus transmission in vitro. Science 1987; 237:886–893.

25. Strebel K, Daugherty D, Clouse K, Cohen D, Folks T, Martin M. The HIV "A" (*sor*) gene product is essential for virus infectivity. Nature 1987; 328: 728–730.

26. Cohen EA, Terwillinger EF, Sodroski JG, Haseltine WA. Identification of a protein encoded by the *vpu* gene of HIV-1. Nature 1988; 334:532–534.

27. Franchini G, Rusche JR, O'Keeffe TJ, Wong-Staal F. The human immunodeficiency virus type 2 (HIV-2) contains a novel gene encoding a 16kD protein associated with mature virions. AIDS Res Hum Retroviruses 1988; 4:243–250.

28. Henderson LE, Sowder RC, Copeland TD, Benveniste RE, Oroszlan S. Isolation and characterization of a novel protein (X-ORF product) from SIV and HIV-2. Science 1988; 241:199–202.

29. Kappes JC, Morrow CD, Lee S-W, Jameson BA, Kent SBH, Hood LE, Shaw GM, Hahn BH. Identification of a novel retroviral gene unique to human immunodeficiency virus type 2 and simian immunodeficiency virus SIV$_{mac}$. J Virol 1988; 62:3501–3505.

30. Starcich BR, Hahn BH, Shaw GM, McNeely PD, Modrow S, Wolf H, Parks ES, Parks WP, Josephs SF, Gallo RC, Wong-Staal F. Identification and characterization of conserved and variable regions in the envelope gene of HTLV-III/LAV, the retrovirus of AIDS. Cell 1986; 45:637–648.

31. Putney SD, Matthews JJ, Robey WG, Lynn DL, Robert-Guroff M, Mueller WT, Langlais AJ, Ghrayeb J, Petteway SR Jr., Weinhold KJ, Fischinger PJ Wong-Staal F, Gallo RC, Bolognesi D. HTLV-III/LAV—Neutralizing antibodies to an *E. coli*-produced fragment of the virus envelope. Science 1986; 234:1392–1395.

32. Goudsmit J, Debouck C, Meloen RH, Smit L, Bakker M, Asher DM, Wolff AV, Gibbs CJ Jr, Gajdusek DC. Human immunodeficiency virus type 1 neutralization epitope with conserved architecture elicits early type-specific antibodies in experimentally infected chimpanzees. Proc Natl Acad Sci USA 1988; 85:4478–4482.

33. Matsushita S, Robert-Guroff M, Rusche J, Koito A, Hattori T, Hoshino H, Javaherian K, Takatsuki K, Putney S. Characterization of a human immunodeficiency virus neutralizing monoclonal antibody and mapping of the neutralizing epitope. J Virol 1988; 62:2107–2114.

34. Ho DD, Sarngadharan MG, Hirsch MS, Schooley RT, Rota TR, Kennedy RC, Chanh TC, Sato VL. Human immunodeficiency virus neutralizing antibodies recognize several conserved domains on the envelope glycoproteins. J Virol 1987; 61:2024–2028.

35. Dalgleish A, Beverley P, Clapham P, Crawford D, Greaves M, Weiss R. The CD4 (T4) antigen is an essential component of the receptor for the AIDS retrovirus. Nature 1984; 312:763–766.

36. Klatzmann D, Champagne S, Gruest J, Guetard D, Hercend T, Gluckman JC, Montagnier L. T-lymphocyte T4 molecule behaves as the receptor for human retrovirus LAV. Nature 1984; 312:767–768.

37. Lasky LA, Nakamura G, Smith DH, Fennie C, Shimasaki C, Patzer E, Berman P, Gregory T, Capon DJ. Delineation of a region of the human immunodeficiency virus type 1 gp120 glycoprotein critical for interaction with the CD4 receptor. Cell 1987; 50:975–985.

38. Gallagher WR. Detection of fusion peptide sequence in the transmembrane protein of human immunodeficiency virus. Cell 1987; 50:327–328.

39. Kowalski M, Potz J, Basiripour L, Dorfman T, Goh WC, Terwilliger E, Dayton A, Rosen C, Haseltine W, Sodroski J. Functional regions of the envelope glycoprotein of human immunodeficiency virus type 1. Science 1987; 237:1351-1355.

40. Bosch M, Earl PC, Fargnoli K, Picciafuoco S, Giombini F, Wong-Staal F, Franchini G. Identification of the fusion peptide of primate immunodeficiency viruses. Science 1989; 244:694-697.

41. Alter JH, Eichberg JW, Masur H, Saxinger WC, Gallo R, Macher AM, Lane HC, Fauci AS. Transmission of HTLV-III infection from human plasma to chimpanzees: an animal model for AIDS. Science 1984; 226:549-552.

42. Francis DP, Feorino PM, Broderson JR, McClure HM, Getchell JP, McGrath CR, Swenson B, McDougal JS, Plamer EL, Harrison AK, Barre-Sinoussi F, Chermann J-C, Montagnier L, Curran JW, Cabradilla CD, Kalyanaraman VS. Infection of chimpanzees with lymphadenopathy-associated virus. Lancet 1984; 2:1276-1277.

43. Gajdusek DC, Gibbs CJ Jr, Rodgers-Johnson P, Amyx HL, Asher DM, Epstein LG, Sarin PS, Gallo RC, Maluish A, Arthur LO, Montagnier L, Mildvan D. Infection of chimpanzees by human T-lymphotropic retroviruses in brain and other tissues from AIDS patients. Lancet 1985; 2:55-56.

44. Nara PL, Robey WG, Arthur LO, Gonda MA, Asher DM, Yanagihara R, Gibbs CJ, Gajdusek DC, Fischinger PJ. Simultaneous isolation of simian foamy virus and HTLV-III/LAV from chimpanzee lymphocytes following HTLV-III or LAV inoculation. Arch Virol 1987; 93:183-184.

5

Genetic Variability in Human Immunodeficiency Viruses

Beatrice H. Hahn and George M. Shaw
University of Alabama at Birmingham
Birmingham, Alabama

INTRODUCTION

Genetic diversity is a hallmark of human and simian immunodeficiency viruses. This was first recognized when HIV-1-infected cell cultures were analyzed by Southern blot hybridization and found to exhibit considerable differences in restriction enzyme cleavage patterns (1-4). Subsequently, molecular cloning and sequence analysis demonstrated that every HIV-1 virus was unique and readily distinguishable from others varying in up to 10% overall nucleotide sequence (5). Genetic variation was also demonstrated among HIV-1 isolates obtained sequentially from the same individual over time (6), among HIV-1 viruses from donor-recipient transfusion cases (7), and among isolates from mother-child transmission pairs (S. Wolinsky, J. Sninsky, S. Kwok, studies in progress). Most recently, molecular cloning and mapping studies (8,9) as well as nucleotide sequence analysis of PCR amplified proviral fragments (10,36) have uncovered still another dimension of HIV variability: by demonstrating the coexistence of closely related, yet distinguishable genotypes within the same infected individual, these studies have identified HIV "isolates" as heterogeneous virus mixtures of unprecedented genetic complexity (8-10,36).

While most data on genetic variability thus far has been the result of studies involving HIV-1, the propensity for genetic change has also been confirmed for HIV-2 and SIV viruses. To date, complete and partial nucleotide sequence data are available for a number of HIV-2 viruses (11-14), as well as for several strains of SIV, including SIV_{mac} (15-18), SIV_{sm} (42) and SIV_{agm} 19,20). Analysis of these sequences revealed that SIV_{sm} and SIV_{mac} are approximately 85% similar to each other, that each is approximately 75% similar to HIV-2, and that clones of SIV obtained from wild-caught African green monkeys differ from SIV_{mac}, HIV-2, and HIV-1 by approximately 50% (19,20). Most recently, still another member of the SIV/HIV group has been identified in wild-caught mandrills (21). Molecular studies revealed cross-hybridization between SIV_{mnd} and all other HIV/SIV viral strains only under low stringency conditions (21). Thus, several nonhuman primate species in Africa appear to be naturally infected with evolutionarily quite different SIV strains.

While considerable progress has been made characterizing HIV/SIV viruses molecularly, many questions remain regarding the biological importance and clinical relevance of their genetic differences. In particular, it is presently unknown whether or not the generation of genotypic variants during persistent viral infection influences and/or determines the clinical outcome; whether genetic changes can result in the generation of highly pathogenic versus more attenuated HIV/SIV viruses; whether future treatment protocols need to take into consideration the existence and degree of genetic diversity within individual patients; and most importantly, whether genetic variation will render traditional approaches to vaccine development unsuccessful. In this paper, we will review current knowledge pertaining to HIV/SIV genetic variation. We will describe mechanisms by which this divergence is believed to be generated, and we will discuss some of the still unresolved questions of HIV/SIV genetic variability in the context of recent data and current research efforts designed to resolve them.

HIV ISOLATES ARE GENETICALLY HIGHLY POLYMORPHIC AND REPRESENT A RAPIDLY EVOLVING MIXTURE OF GENOTYPIC VARIANTS

One of the most significant findings regarding genetic variation of HIV was the recent discovery of coexisting genotypic variants within single "isolates" in vitro as well as individual patients in vivo (8-10,36). That isolates of HIV-1 are actually comprised of complex mixtures of closely related, yet distinguishable genotypes was first identified when three HIV-1 cultures established from two independent patients were molecularly "dissected" by lambda phage cloning (8). In contrast to previous studies, where generally only a handful of molecular clones were isolated and characterized, Saag and coworkers obtained a total of 62 full-length HIV-1 clones from three different genomic libraries and detail mapped each clone using 11 restriction endonucleases. Surprisingly, 17 of 27 clones representing the first isolate, 9 of 17 clones representing the second isolate, and 13 of 18 clones representing the third isolate were each distinguish-able and characterized by a unique set of restriction enzyme cleavage sites.

While the restriction pattern of the most prevalent clone corresponded to the restriction pattern of the primary isolate DNA, the existence of additional minor genotypes was not readily identifiable on the original blot and thus had previously gone unrecognized. Although clearly distinguishable by restriction enzyme site polymorphisms, the clones comprising each library were considerably more similar to each other than to other clones obtained from unrelated individuals. Two of the isolates were derived from PBMC cultures of the same individual cultured 16 months apart. As expected, the extent of genetic similarity between these two groups of viruses was greater as compared to unrelated viruses, however, none of the genotypic variants identified in the first culture was present in the later isolate. Taken together, these studies (8) as well as others (9) showed that a remarkably large number of related but distinguishable genotypic variants evolve in parallel and coexist during chronic infection, and that "isolates" of HIV-1, unless molecularly or biologically cloned, generally consist of complex mixtures of genotypically distinguishable viruses.

While Saag et al. used molecular cloning and restriction enzyme mapping to identify coexisting variants, other investigators took a different approach to molecularly characterize HIV-1 "isolates." Using the polymerase chain reaction (PCR) to amplify and subsequently sequence HIV-1 *gag* and *env* regions, Goodenow, Wain-Hobson, and colleagues analyzed seven different HIV-1 cultures for their genetic composition (10). The data obtained not only confirmed the concept of HIV isolates comprising mixtures of genotypic variants, but further extended this concept by demonstrating an unexpected genetic complexity, where no two viral sequences were found to be identical. Sequence analysis of up to 25 individual *env*- or *gag*-containing M13 clones per isolate revealed a predominant sequence within each isolate, but also the presence of additional variants that differed from this master sequence in point mutations, insertions, deletions, translational stop codons, as well as frame shift mutations. Interestingly, not every HIV-1 isolate revealed the same degree of complexity. The relative abundance of the master sequence ranged between 40% and 95%, whereas additional variants ranged in frequency between 4% and 30%. Certain cultures therefore appeared to comprise a rather homogeneous group of genotypic forms, while others seemed to harbor very divergent sets of genotypes. Finally, a surprisingly high number of variants were identified to be replication defective since they contained translational stop codons and/or frame shift mutations in critical viral genes. In view of such complexity, the authors proposed to redefine the term "virus isolate" as a collection of genomes isolated from a single seropositive individual (10).

Given this extent of diversity, the question arose whether in vitro cultivation per se selected certain viral forms over others, and thereby resulted in the isolation of only a fraction of the genotypic variants that were present in vivo.

To address this, several investigators began to utilize the powerful PCR technique to amplify HIV sequences directly from uncultured, infected PBMC, thereby circumventing potential selection pressures posed by in vitro cultivation. The data confirmed the coexistence of viral variants in vivo (36, Wolinsky and coworkers, studies in progress), however, the data also revealed that the viral genotypes present in cultured PBMC did not resemble the predominant viral genotypes present in uncultured PBMC from the same patient (36). Moreover, defective viral genomes were found in high frequency in all uncultured patient material studied.

Taken together, these results have significant theoretical and obvious practical implications relevant to AIDS pathogenesis and research. Most importantly, they define the biological phenotype of any given HIV isolate as the weighted sum of the biological properties of *all* existing variants within that isolate. Moreover, they point toward an enormous potential for rapid adaptation and functional alterations in response to in vivo or in vitro pressures, as has been observed for other RNA viruses (23). The presence of defective genomes in vitro and in vivo further complicates the picture. Although their biological function is presently unclear, they could play an important role in viral pathogenesis, as has been suggested for feline leukemia virus-induced immunodeficiency (24).

GENOTYPIC VARIATION IS, AT LEAST IN PART, THE RESULT OF ERRORS IN HIV REVERSE TRANSCRIPTION

Because retroviral replication is unique, genetic changes may evolve during one or all of several steps in the viral life cycle (25). These include: reverse transcription (RNA to DNA), proviral replication (DNA to DNA), and proviral transcription (DNA to RNA). While the host cell's replication machinery is responsible for proviral replication and transcription, the first step in HIV replication is performed by a virally encoded enzyme, the reverse transcriptase (RT). This enzyme polymerizes deoxyribonucleotides using viral RNA as a template and also acts as a DNA polymerase in converting the resulting minus strand DNA in double-stranded DNA (26,27). While the error rate of all retroviral reverse transcriptases is believed to be high, because of the lack of proofreading mechanisms (28,29), proviral replication is not believed to be very error prone (30) because replication is achieved by the more accurate host cell DNA polymerase a (31). Thus, two independent groups of investigators have recently focused on the HIV-1 reverse transcriptase as a potential source for genetic diversity (32,33).

Using a variety of experimental approaches, both groups concluded that the accuracy of the HIV-1 reverse transcriptase is exceptionally poor with estimated error rates for base pair substitutions ranging between 1 in 1700 and 1 in 4000 polymerized nucleotides (32,33). This was found to be true for RT isolated from virus particles as well as for prokaryotically expressed enzyme. Analysis of mutations generated by the HIV-1 reverse transcriptase in these assays revealed a similar spectrum of genetic alterations, including base substitutions, additions, and deletions, which had previously been seen in divergent proviruses (6,34). These studies also revealed that certain positions in the template sequence represented mutational hot spots with error rates as high as 1 in 70 polymerized nucleotides, demonstrating a nonrandom distribution of mutations within the target sequence (32). Overall, the HIV-1 reverse transcriptase was identified to be the least accurate polymerase described to date and to differ in fidelity from the avian myeloblastosis virus or murine leukemia virus reverse transcriptase by one order of magnitude (32).

Taken together, these data strongly suggest that the viral reverse transcriptase is, at least in part, responsible for the observed hypermutability of HIV viruses. Forward transcription (DNA to RNA), copy choice misreading of the viral RNA template, and recombination between different retroviral sequences are also theoretical possibilities (35), however, no experimental evidence demonstrating that these mechanisms actually contribute to HIV/SIV genetic diversity in a major way has been reported thus far.

MOLECULAR EVOLUTION OF HUMAN AND SIMIAN IMMUNODEFICIENCY VIRUSES

An understanding of the molecular evolution of human and simian AIDS viruses and the determination of their origins are of obvious importance. A detailed knowledge of their in vivo mutation rates would allow us to better follow these viruses' molecular epidemiology, their pattern of spread, and ultimately would enable us to better understand their pathogenic potential.

Clinically, AIDS was first recognized in the United States in 1981, a few years after the virus was introduced into the population, and blood samples collected in the United States and Europe before the mid-1970s generally lacked evidence of anti-HIV-1 antibodies. Serologic and clinical evidence suggests that HIV-1 infection began to spread epidemically in urban areas of Central Africa during the mid- and late 1970s, and in retrospect, cases of AIDS in African individuals from that period are now recognized (37–40). In contrast, the spread of HIV-1 in rural areas of Africa appears not to have changed substantially during the same time period. For example, there was a 10-fold increase in HIV-1 seroprevalence documented in pregnant women in an urban area of Zaire between 1970 and 1980, but the prevalence of HIV-1 antibodies in the rural area of the same country remain unchanged at 0.8% between 1976 and 1986 (41). These data provide evidence for HIV-1 having existed in Central Africa for a long time and for transmission rates of HIV-1 to be related to social and economic factors and the disruption of traditional lifestyles. Once introduced into populations where individuals were likely to have multiple sexual partners or to be exposed to blood products, the virus most likely spread rapidly and became clinically apparent.

Nucleic acid sequence analyses and comparisons of molecular clones of HIV-1 from Zaire, Haiti, Europe, and the United States have allowed the construction of phylogenetic trees for these viruses (5). This type of analysis is highly reliable and intelligibly reflects the geographical and temporal features of the respective viruses analyzed. For example, U.S. HIV-1 isolates cluster closer together than do African HIV-1 viruses. Viruses isolated more recently are phylogenetically more related than viruses from a single specimen obtained 20 years ago. Tree analysis also revealed that HIV-2 and SIV_{mac} viruses must have evolved from a common progenitor more recently than did this progenitor from HIV-1 (47).

While phylogenetic trees yield evolutionary distances, they do not provide information about the time required for this evolution to occur. In order to approach this question, mutation rates and estimated times of divergence have been calculated for HIV/SIV viral strains (43–46), however, these values have to be evaluated with appropriate caution. A major assumption in these calculations is mutation rate constancy. Since mutation is a function of viral replication, this means that the replication rates in HIV and SIV viruses are assumed to be constant over time. There is presently no experimental evidence indicating whether or not this is the case. Moreover, it is not known whether HIV-2 and SIV viruses replicate to the same extent in vivo or in vitro as does HIV-1. Thus, if the replicative and mutational processes were found not to be linear, all tree analyses published to date would not be satisfactorily calibrated with time, although the branching order would remain valid.

An alternative way to estimate mutation rates in HIV/SIV viruses is to calculate the number of base pair substitutions per replication cycle. Using an avian retroviral vector (spleen necrosis virus), Dougherty and Temin determined that the mutation rate for a single base pair substitution per replication cycle was 2×10^{-5} per base pair per cycle (48). Utilizing misincorporation data from in vitro studies involving the HIV-1 reverse transcriptase, Roberts and colleagues estimated 5–10 substitutions per HIV-1 genome per replication cycle (32), while Goodenow and Wain-Hobson estimated more than one mutation per genome per round of replication (10). These values for HIV-1 appear to be greater than mutation rates of certain other retroviruses (48). Obviously, more information on the extact mechanisms of HIV/SIV replication in vivo is required before the number of mutations per cycle can be used to accurately calculate times of divergence for HIV and SIV viruses.

BIOLOGICAL SIGNIFICANCE OF HIV/SIV GENETIC VARIATION

One of the most important questions, of course, is whether the extensive genetic variability seen in HIV/SIV viruses is of pathophysiologic and clinical relevance, and whether it represents a prerequisite for viral persistence in vivo. If the latter was true, one would have to assume that the produced variability is designed to allow the virus to evade host defense mechanisms. It is presently unknown whether truly potent and protective defense mechanisms actually exist in vivo. Neutralizing antibodies, present in most seropositive individuals, are generally of low titer and apparently not sufficient to rid the body of HIV infection (49-52). On the other hand, neutralizing antibodies of high titer and specificity can be produced in laboratory animals (53), and a major neutralizing epitope has been identified in the envelope glycoprotein of HIV-1 (54,55). Thus, it is conceivable that type-specific and protective neutralizing antibodies are being produced in vivo, but that novel virus populations with altered antigenicity are constantly generated during infection which can no longer be successfully eliminated by these antibodies. All neutralization studies described to date have either used cell cultures of uncloned virus (which as we now know are comprised of genotypic mixtures), or molecularly derived virus strains in combination with sera from unrelated patients. Interestingly, in the latter study even minor amino acid sequence differences resulted in dramatic differences of neutralizability (56). Moreover, virus cultivation in the presence of neutralizing sera resulted in the rapid generation of a neutralization-resistant variant with genetic alterations in the viral envelope gene (57). Thus, patient sera could contain neutralizing antibodies which are protective against certain viral strains. The other alternative is that neutralizing antibodies are generally not protective, possibly because of low affinity toward the envelope glycoprotein, but are able to cause enough selective pressure to significantly alter the genetic composition of the virus populations in vivo.

Like neutralizing antibodies, cellular immunity seems to be highly sequence specific (58). In a recent paper which analyzed primary T-cell responses to HIV-1, it was found that the interaction of gp120 epitopes with T-cell receptors and MHC molecules is precise and poorly cross-reactive. Even one conservative amino acid substitution drastically reduced T-cell recognition (58). It was suggested that naturally occurring sequence variation could markedly affect recognition by T-cell clones and result in a decrease or complete loss of responsiveness to the evolving variants. Moreover, it was proposed that even minor degrees of sequence variation may be sufficient to allow the virus to evade an ongoing T-cell response via the selection of variants with amino acid changes in T-cell epitopes (58). Again, it is presently unknown whether T-cell immunity against

HIV/SIV viruses is truly protective, or whether it only contributes to the selection of variants without having a major impact on the potency of the host's immune defense.

The net frequency of variation that we observe in HIV/SIV virus populations must be a function of both the viral mutation rates and the host's in vivo selective forces. While immunologic pressures might comprise one form of the selection force, other parameters could also greatly influence the selection of viral variants in vivo. These include mutations that affect the replication rate, the ability to spread cell-free or cell-to-cell, the tropism for certain cell types, as well as the ability to establish latency. Mutations in virtually every gene product or combination of gene products could alter the biological phenotype and, possibly, the pathophysiologic potential of HIV/SIV viruses in vivo. In addition, the number of genetic variants at any one point in time might critically influence the virus's flexibility to respond in a timely fashion to changing in vivo pressures.

There is some experimental evidence suggesting that genetic variability could be responsible for differences in disease manifestation. Recent data by Koanagi and Chen indicate the genetic variation in vivo may result in altered cell tropism (59). These investigators showed that two viruses isolated from brain and cerebral spinal fluid from the same patient could both replicate in PBL, but only virus from the brain could efficiently infect macrophage/monocytes (59). Similarly, Popovic and colleagues reported that not every HIV-1 isolate is able to infect macrophage/monocytes (60). Since there is increasing evidence that these cells are primarily responsible for the persistence of the virus in the brain, genomic variability could play a role in determining which strains of HIV are able to induce brain infection (60). In still another study, sequential isolates of HIV-1 were obtained from four individuals at different time points during their infection (61). The development of the disease in these individuals appeared to correlate with the emergence of HIV-1 variants that were more cytopathic in vitro. These newly emerged viruses were reported to replicate more efficiently and to higher titers in a wider variety of different human cells (61). In light of the genetic complexity of viral isolates (8–10), it will be important to determine whether cultures obtained later in disease actually comprise a greater number of genetically distinct variants with a broader spectrum of biological properties. If this was the case, the emergence of "more cytopathic variants" (61–63) late in infection could be the result of a greater number of variants rather than the de novo generation of particular cytopathic forms.

Biological diversity has also been observed among isolates of HIV-2. Although HIV-2 can cause fatal immunodeficiency (64,65), epidemiologic studies suggested that many West African individuals infected with HIV-2 may develop less severe immunodeficiency than individuals infected with HIV-1 (66). Interestingly, virus isolation studies done independently by two groups of investigators resulted in the identification of strains of HIV-2 which do not cause cell death or induce fusion with CD4-bearing T cells in vitro (67,68). The molecular basis for the attenuated virulence of these viruses is not yet known. Differences in envelope properties which affect viral spread, differences in envelope/CD4 interactions, or mutation which affect their ability to replicate might be responsible. More important, it is not known whether these viruses have attenuated virulence in vivo. Long-term follow-up studies on the individuals from whom these viruses were isolated are necessary to address this question. Nevertheless, the possibility that genetic changes could render HIV/SIV viruses less pathogenic is intriguing and will have to be investigated further.

FUTURE DIRECTIONS

Variation of HIV parallels that of other lentiviruses, including equine infectious anemia virus (EIAV) and visna virus (69–71). For EIAV it is clear that genotypic changes are responsible for biologically important alterations in viral antigenicity which allow the virus to evade host immune defenses (69,72). For visna, the significance of antigenic variation is less clear (71). In the SIV system, a virus strain was recently isolated from a pig-tailed macaque that possesses altered biological and antigenic properties leading to a broader host range and a rapid, fatal immunodeficiency syndrome several days after inoculation (73). As outlined above, there are indications that genotypic varriants of HIV-1 and HIV-2 might be similarly associated with potentially important biological differences.

The exact pathophysiologic processes of HIV/SIV infection that ultimately lead to immunodeficiency and death have still to be determined. The impact of genetic variability on these processes is similarly unclear, yet has considerable practical implications: If a rapid evolution of divergent genomes does, in fact, contribute to viral pathogenicity in a major way, one might consider a therapeutic strategy which controls viral replication early in infection. If genotypic strains exist which differ dramatically in their pathogenic potential, molecular determinants of cytopathicity should be evaluated. If certain individuals are infected with more attenuated HIV viruses, their disease prognosis and resulting therapy might differ from individuals infected with a more cytopathic strain. Finally, if variability allows the virus to outrun host immune responses, traditional vaccination efforts might not be successful.

While a combination of different experimental approaches will be required to begin to address these issues, one technique will be particularly useful for these studies (22). This technique utilizes the polymerase chain reaction (PCR) to amplify and subsequently analyze the genomes of HIV and SIV viruses directly, without culture or molecular cloning. It is expected that PCR will eventually allow investigators to routinely amplify up to 5000 or more base pairs. PCR can be used to evaluate infection, to compare cultured and uncultured virus populations, to determine predominant viral forms in different tissues (brain, lymphoid tissue, etc.), and to closely monitor the generation of new variants during the course of infection. PCR-amplified sequences can also be tested biologically by inserting them back into transfection competent proviruses.

In summary, much has been learned about the nature and extent of genetic and biological diversity of HIV/SIV viruses since their identification as the etiologic agents of immunodeficiency. The impact of this diversity on the host's immune response must be understood. Such knowledge is critically needed to devise more rational strategies for vaccination, to develop better approaches to therapy, and to ultimately understand viral pathogenesis.

ACKNOWLEDGMENTS

We thank Drs. M. Goodenow, S. Wain-Hobson, and S. Wolinsky for providing PCR sequence data prior to publication, Dr. G. Myers for valuable discussions and suggestions, and Miss Jan Nicholson for preparation of the manuscript. This work was supported in part by grants from the NIH, the U.S. Army Medical Research Acquisition Activity, and the Life and Health Insurance Medical Research Fund. B.H.H. is a Special Fellow of the Leukemia Socity of America, and G.M.S. is a Pew Scholar in the Biomedical Sciences.

REFERENCES

1. Hahn BH, Shaw GM, Arya SK, Popovic M, Gallo RC, Wong-Staal F. Molecular cloning and characterization of the HTLV-III virus associated with AIDS. Nature 1984; 312:166–9.
2. Shaw GM, Hahn BH, Arya SK, Groopman JE, Gallo RC, Wong-Staal F. Molecular characterization of human T-cell leukemia (lymphotropic) virus type III in the acquired immune deficiency syndrome. Science 1984; 226: 1165–71.
3. Wong-Staal F, Shaw GM, Hahn BH, Salahuddin SZ, Popovic M, Markham PD, Redfield R, Gallo RC. Genomic diversity of human lymphotropic virus type III (HTLV–III). Science 1985; 229:759–62.
4. Benn S, Rutledge R, Folks T, Gold J, Baker L, McCormick J, Feorino P, Piot P, Quinn T, Martin M. Genomic heterogeneity of AIDS retroviral isolates from North America and Zaire. Science 1985; 230:949–51.
5. Myers G, Rabson AB, Josephs SF, Smith TF, Wong-Staal F, Berzofsky JA. Human retroviruses and AIDS, a compilation and analysis of nucleic acid and amino acid sequences. In Human Retroviruses and AIDS, 1989. Los Alamos National Laboratory, Los Alamos, NM.
6. Hahn BH, Shaw GM, Taylor ME, Redfield RR, Markham PD, Salahuddin SZ, Wong-Staal F, Gallo RC, Parks ES, Parks WP. Genetic variation in

HTLV–III/LAV over time in patients with AIDS or at risk for AIDS. Science 1986; 232:1548–53.

7. Srinivasan A, York D, Raganathan P, Ferguson R, Butler D Jr, Feorino P, Kalyanaraman V, Jaffe H, Curran J, Anand R. Transfusion-associated AIDS: Donor-recipient human immunodeficiency virus exhibits genetic heterogeneity. Blood 1987; 99:1766–70.

8. Saag MS, Hahn BH, Gibbons J, Li Y, Parks ES, Parks WP, Shaw GM. Extensive variation of human immunodeficiency virus type-1 in vivo. Nature 1988; 334:440–4.

9. Sakai K, Dewhurst S, Ma X, Volski DJ. Differences in cytopathogenicity and host cell range among infectious molecular clones of human immunodeficiency virus Type 1 simultaneously isolated from an individual. J Virol 1988; 62:4078–85.

10. Goodenow M, Huet T, Saurin W, Kwok S, Sninsky J, Wain-Hobson S. HIV-1 isolates are rapidly evolving quasispecies: Evidence for viral mixtures and preferred nucleotide substitutions, JAIDS 1989; 2:344–52.

11. Franchini G, Fargnoli KA, Giombini F, Jagodzinsky L, De Rossi A, Bosch M, Biberfeld G, Fenyo EM, Albert J, Gallo RC, Wong-Staal F. Molecular and biological characterization of a replication competent human immunodeficiency type-2 (HIV-2) proviral clone. Proc Natl Acad Sci USA 1989; 86:2433–7.

12. Zagury JF, Franchini G, Reitz M, Collalti E, Starcich B, Hall L, Fargnoli K, Jagodzinski L, Guo H-G, Laure F, Arya SK, Josephs S, Zagury D, Wong-Staal F, Gallo RC. Genetic variability between isolates of human immunodeficiency virus type 2. is comparable to the variability among HIV type 1. Proc Natl Acad Sci USA 1988; 85:5941–5.

13. Guyader M, Emerman M, Sonigo P, Clavel F, Montagnier L, Alizon M. Genome organization and transactivation of the human immunodeficiency virus type 2. Nature 1987; 326:662–9.

14. Kumar P, Hui H, Kappes JC, Parkin JS, et al. Molecular characterization and complete nucleotide sequence analysis of an attenuated isolate of HIV-2. J Virol (in press).

15. Chakrabarti L, Guyader M, Alizon M, Daniel MD, Desrosiers RC, Tiollais P, Sonigo P. Sequence of simian immunodeficiency virus from macaque and its relationship to other human and simian retroviruses. Nature 1987; 328: 543–7.

16. Hirsch V, Riedel N, Mullins J. The genome organization of STLV-3 is similar to that of the AIDS virus except for a truncated transmembrane protein. Cell 1987; 49:307–19.

17. Franchini G, Gurgo C, Guo HG, Gallo RC, Collalti E, Fargnoli KA, Hall LF, Wong-Staal F, Reitz MS Jr. Sequence of simian immunodeficiency virus and its relationship to the human immunodeficiency viruses. Nature 1987; 328: 539–43.

18. Hahn BH, Kong LI, Lee S-W, Kumar P, Taylor ME, Arya SK, Shaw GM. Relation of HTLV-4 to simian and human immunodeficiency-associated viruses. Nature 1987; 330:184–6.

19. Fukasawa M, Miura T, Hasegawa A, Morkawa S, Tsujimoto H, Miki K, Kitamura T, Hayami M. Sequence of simian immunodeficiency virus from African green monkey, a new member of the HIV/SIV group. Nature 1988; 333:457–61.

20. Daniel MD, Li Y, Naidu YM, Durda PJ, Schmidt DK, Troup CD, Silva DP, Mackey JJ, Kestler HW III, Sehgal PK, King MS, Ohta Y, Hayami M, Desrosiers RC. Simian immunodeficiency virus from African green monkeys. J Virol 1988; 62:4123–8.

21. Tsujimoto H, Cooper RW, Toshiaki K, Masashi F, Tomoyuki M, Ohta Y, Ishikawa K-I, Nakai M, Frost E, Roelants GE, Roffi J, Hayami M.Isolation and characterization of simian immunodeficiency virus from mandrills in Africa and its relationship to other human and simian immunodeficiency viruses. J Virol 1988; 62:4044–50.

22. Kwok SD, Mack H, Mullis KB, Poiesz B, Ehrlich G, Blair D, Friedman-Kien A, Sninsky JJ. Identification of human immunodeficiency virus sequences by using in vitro enzymatic amplification and oligomer cleavage detection. J Virol 1987; 61:1690–4.

23. Domingo E, Martinez-Salas E, Sobrino F, de la Torre JC, Portela A, Ortin J, Lopez-Galindez C, Perez-Brena P, Villanueva N, Najera R, VandePol S, Steinhauer D, DePolo N, Holland J. The quasispecies (extremely heterogeneous) nature of viral RNA genome populations: biological relevance—a review. Gene 1985; 40:1–8.

24. Overbaugh J, Donahue PR, Quackenbush SL, Hoover EA, Mullins JI. Molecular cloning of a feline leukemia virus that induces fatal immunodeficiency disease in cats. Science 1988; 239:906–10.

25. Weiss R, Teich N, Varmus H, Coffin J, Eds. RNA Tumor Viruses, Supplements and Appendixes 1985; 2:75–134.

26. Verma IM. Reverse transcriptase. Enzymes 1981; 14:87–103.

27. Hoffman AD, Banapour B, Levy JA. Characterization of the AIDS-associated retrovirus reverse transcriptase and optimal conditions for its detection in virions. Virology, 1985; 147:326–35.

28. Steinheuer DA, Holland JJ. Rapid evolution of RNA viruses. Ann Rev Microbiol 1987; 41:409–17.

29. Temin HM. Evolution of cancer genes as a mutation-driven process. Cancer Res 1988; 48:1697–1701.

30. Jolly DJ, Willis RC, Friedmann T. Variable stability of a selectable provirus after retroviral vector gene transfer into human cells. Mol Cell Biol 1986; 6: 1141–7.

31. Reyland ME, Loeb LA. On the fidelity of DNA replication: Isolation of high fidelity DNA polymerase-primase complexes by immunoaffinity chromatography. J Biol Chem 1987; 262:10824–30.

32. Roberts JD, Bebenek K, Kunkel TA. The accuracy of reverse transcriptase from HIV-1. Science, 242:1171–3.

33. Preston BD, Poiesz BJ, Loeb LA. Fidelity of HIV-1 reverse transcriptase. Science 1988; 242:1168–71.

34. Starcich BR, Hahn BH, Shaw GM, McNeely PD, Modrow S, Wolf H, Parks ES, Parks WP, Josephs SF, Gallo RC, Wong-Staal F. Identification and characterization of conserved and variable regions in the envelope gene of HTLV-III/LAV, the retrovirus of AIDS. Cell 1986; 45:637-48.
35. Coffin JM. Genetic variation in AIDS viruses. Cell 1986; 46:1-4.
36. Meyerhans A, Cheynier R, Albert J, Seth M, Kwok S, Sninsky J, Morfeldt-Manson L, Asjö B, Wain-Hobson S. Temporal fluctuations in HIV quasi-species in vivo are not reflected by sequential HIV isolations. Cell 1989; 58:901-10.
37. Piot P, Plummer LFA, Mhalu FS, Lamboray JL, Chin J, Mann JM. AIDS: an international perspective. Science 1988; 239:573-9.
38. Quinn TC, Mann JM, Curran JW, Piot P. AIDS in Africa: an epidemiologic paradigm. Science 1986; 234:955-63.
39. Bygbjerg C. Aids in Danish surgeon (Zaire, 1976). Lancet 1983; 1:925.
40. Vandepitte J, Verwilghen R, Zachee P. AIDS and cryptococcosis (Zaire, 1977). Lancet 1983; 1:925-6.
41. Nzilambi N, Decock KM, Forthal DN, Francis H, Ryder RW, Malebe I, Getchell J, Laga M, Piot P, McCormick JB. The prevalence of infection with HIV over a 10-year period in rural Zaire. N Engl J Med 1988; 318:276-9.
42. Hirsch VM, Olmsted RA, Murphey-Corb M, Purcell RH, Johnson PR. An African primate lentivirus (SIV_{sm}) closely related to HIV-2. Nature 1989; 339:389-92.
43. Smith TF, Srinivasan A, Schochetman G, Marcus M, Myers G. The phylogenetic history of immunodeficiency viruses. Nature 1988; 333:573-5.
44. Li W-H, Tanimura M, Sharp PM. Rates and dates of divergence between AIDS virus nucleotide sequences. Mol Biol Evol 1988; 5(4):313-30.
45. Sharp PM, Li W-H. Understanding the origins of AIDS viruses. Nature 1988; 336:315-6.
46. Yokoyama S, Chung L, Gojobori T. Molecular evolution of the human immunodeficiency and related viruses. Mol Biol Evol 1988; 5(3):237-51.
47. Smith TF, Marcus M, Myers G. Phylogenetic analysis of HIV-1 and HIV-2. In: Ginsberg H, ed. Vaccines 88. Cold Spring Harbor NY: Cold Spring Harbor Laboratory, 1988;317-21.
48. Dougherty JP, Temin HM. Determination of the rate of base-pair substitution and insertion mutations in retrovirus replication. J Virol 1988; 62:2817-22.
49. Weiss RA, Clapham PR, Cheingsong-Popov R, Dalgleish AG, Carne CA, Weller IVD, Tedder RS. Neutralization of human T-lymphotropic virus type III by sera of AIDS and AIDS-risk patients. Nature 1985; 324:69-72.
50. Weiss RA, Clapham PR, Weber JN, Dalgleish AG, Lasky LA, Berman PW. Variable and conserved neutralization antigens of human immunodeficiency virus. Nature 1986; 324:572-5.
51. Wendler I, Beinzle U, Hunsmann G. Neutralizing antibodies and the course of HIV-induced disease. AIDS Research and Human Retroviruses 1987; 3:157-63.

52. Groopman JE, Benz PM, Ferriani R, Mayer K, Allan JD, Weymouth LA. Characterization of serum neutralization response to the human immunodeficiency virus (HIV). AIDS Research and Human Retroviruses 1987; 3: 71-85.

53. Nara PL, Robey WG, Pyle SW, Hatch WC, Dunlop NM, Bess JW Jr, Kelliher JC, Arthur LO, Fischinger PJ. Purified envelope glycoproteins from human immunodeficiency virus type 1 variant induce individual, type-specific neutralizing antibodies. J Virol 1988; 62:2622-8.

54. Rusche JR, Javaherian K, McDanal C, Petro J, Lynn DL, Grimaila R, Langlois A, Gallo RC, Arthur LO, Fischinger PJ, Bolognesi DP, Putney SD, Matthews TJ. Antibodies that inhibit fusion of human immunodeficiency virus-infected cells bind a 24-amino acid sequence of the viral envelope, gp120. Proc Natl Acad Sci USA 1988; 85:3198-202.

55. Goudsmit J, Debouck C, Meloen RH, Smit L, Bakker M, Asher DM, Wolff AV, Gibbs CJ Jr, Gajdusek DC. Human immunodeficiency virus type 1 neutralization epitope with conserved architecture elicits early type-specific antibodies in experimentally infected chimpanzees. Proc Natl Acad Sci USA 1988; 85:4478-82.

56. Looney DJ, Fisher AF, Putney SD, Rusche JR, Redfield RR, Burke DS, Gallo RC, Wong-Staal F. Type-restricted neutralization of molecular clones of human immunodeficiency virus. Science 1988; 241:357-9.

57. Reitz MS Jr, Wilson C, Naugle C, Gallo RC, Robert-Guroff M. Generation of a neutralization-resistant variant of HIV-1 is due to selection for a point mutation in the envelope gene. Cell 1988; 54:57-63.

58. Siliciano RF, Lawton T, Knall C, Karr RW, Berman P, Gregory T, Reinherz EL. Analysis of host-virus interactions in AIDS with anti-gp120 T cell clones: Effect of HIV sequence variation and a mechanism for $CD4^+$ cell depletion. Cell 1988; 54:561-75.

59. Koyanagi Y, Miles S, Mitsuyasu RT, Merrill JE, Vinters HV, Chen ISY. Dual infection of the central nervous system by AIDS viruses with distinct cellular tropisms, Science 1987; 236:819-22.

60. Popovic M, Mellert W, Erfle V, Gartner S. Role of mononuclear phagocytes and accessory cells in human immunodeficiency virus type I infection of the brain. Annals of Neurology 1988; 23(suppl):S74-7.

61. Cheng-Mayer C, Seto D, Tateno M, Levy JA. Biologic features of HIV-1 that correlate with virulence in the host. Science 1988; 240:80-2.

62. Asjo B, Morfeldt-Manson L, Albert J, Biberfeld G, Karlsson A, Lidman K, Fenyo EM. Replicative capacity of human immunodeficiency virus from patients with varying severity of HIV infection. Lancet 1986; 2:660-2.

63. Fenyo EM, Morfeldt-Manson L, Chiodi F, Lind B, von Gegerfelt A, Albert J, Olausson E, Asjo B. Distinct replicative and cytopathic characteristics of human immunodeficiency virus isolates. J Virol 1988; 62:4414-0.

64. Clavel F, Guetard D, Brun-Vezinet F, Chamaret S, Rey MA, Santos-Ferreira MO, Laurent AG, Dauguet C, Katlama C, Rouzioux C, Klatzmann D, Champalimaud JL, Montagnier L. Isolation of a new human retrovirus from West African patients with AIDS. Science 1986; 233:343-6.

65. Clavel F, Mansinho K, Chamaret S, Guetard D, Favier V, Nina J, Santos-Ferreira MO, Champalimaud JL, Montagnier L. Human immunodeficiency virus type 2 infection associated with AIDS in West Africa. N Engl J Med 1987; 316:1180–5.

66. Kanki PJ, M'Boup S, Ricard D, Barin F, Denis F, Boye C, Sangare L, Travers K, Albaum M, Marlink R, Romet-Lemonne J-L, Essex M. Human T-lymphotropic virus type 4 and the human immunodeficiency virus in West Africa. Science 1987; 236:827–31.

67. Evans LA, Moreau J, Odehouri K, Legg H, Barboza A, Cheng-Mayer C, Levy JA. Characterization of a noncytopathic HIV-2 strain with unusual effects on CD4 expression. Science 1988; 240:1522–9.

68. Kong LI, Lee SW, Kappes JC, Parkin JS, Decker D, Hoxie JA, Hahn BH, Shaw GM. West African HIV-2 related human retrovirus with attenuated cytopathicity. Science 1988; 240:1525–1529.

69. Payne S, Salinovich O, Nauman S, Issel CJ, Montelara RC. Course and extent of variation of equine infectious anemia virus during parallel persistent infections. J Virol 1987; 61:1266–70.

70. Montelaro RC, Parekh B, Orrego A, Issel CJ. Antigenic variation during persistent infection by equine infectious anemia virus, a retrovirus. J Biol Chem 1984; 259:10539–44.

71. Thormar H, Barshatzky MR, Arnesen K, Kozlowski PB. The emergence of antigenic variants is a rare event in long-term visna virus infection in vivo. J Gen Virol 1983; 64:1427–32.

72. Payne SL, Fang F-D, Liu C-P, Dhruva BR, Rwambo P, Issel CJ, Montelaro RC. Antigenic variation and lentivirus persistence: variations in envelope gene sequences during EIAV infection resemble changes reported for sequential isolates of HIV. Virology 1987; 161:321–31.

73. Fultz PN, McClure HM, Anderson DC, Switzer WM. Identification and biologic characterization of an acutely lethal variant of simian immunodeficiency virus from sooty mangabeys (SIV/SMM). AIDS Res Hum Retroviruses 1989; 5:397–409.

CELLULAR IMMUNE RESPONSE RELEVANT TO VACCINE DEVELOPMENT

6

T-Cell Immunity and Vaccine Engineering
Application to the AIDS Virus

Kemp B. Cease
University of Michigan Medical School
Ann Arbor, Michigan

Jay A. Berzofsky
National Cancer Institute
National Institutes of Health
Bethesda, Maryland

VACCINES AND IMMUNE PROTECTION

Protective immunity against the AIDS virus is the goal of all current AIDS vaccine research. However, even the possibility of such immunity remains hypothetical as it is yet to be demonstrated in man under any circumstances (1,2). Thus, we are confronted with the unprecendented challenge of developing a safe and effective vaccine for a disease for which the immunologic prerequisites of protection are unknown. The difficulty is compounded by the fact that HIV is a highly variable retrovirus that is transmitted by infected cells as well as by free virus, and that devastates the immune system. Never in the history of vaccine development has such a formidable foe been confronted.

With all diseases where vaccines have been successfully developed previously, disease experience itself confers at least some degree of protection. Thus, the goal of the vaccine was to simulate that experience in a way sufficient for acquisition of protective immunity. Jenner was able to achieve this for smallpox virus with a live, related virus from cowpox. In the nearly 200 years since that time, other more sophisticated strategies have been used effectively to simulate disease experience and achieve protective immunity. These have included use of live attenuated virus, killed virus, purified subunits, toxoids, and more recently subunits produced using the methods of modern molecular genetics. Though safer variants of HIV are being developed, interest in live attentuated virus, killed virus, and purified native subunit vaccines for widespread clinical use has been dampened by issues of safety and practicality (3). Consequently there has been considerable interest in vaccines based on recombinant proteins and synthetic peptides. These constructs would include only a selected subset of the potential antigenic information of the virus, and thus a molecular-level understanding of the immune response to the virus is a prerequisite for the rational development of such vaccines.

While the elements of human immunologic protection are unknown, there are several lines of evidence that may direct us toward those elements. With regard to humoral immunity, it is well known that patients with AIDS have progressive disease in spite of making antibodies to the whole panoply of AIDS viral proteins (1,2). Clearly much of that response is an epiphenomenon with no relevance to protection. Neutralizing antibodies may be more important. Initial reports indicated that neutralizing antibodies were infrequent in patients seropositive for HIV but were more likley to be present in healthy seropositives and AIDS-related complex (ARC) patients than in patients with frank AIDS (4–6). Subsequent studies have shown that titer of neutralizing antibody is a predictor of clinical course in at least some risk groups (7). The titer of such antibodies may have both quantitative and qualitative importance. It has been found that group-specific activity may be seen only in high-titer AIDS sera whereas only type-specific neutralizing activity is seen in low-titer AIDS sera (8,9). Additionally, it is possible that high-titer sera will possess effective antiviral activity in vivo while low-titer serum is not only ineffective but may actually facilitate entry of virus into Fc receptor-bearing cells similar to the situation with Dengue virus (10). Thus, induction of the highest possible titer of neutralizing antibodies would appear to be important for protective humoral immunity.

Cellular immunity would also appear to be a critical component of protective immunity. Not only would potent T-cell help be needed to achieve the strong humoral immunity discussed above, but it would also be needed to support cytotoxic T cells, activated macrophages, LAK cells, and NK cells that may be participating in the response to virus or infected cells (11). Experimental support for the importance of T-cell immunity in protection comes from human and chimpanzee studies. In man, it is difficult to reproducily demonstrate HIV-specific T-cell immunity in HIV-exposed patients and protective immunity does not develop (12). However, in chimpanzees, HIV-specific T-cell immunity is readily demonstrated, and the animals do not develop clinical disease (13). Thus, induction of potent T-cell immunity specific for HIV may be a prerequisite for prevention of disease.

EXPERIMENTAL DESIGN IN SUBUNIT VACCINE DEVELOPMENT

When considering immunologic experiments involving synthetic peptides, whether involving antibodies or T cells, the type of experimental design is critical to the interpretation and should be kept clearly in mind. One can use either a native antigen or peptide as the immunogen or inducing antigen and can similarly test with either native antigen or peptide. Thus, four experimental designs result with mnemonic designations as follows: *native* immunogen, *native* test antigen (NN design); *native* immunogen, *peptide* test antigen (NP design); *peptide* immunogen, *native* test antigen (PN design); and *peptide* immunogen, *peptide* test antigen (PP design). Recombinant proteins can generally be operationally classified as native or peptide within a given experimental system. An example of an NN experiment would be immunization with a native protein from one isolate and testing with the native protein from second isolate or variant. An NP experiment uses a peptide to probe the specificity of a response to the native immunogen. In distinction to this, a PN experiment examines the ablity of a specific peptide to induce an immune response to the native protein. A PP experiment simply examines the immunogenicity of a specific peptide without regard for its parent native protein. This shorthand designation with a two-letter mnemonic indicating the immunogen followed by the test antigen will be used in the remainder of this chapter.

MOLECULAR ANALYSIS OF THE ANTIBODY RESPONSE TO HIV

Several studies have shown that purified native envelope protein as well as recombinant envelope proteins can elicit neutralizing antibodies (14-16). The sites within the gp160 precursor envelope glycoprotein that are recognized by antibody, have been extensively studied using synthetic peptides and recombinant proteins in NP and PN studies. Kennedy et al. reported that a peptide encompassing residues 735-752 of gp160, falling within the gp41 segment, was recognized by AIDS sera (NP experiment) (17). Furthermore, they found that when it was conjugated to a carrier, it could induce antibodies reactive with gp160 in enzyme immunosorbant assays (EIAs) and by radioimmunoprecipitation (RIP). These latter PN experiments demonstrated the type of immunogenic potential that would be necessary though not sufficient for utility in a vaccine. Wang et al. identified a second site in the 586-606 segment within gp41 that reacted with AIDS sera in NP design experimnts (18). Rosen et al. (19) and Gnann et al. (20) independently identified this site and contributed to the definition of the core residues. The activity of this site in PN experiments was not reported. Chanh et al. identified a third antibody site, this time at the gp120-gp41 junction within the segment 503-532 (21). In addition to being recognized by AIDS sera in NP experiments, when coupled to a carrier and used as immunogen in PN experiments it was able to elicit neutralizing antibodies. Palker et al. independently identified this site using a peptide termed SP-22 representing residues 504-518 in gp120 (22). They found that while 70% of the antibodies in AIDS sera are specific for this site, those antibodies fail to neutralize virus. Thus, while an antibody response directed at this site has the potential to be neutralizing, at least in rabbits, the actual response to this site in infected patients appears to fail in this regard. Ho et al. performed PN studies using a panel of synthetic peptides using neutralization as the read-out (23). These studies revealed four additional sites whose peptides could induce neutralizing antibody, 298-314, 616-632, 728-751, and 458-484. Palker et al. identified a peptide termed SP-10 representing residues 303-321 which elicits type-specific neutralizing antibodies in PN experiments when conjugated to an appropriate carrier (24). This peptide overlaps the 298-314 peptide mentioned above. Rusche et al. found that antibodies capable of inhibiting cell fusion bound to a peptide representing residues 307-330 (25). The core segment of this site would thus appear to lie within the center of the variable region 3 loop.*

Thus seven antibody sites within gp160 have been reported to date: three within gp120 and four within gp41. Six of these are known to have activity in PN experiments, and at least five have some potential for eliciting neutralizing antibody. The site focused on residues 307-314 appears the most promising in this regard, although it is in a region of sequence variability among different isolates.

ANALYSIS OF HIV-SPECIFIC T-CELL RESPONSES

While substantial activity in studying the antibody response has led to the detailed understanding outlined above, the T-cell response to this virus has been explored only more recently, and our knowledge is considerably less developed. While the presence of antibodies implied that specific T helper cells were elicited to help that response, data documenting specific cell mediated immunity to any HIV antigen was not forthcoming until Zarling et al. demonstrated HIV-specific T-cell immunity in macaques infected with a recombinant vaccinia virus expressing the gp120 envelope protein (26). They demonstrated both helper and cytolytic T-cell responses. Later that year Walker and colleagues provided evidence for CD8$^+$ T cell participation in the specific immune response to HIV with these cells acting to suppress viral replication (27). In a study examining the major histocompatibility restriction of the response, HIV envelope proteins were found to be immunogenic for T-cell responses in three of four murine MHC haplotypes studied, an indication of a potential for broad MHC-restricted responsiveness

---

*Recent studies have shown that the GPG sequence and adjacent residues form the core of this site, which is the major segmental neutralizing antibody site of gp120 (73,74).

(28). Cellular immunity was demonstrated in goats as well (29). However, while these studies indicated that HIV antigens were certainly recognizable by the immune system, early indications were that HIV seropositive individuals exhibited minimal and inconsistent cellular immunity to this virus (30,75) even when they were in asymptomatic pre-ARC stages of the infection. These preliminary observations were substantiated by Wahren and colleagues (12), who showed that of the 40 seropositive patients they studied, only 9 had reactivity to HIV virion, and these tended to be the earlier stage patients. Thus, a proliferative/helper T-cell response to HIV proteins could be demonstrated in man but was limited, and the broad, strong responsiveness seen in the animal studies was lacking. Cytotoxic T-cell immunity was subsequently demonstrated in seropositive individuals in both peripheral blood and bronchoalveolar lavage mononuclear cells (31,32). Walker et al. could demonstrate HIV envelope protein-specific CTL in eight of eight seropositive individuals suggesting that such a CTL response was highly prevalent in the seropositive population (31). The same group more recently demonstrated polymerase specific CTL as well (33). These studies employed autologous and heterologous target cells that were first immortalized with EBV and subsequently infected with a recombinant vaccinia virus. This elegant experimental system clearly demonstrated antigen-specific, MHC-restricted CTL responses to HIV. However, the strength of that response is more difficult to ascertain. The fact that such seropositive individuals ultimately develop AIDS indicates that this response to natural HIV infection is qualitatively or quantitatively insufficient for protection.

Thus, individuals infected with HIV exhibited significant antibody and cytolytic T-cell responses and even had $CD8^+$ T cells capable of down-regulating HIV replication. Nonetheless, their helper T-cell response to HIV appeared specifically deficient in both prevalence and strength even when responses to other antigens were intact. In contrast to this limited helper T-cell response to HIV observed in humans infected with the virus, chimpanzees were found to develop strong cellular immunity (13). While susceptible to infection with HIV, the chimpanzee does not develop clinical AIDS. These results thus demonstrated that strong T-cell immunity was associated with protective immunity in this species, though cause and effect could not be confidently assigned. Since natural infection in man neither induces strong T-cell immunity nor leads to protective immunity, the implication is that enhanced HIV-specific helper T-cell immunity may be critical for protective immunity in man. It has been possible to elicit T-cell immunity in noninfected human volunteers by immunization with a recombinant vaccinia virus expressing the HIV envelope gene (34,35). However, it is not known yet whether this response is protective. Optimization of protective T-cell immunity in humans is likely to require detailed knowledge of the basic molecular immunology of the helper T-cell response to HIV.

T-CELL SITE IDENTIFICATION IN AIDS VIRUS PROTEINS

A major focus of our studies has been the identification and immunologic characterization of AIDS virus protein sites recognized by T cells so as to understand the basic molecular immunology of the response that now appears essential for the engineering of optimized HIV vaccines.

T cells recognize small segments of protein antigen after appropriate processing and presentation on a presenting cell surface in association with an appropriate major histocompatibility complex (MHC) molecule—generally class II for TH and class I for CTL (36). Consequently, it has been possible to use small synthetic peptides as probes of T-cell antigen recognition. Careful studies with a number of different antigens have revealed that for any given antigen, the T-cell response is focused on a relatively limited number of immunodominant sites (37). Furthermore, the segments within proteins recognized by helper T cells frequently have amino acid sequences that would allow them to fold as amphipathic helicies (38,39). Thus, our approach was to use a computer algorithm we developed entitled AMPHI to examine the sequence of HIV isolates for segments that displayed a periodicity of amino acid side chain hydrophobicity such that if the segment were folded into an alpha helix, the helix would be amphipathic, with hydrophobic side chains on one side and hydrophilic on the opposite side (40,41). In an alpha helix there are 3.6 residues per turn of the helix, and consequently an amphipathic alpha helix would display sinusoidal variation in hydrophobicity along the sequence with a period of 3.6 residues per cycle and a frequency of $100°$ per residue ($360°/3.6 = 100°$ progression around the helix). Segments with these properties can be identified using discrete Fourier analysis or least squares fitting of a sinusoidal function. We have found the latter to be superior for analyzing short segments of protein sequence information, and thus it is employed by the AMPHI program. AMPHI analyzes a protein sequence by examining overlapping blocks of 11 residues (residues 1-11, 2-12, 3-13, etc.) and computing parameters reflecting their potential to form an amphipathic helix as evidenced by their periodicity of hydrophobicity. For each 11-residue block, a maximum in the frequency spectrum between $80°$ and $130°$ is considered consistent with amphipathic helix formation, and a computed parameter called the Amphipathic Index reflects the degree of fit. Consecutive overlapping blocks exhibiting the favorable helical amphipathicity characteristics combine to define an amphipathic segment. As mentioned above such sites appear to be preferentially presented to and recognized by class II restricted TH cells. The AMPHI algorithm correctly identifies 18 of the 23 immunodominant TH sites in our data base of 12 proteins with a high significance ($p < 0.001$).

When we performed AMPHI analysis on the HIV gp120 envelope protein, we identified several candidate T-cell sites within the protein (28). Sites were ranked according to the apparent strength of helical amphipathicity as reflected in an Amphipathic Index, and the locations of the maxima in the frequency spectra were examined for consistency with helical structure. Segments were also examined for conservation in the available HIV sequences and for absence of N-linked glycosylation sites that might mask an epitope that would otherwise be recognized. We selected peptides encompassing each segment and in our initial studies focused on the two most promising sites termed *env* T1 and *env* T2. We prepared the appropriate peptides using solid phase peptide synthesis for use as probes of T-cell specificity. The TH cell response to gp120 was then studied using lymph node proliferation assays performed employing these peptides along with recombinant envelope proteins and purified gp120. After immunization with the large recombinant fragment R10, significant responses were seen to native gp120 (NN experimental design, see above) as well as to the *env* T1 and *env* T2 peptides (NP design) which indicated that they did in fact represent sites seen as part of the response to a large (425 residue) fragment. Conversely, immunization with the 16-residue *env* T1 peptide induced T-cell immunity to native gp120 (PN design). As mentioned above we found that three of the four MHC haplotypes examined were responders to the *env* T1 site, which suggested that broad responsiveness would be expected in an outbred population. The proliferative response is abrogated by T-cell depletion and the responding cells are making lymphokines (IL2 and/or IL4; Cease and Berzofsky, unpublished), consistent with a helper T-cell dependent response. Thus the *env* T1 site is a helper T-cell site within the gp120 envelope protein of HIV that can be encompassed within a small synthetic peptide that has the important properties of 1) broad MHC-restricted immunogenic activity, and 2) the ability to induce immunity to the native protein. These properties would appear critical for general utility of a T-cell site in synthetic peptide and recombinant vaccine constructs.

The *env* T1 site as the first and most well-characterized helper T-cell site in HIV has already found application in prototype vaccine development. Palker et al. recently reported studies using a bivalent synthetic peptide vaccine construct incorporating the *env* T1 site for T-cell help and the SP-10 B cell site described above for antibody responses (42). This construct, without an additional carrier, was able to elicit high-titer type-specific antibody against gp120 in goats. The antiserum both neutralized HIV and inhibited HIV-induced syncitia formation in vitro. The powerful role of molecular immunology in modern vaccine development is underscored by this simple result and is discussed further below.

Recent studies have also confirmed the importance of the *env* T1 site in the human response to gp120 in volunteers immunized with a recombinant vaccinia virus encoding the gp120 envelope protein of HIV (43). When these individuals were boosted with recombinant gp120 protein, immunity specific for the *env* T1 site was observed as demonstrated by responsiveness to the 16-residue synthetic peptide. The response following boosting reached a peak around day 14 and gradually fell to a plateau around twice background, which is maintained in excess of 7 weeks.

Aside from the immunologic properties of the *env* T1, this site has also been found to be of critical importance to the virus for binding to its cellular receptor, CD4. Lasky et al. (44) studied the binding of recombinant gp120 to recombinant CD4 using monoclonal antibodies to gp120 that inhibit the binding. One of these inhibitory antibodies was used to prepare an affinity column and was found to bind a 43-residue cleavage peptide from gp120 which spanned the *env* T1 site. They next showed that a 12-residue deletion abrogated CD4 binding without grossly altering the overall protein structure. Eleven of the 12 amino acids deleted fall at the C-terminus of the *env* T1 site. Additionally, site directed mutagenesis of an alanine residue, which falls within the *env* T1 site, to an aspartic acid greatly reduced gp120 binding to CD4. Why this site should be critical for binding to CD4 as well as preferentially recognized by T cells is unknown but could relate to its protential for assuming amphipathic alpha helical structure. From a practical standpoint, these data make the *env* T1 site an even more attractive subject for immune targeting since this segment appears to serve an indispensable function for the virus and thus variation under immune pressure may be constrained.*

While the AMPHI program was developed to identify TH sites, it may be useful for identifying the CTL sites as well (77). However, a careful assessment of the utility of AMPHI for identifying CTL sites must await characterization of additional sites at the peptide level.

CTL has been demonstrated in HIV seropositive individuals. As mentioned above, a response was initially demonstrated against envelope and more recently against the polymerase. However, little was known about the potential or actual CTL response with regard to the fine specificity of the response. To explore this, Takahashi et al. developed an experimental system for eliciting and characterizing CTL specific for gp160 in mice (45). Mice were first immunized with a recombinant vaccinia virus encoding the gp160 protein. Several weeks later spleen cells from these mice were boosted with either vaccinia-infected cells or cells transfected with an expression vector containing the same gp160 insert. The responding cells were then assayed not only on vaccinia-infected or transfected targets, but also with normal cells in the presence of selected peptides from gp160. This system enabled induction of a gp160-specific CTL response in vivo using a recombinant vaccinia, with subsequent selective boosting of the gp160-specific response in vitro using a transfectant. The CTL induced were shown to be conventional CD8$^+$, CD4$^-$ T cells. The gp160-specific CTL response could

---

*Recent studies have demonstrated additional multideterminant regions of gp160 recognized by gp160-immune T cells from mice of multiple MHC types (76).

then be characterized at the molecular level using synthetic peptides by the method of Townsend et al. (46). It was found that H-2^d was a CTL high responder haplotype whereas H-2^k was a low responder under these conditions. Studies employing 41 peptides yielded only one major immunodominant CTL antigenic site and a few minor sites. The site identified did in fact have some amphipathic alpha helical potential but also contained a strong helix-breaking turn segment in the middle. Surprisingly, the site was localized to 315–329, the same segment as the 303–330 B-cell site discussed above, a highly variable region of gp160. It is not clear whether the variability is selected by immune pressure from neutralizing antibodies or human CTL.* It was shown that T cells recognize the peptide in association with the D^d class I MHC molecule. This study suggests that the potential repertoire of gp160-specific CTL may be extremely limited, as only 1 of 5 class I molecules examined appeared to be used, and with that one, only one major antigenic site was identified. Consequently, knowledge of the location and characteristics of such sites becomes all the more critical to successful vaccine development.

Initial work by ourselves and others has focused on the envelope proteins for several reasons. In feline and murine retrovirus models the antibody response to envelope proteins has been critical to protection (47). The interest in studying the antibody response to HIV envelope proteins has resulted in the availability of essential envelope reagents enabling the studies discussed. It is clear that T-cell responses to internal proteins may be as important as the response to envelope proteins if not more so (48–53). The critical internal protein reagents from HIV are increasingly available and will facilitate the study of these responses.

MOLECULAR IMMUNOLOGY AND MODERN VACCINE DEVELOPMENT

Just as structure-activity relationships have been central to conventional pharmaceutical development, a molecular-level knowledge of the potential and actual immune response to a given antigen will become increasingly central to modern vaccine development. Unlike live virus, killed virus, and major subunit vaccines where whole virions or intact native proteins are used, recombinant protein and synthetic peptide vaccines generally require conscious decisions regarding what segments of protein are to be included or excluded. While convenience (e.g., locations of restriction enzyme sites within DNA or the synthetic difficulty or solubility of a given peptide) can weigh heavily in such decisions, knowledge of the immunological properties of various segments can provide a more rational basis for decision. For example one or more copies of selected helper T-cell sites may be included to enhance T-cell help of a given specificity. Cytolytic T-cell

---

*Recent results indicate that within this site the virus mutates both residues interacting with the T cell receptor and residues interacting with the class I MHC molecule presenting the peptide (78, 79). Such changes may allow HIV to escape control by CTL (80).

sites would be selectively retained in vaccine constructs intended to induce such responses, whereas sites that induce suppressor T cells might be excluded (54). Sites responsible for potentially undesirable autoimmune cross-reactions with human proteins might be excluded, such as the neuroleukin homology site in HIV (55,56) or the MHC homology site in CMV (57) or in HIV (81). B-cell sites may be included to selectively induce antibody responses of the desired specificity. The result would be a highly engineered recombinant protein or synthetic peptide vaccine construct with selected immunological activity.

Several examples from the literature illustrate the application of these principles. The hepatitis B virus is the first pathogen for which a recombinant vaccine has been developed. This vaccine is composed primarily of recombinant surface antigen encoded by the "S" region. However Milich et al. found that nonresponsiveness to the S region due to lack of helper T-cell sites was overcome in a longer peptide that brings in an immunodominant T-cell site in the pre-S2 region of the protein (58). This suggests that inclusion of this region would be an important enhancement for the next generation of recombinant HBV vaccine. Several examples of synthetic peptide constructs containing T-cell and B-cell sites have been reported. A bivalent peptide combining the *env* T1 site and the SP10 site from HIV has been reported as described in detail above (42). Bivalent peptide vaccine constructs with T-cell and B-cell sites have also been reported by Good et al. for malaria (59), Klipstein et al. for enterotoxigenic *E. coli* (60), Francis et al. for foot and mouth disease virus (61), Minden et al. for *Mycobacterium bovis* (62), and Milich et al. for the HBV pre-S region and core antigen (63). The T-cell site and B-cell site need not even come from the same protein as demonstrated by Milich et al., who used a T-cell site from the HBV core protein and a B-cell site from the surface or envelope protein (63). This point is further underscored by other studies of Francis et al. in which they employed helper T-cell sites from non–pathogen-associated model proteins such as sperm whale myoglobin and ovalbumin, along with a B-cell site from FMDV (64). In a FMDV-peptide low responder strain (H-2^d), they were able to elicit responses to FMDV by including the appropriate T-cell site.

While inclusion of the appropriate T-cell and B-cell sites in a vaccine construct is certainly necessary for their immunological activity, it in no way guarantees it. This problem almost certainly relates to the tertiary structure assumed by the construct and has been of greater concern for B-cell sites than for T-cell sites since T cells recognize processed antigen. Two mechanisms may be important: 1) a segment may not assume the conformation required for activity, or 2) certain segments may assume conformations that hinder the recognition of other segments. We might refer to such hindering structures as "hindratopes" (65). The first mechanism represents a common problem in the production of anti-peptide antibodies that bind the native antigen. In such cases conformation is critical, and factors such as the end of the peptide used for coupling, the types and number of spacer residues between peptide and carrier, as well as the specific carrier used can dramatically alter the properties of the antibodies elicited (66,67). The second mechanism, interference by hindratopes, can be important for both T-cell and B-cell sites (65,68). Brett et al. recently demonstrated the importance of this phenomenon in antigen presentation and T-cell receptor recognition (65). They provided evidence supporting the presence of hindratopes exerting an MHC-specific inhibitory effect on the recognition of a given site within a specific antigen. Furthermore, this effect was neither due to classical determinant selection nor to a hole in the T-cell repertoire and thus represents a novel Ir gene-related phenomenon. Hindratopes can interfere with antibody recognition as well. A hindratope effect might explain the finding of Francis et al. that the FMDV peptide coupled to 323-339 of ovalbumin or 132-148 of sperm whale myoglobin induced neutralizing antibodies in B10.D2 mice, whereas when coupled to the 105-121 site of sperm whale myoglobin, such antibodies were not elicited in this strain (64). All three sites are well characterized $H\text{-}2^d$-restricted helper T cell sites. This observation is consistent with a hindratope introduced by the 105-121 T-cell site perturbing the segment available for antibody recognition and thereby skewing the response with resultant loss of neutralizing activity. It has been suggested that the variable regions of the HIV gp120 envelope protein may function as hindratopes or "umbrellas" preventing antibody binding to critical structural sites with the protein (69). When engineering a peptide or recombinant protein immunogenic construct, the creation of undesirable hindratopes is always a possibility. As tertiary folding cannot be predicted accurately, only empiric experimentation can assure that immunological activity is not compromised by hindratopes in a given construct. The trivalent peptide construct reported by Beachey et al. illustrates this point (70). They were concerned that antibody recognition of the middle site in the construct would be hindered by flanking residues in the folded peptide. Their experiments showed that for this construct, significant interference was not seen. Potential hindratope effects may be especially important in more complex multivalent and polymeric constructs (60,70-72).

The development of a safe and effective vaccine for AIDS is clearly one of the most difficult vaccine challenges in history. However, it comes at a time when the powerful insights and methods of modern molecular immunology can be brought to bear on the problem. The T-cell response to a given antigen is essential to immunogenicity and specificity. Consequently, an understanding of this response at the molecular level is essential to vaccine engineering as it allows one to develop highly immunogenic constructs that elicit pathogen-specific T-cell responses and that at the same time avoid the use of an irrelevant carrier protein. This platform of T-cell help can then support the addition of desired B-cell sites or possible CTL sites. Sites responsible for undesirable cross-reactions would be excluded by design, while hindratope effects must be empirically discovered and engineered out. Such rational vaccine development is being pursued in a number of laboratories currently and may in fact represent the critical path to a safe and effective AIDS vaccine.

REFERENCES

1. Koenig S, Rosenberg ZF. Immunology of infection with the human immunodeficiency virus (HIV): A view from the III international conference on AIDS. Ann of Int Med 107: 409–412 (1987).
2. Seligmann M, Pinching AJ, Rosen FS, Fahey JL, Khaitov RM, Klatzmann D, Koenig S, Nkandu L, Ngu J, Riethmuller G, Spira TJ. Immunology of human immunodeficiency virus infection and the acquired immunodeficiency syndrome. Ann Int Med 107: 234–242 (1987).
3. Weiss SH, Goedert JJ, Gartner S, Popovic M, Waters D, Markham P, Veronese FDM, Gail MH, Barkley WE, Gibbons J, Gill FA, Leuther M, Shaw GM, Gallo RC, Blattner WA. Risk of human immunodeficiency virus (HIV-1) infection among laboratory workers. Science 239: 68–71 (1988).
4. Clavel F, Klatzmann D, Montagnier L. Deficient LAV1 neutralising capacity of sera from patients with AIDS or related syndromes. Lancet, 1: 879–880 (1985).
5. Weiss RA, Clapham PR, Cheingsong-Popov R, Dalgleish AG, Carne CA, Weller IVD, Tedder RS. Neutralization of human T-lymphotropic virus type III by sera of AIDS and AIDS risk patients. Nature, 316: 69–72 (1985).
6. Robert-Guroff M, Brown M, Gallo RC. HTLV–III-neutralizing antibodies in patients with AIDS and AIDS-related complex. Nature, 316: 72–74 (1985).
7. Robert-Guroff M, Giardina PJ, Robey WG, Jennings AM, Naugle CJ, Akbar AN, Grady RW, Hilgartner MW. HTLV–III neutralizing antibody development in transfusion-dependent serpositive patients with beta-thalassemia. J Immunol, 138: 3731–3736 (1987).
8. Levy JA, Evans L, Pan L-Z, Tateno M, Reed MF, Walker C, Homsy J, Cheng-Mayer C. Biologic heterogeneity of HIV and host immune response during HIV infection. In Chanock, R. M., Lerner, R. A., Brown, F., and H. Ginsberg, eds. Vaccines 87—Modern approaches to new vaccines: Prevention of AIDS and other viral, bacterial, and parasitic diseases. Cold Spring Harbor, New York: Cold Spring Harbor Laboratory, 1987:168–173.
9. Geffin R, Parks ES, Parks WP, Hahn B, Shaw GM. AIDS retrovirus neutralization: Group- and type-specific reactions. In Chanock, R. M., Lerner, R. A., Brown, F., and H. Ginsberg, eds. Vaccines 87—Modern approaches to new vaccines: Prevention of AIDS and other viral, bacterial, and parasitic diseases. Cold Spring Harbor, New York: Cold Spring Harbor Laboratory, 1987:159–163.
10. Halstead SB. Pathogenesis of dengue: Challenges to molecular biology. Science, 240:476–481 (1988).

11. Ruscetti FW, Mikovits JA, Kalyanaraman VS, Overton R, Stevenson H, Stromberg K, Herberman RB, Farrar WL, Ortaldo JR. Analysis of effector mechanisms against HTLV-I and HTLV-V-III/LAV-infected lymphod cells. J Immunol, 136: 3619 (1986).

12. Wahren B, Morfeldt-Mansson L, Biberfeld G, Moberg L, Sonnerberg A, Ljungman P, Werner A, Durth R, Gallo R, Bolognesi D. Characteristics of the specific cell-mediated immune response in human immunodeficiency virus infection. J Virol, 61: 2017–2023 (1987).

13. Eichberg JW, Zarling JM, Alter HJ, Levy JA, Berman PW, Gregory T, Lasky LA, McClure J, Cobb KE, Moran PA, Hu S-L, Kennedy RC, Chanh TC, Dreesman GR. T-Cell Responses to Human Immunodeficiency Virus (HIV) and Its Recombinant Antigens in HIV-Infected Chimpanzees. J Virol, 61: 3804–3808 (1987).

14. Lasky LA, Groopman JE, Fennie CW, Benz PM, Capon DJ, Dowbenko DJ, Nakamura GR, Nunes WM, Renz ME, Berman PW. Neutralization of the AIDS Retrovirus by Antibodies to a Recombinant Envelope Glycoprotein. Science, 233: 209–212; (1986).

15. Robey WG, Arthur LO, Matthews TJ, Langlois A, Copeland TD, Lerche NW, Oroszlan S, Bolognesi DP, Gilden RV, Fischinger PJ. Prospect for Prevention of Human Immunodeficiency Virus Infection: Purified 120-kDa Envelope Glycoprotein Induces Neutralizing Antibody. Proc Natl Acad Sci USA, 83: 7023–7027, (1986).

16. Putney SD, Matthews TJ, Robey WG, Lynn DL, Robert-Guroff M, Mueller WT, Langlois AJ, Ghrayeb J, Petteway SR Jr, Weinhold KJ, Fischinger PJ, Wong-Staal F, Gallo RC, Bolognesi DP. HTLV-III/LAV-neutralizing antibodies to an *E. coli*-produced fragment of the virus envelope. Science, 234: 1392–1395 (1986).

17. Kennedy RC, Genkel RD, Pauletti D, Allan JS, Lee TH, Essex M, and Dreesman GR. Antiserum to a synthetic peptide recognizes the HTLV-III envelope glycoprotein. Science 231: 1556–1559 (1986).

18. Wang JJG, Steel S, Wisniewolski R, Wang CY. Detection of antibodies to human T-lymphotropic virus type III by using a synthetic peptide of 21 amino acid residues corresponding to a highly antigenic segment of gp41 envelope protein. Proc Natl Acad Sci USA, 83: 6159–6163 (1986).

19. Rosen J, Hom Y-L, Whalley A, Smith R, Naso RB. Detection of antibodies to HIV using synthetic peptides derived from the gp41 envelope protein. In Chanock, R. M., Lerner, R. A., Brown, F., and H. Ginsberg, eds. Vaccines 87—Modern approaches to new vaccines: Prevention of AIDS and other viral, bacterial, and parasitic diseases. Cold Spring Harbor, New York: Cold Spring Harbor Laboratory, 1987:188–193.

20. Gnann JW Jr, Neslon JA, Oldstone MBA. Fine mapping of an immuno-dominant domain in the transmembrane glycoportein of human immuno-deficient virus. J Virol 61: 2639–2641 (1987).

21. Chanh TC, Dreesman GR, Kanda P, Linette GP, Sparrow JT, Ho DD, Kennedy RC. Induction of anti-HIV neutralizing antibodies by synthetic peptides. EMBO J, 5: 3065–3071 (1986).

22. Palker TJ, Matthews TJ, Clark ME, Cianciolo GJ, Randall RR, Langlois AJ, White GC, Safai B, Snyderman R, Bolognesi DP, Haynes BF. A conserved region at the COOH terminus of human immunodeficiency virus gp120 envelope protein contains an immunodominant epitope. Proc Natl Acad Sci USA, 84: 2479–2483 (1987).
23. Ho DD, Sarngadharan MG, Hirsch MS, Schooley RT, Rota TR, Kennedy RC, Chanh TC, Sato VL. Human immunodefieincy virus neutralizing antibodies recognize several conserved domains on the envelope glycoproteins. J Virol, 61:2024–2028 (1987).
24. Palker TJ, Clark ME, Langlois AJ, Matthews TJ, Weinhold KJ, Randall RR, Bolognesi DP, Haynes BF. Type-specific neutralization of the human immunodeficiency virus with antibodies to env-encoded synthetic peptides. Proc Natl Acad Sci USA, 85: 1932–1936 (1988).
25. Rusche JR, Javaherian K, McDanal C, Petro J, Lynn DL, Grimaila R, Langlois A, Gallo RC, Arthur LA, Fischinger PJ, Bolognesi DP, Putney SD, Matthews TJ. Antibodies that inhibit fusion of HIV infected cells bind a 24 amino acid sequence of the viral envelope, gp120. Proc Natl Acad Sci USA, 85, 3198–3202 (1988).
26. Zarling JM, Morton W, Moran PA, McClure J, Kosowski SG, Hu S-L. T-cell responses to human AIDS virus in macaques immunized with recombinant vaccinia viruses. Nature, 323: 344–346 (1986).
27. Walker CM, Moody DJ, Stites DP, Levy JA. CD8+ lymphocytes can control HIV infection in vitro by suppressing virus replication. Science, 234: 1563–1566 (1986).
28. Cease KB, Margalit H, Cornette JL, Putney SD, Robey WG, Ouyang C, Streicher HZ, Fischiner PJ, Gallo RC, DeLisi C, Berzofsky JA. Helper T cell site identification in the AIDS virus gp120 envelope protein and induction of immunity in mice to the native protein using a 16-residue synthetic peptide. Proc Natl Acad Sci USA, 84: 4249 (1987).
29. Krohn K, Robey WG, Putney S, Arthur L, Nara P, Fischinger P, Gallo RC, Wong-Staal F, Ranki A. Specific cellular immune response and neutralizing antibodies in goats immunized with native or recombinant envelope proteins derived from human T-lymphotropic virus type IIIB and in human immunodeficiency virus-infected men. Proc Natl Acad Sci USA, 84: 4994–4998 (1987).
30. Wahren B, Morfeldt-Mansson L, Biberfeld G, Boberg L, Ljungman P, Nordlund S, Bredberg-Raden U, Werner A, Lower J, Kurth R. Impaired specific cellular response to HTLV–III before other immune defects in patients with HTLV–III infection. (letter), N Eng J Med, 315: 393–394 (1986).
31. Walker BD, Chakrabarti S, Moss B, Paradis TJ, Flynn T, Durno AG, Blumberg RS, Kaplan JC, Hirsch MS, Schooley RT. HIV-specific cytotoxic T lymphocytes in seropositive individuals. Nature, 328: 345–348 (1987).

32. Plata F, Autran B, Martins LP, Wain-Hobson S, Raphael M, Mayaud C, Denis M, Guillon J-M, Debré P. AIDS virus-specific cytotoxic T lymphocytes in lung disorders. Nature, 328: 348–351 (1987).

33. Walker BD, Flexner C, Paradis TJ, Fuller TC, Hirsch MS, Schooley RT, Moss B. HIV-1 reverse transcriptase is a target for cytotoxic T lymphocytes in infected individuals. Science, 240: 64–66 (1988).

34. Zagury D, Leonard R, Rouchard M, Reveil B, Bernard J, Ittele D, Cattan A, Zirimwabagabo L, Kalumbu M, Justin W, Salaun J-J, Boussard B. Immunization against AIDS in humans. Nature, 326: 249–250 (1987).

35. Zagury D, Bernard J, Cheynier R, Desportes I, Leonard R, Fouchard M, Reveil B, Ittele D, Zirimwabagabo L, Mbayo K, Wane J, Salaun J-J, Goussard B, Dechazal L, Burny A, Nara P, Gallo RC. A group specific anamnestic immune reaction against HIV-1 induced by a candidate vaccine against AIDS. Nature, 332: 728–731 (1988).

36. Berzofsky JA. IrGenes: Antigen-specific genetic regulation of the immune response. In Sela M, ed. The Antigens, Vol. VII. New York, Academic Press, 1988: 1–146.

37. Berzofsky JA. Structural features of protein antigenic sites recognized by helper T cells: What makes a site immunodominant? In Cruse, J. M., and R. E. Lewis, Jr., eds. The Year in Immunology, Basel S. Karger, 1986: 28–38.

38. DeLisi C, Berzofsky JA. T-cell antigenic sites tend to be amphipathic structures. Proc Natl Acad Sci USA, 82: 7048–7052 (1985).

39. Spouge JL, Guy HR, Cornette JL, Margalit H, Cease KB, Berzofsky JA, DeLisi C. Strong conformational propensities enhance T-cell antigenicity. J Immunol, 138: 204–212 (1987).

40. Cornette JL, Cease KB, Margalit H, Spouge JL, Berzofsky JA, DeLisi C. Hydrophobicity scales and computational techniques for detecting amphipathic structures in proteins. J Mol Biol, 195: 659–685 (1987).

41. Margalit H, Spouge JL, Cornette JL, Cease KB, DeLisi C, Berzofsky JA. Prediction of immunodominant helper T-cell antigenic sites from the primary sequence. J Immunol, 138: 2213–2229 (1987).

42. Palker TJ, Matthews TJ, Langlois A, Tanner ME, Martin ME, Scearce RM, Kim JE, Berzofsky JA, Bolognesi DP, Haynes BF. Polyvalent human immunodeficiency virus synthetic immunogen comprised of envelope gp120 T helper cell sites and B cell neutralization epitopes. J Immunol, 142:3612–3619 (1989).

43. Berzofsky JA, Bensussan A, Cease KB, Bourge JF, Cheynier R, Zirimwabagabo L, Salaun J-J, Gallo RC, Shearer GM, Zagury D. Antigenic peptides recognized by T lymphocytes from AIDS viral envelope-immune humans. Nature, 334: 706–708 (1988).

44. Lasky LA, Nakamura G, Smith DH, Fennie C, Shimasaki C, Patzer E, Berman P, Gregory T, Capon DJ. Delineation of a region of the human immunodeficiency virus type 1 gp120 glycoprotein critical for interaction with the CD4 receptor. Cell, 50: 975–985 (1987).

45. Takahashi H, Cohen J, Hosmalin A, Cease KB, Houghten R, Cornette JL, DeLisi C, Moss B, Germain RN, Berzofsky JA. An immunodominant epitope of the HIV gp120 envelope glycoprotein recognized by class I MHC molecule-restricted murine cytotoxic T lymphocytes. Proc Natl Acad Sci USA, 85: 3105–3109 (1988).

46. Townsend ARM, Rothbard J, Gotch FM, Gahadur G, Wraith D, McMichael AJ. The epitopes of influenza nucleoprotein recognized by cytotoxic T lymphocytes can be defined with short synthetic peptides. Cell, 44: 959–968 (1986).

47. Thiel HJ, Schwarz H, Fischinger P, Bolognesi D, Schafer W. Role of antibodies to murine leukemia virus p15E transmembrane protein in immunotherapy against AKR leukemia: A model for studies in human acquired immunodeficiency syndrome. Proc Natl Acad Sci USA, 84: 5893–5897 (1987).

48. Townsend ARM, Skehel JJ. Influenza A specific cytotoxic T-cell clones that do not recognise viral glycoproteins. Nature, 300: 655–657 (1982).

49. Townsend ARM, Skehel JJ. The influenza A virus nucleoprotein gene controls the induction of both subtype specific and crossreactive cytotoxic T cells. J Exp Med, 160: 552–563 (1984).

50. Tevethia SS, Lewis AJ, Campbell AE, Tevethia MJ, Rigby PWJ. Simian virus 40 specific cytotoxic lymphocyte clones localize two distinct TSTA sites on cells synthesizing a 48 kD T antigen. Virol, 133:443–447 (1984).

51. Yewdell JW, Bennink JR, Mackett M, Lefrancois L, Lyles DS, Moss B. Recognition of cloned vesicular stomatitis virus internal and external gene products by cytotoxic T lymphocytes. J Exp Med, 163: 1529–1538 (1986).

52. Yewdell JW, Bennink JR, Smith GL, Moss B. Influenza A virus nucleoprotein is a major target antigen for cross-reactive anti-influenza A virus cytotoxic T lymphocytes. Proc Natl Acad Sci USA, 82: 1785–1789 (1985).

53. Bangham CRM, Openshaw PJM, Ball LA, King AMQ, Wertz GW, Askonas BA. Human and murine cytotoxic T cells specific to respiratory syncytial virus recognize the viral nucleoprotein (N), but not the major glycoprotein (G), expressed by vaccinia virus recombinants. J Immunol, 137: 3973–3977 (1986).

54. Krzych U, Fowler AV, Miller A, Sercarz EE. Induction of helper and suppressor T cells to nonoverlapping determinants on the large protein antigen, β-galactosidase. FASEB J, 2: 141–145 (1988).

55. Gurney ME, Heinrich SP, Lee MR, Yin HS. Molecular cloning and expression of neuroleukin, a neurotrophic factor for spinal and sensory neurons. Science, 234: 566–574 (1986).

56. Gurney ME, Apatoff BR, Spear GT, Baumel MJ, Antel JP, Bania MB, Reder AT. Neuroleukin: A lymphokine product of lectin-stimulated T cells. Science, 234: 574–581 (1986).

57. Beck S, Barrell BG. Human cytomegalovirus encodes a glycoprotein homologous to MHC Class-I antigens. Nature, 331: 269–272 (1988).

58. Milich DR, Thornton GB, Neurath AR, Kent SB, Michel M-L, Tiollais P, Chisari FV. Enhanced immunogenicity of the pre-S region of hepatitis B surface antigen. Science, 228: 1195–1199 (1985).

59. Good MF, Maloy WL, Lunde MN, Margalit H, Cornette JL, Smith GL, Moss B, Miller LH, Berzofsky JA. Construction of synthetic immunogen: Use of new T-helper epitope on malaria circumsporozoite protein. Science; 235: 1059–1062 (1987).

60. Klipstein FA, Engert RF, Houghten RA. Immunisation of volunteers with a synthetic peptide vaccine for enterotoxigenic *Escherichia coli*. Lancet, i: 471–473 (1986).

61. Francis, MJ, Fry CM, Clarke BE, Rowlands DJ, Brown F, Bittle JL, Houghten RA, Lerner RA. A foot-and-mouth disease virus synthetic peptide containing B- and T-cell determinants. In Chanock, R. M., Lerner, R. A., Brown, F., and H. Ginsberg, eds. Vaccines 87—Modern approaches to new vaccines: Prevention of AIDS and other viral, bacterial, and parasitic diseases. Cold Spring Harbor, New York: Cold Spring Harbor Laboratory, 1987: 60–67.

62. Minden P, Houghten RA, Spear JR, Shinnick TM. A chemically synthesized peptide which elicits humoral and cellular immune responses to mycobacterial antigens. Infection and Immunity, 53: 560–564 (1986).

63. Milich DR, Hughes JL, McLachlan A, Thornton GB, Boriarty A. Hepatitis B synthetic immunogen comprised of nucleocapsid T-cell sites and an envelope B-cell epitope. Proc Natl Acad Sci USA, 85: 1610–1614 (1988).

64. Francis MJ, Hastings GZ, Syred AD, McGinn B, Brown F, Rowlands DJ. Non-responsiveness to a foot-and-mouth disease virus peptide overcome by addition of foreign helper T-cell determinants. Nature, 330: 168–170 (1987).

65. Brett SJ, Cease KB, Berzofsky JA. Influences of antigen processing on the expression of the T cell repertoire: Evidence for MHC-specific hindering structures on the products of processing. J Exp Med, 168: 357–373 (1988).

66. Dryberg T, Oldstone MBA. Orientation of peptide antigens relative to carrier proteins influence antibody specificity. In Chanock, R. M., Lerner, R. A., Brown, F., and H. Ginsberg, eds. Vaccines 87—Modern approaches to new vaccines: Prevention of AIDS and other viral, bacterial, and parasitic diseases. Cold Spring Harbor, New York: Cold Spring Harbor Laboratory, 1987: 38–43.

67. Jacob CO, Arnon R, Sela M. Effect of carrier on the immunogenic capacity of synthetic cholera vaccine. Mol Immunol, 22: 1333–1339 (1985).

68. Nicolaisen-Strouss K, Kumar HPM, Fitting T, Grant CK, Elder JH. Natural Feline leukemia virus variant escapes neutralization by a monoclonal antibody via an amino acid change outside the antibody-binding epitope. J Virol, 61: 3410–3415 (1987).

69. Coffin JM. Genetic variability of the AIDS virus: Nucleotide sequence analysis of two isolates from African patients. Cell, 46: 63–74 (1986).

70. Beachey EH, Seyer JM, Dale JB. Protective immunogenicity and T lympho-cyte specificity of a trivalent hybrid peptide containing NH2-terminal sequences of types 5, 7, and 24 M proteins synthesized in tandem. J Exptl Med, 166: 647–656 (1987).
71. Patarroyo, ME, Romero P, Torres ML, Clavijo P, Moreno A, Martinez A, Rodriguez R, Guzman F, Cabezas E. Induction of protective immunity against experimental infection with malaria using synthetic peptides. Nature, 328: 629–632 (1987).
72. Patarroyo ME, Amador R, Clavijo P, Moreno A, Guzman F, Romero P, Tascon R, Franco A, Murillo LA, Ponton G, Trujillo G. A synthetic vaccine protects humans against challenge with asexual blood stages of *Plasmodium falciparum* malaria. Nature, 332: 158-161 (1988).

REFERENCES ADDED IN PROOF

73. Goudsmit J, et al. Human immunodeficiency virus type 1 neutralization epitope with conserved architecture elicits early type-specific antibodies in experimentally infected chimpanzees. Proc Natl Acad Sci USA, 85: 4478-4482 (1988).
74. Javaherian K, et al. Principal neutralizing domain of the human immuno-deficiency virus type 1 envelope protein. Proc Natl Acad Sci USA, 86: 6768–6772 (1989).
75. Clerici M, et al. Interleukin-2 production used to detect antigenic peptide recognition by T-helper lymphocytes from asymptomatic HIV seropositive individuals. Nature, 339: 383–385 (1989).
76. Hale PM, et al. T cell multideterminant regions in the human immunodefi-ciency virus envelope: toward overcoming the problem of major histocom-patibility complex restriction. Internat Immunol, 1: 409–415 (1989).
77. Cornette JL, et al. Concepts and methods in the identification of T cell epitopes and their use in the construction of synthetic vaccines. Methods Enzymol, 178: 611–634 (1989).
78. Takahashi H, et al. A single amino acid interchange yields reciprocal CTL specificities for HIV gp160. Science, 246: 118-121 (1989).
79. Takahashi H, et al. Structural requirements for class-I MHC molecule-mediated antigen presentation and cytotoxic T-cell recognition of an immunodominant determinant of the HIV envelope protein. J Exp Med, 170, in press (1989).
80. Tsubota H, et al. A cytotoxic T lymphocyte inhibits acquired immunode-ficiency syndrome virus replication in peripheral blood lymphocytes. J Exp Med, 169: 1421-1434 (1989).
81. Golding H, et al. Identification of homologous regions in human immuno-deficiency virus I gp41 and human MHC class II β 1 domain I. Monoclonal antibodies against the gp41-derived peptide and patients' sera react with native HLA class II antigens, suggesting a role for autoimmunity in the pathogenesis of acquired immune deficiency syndrome. J Exp Med, 167: 914–923 (1988).

7

Anti-HIV-1 ADCC

H. Kim Lyerly, Douglas S. Tyler, Chet L. Nastala, and Kent J. Weinhold
Duke University Medical Center
Durham, North Carolina

INTRODUCTION

A comprehensive approach to the development of preventive or interventive anti-HIV-1 therapeutic strategies must incorporate elements capable of eliciting widely diverse immune reactivities. In addition to virus neutralizing antibodies, a candidate vaccine, for example, should stimulate virus-specific cytotoxic activities capable of destroying HIV-1-infected cells. Such activities include: 1) HLA-restricted and -unrestricted cytotoxic T-lymphocytes (CTL), 2) cytolytic antibodies, 3) antibody-dependent cellular cytotoxicity (ADCC), and perhaps 4) cytotoxic macrophages, 5) natural killer (NK) cells, and 6) lymphokine-activated killer (LAK) cells. The purpose of this chapter is to provide an overview of our current understanding of various forms of ADCC as they relate to HIV-1-specific protective and pathogenic responses, with particular emphasis on recent findings in our own laboratory. As a means of organizing this presentation we will discuss, under separate headings, the specific areas of ADCC target antigens, the specificity and ontogeny of antibodies directing ADCC, effector cells, direct forms of ADCC in HIV-1-infected individuals, and therapeutic approaches based on augmentation of ADCC reactivities.

TARGET ANTIGENS AND ANTIBODY SPECIFICITIES FOR ADCC

Because of its potential utility in both preventive and interventive therapeutic strategies, the elements which comprise anti-HIV-1 ADCC have recently come under close experimental scrutiny. A central issue in many of these studies relates to the targets for ADCC reactivities. This can be examined at two interrelated levels, namely: 1) which HIV-1 antigens expressed on cells confer lytic susceptibility to ADCC? and 2) what is the specificity of antibodies which direct ADCC? Our current understanding of anti-HIV-1 ADCC reactivities is based largely on the reports listed in Table 1. These studies will provide a framework to discuss the numerous approaches to the measurement of ADCC in HIV-1-infected individuals.

Target Antigens for ADCC

From a technical standpoint, the single most important aspect in determining ADCC activity is the selection of an appropriate target cell population. This, in itself, has been a formidable obstacle for many investigators, since most of the established human cell lines that are susceptible to HIV-1 infection are likewise highly susceptible to lysis by natural killer (NK) cells. These cell lines include H-9, HUT-78, Molt 4, U937, and CEM, to name but a few. Thus, the normal peripheral blood mononuclear cells (PBMC) employed as effectors in most ADCC assays contain high lytic activities against both noninfected and HIV-1-infected cells in the absence of antibodies, indicative of NK reactivity. In many cases, addition of patient sera results in only slight increases in specific lysis. In this manner, normal NK reactivity can mask HIV-1-specific ADCC. To overcome this problem, our laboratory sought to obtain NK-resistant cell lines susceptible to HIV-1 infection. In 1985, Howell and coworkers reported that NK-resistant sublines of human T lymphoblastoid cells could be derived by repeated co-cultivation in the presence of normal PBMC (8). Adopting this strategy, it was possible to obtain an NK-resistant variant of the CEM line, which we referred to as CEM.NKR. Whereas the standard CEM line was highly susceptible to NK lysis

Table 1 Anti-HIV-1 Antibody-Dependent Cellular Cytotoxicity (ADCC)

Antigen	Target cells	References
env (gp120)	Normal CD4$^+$ lymphocytes + gp120 CEM.NKR + gp120 CEM.NKR/HIV-1	1–3
env (?)	Molt 4/HIV-1 CEM6hiv-1	4
env (?)	U937/HIV-1	5
env (gp41)	H-9/HIV-1	6
gag (?)	A3.01/HIV-1	7

(i.e., 50-70% lysis at 50:1 E:T ratio), the immunoselected CEM.NKR subline was nearly refractory to lysis by NK cells (i.e., 1-5% lysis at 50:1 E:% ratio). For the first time, measurements of ADCC reactivity could be made without the complication of high NK lysis.

Like the parental CEM line, the CEM.NKR subline exhibited high expression of OKT4A-defined cell surface CD4 epitopes. In addition, this line retained its high susceptibility to infection by various prototypic and field strains of HIV-1. Both the CEM and CEM.NKR target lines are extremely sensitive to the cytopathic effects of HIV-1. In order to obtain a stably infected population of targets, CEM.NKR cells are acutely infected with HIV-1, which results in death of >99% of cells within 7-14 days. By day 21, a subpopulation of "grow through" cells becomes apparent. In the majority of cases, these cells are infected with HIV-1 and express cell surface viral antigens. They retain this expression for 4-6 weeks during which time they are excellent targets for ADCC. Eventually, this subpopulation loses cell surface viral expression and becomes refractile to any form of anti-HIV-1 cytolysis. Therefore, new "grow through" lines must be continually established.

An alternative approach to using infected cell lines as ADCC targets takes advantage of the high affinity interaction between cell surface CD4 and the HIV-1 envelope glycoprotein gp120 (9,10). In this scheme, highly purified HIV-1 gp120 is incubated with CEM. NKR cells under conditions that will saturate all available CD4 molecules. Since the number of CD4 molecules on these cells remains relatively stable, the quantity of gp120 adsorbed onto the surface of CEM.NKR cells is fairly constant. This, in turn, minimizes the major variable contributing to assay-to-assay variation—quantities of relevant antigen expressed on the surface of target cells.

A second, and perhaps equally important, aspect of cells bearing passively adsorbed gp120 is their utility in examining the role of the major envelope glycoprotein as a target antigen in the absence of other HIV-1 structural components which may be present on the surface of infected cells. Our laboratory has screened several hundred sera for ADCC activity against HIV-1-infected versus gp120-adsorbed CEM.NKR targets. We have yet to identify a serum which directs the lysis of infected targets but fails to behave similarly against gp120-adsorbed cells. These observations strongly suggest that epitopes contained in gp120 represent the major targets for ADCC.

Antibody Specificities

The specificity of the antibodies which direct ADCC against HIV-1-infected targets can also be utilized to map epitopes which serve as targets for ADCC. In one of the first reports of anti-HIV-1 ADCC, Rook and coworkers (7) concluded, "antibody reactivity with the p24 protein of HTLV-III/LAV correlated with higher levels of ADCC activity than did reactivity with Gp120/160." While this correlation may exist in certain groups, it is not likely to be indicative of anti-p24 antibodies directing ADCC. To date no laboratory, including our own, has been able to demonstrate conclusively that anti-p24 antibodies can direct anti-HIV-1 ADCC. Although nonenvelope structural antigens have been shown, in murine systems, to serve as ADCC targets (11), there is still a great deal of speculation concerning the presence of p24 antigens on the surface of infected cells.

Such uncertainty does not, however, exist concerning the role of gp120 epitopes as ADCC targets. Ojo-Amaize and coworkers reported that patient sera devoid of detectable anti-gp120 reactivities (determined by radioimmunoprecipitation assays) failed to direct ADCC even though these same sera contained anti-p24 and anti-p55 activities (4). Serologic evidence from our own laboratory revealed that following passage of sera from infected patients over a gp120 affinity column, highly reactive ADCC antibodies were contained in the column eluates (2). Repeated passage of the effluent material over the gp120 column failed to remove all of the ADCC antibodies active against gp120-coated targets, most likely indicating that both high affinity (eluate) and low affinity (effluent) anti-gp120 antibodies can direct ADCC or another *env* target antigen (i.e., gp41) exists.

Antibodies that direct virus neutralization are also directed against gp120 epitopes. An important aspect in understanding the host immune response with particular relevance to vaccine strategies would be to consider epitopes of gp120 that are targets for both viral neutralization and ADCC. In early studies, we compared the viral neutralizing activity, the ADCC activity, and the ability of serum to block the gp120/CD4 interaction leading to cell fusion in 37 patient sera (12). Neutralizing titers were plotted against both fusion blocking and ADCC titers. Linear regression analysis revealed a coefficient of correlation of 0.85 between viral neutralizing and cell fusion blocking activity, indicating a high degree of correlation. However, a coefficient of correlation of only 0.05 was found between viral neutralizing activity and ADCC activity, indicating a low degree of correlation. These studies suggest that epitopes acting as ADCC targets may be distinct from neutralizing epitopes.

Studies aimed at mapping the fine specificity of ADCC epitopes within the gp120 molecule are the focus of ongoing efforts in a number of laboratories. We have adopted the approach of coupling recombinant or synthetic peptides of known amino acid composition to solid supports in order to bind antibodies contained in polyspecific patient sera. Eluates from such columns are subsequently assayed for their ability to direct ADCC. Using this strategy, we found that antibodies which bind to the recombinant peptide pEnv 9 (2) efficiently direct ADCC. This peptide represents the carboxyl end (46 amino acids) of gp120 and extends beyond the midportion of gp41 (13). Blumberg and coworkers have recently reported that mice immunized with synthetic peptides representing regions within gp41 produce antibodies capable of directing ADCC against HIV-1-infected targets (6). A comprehensive analysis of human seroreactivity against regions within this portion of the HIV-1 envelope gene product using synthetic peptide octomers is the focus of future studies.

Perhaps two of the most distinctive features of anti-HIV ADCC are the relatively high titers of ADCC antibodies found in patient sera as well as their broad cytolytic reactivity. The great majority of sera analyzed for ADCC activities against gp120-adsorbed targets exhibit optimal lytic activities at dilutions of 10^{-3}-10^{-5}. Our laboratory has also analyzed large numbers of patient sera in assays against CEM.NKR targets infected with HTLV-III$_B$, HTLV-III$_{MN}$, and HTLV-III$_{RF}$ isolates of HIV-1. These studies revealed that over 80% of patient sera exhibited nearly equivalent lysis of all three infected cell lines, indicating broad cytolytic reactivity. The remaining 20% of sera exhibited preferential cytolytic reactivity against targets infected with one of the prototypic isolates with lower but detectable activity against the other target lines. In no case was absolute isolate specificity observed. It should be stressed here that we do not know the extent to which this broad prototypic reactivity carries over to individual patient isolates. However, within the context of the prototypic isolates, this broad specificity could result from antibody reactivities againt conserved epitopes shared among the three isolates or from type-specific reactivity against each of the isolates. To examine these possibilities, broadly reactive sera from two patients was passed over an affinity column comprised of purified HTLV-III$_B$ gp120 coupled to Sepharose 4B. If group reactivity was due to a combination of individual type specificities, the eluates from the HTLV-III$_B$ gp120 column should direct HTLV-III$_B$-specific ADCC. As shown in Figure 1, gp120 eluates retain their group reactivity in lysing HTLV-III$_B$ and HTLV-III$_{RF}$ targets, thus indicating specificity against conserved epitopes within the gp120 molecule. In contrast, the virus-neutralizing activity of the column eluate remained highly type-specific for HTLV-III$_B$—again reaffirming our contention that epitopes other than those associated with virus neutralization can serve as ADCC targets.

Antibodies which direct ADCC might show anticarbohydrate specificity for the heavily glycosylated gp120 molecule. Carbohydrate moieties have been demonstrated to play a large role in the ability of gp120 to bind to the CD4 molecule. Purified gp120 which has been deglycosylated has been shown to be ineffective in binding to CD4 (9). Furthermore, cells infected with HIV-1 isolates and grown in the presence of castanospermine (CAST), an alpha-glucosidase inhibitor, lose their ability to produce both infectious virus and participate in cell fusion with CD4-bearing cells, presumably due to the alterations in the gp120. Target cells infected with isolates of HIV-1 and cultured in the presence

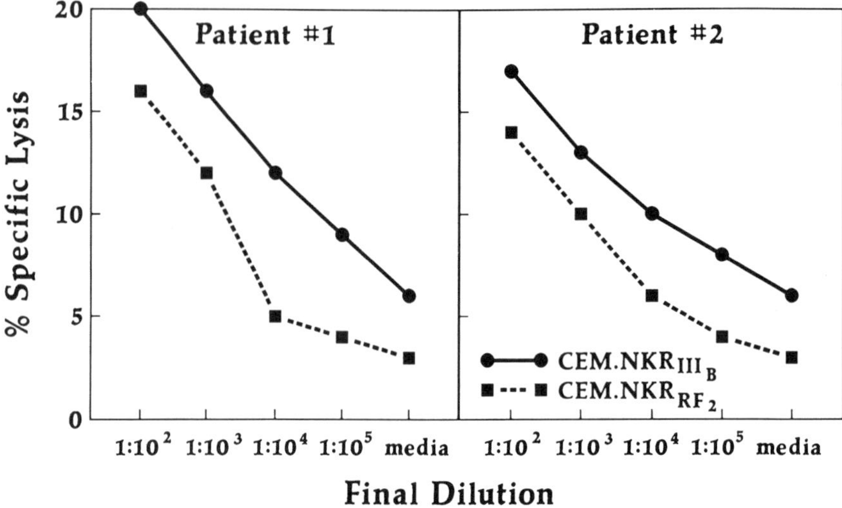

Figure 1 ADCC activity of antibody eluates from an HTLV–III$_B$ gp120 column tested against targets infected with the widely diverse HTLV–III$_B$ and HTLV–III$_{RF2}$ isolates of HIV-1.

of CAST at concentrations which alter the gp120 by Western blot analysis remain susceptible to ADCC. Furthermore, antibodies contained in the eluates of serum passed over gp120 columns retain the ability to direct the lysis of cells infected with divergent HIV-1 isolates despite alteration in the gp120 glycosylation. Thus, anticarbohydrate reactivities do not appear to play a major role in ADCC. Finally, it should be noted that although sera from HIV-1–infected individuals exhibit broad reactivity against HIV-1 isolates, this specificity apparently does not include HIV-2 antigens since Ljunggren and coworkers have reported a lack of ADCC cross-reactivity between HIV-1 and HIV-2 isolates (14).

Many of the patient sera analyzed for anti-HIV ADCC exhibit a distinct "prozone" of suboptimal lytic activity at high serum concentrations. Routinely, this prozone extends through the serum dilutions against gp120 adsorbed cells. This phenomenon is illustrated in Figure 2 using a representative serum. The basis for this "prozone" reactivity remains elusive, but may involve "blocking" antibodies or immune complexes. Further studies of this phenomenon are underway.

Antibody Isotypes Directing ADCC

Several studies have attempted to identify the isotype of antibodies mediating ADCC, as the selection of IgG isotype does not appear to occur at random and isotypes vary widely in their biological activity. We have shown that antibodies which mediate HIV-specific ADCC are primarily of the IgG_1 isotype (15). This conclusion is based on studies in which anti-isotype monoclonal antibodies were used to inhibit gp120-specific ADCC. As shown in Figure 3, anti-IgG_1 antibodies were found to preferentially inhibit ADCC when compared to anti-IgG_2, anti-IgG_3, and anti-IgG_4 antibodies. However, the antibody response to the envelope proteins, in general, has also been reported to be confined to the IgG_1 isotype (16,17), indicating that anti-*env* IgG_2, IgG_3, and IgG_4 antibody isotypes may not be present in patient sera. Therefore, it still remains to be determined whether antibodies of other isotypes could direct ADCC against HIV-1-expressing targets.

ONTOGENIC ASPECTS OF ADCC REACTIVITIES

As discussed in the previous sections, sera from infected individuals contains high titers of broadly reactive antibodies capable of directing ADCC against HIV-1 *env* gene products. A number of issues relating to the events which lead to the establishment of this activity merit further attention. Two questions of particular relevance to the development of preventive therapeutic strategies are: 1) is the appearance of broadly reactive antibodies preceded by isolate-specific ADCC early in infection? and 2) does the appearance of ADCC-directing antibodies coincide temporally with the development of neutralizing antibodies? Information relating to these two issues can be readily obtained from animals or

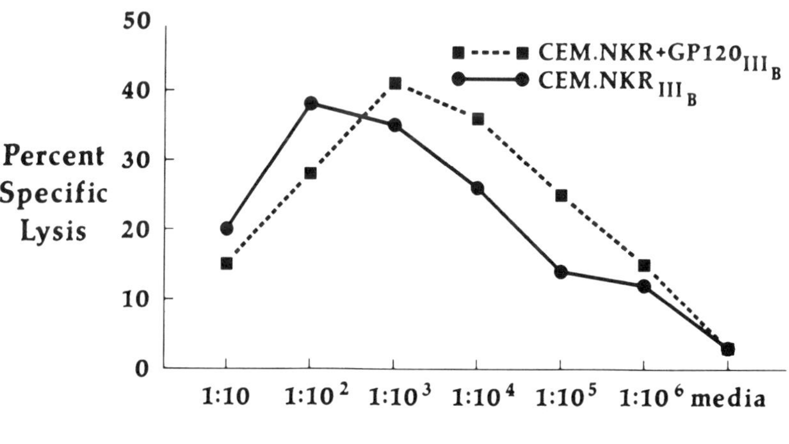

Figure 2 ADCC activity directed by serum from a representative HIV-1-infected patient tested against HTLV-III$_B$-infected and gp120-adsorbed targets.

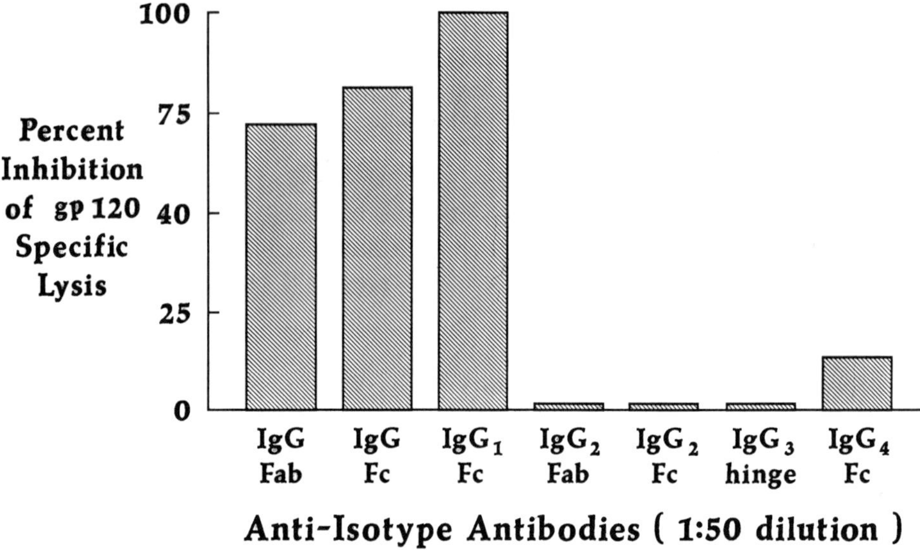

Figure 3 Inhibition of gp120-specific ADCC by antibodies directed against human Ig fragments and isotypes.

patients infected with known isolates of HIV-1 in whom serum samples were taken during the early postinfection period. In this section, we will summarize the pertinent information obtained from infected chimpanzees and from a laboratory worker accidentally exposed to the HTLV-III$_B$ isolate of HIV-1. We will also discuss the status of ADCC antibodies in infected individuals at various disease states.

Infected Chimpanzees

The chimpanzee has been utilized extensively as a model for HIV-1 infection. Although no apparent disease has been observed following HIV-1 inoculation, a stable HIV-1 infection is readily established in infected animals. Infected chimpanzees produce antibodies capable of directing HIV-1 ADCC. As can be seen in Figure 4, ADCC activity against HTLV-III$_B$ infected cells is apparent within 2 months (Bleed #2) after inoculation of HTLV-III$_B$, and activity continues to rise rapidly thereafter. Although not shown in this figure, the cytolytic reactivity against target cells infected with the HTLV-III$_{RF}$ isolate of HIV-1 parallels the lysis of HTLV-III$_B$ infected targets. Thus, isolate restricted ADCC is not apparent in infected chimps at any point during the early postinfection period. This is in marked contrast to the neutralizing antibodies produced in infected chimps which exhibit highly isolate restricted activities in the early postinfection period.

Infected Laboratory Worker

A major problem in sorting out the ontogeny of isolate versus broadly reactive ADCC activities in infected individuals is the possibility that infection with more than one isolate could have occurred. Therefore, even sera obtained shortly after infection could contain multiple isolate specificities which mimic broad reactivity. One group of individuals where such concerns are eliminated are laboratory workers accidentally infected with a single known isolate of HIV-1. In conjunction with Dr. William Blattner and his colleagues, our laboratory has studied the anti-HIV-1 serologic activities of serial samples obtained from such an individual at various intervals following exposure to and infection by the HTLV-III$_B$ isolate of HIV-1. These studies revealed that antibodies capable of directing ADCC appeared prior to all other functional reactivities including virus neutralization, fusion inhibition, and blockade of gp120/CD4 interactions. In this individual, ADCC antibodies were detected prior to seropositivity by Western blot analysis. This observation could be consistent with the development of antibodies to the region of gp120/41 represented by pEnv 9 (12). Finally, in a manner which paralleled the observations made with infected chimps, the ADCC reactivity was broadly reactive from the onset—thus reinforcing the notion that isolate restricted ADCC activities if they indeed exist, may be difficult to detect since they can be easily masked by the early broad reactivity.

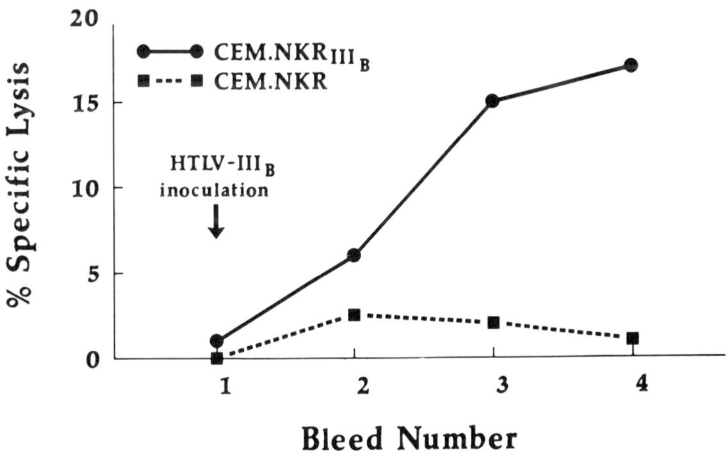

Figure 4 Ontogeny of ADCC directing antibodies in the serum of a chimpanzee inoculated with HTLV-III$_B$. The interval between each bleed is 2 months.

ADCC vs. Stage of Disease

From the studies highlighted in the previous section, it is apparent that ADCC reactivity appears early after infection with titers increasing progressively thereafter. However, a major question remained concerning whether these levels persisted with progression of disease or declined in a manner similar to that reported for anti-p24 antibodies (18). To address this question, serum samples were obtained from a cohort of patients established by Dr. Robert Redfield at the Walter Reed Army Hospital. Sera from a total of 137 patients at various Walter Reed stages of disease were tested for ADCC activity. As shown in Figure 5, no significant difference existed in the mean level (closed squares) of lysis by sera from infected patients at various stages. This implies, from a random sampling, that ADCC activity in patient sera does not vary significantly with disease progression. Confirmatory longitudinal surveys of individual patient sera are currently underway.

EFFECTOR CELLS MEDIATING ADCC

By definition, ADCC is a *serologic* measurement of the capacity of antibodies to direct the lysis of target cells by normal NK/K cells effectors. Thus, the normal donor PBMC routinely used as effector cells in ADCC assays is simply

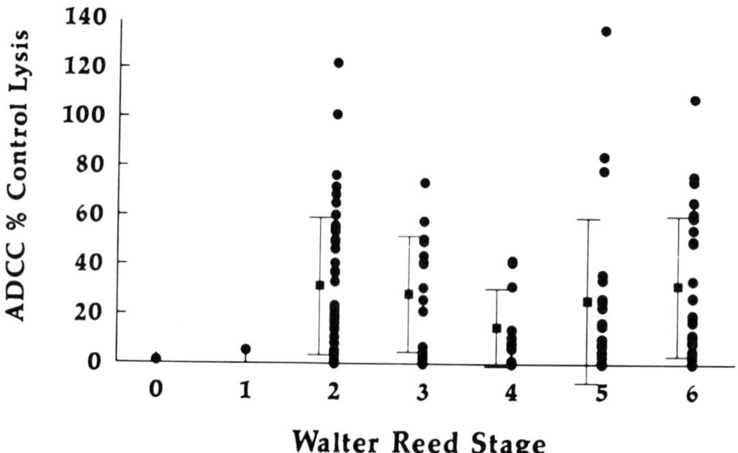

Figure 5 ADCC-directing antibodies in a cohort of infected individuals at various stages of disease. All sera were tested at a final 1:1000 dilution against gp120-adsorbed targets. Control lysis was derived from a preselected reference serum from an HIV-1–infected individual.

a reagent used to make this measurement. If ADCC is defective in HIV-1-infected individuals, the defect could occur at the level of effector cells. This possibility will be addressed in the latter sections of this chapter. However, the ability of sera from infected individuals to direct target cell lysis by normal PBMC has great relevance to a number of scenarios which either exist naturally or are being considered as possible therapeutic strategies. Three such settings where anti-HIV antibodies would interact with "normal" effectors include: 1) active immunization of noninfected individuals as a vaccine strategy, 2) passive administration of high-titered anti-HIV IgG immediately following exposure to the virus, and 3) placental transfer of immunoglobulin from mother to fetus.

Although it was originally thought that the effector cells which mediate ADCC, termed K cells, were a discrete population distinct from natural killer (NK) cells, current evidence suggests that NK lysis and ADCC are mediated by identical or largely overlapping populations (19-21). The Fc receptor (FcR) present on NK/K cells (22) binds selected subclasses of immunoglobulin, and, in doing so, the cell acquires its antigen receptor. Extensive characterization of NK/K cell effectors reveals their phenotypic pattern to be $CD2^-$, $CD3^-$, $Leu7^+$, $Leu19^+$. Of these markers, CD16 defines the Fc receptor (22). Even though this cell population is phenotypically homogenous, functional defects can be selective. In this regard, Katz and coworkers have recently reported that NK/K cells obtained from AIDS patients may be defective in triggering NK cytolysis but possess intact lytic activities when triggered by the FcR for ADCC (23).

It has been shown previously that NK activity can be augmented by various agents, including interleukin-2 (IL-2) and gamma interferon (IFN) (24). In a series of in vitro studies, we examined the effect of IL-2 on anti-HIV ADCC. We found that a standard dose of 5 BRMP units/ml of IL-2 added at the beginning of the 4-hour assay dramatically augmented the cytolysis of $HTLV-III_B$-infected and gp120-adsorbed target cells in the presence of normal donor effector cells (25). These findings may have important ramifications in the design of multimodal approaches to anti-HIV therapy. These approaches will be discussed further later in this chapter.

GP120 SPECIFIC CELL-MEDIATED CYTOTOXICITY (CMC)

Examination of the various cellular reactivities present in HIV-1-infected individuals has revealed a gp120-specific cytotoxic response that mediates lysis via a form of ADCC. The following section will provide a characterization of this gp120-specific cell-mediated cytotoxicity (CMC) and a comparison of how this activity correlates with the anti-gp120 ADCC activities described in the previous sections.

Characterization

Fresh peripheral blood mononuclear cells (PBMC) isolated from HIV-1-infected individuals have been shown to lyse autologous and heterologous CD4$^+$ lymphocytes coated with free gp120 purified from the III$_B$ strain of HIV-1 in short-term ^{51}Cr release assays (26,27). This non-MHC–restricted cytolytic response is greatest in asymptomatic HIV-1-seropositive individuals and declines significantly with disease progression into ARC and AIDS. The ability of each patient's effector cells to lyse targets coated with gp120 from the III$_B$ strain, which would be different from the gp120 of their own HIV-1 isolate, suggested the presence of a broad cytolytic reactivity against gp120. This characteristic was confirmed when freshly isolated PBMC from seropositive individuals were found to have equivalent lytic activities against targets coated with gp120 purified from either the HTLV–III$_B$ or HTLV–III$_{RF2}$ isolate of HIV.

In addition to the broad reactivity, the lack of MHC-restricted killing suggested that the effector cell mediating this cytolytic response was not a classical CD8$^+$ or CD4$^+$ CTL. Subsequent studies employing cytotoxic depletion of effector cells with monoclonal phenotyping antibodies and complement revealed the killer cells mediating this response to be CD16$^+$, Leu7$^+$, CD15$^-$, CD4$^-$, CD3$^-$ NK/K cells and not T cells. This phenotype was identical to that of the seronegative effector cells in the ADCC assays described in previous sections. Although NK/K cells in seronegative individuals are classically known for their ability to spontaneously lyse a number of malignant and nonneoplastic target cells, they do not preferentially lyse gp120 expressing cells. Cold target competition assays using unlabeled target cells coated with free gp120 revealed that the form of NK/K cell cytloysis present in HIV-1-infected individuals was specifically directed at gp120. This observation suggested that gp120-specific CMC involved an antigen receptor distinct from the putative NK/K cell receptor and unique to the NK/K cells of HIV-1-infected individuals.

To confirm that gp120-specific CMC was mediated via a different receptor than the putative NK/K cell receptor and to see if the effector cells mediating this response could lyse virally infected targets in addition to those coated with free gp120, the CEM.NKR cell line was used. The effector cells isolated from HIV-1-infected patients exhibited significant lytic activities against both the gp120-adsorbed and targets infected with widely divergent HIV-1 isolates (III$_B$, MN, RF) but not CEM.NKR cells, which do not express gp120. Lymphocytes from uninfected individuals show no significant lytic activity against CEM.NKR cells regardless of their gp120 expression.

As a means of determining whether the same epitopes on gp120 were being recognized by effector cells against infected versus adsorbed targets, cold target competition assays were again employed. Not only could unlabeled infected targets compete for killing of gp120 adsorbed cells, but also unlabeled targets bearing adsorbed gp120 on their surface competed for killing of virally infected targets. These observations add further support to the contention that gp120 is the predominant CMC target in seropositive individuals regardless of its orientation on the target cell surface. The amount of surface expression necessary to render a given target cell susceptible to cytolysis via gp120-specific CMC is currently under investigation. However, recent evidence using various concentrations of free gp120 would suggest that lysis via this mechanism can occur at sub-saturating levels of gp120 when many potential CD4 binding sites on a target cell are not occupied (K. Weinhold, unpublished observation).

Antigen Receptors

Many similarities exist between gp120-specific CMC and anti-gp120 ADCC. These similarities, including broad cytolytic reactivity, non–MHC–restricted killing and the phenotypic populations of NK/K cells mediating the cytolysis, suggested that gp120-specific CMC could represent a form of ADCC mediated via anti-gp120 antibodies bound directly to the surface of NK/K cells. This concept, depicted in Figure 6, was supported by studies in which F(ab′)₂ fragments

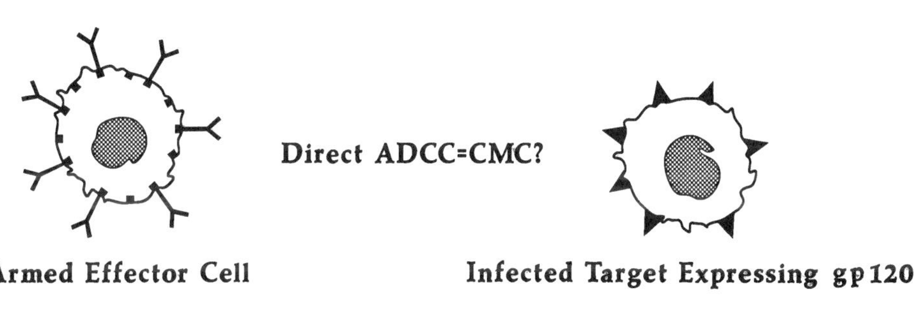

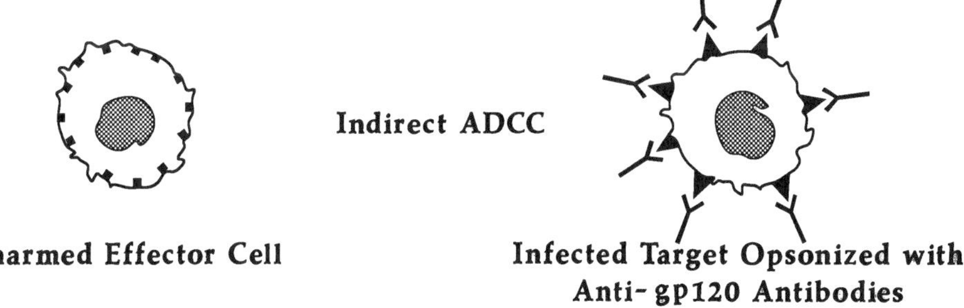

Figure 6   Schematic representation of direct versus indirect ADCC.

of anti-immunoglobulin directed against the F(ab')$_2$ and Fc portion of human IgG were used in attempts to block gp120-specific CMC. Significant inhibition over a broad range of antibody dilutions was seen with both the anti-F(ab')$_2$ and anti-Fc fragments, as shown in Figure 7. No significant inhibition was seen using an F(ab')$_2$ fragment of antialbumin as a control. None of the three fragments showed any inhibitory effect on NK activity against K562 targets (28, 29). Subsequent studies showed that anti-IgG$_1$ isotype antibodies and not antibodies against IgG$_2$, IgG$_3$, or IgG$_4$ could significantly inhibit gp120-specific CMC (15). Taken together, the marked inhibition of gp120-specific CMC by anti-immunoglobulin antibodies and fragments strongly suggests that antibodies of the IgG$_1$ isotype directed against gp120 act as antigen receptors during cytolysis.

While anti-F(ab')$_2$ fragments would be expected to inhibit gp120-specific CMC by interfering with the interaction between the cytophilic antibody acting as antigen receptor and gp120, it is somewhat surprising that such marked inhibition of CMC can be obtained using an anti-Fc fragment. In addition, the anti-Fc receptor (FcR) antibody (Leu 11b) can also significantly inhibit gp120-specific CMC but not NK activity against K562 targets. The marked inhibition of gp120-specific CMC seen with both anti-Fc and anti-FcR antibodies most likely reflects the relative differences in affinities of these blocking antibodies for their target structures versus that of cytophilic antibody for the FcR on NK/K cells. As shown in Figure 8, the binding between cytophilic IgG and the FcR on NK/K cells is an apparently low affinity interaction. The affinities of

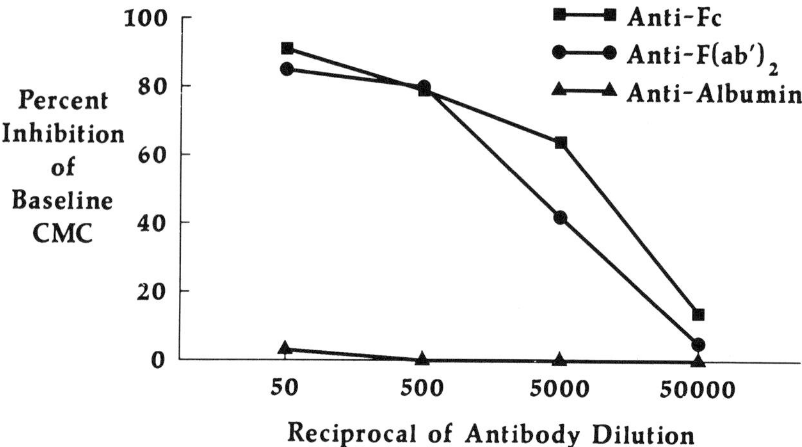

Figure 7 Inhibition of gp120-specific CMC by F(ab')$_2$ fragments of antihuman Fc and F(ab')$_2$ antibodies.

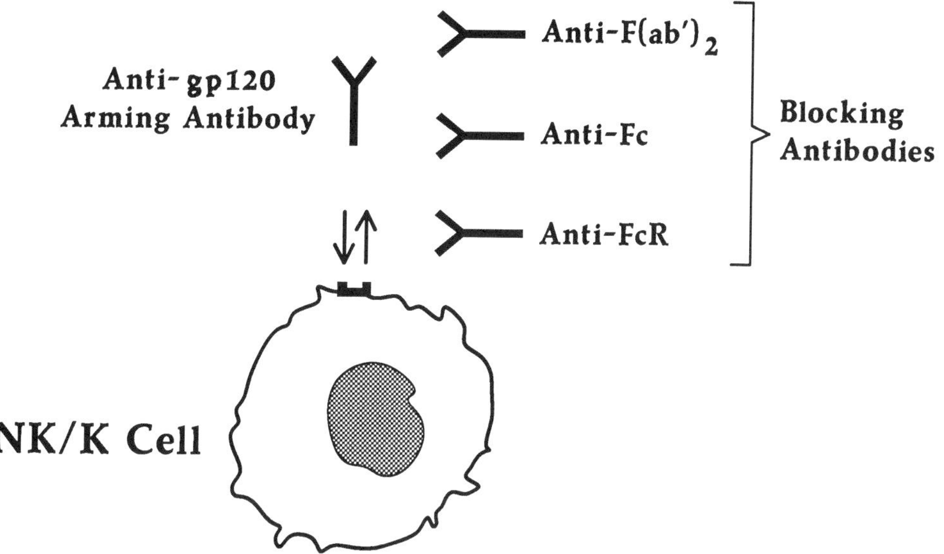

Figure 8 Speculated mechanism by which blocking antibodies inhibit gp120-specific CMC.

anti-Fc and anti-FcR antibodies for their target structures are high. Cytophilic antibodies, by virtue of their low affinity for the NK/K cell FcR, readily dissociate from the cell surface. These antibodies may be prevented from reassociating with the membrane either through their high affinity interaction with anti-Fc antibodies or through the high affinity interaction of the vacant FcR with anti-Leu 11b.

Studies to determine the origin of the anti-gp120 antibodies acting as antigen receptor for gp120-specific CMC in short-term ^{51}Cr release assays suggested that NK/K cells circulate in vivo with these antibodies bound to their surface. If B cells are removed from anti-gp120 cytotoxicity assays using complement depletion, no significant decrease in gp120-specific CMC is observed, indicating that antibodies secreted during the course of the assay play no role in the cytolytic response. In addition, after selective entrichment, anti-gp120 cytophilic antibodies that mediate ADCC can be isolated from the surface of freshly isolated NK/K cells using a short 30-minute, 56°C incubation (28). With this same method, no significant gp120-specific ADCC-mediating antibodies can be recovered from the surface of B cells or monocytes/macrophages. Staphylococcal protein A (SPA) can bind greater than 90% of the anti-gp120 cytophilic antibodies released from the surface of NK/K cells confirming that these antibodies are IgG (29). The fact that NK/K cells bind predominantly antibodies of the IgG_1 and IgG_3 isotypes, and of these two isotypes, SPA binds only IgG_1, supported earlier blocking studies which suggested that the anti-gp120 antibodies acting as antigen receptors during gp120-specific CMC were of the IgG_1 isotype.

Correlation Between Anti-gp120 CMC and ADCC Activities

Although gp120-specific CMC and anti-gp120 ADCC share many similarities, as outlined in Table 2, the interrelationship between the two activities remains to be determined. Serum from HIV-1–infected individuals contains antibodies which can arm lymphocytes from seronegative donors to be cytotoxic for HIV-1–expressing targets after only a short (i.e., 3-hour) incubation (30). There is a highly significant positive correlation between the anti-gp120 ADCC activity of a given serum and how well that serum can arm seronegative lymphocytes to lyse gp120-expressing targets (D. Tyler, unpublished observation). The statistical significance of this correlation is apparently lost with disease progression into ARC and AIDS, suggesting that some factor(s) eventually interferes with the ability of these antibodies to arm NK/K cells.

Interestingly, there is no apparent correlation between the presence of anti-gp120-directing antibodies and gp120-specific CMC. The finding that gp120-specific CMC declines rapidly with disease progression, whereas anti-gp120 ADCC antibody titers and the number of NK/K cells stays relatively stable, suggests that a functional NK/K cell defect occurs early during disease progression.

Table 2 Summary of Anti-HIV-1 ADCC Activities

	Indirect ADCC	Direct ADCC (CMC)
Activity in HIV^+ individuals:		
Asymptomatic	Present	Present (high)
symptomatic	Present	Present (low)–absent
Specificity:		
Target antigen(s)	Gp120 (gp41?)	Gp120
HIV-1 isolate reactivity	Broad	Broad
Antibody isotype	IgG_1	IgG_1, IgG_4 (?)
Effector cells:		
Identity	$CD3^-$, $CD16^+$	$CD3^-$, $CD16^+$, $Leu7^+$
MHC restriction	Absent	Absent
Augmentation:		
Interleukin-2	Positive	Positive

Further support for defective NK/K cell function comes from the inability to increase low levels of gp120-specific CMC mediated by the NK/K cells of either symptomatic or asymptomatic patients by preincubating cells with sera that effectively arm lymphocytes from seronegative donors. This NK/K cell defect, which may be a further manifestation of the NK defect described by Katz and coworkers (23), appears to be related to the cell's lytic mechanism triggered via the Fc receptor and may explain why gp120-specific CMC declines early in the course of infection. As the HIV-1 infection advances on through symptomatic stages, the uncharacterized humoral defects that decrease the arming ability of a patient's sera help compound the inability of a patient's NK/K cells to lyse targets expressing gp120 via the mechanism of ADCC.

Gp120-Specific CMC and Interleukin-2

Currently efforts are underway to see if immune modulators can restore gp120-specific CMC. Recombinant interleukin-2 (IL-2) can significantly augment gp120-specific CMC in short-term assays (26,27). However, this augmentation is closely related to the baseline gp120-specific CMC, such that patients who have high levels of activity augment well, whereas those with low levels of activity augment poorly. This observation suggests that while short-term administration of IL-2 renders gp120-specific CMC more effective, it does little to correct any cellular defect in the NK/K cell lytic mechanism. Studies to examine whether defective NK/K cell ADCC activity can be restored after more prolonged administration of IL-2 in vitro and/or in vivo are presently underway.

THERAPEUTIC APPROACHES

The exact role of antibody-dependent cellular cytotoxicity in HIV-1 infection is currently unclear and may not be resolved until a suitable animal model of HIV-1 infection is developed. Theoretically, the fact that virally infected target cells expressing gp120 can be destroyed effectively by either direct or indirect ADCC suggests that this form of cytolytic reactivity may be beneficial in limiting the spread of virus and slowing disease progression. Conversely, the phenomenon of ADCC could conceivably accelerate disease progression via a process of noninfectious lympholysis. This process, which may be a contributing factor in the overwhelming lymphopenia seen in HIV-1 infection, occurs when gp120 liberated from HIV-1–infected cells binds to the CD4 molecule on uninfected lymphocytes thereby making them a target for both indirect and direct ADCC.

While the value of ADCC in infected individuals is still uncertain, this form of anti-HIV-1 cytolytic reactivity may be of great importance to an individual at the point of infection. Since current evidence suggests that HIV-1 transmission occurs through a combination of free virus and virally infected allogeneic cells, neutralizing antibodies may not by themselves be able to prevent infection. Antibodies that mediate ADCC, however, could facilitate the removal of allogeneic cells expressing gp120 from a wide variety of viral isolates and thus would be a valuable adjunct, in conjunction with neutralizing antibodies, to any vaccine strategy.

Currently efforts are underway to further define epitopes on gp120 which serve as targets for ADCC. As such epitopes are identified, they must be carefully screened to make sure that they are not epitopes which would enhance viral entry into FcR-bearing cells (i.e., macrophages, monocytes). A further understanding of the differences between indirect and direct ADCC and which mechanisms are operative in vivo at all stages of disease is also important. Through this understanding, a more rational approach to incorporating ADCC into future vaccine efforts as well as maximizing its therapeutic benefit can be attained.

SUMMARY

Antibody-dependent cellular cytotoxicity (ADCC) is an effective mechanism whereby gp120-expressing targets are lysed in vitro either directly by antibody armed NK/K cells or indirectly by NK/K cells after the gp120 has been bound by anti-gp120 antibodies. Both forms of ADCC exhibit lytic activities against gp120-expressing targets from widely divergent HIV-1 isolates in a non–MHC-restricted fashion. Although the antibodies which mediate anti-HIV-1 ADCC are present in high titers soon after infection, the effectiveness of ADCC in vivo and its role in the pathogenesis of HIV-1 infection still remain to be determined. Classically, the antiviral CTL has held a dominant position as the major cytolytic effector population capable of controlling disease progression. The level of in vitro ADCC activities (both direct and indirect) described herein are, at the very least, on a par with those of anti-HIV-1 CTL. In an arena of high titers of antibodies and continuously circulating effector cells, ADCC could thus be viewed at a level comparable to that of the CTL. Ultimately, the relative contribution of these two effector mechanisms to either disease progression or pathogenesis will need to be assessed.

ACKNOWLEDGMENTS

The authors of this chapter gratefully acknowledge the valuable scientific input by Dr. D. P. Bolognesi as well as the excellent technical contributions of S. D. Stanley, C. Compton, and J. Pratz. We also thank Dr. T. J. Matthews for his gifts of gp120 and Ms. V. Gibson for preparing this manuscript. This research was supported by National Cancer Institute Grant #5P01-CA43447-03, National

Institutes of Health Contract #8U01-AI26054-02, Frederick Cancer Research Facility-NIH Contract #FOD-0759 and #FOD-0758, and U.S. Army Medical Research Acquisition Activity Contract #DAMD17-87-C7173.

REFERENCES

1. Lyerly HK, Matthews TJ, Langlois AJ, Bolognesi DP, Weinhold KJ. Human T-cell lymphotorpic virus III$_B$ glycoprotein (gp120) bound to CD4 determinants on normal lymphocytes and expressed by infected cells serves as a target for immune attack. Proc Natl Acad Sci 1987; 84:4601–5.

2. Lyerly HK, Reed DL, Matthews TJ, Langlois AJ, Ahearne PA, Petteway SR Jr, Weinhold KJ. Anti-gp120 antibodies from HIV seropositive individuals mediate broadly reactive anti-HIV ADCC. AIDS Res and Human Retroviruses 1987; 3:409–22.

3. Lyerly HK, Matthews TJ, Langlois AJ, Bolognesi DP, Weinhold KJ. HIV gp120 serves as a target for antibody dependent cellular cytotoxicity. In: Bolognesi DP, ed. Human retroviruses, cancer, and AIDS: Approaches to prevention and therapy. UCLA Symposia on Molecular and Cellular Biology, Volume 71. New York: Alan R. Liss, In., 1988: 229–40.

4. Ojo-Amaize EA, Nishanian P, Keith DE Jr, Houghton RL, Heitjan DF, Fahey JL, Giorgi JV. Antibodies to human immunodeficiency virus in human sera induce cell-mediated lysis of human immunodeficiency virus-infected cells. J Immunol 1987; 139:2458–63.

5. Ljunggren K, Bottinger B, Biberfeld G, Karlson A, Fenyo E-M, Jondal M. Antibody-dependent cellular cytotoxicity-inducing antibodies against human immunodeficiency virus: Presence at different clinical stages. J Immunol 1987; 139:2263–7.

6. Blumberg, RS, Paradis T, Hartshorn KL, Vogt M, Ho DD, Hirsch MS, Leban J, Sato VL, Schooley RT. Antibody-dependent cell-mediated cytotoxicity against cells infected with the human immunodeficiency virus. J Infect Dis 1987; 156:878–84.

7. Rook AH, Lane HC, Folks T, McCoy S, Alter H, Fauci AS. Sera from HTLV–III/LAV antibody positive individuals mediate antibody-dependent cellular cytotoxicity against HTLV–III/LAV-infected T cells. J Immunol 1987; 138:1064–7.

8. Howell DN, Andreotti PE, Dawson JR, Cresswell P. Natural killing target antigens as inducers of interferon: Studies with an immunoselected, natural killing-resistant human T lymphoblastoid cell line. J Immunol 1985; 134: 971–6.

9. Matthews TJ, Weinhold KJ, Lyerly HK, Langlois AJ, Wigzell H, Bolognesi DP. Interaction between the human T-cell lymphotropic virus type III$_B$ envelope glycoprotein gp120 and the surface antigen CD4: Role of carbohydrate in binding and cell fusion. Proc Natl Acad Sci USA 1987; 84: 5424–8.

10. Lasky, LA Nakamura G, Smith DH, Fennie C, Shimasaki C, Patzer E, Berman P, Gregory T, Capon DJ. Delineation of a region of the human immunodeficiency virus type 1 gp120 glycoprotein critical for interaction with CD4 receptor. Cell 1987; 50:975–85.

11. Peters CJ, Theofilopoulos AN. Antibody-dependent cellular cytotoxicity against murine leukemia viral antigens: Studies with human lymphoblastoid cell lines and human peripheral lymphocytes as effector cells comparing rabbit, goat, and mouse antisera. J Immunol 1977; 119:1089–96.

12. Lyerly HK, Pratz JE, Tyler DS, Matthews TJ, Langlois AJ, Bolognesi DP, Weinhold KJ. Discordant virus neutralization and anti-HIV ADCC activity in HIV-seropositive patient sera. In Vaccines 88. Cold Spring Harbor, NY: Cold Spring Harbor Laboratory, 1988: 323–6.

13. Kenealy W, Reed D, Cybulski R, Tribe D, Taylor P, Stevens C, Matthews T, Petteway S. Analysis of human serum antibodies to human immunodeficiency virus (HIV) using recombinant *env* and *gag* antigens. AIDS Res and Human Retroviruses 1987; 3:95–105.

14. Ljunggren K, Chiodi F, Biberfeld G, Norrby E, Jondal M, Fenjo E-M. Lack of cross-reaction in antibody-dependent cellular cytotoxicity between human immunodeficiency virus (HIV) and HIV-related West African strains. J Immunol 1988; 140:602–5.

15. Nastala CL, Tyler DS, Lyerly HK, Matthews TJ, Bolognesi DP, Weinhold KJ. Antibody isotypes directing anti-gp120 antibody-dependent and cell-mediated cytotoxicities. In Proceedings of the Fourth International Conference on AIDS 1988; 1:2102.

16. Khalife J, Guy B, Capron M, Kieny MP, Ameisen JC, Montagnier L, Lecocq JP, Capron A. Isotypic restriction of the antibody response to human immunodeficiency virus. AIDS Res and Human Retroviruses 1988; 4:3–9.

17. Klasse J, Blomberg J. Patterns of antibodies to human immunodeficiency virus proteins in different subclasses of IgG. J Inf Dis 1987; 156:1026–30.

18. Allain J-P, Laurian y, Paul DA, Verroust F, Leuther M, Gazengei C, Senn D, Larrieu M-J, Bosser C. Long-term evaluation of HIV antigenemia and antibodies to p24 and gp41 in patients with hemophilia. N Engl J Med 1987; 317:1114–21.

19. Kay HD, Bonnard GD, West WH, Herberman RB. A functional comparison of human Fc-receptor-bearing lymphocytes active in natural cytotoxicity and antibody-dependent cellular cytotoxicity. J Immunol 1977; 118:2058–66.

20. Abo T, and Balch CM. A differentiation antigen of human NK and K cells identified by a monoclonal antibody (HNK-1). J Immunol 1981; 127:1024–9.

21. Bradley TP, Bonavida B. Mechanism of cell-mediated cytotoxicity at the single cell level. IV. Natural killing and antibody-dependent cellular cytotoxicity can be mediated by the same human effector cell as determined by the two-target conjugate assay. J Immunol 1982; 129:2260–5.

22. Perussia B, Trinchieri G, Jackson A, Warner NL, Faust J, Rumpold H, Kraft D, Lanier LL. The Fc receptor for IgG on human natural killer cells: phenotype, functional, and comparative studies with monoclonal antibodies. J Immunol 1984; 133:180–9.

23. Katz JD, Mitsuyasu R, Gottlieb MS, Lebow L, Bonavida B. Mechanism of defective NK cell activity in patients with acquired immunodeficiency syndrome (AIDS) and AIDS-related complex. II. Normal antibody-dependent cellular cytotoxicity (ADCC) mediated by effector cells defective in natural killer (NK) cytotoxicity. J Immunol 1987; 139:55–60.

24. Wright SC, Bonavida B. Studies of the mechanism of natural killer cell-mediated cytotoxicity. III. Interferon-pretreatment of effector cells augments the lytic activity of natural killer cytotoxic-factors (NKCF). J Immunol 1983; 130:2960–4.

25. Lyerly HK, Matthews TJ, Ahearne PM, Langlois AJ, Bolognesi DP, Weinhold KJ. Augmentation of anti-HIV ADCC with interleukin 2. In American College of Surgeons: Surgical Forum Volume 38, 1987: 425–8.

26. Weinhold KJ, Lyerly HK, Matthews TJ, Tyler DS, Ahearne PM, Stine KC, Langlois AJ, Durack DT, Bolognesi DP. Cellular anti-gp120 cytolytic reactivities in HIV-1 seropositive individuals. Lancet 1988; 1:902–5.

27. Weinhold KJ, Lyerly HK, Matthews TJ, Tyler DS, Nastala CL, Bolognesi DP. Specific cell-mediated cytotoxciity against HIV-1 envelope glycoprotein coated CD4 cells. In Andrieu J-M et al., eds. Autoimmune Aspects of HIV Infection. Royal Society of Medicine Services International Congress and Symposium Series No. 141, 1988: 143–51.

28. Tyler DS, Nastala CL, Stanley SD, Matthews TJ, Lyerly HK, Bolognesi DP, Weinhold KJ. Gp120 specific cellular cytotoxicity in HIV-1 seropositive individuals: Evidence for circulating CD16 positive effector cells armed *in vivo* with cytophilic antibody (Submitted).

29. Tyler DS, Nastala CL, Lyerly HK, Matthews TJ, Bolognesi DP, Weinhold KJ. Direct ADCC: Evidence of circulating antibody armed cytotoxic CD16$^+$ K cells in patients infected with HIV-1. Surgical Forum (in press).

30. Tyler DS, Stnaley SD, Nastala CL, Lyerly HK, Matthews TJ, Bolognesi DP, Weinhold KJ. Antibody directed anti-HIV-1 cellular cytotoxicity: The role of NK/K cells armed with gp120 specific antibodies in therapeutic and vaccine strategies. In: Vaccines 89: Modern Approaches to New Vaccines. Cold Spring Harbor, NY: Cold Spring Harbor Laboratory, 1989 (in press).

8

Cytotoxic T-Lymphocyte Responses to HIV-1 in Infected Individuals

Bruce D. Walker
*Harvard Medical School
and Massachusetts General Hospital
Boston, Massachusetts*

INTRODUCTION

One and a half to two million persons in the U.S. alone are presumed to be infected with the human immunodeficiency virus I (HIV-1), the causative agent of AIDS and related syndromes (1,2). The disease is associated with a persistent viremia, with virus readily cultured from the peripheral blood of infected individuals (3). Despite this, most individuals remain asymptomatic for years after infection, suggesting that a virus-specific host immune response might play a role in keeping these people healthy in the face of ongoing exposure to the virus. The role of the cell mediated immune response may be particularly important in this infection, since HIV is thought to be predominantly cell associated and therefore not readily accessible to neutralizing antibodies. This discussion will focus on our studies of the cytotoxic T-lymphocyte (CTL) response to HIV in infected individuals.

HISTORICAL PERSPECTIVE

Virus-specific CTL are thought to be a major host defense in a number of viral infections (for review, see 4,5). These CTL are generated in response to viral infection and characteristically mediate lysis of infected cells by recognition of viral antigen in conjunction with an appropriate "self" major histocompatibility complex (MHC) molecule (6,7). CTL of both the CD4 and CD8 phenotype have been identified. $CD4^+$ lymphocytes typically recognize exogenous antigens which are endocytosed by antigen-presenting cells, processed in phagolysosomes, and presented at the cell surface in conjunction with HLA class II (D locus) antigens. In contrast, $CD8^+$ lymphocytes are thought to recognize endogenous antigen synthesized in the cytoplasm of an infected cell and presented at the cell surface in conjunction with HLA class I (A, B, C) antigens (8-10).

Evidence suggests that virus-specific CTL are generated early on in viral infections, recognize external and internal viral antigens, and may serve as an important protective host defense. For example, in mice inoculated with influenza A virus, virus-specific CTL could be detected in lung, spleen, cervical lymph node, and blood, with peak activity 6 days after virus inoculation—before the production of significant levels of antibody (11). Adoptive transfer of these influenza-specific CTL to mice subsequently inoculated with influenza A resulted in a significant decrease in pulmonary titers of virus, as well as in decreased mortality, but only if the recipient mice were histocompatible at MHC class I loci. Similar results have been obtained using adoptively transferred mouse CTL clones, which protected syngeneic recipients and resulted in reduced viral titers in mice challenged with heterologous type A influenza virus (12). Lymphocytic choriomeningitis virus (LCMV)-specific CTL have also been shown in mice to play a protective role as a host defense. Adoptive transfer of these cells to mice inoculated one day previously with LCMV resulted in total clearance of virus from the spleens of syngeneic but not allogeneic animals (13), again reflecting the necessity of an appropriate MHC antigen. Virus-specific CTL are also generated in response to murine retroviral infections such as murine leukemia virus (MuLV), and this cellular immune response has been shown to play a protective role (14,15). The mechanism by which antiviral CTL mediate protection may be due to lysis of infected cells before infectious virus progeny is assembled (16).

In the human host, evidence indicates that virus-specific CTL are an important host defense. For example, recovery from CMV infection in bone marrow transplant recipients has been shown to correlate with development of CMV-specific CTL, suggesting that these cells mediate recovery from infection (17). Similarly, CTL have been shown to contribute to recovery from influenza A virus infection in humans (18), and such CTL have been shown to be cross-reactive for different subtypes of influenza A virus.

While the hallmark of HIV infection is progressive and profound immunosuppression, it is noteworthy that the mean incubation period is 8 years or more (19), during which time persons may remain asymptomatic. Despite lack of clinical expression of infection, virus is readily cultured from the peripheral blood of these individuals, suggesting that the host immune response might play a role in keeping these persons healthy. The demonstration of antiviral CTL in other viral and retroviral infections led us to investigate whether such cells might be a component of the host response to HIV infection.

CYTOTOXICITY ASSAY

The assay system we have used to detect human HIV-1–specific CTL utilizes recombinant vaccinia vectors to express HIV-1 gene poducts in EBV-immortalized B-lymphoblastoid target cells (20,21). This system is an adaptation of a system already shown to demonstrate CTL activity in influenza virus infection (22). Vaccinia viruses are particularly advantageous as a means of recombinant antigen expression, as they have a wide host range, readily infect EBV-immortalized B cells, and the recombinant antigens are normally processed and glycosylated (23).

Three vaccinia-HIV-1 recombinant vectors have been used in these studies, all constructed from a proviral clone of the HTLV–IIIB viral isolate. VAC/lac (also known as VCS-8) is the designation for a recombinant expressing the *E. coli* β-galactosidase gene product, and is used as a control. The VAC/env (also called VSC-25) vector results in production of the HIV-1 envelope gene products gp160, gp120, and gp41 when used to infect susceptible cells. The envelope gene product so produced is biologically active, as demonstrated by syncytia formation when envelope-expressing target cells are co-cultivated with CD4-positive lymphocytes (24). VAV/gag (also called VSC-40) is the designation for a recombinant vector which results in production of the HIV-1 *gag* gene product p55, although no further processing to p24 is seen with this vector. A representative radioimmunoprecipitation of EBV blasts infected with these recombinant vaccinia viruses is shown in Figure 1. Recently, we have also been investigating HIV-specific CTL directed against the viral reverse transcriptase (RT) protein. The vector used for these experiments is designated VAC/pol (also called CFv21) and results in production of the reverse transcriptase protein p65, with a minor p51 product. In addition, biologically active reverse transcriptase is detectable in lysates of cells infected with this vector (25).

These vaccinia viruses are used to express the selected HIV-1 antigens in target cells. An EBV-immortalized B-cell line is established for each subject to be studied. These B-cell lines grow continuously in culture, express both class I and class II antigens, and are readily infectable with the recombinant vaccinia viruses. The assay used to detect CTL is shown diagrammatically in Figure 2. Infection with the above described vaccinia vectors is carried out at a low multiplicity of infection (1-10 pfu/cell). These cells are harvested after a 16-hour incubation, chromium labeled, and used as target cells in a 6-hour chromium release assay. Despite the fact that vaccinia produces a lytic infection, cells typically are 80-90% viable at the time of chromium labeling, and virtually all cells are infected with vaccinia, as detected by immunofluorescence.

Fresh autologous PBMC are used as effector cells in our system. Detection of CTL activity in most viral systems requires an in vitro stimulation phase in which memory cells expand in response to added viral antigen. In contrast, we have

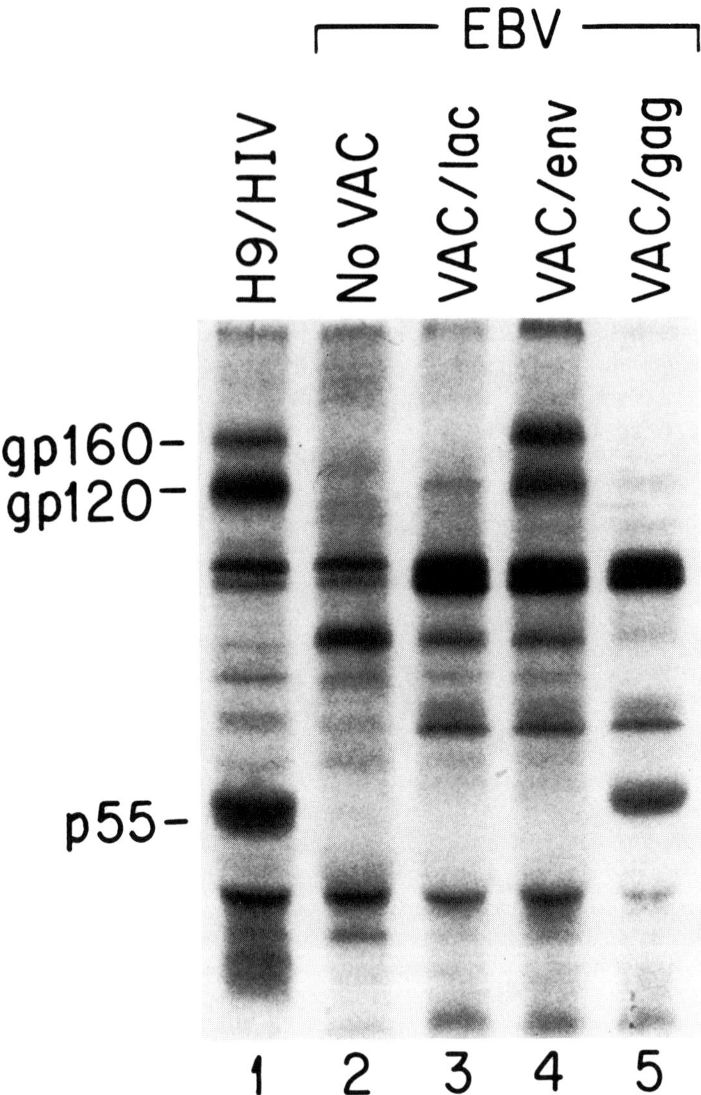

Figure 1 Radioimmunoprecipitation of EBV lymphoblasts infected with recombinant vaccinia-HIV vectors. Lane 1, HIV-infected H9 cells; lane 2, uninfected EBV lymphoblasts; lane 3, lymphoblasts infected with a control vaccinia vector; lane 4, lymphoblasts infected with the VAC/env vector; lane 5, lymphoblasts infected with the VAC/gag vector.

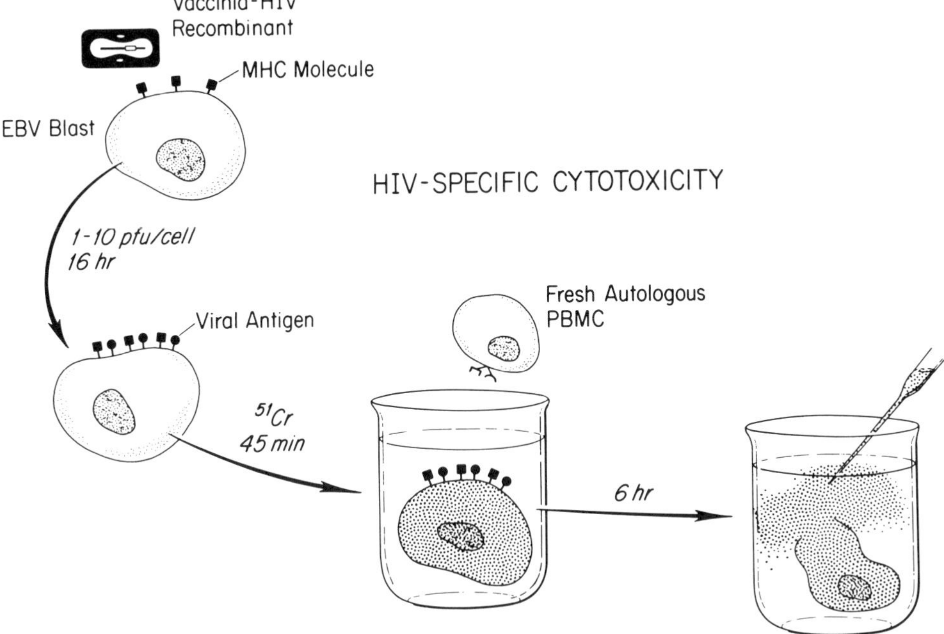

Figure 2 Cytotoxicity assay utilizing vaccinia-HIV-1 recombinant vectors to express viral antigen.

found that HIV-specific CTL can be detected using fresh PBMC from infected individuals, presumably reflecting ongoing in vivo stimulation of the effector cell population. This is perhaps not unexpected, given the persistent viremia and intermittent viral antigenemia associated with this disease.

HIV-1 ENVELOPE, GAG AND RT-SPECIFIC CTL

Utilizing the assay system described above, we have now detected HIV-1-specific CTL in 22 of 22 seropositive subjects, in all stages of clinical illness. Envelope-specific CTL have been present in all seropositive subjects assayed, although activity has been observed to drop in subjects with clinical disease progression. CTL which recognize the viral reverse transcriptase protein have been present in 12 of 14 subjects studied, shown in Figure 3 at a representative effector:target (E:T) ratio of 50:1. In some instances the relative magnitude of the RT-specific cytotoxicity has been higher than the observed envelope-specific cytotoxicity.

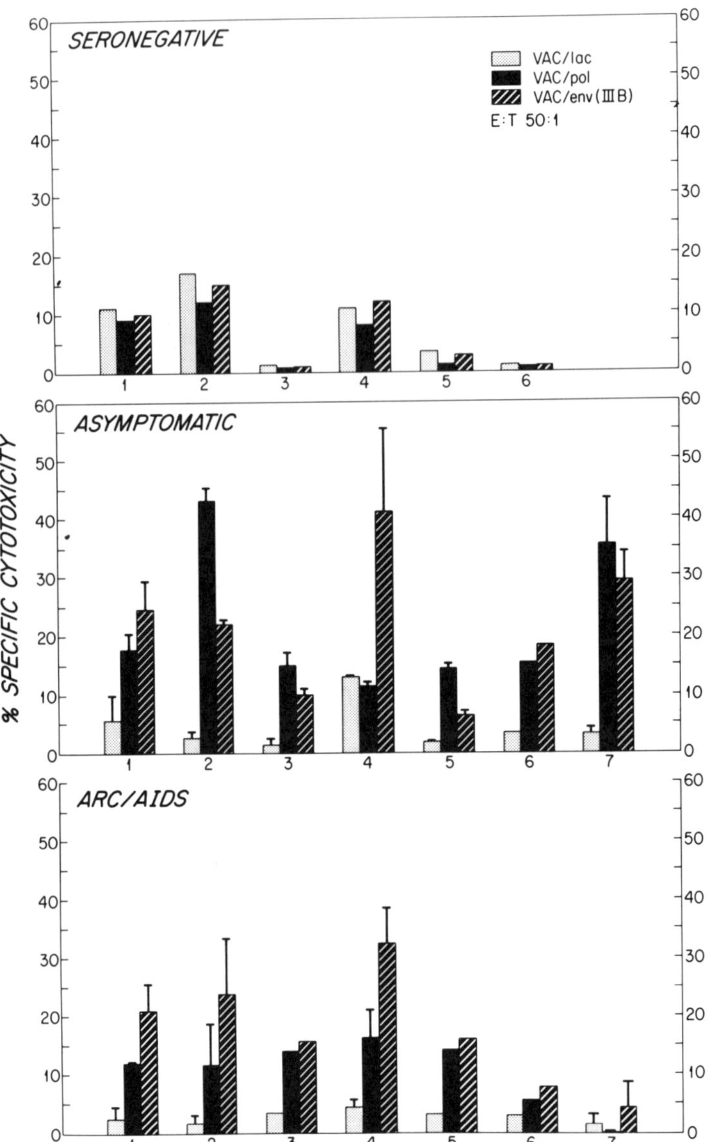

Figure 3 HIV-1 envelope–specific and RT-specific cytotoxicity.

Interestingly, *gag*-specific CTL have been infrequently detected using this system. Of the 22 subjects evaluated, only four demonstrated *gag*-specific CTL, and this was always observed at low levels compared to the envelope and RT-specific CTL (20,21). Whether this lack of activity reflects a relative absence of *gag*-specific CTL or whether a defect in processing of the *gag* gene product with the vaccinia recombinant utilized prevents these cells from being recognized as target cells is not presently known. Thus far we have been unable to correlate the relative magnitude of HIV-specific CTL activity with clinical disease stage, although the number of subjects studied is small.

CHARACTERISTICS OF THE HIV-1–SPECIFIC CYTOTOXIC EFFECTOR CELL POPULATION

The presence of a persistent vigorous CTL response detectable in fresh peripheral blood of infected individuals is unprecedented and raises questions as to whether the cells mediating this response are phenotypically analogous to CTL seen in other viral infections after secondary in vitro stimulation. Classically antiviral CTL of the CD8 phenotype and CD4 phenotype have been detected, although the role of the latter as a host-protective response is unclear.

In initial analysis of the phenotype characteristics of the effector cells, monoclonal antibodies to the CD3, CD4, and CD8 cell surface proteins were used to attempt to block the cytotoxic activity. The CD3-specific monoclonal antibody 12F6 in each case inhibited the RT-specific CTL activity of fresh PBL, although results were less consistent with similar concentrations of OKT3 (21). In each subject tested, CD8-specific monoclonal antibody also abrogated the response, whereas no inhibition was observed with OKT4. Inhibition of envelope-specific cytotoxicity has also been observed in the presence of 12F6 (20) and CD8-specific monoclonal antibody, but not CD4-specific monoclonal antibody (unpublished observations). These results have lead to the conclusion that the major effector cell of this virus-specific CTL response is a CD3$^+$, CD8$^+$ lymphocyte.

In a second set of experiments to analyze the effector cell population, monoclonal antibody and complement were used to specifically remove cells of certain phenotypes from fresh PBMC. As shown in Figure 4, removal of either CD3$^+$ or CD8$^+$ lymphocytes, but not CD4$^+$ lymphocytes, resulted in abrogation of the envelope-specific CTL responses, again indicating that CD8$^+$ lymphocytes are the antiviral population in this system.

The issue of effector cell phenotype has also been addressed by culturing CD4- or CD8-enriched lymphocytes from seropositive subjects in interleukin-2 (IL-2). As seen in Figure 5, CD8-enriched lymphocytes from an asymptomatic subject readily lyse cells expressing HIV-1 viral proteins, whereas CD4-enriched lymphocytes mediate equivalent lysis of all vaccinia-infected target cells, regardless of whether HIV antigens are expressed. These data again suggest that, at

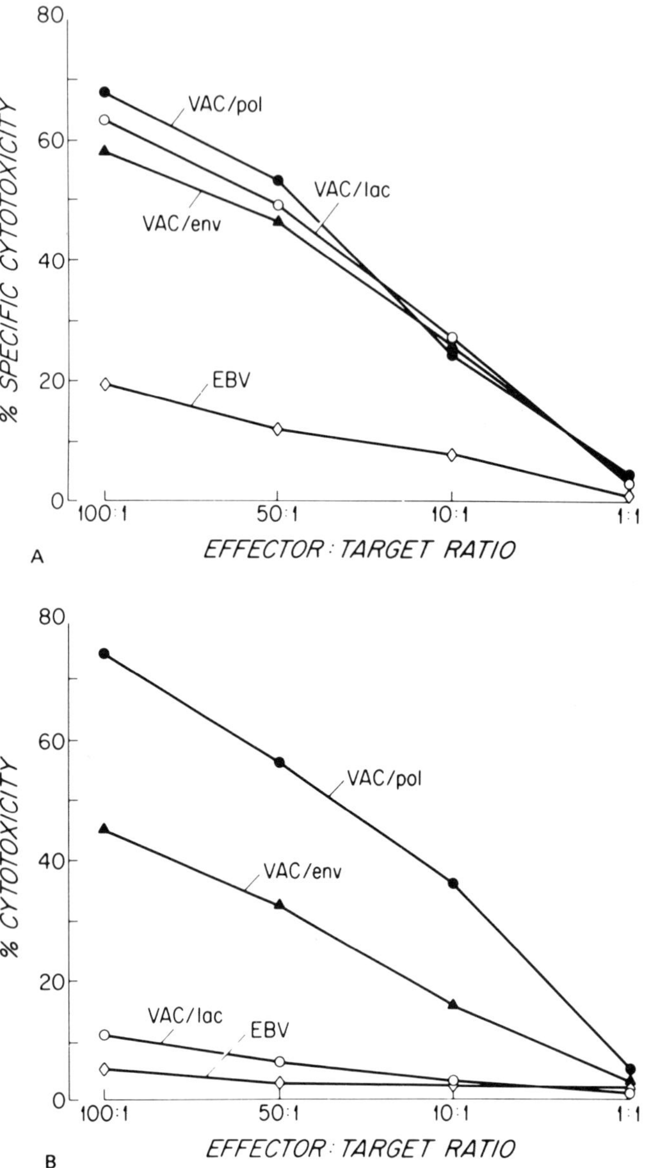

Figure 4 HIV-1–specific cytotoxicity mediated by cultured lymphocytes from a seropositive subject. A: CD-4 enriched lymphocytes. B: CD-8 enriched lymphocytes.

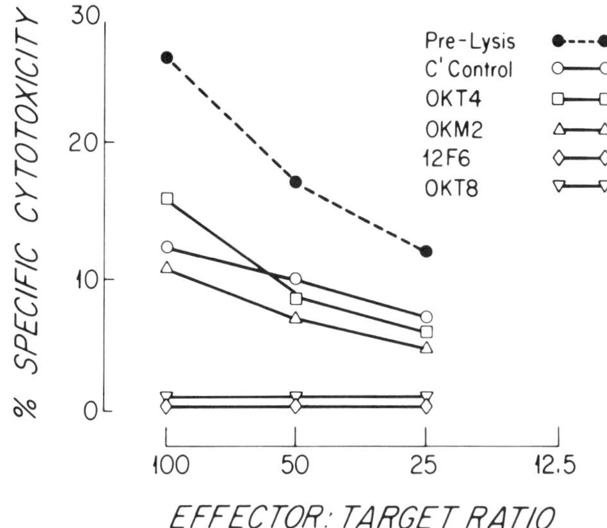

Figure 5 HIV-1 envelope–specific lysis following monoclonal antibody and complement-mediated lysis.

least in this in vitro system, virus-specific CTL activity is predominantly medi-ated by cells of the CD8 phenotype.

If these effector cells are classic CD8[+] lymphocytes, then one would expect to find that the response is restricted by HLA class I antigens. In the case of envelope-specific CTL, we have observed a preferential lysis of autologous target cells in some subjects but have been unable to demonstrate a clear restricting role of HLA antigens in this response (20). Alternatively, RT-specific CTL are clearly restricted by HLA class I antigens, as shown for two subjects in Table 1. The reason that the role of MHC in the RT-specific response is clearer than in the envelope-specific response is not known, but may relate to differences in antigen processing. The RT protein has no leader sequence or transmembrane region, and therefore all that is expressed at the surface must be degraded proteins which get there through a class I pathway. Alternatively, the gp120/ gp41 complex is expressed on the surface of cells infected with the vaccinia-HIV-1 envelope construct. In addition, presumably degraded envelope proteins are also presented at the cell surface in conjunction with HLA class I molecules. Surface expression of full-length envelope may alter the membrane characteris-tics in such a way that strict HLA restriction is not observed; alternatively, other

Table 1 RT–Specific Lysis by PBMC from Two Seropositive Subjects Is HLA Class I Restricted

Subject	Shared HLA antigens	RT-specific lysis
A	Autologous	38.1
	A1, A11	9.5
	A1, A11, DRw52, DQw2	6.9
	A1, C24, DRw52	1.1
	A1, B8, DR3, DRw52	4.5
	A1, DRw52	1.5
	A1, DQw2	0
	A1, B8, DR3, DRw52, DQw2	1.9
	Bw62, DRw52	20.1
	BW62	18.1
	Cw4	1.1
	DQw2	0.7
	DRw52	1.2
	DRw52	0
	DRw52	2.2
B	Autologous	16
	A1, A29, DR1, DQw1	0.1
	A1, DQw2	0
	A1, DQw1	0
	A1	0
	A1, DQw2	2.3
	B44, Cw5, DR1, DQw1	11.6
	B44, Cw5, DRw53	9.1
	A1, B44, Cw5, DR7, DRw53	10.9
	A29, B44, DR7, DRw53, DQw2	3.8
	DQw1	0
	DR7, DRw53, DQw2	0
	DQw1	0

Results are given at an E:T of 50:1. RT-specific lysis is defined here as % lysis of VAC/RT target - % lysis of VAC/lac control target.

effector cells besides HLA class I restricted CD8$^+$ lymphocytes may be present (26). However, we (unpublished observations) and others (27) have found that both RT and envelope-specific CTL clones derived from seropositive subjects are MHC class I restricted. Others have reported the in vitro generation to CD4$^+$ HLA class II restricted HIV-specific CTL from seronegative subjects (28). Whether such cells exist in vivo is not known.

HIV-1-SPECIFIC CTL WITH DISEASE PROGRESSION

Although antiviral CTL have been shown to be a protective host defense in many viral infections, the role of HIV-1-specific CTL remains unclear. In fact, it has been suggested by Plata et al. that HIV-1-specific CTL may contribute to lung disease in infected individuals (29). We have now followed a number of subjects longitudinally and have observed the virus-specific CTL response to be stable in the absence of clinical disease progression. However, in the three subjects studied who progressed from asymptomatic infection to develop AIDS, a marked reduction in HIV-1 envelope-specific CTL activity was seen in each (Table 2). Whether this decrease contributed to disease progression, reflects tissue sequestration of CTL (as has been observed in the lung in experimental influenza infection (30)), or is merely a nonspecific reflection of overall progressive immunologic dysfunction remains to be determined. Interestingly, CD8$^+$ lymphocytes from HIV-infected humans and SIV-infected rhesus macaques have been shown to suppress viral replication in vitro (31,32). Whether this occurs by a virus-specific cytotoxic mechanism, by a soluble factor, or through some other mechanism is not presently known.

Table 2 Envelope-Specific CT1 Decline with Disease Progression

Subject	env-specific lysis[a]	
	Asymptomatic	AIDS
1	35%	10%
2	33%	11%
3	16%	0.3%

[a]env-specific lysis is defined here as % lysis of VAC/env target - % lysis of VAC/lac control target. Results are given at a represetnative E:T ratio of 50:1.

RECENT DEVELOPMENTS

Coincident with our initial report of HIV-specific CTL in the peripheral blood of infected individuals, Plata et al. reported detection of HIV envelope–specific CTL derived by bronchoalveolar lavage from the lungs of seropositive subjects with lymphocytic alveolitis (29). Using as target cells either HIV-infected alveolar macrophages or doubly transfected mouse cells expessing both HLA-A2 and HIV envelope, this group demonstrated the cytotoxic response to be MHC class I restricted and mediated by CD3$^+$, CD8$^+$ lymphocytes. It was postulated that interactions between CTL and infected cells might be directly contributing to the lung pathology in these subjects, although lymphocytes derived from the lungs of seropositive subjects without lung disorders were not tested. Plata's group has now added to these observations using cloned CTL lines established by repeated antigenic stimulation using autologous phytohemagglutinin-stimulated lymphoblasts infected with HIV (33).

These demonstrations of HIV-specific CTL in fresh peripheral blood and lung lymphocytes of seropositive subjects have recently been extended by Sethi et al., who have derived HIV-specific CTL from the cerebrospinal fluid of two AIDS patients suffering from neurologic disorders (34). These bulk CTL were able to lyse target cells coated with either purified HIV-1 envelope glycoprotein, or with UV-inactivated HIV. Cloned CTL were subsequently derived from one subject by culturing cells at limiting dilution in the presence of IL-2 and autologous irradiated PBMC coated with gp120. The major histocompatibility complex was found to restrict cytolysis mediated by these clones, in some instances by HLA class I and some instances by HLA class II antigens. In addition, these authors derived some clones which they interpreted to be dually restricted by both class I and class II antigens. When the cloned CTL were phenotyped, they found considerable heterogeneity, some being CD4$^+$, some CD8$^+$, some CD4$^+$ and CD8$^+$, and some lacking both of these markers. Since these CTL were derived from the CSF of patients with neurologic disorders, the authors suggested that the CTL response might contribute to neurologic dysfunction observed in these patients.

Further data regarding CTL recognition of the HIV core antigen have been provided by Nixon et al. (35). A recombinant vaccinia virus was used to express the HIV-1 *gag* protein in EBV immortalized B cells, and these were used as target cells looking for *gag*-specific CTL in seropositive subjects. Similar to our results, they reported that *gag*-specific CTL were difficult to detect using fresh PBMC. However, when a fraction of the PBMC were stimulated with PHA and co-cultivated for one week with the fresh PBMC, HLA class I restricted *gag*-specific CTL activity was readily observed in 13 of 15 seropositive subjects. Using synthetic HIV-1 peptides, in experiments analogous to those used to identify immunogenic epitopes of influenza (36), a single 16 amino acid *gag* peptide recognized by these CTL in an HLA class I restricted fashion was identified. Such dissection of immunogenic peptides may ultimately facilitate rational design of a subunit vaccine to elicit CTL responses.

Koenig et al. have also used the recombinant vaccinia virus approach for viral antigen expression, and have recently reported findings using both fresh PBMC and cloned CTL from a seropositive subject (27). Envelope-specific cytotoxicity mediated by fresh PBMC was found to be unrestricted by class I antigens, although phenotypic analysis revealed the majority of these effector cells to be CD8$^+$. Using CTL cloned by limiting dilution in the presence of the nonspecific stimulus PHA, CTL to both envelope and reverse transcriptase were found to be HLA class I restricted. In addition, similar lysis of target cells expressing the envelope of divergent viral isolates (HTLV–IIIB and HTLV–IIIRF) was observed, indicating that these cloned CTL recognize conserved epitopes of viral strains.

The issue of the effector cell type mediating cytolysis has also been investigated by Koup et al. (37). Using recombinant vaccinia-HIV vectors to express viral antigen, this group demonstrated HIV-specific CTL in fresh peripheral blood of 88% of hemophiliacs tested. Vigorous responses to both *env* and *gag* proteins were observed. Responses were resistant to natural killer cell (NK) lysis but could consistently be inhibited by monoclonal antibodies to CD3, CD8, and MHC class I antigens, again indicating that the major phenotype mediating the virus-specific cytotoxicity is a classic MHC class I restricted CD8$^+$ T lymphocyte. The reason that *gag*-specific lysis was readily observed by these investigators, while we have infrequently detected *gag*-specific CTL, is not clear and could relate to inherent differences in the HIV-specific immune response in hemophiliacs compared to homosexual men or could be due to differences in the *gag*-expressing vectors used.

SUMMARY AND CONCLUSIONS

Characterization of the host immune response to HIV infection is essential for developing a rational approach to vaccine development. Since the original descriptions of HIV-specific CTL in infected individuals, multiple investigations have documented the existence of vigorous cell mediated immune response to the virus. Virus-specific CTL are readily detected in fresh peripheral blood, indicating that this response is being persistently primed in vivo. Similar to cell mediated immune responses to other viruses, the HIV-specific cytotoxicity is mediated predominantly by MHC class I-restricted CD3$^+$, CD8$^+$ lymphocytes. However, the actual role of these CTL in protection from disease progression remains unclear.

ACKNOWLEDGMENTS

The author wishes to particularly acknowledge the collaborative help of Dr. Robert T. Schooley, Dr. Bernard Moss, Dr. Johnson Wong, Karen Birch-Limberger, and Timothy J. Paradis. I thank Janet Steele for manuscript preparation.

REFERENCES

1. Piot P, Pheumer FA, Mhaln FS, Lamboray JL, Chin J, Mann JM. AIDS: An international perspective. Science 1988; 239:573-9.

2. Curran JW, Jaffe HW, Hardy AM, Morgan WM, Selik RM, Dondero TJ. Epidemiology of HIV infection and AIDS in the United States. Science 1988; 239:610-6.

3. Feorino PM, Jaffe HW, Palmer E, et al. Transfusion-associated acquired immunodeficiency syndrome. Evidence for resistant infection in blood donors. N Engl J Med 1985; 312:1293-6.

4. Pasternack MS. Cytotoxic T-lymphocytes. Adv Intern Med 1988; 33:17-44.

5. Rouse BT, Norley S, Martin S. Antiviral cytotoxic T lymphocyte induction and vaccination. Rev Inf Dis 1988; 10:16-33.

6. Zinkernagel RM and Doherty PC. MHC-restricted cytotoxic T cells: Studies on the biological role of polymorphic major transplantation antigens determining T cell restriction-specificity, function and responsiveness. Adv Immunol 1979; 27:51-177.

7. Zinkernagel RM and Doherty PC. Restriction of in vitro T cell mediated cytotoxicity in lymphocytic choriomeningitis virus within a syngeneic and semiallogeneic system. Nature (London) 1974; 145:644-51.

8. Morrison LA, Lukacher AE, Brachiale VL, Fan DP, Brachiale TJ. Differences in antigen presentation to MHC class I and class II-restricted influenza virus specific cytolytic T lymphocyte clones. J Exp Med 1986; 163:903-21.

9. Germain RN. The ins and outs of antigen processing and presentation. Nature (London) 1986; 322:687-9.

10. Germain RN. Antigen processing and CD4+ T cell depletion in AIDS. Cell 1988; 54:441-4.

11. Yap KL, Ada GL, McKenzie IFC. Transfer of specific cytotoxic T lymphocytes protects mice innoculated with influenza virus. Nature (London) 1978; 273:238-9.

12. Lin YL and Askonas BA. Biological properties of an influenza A virus-specific killer T cell clone. J Exp Med 1981; 154:225-34.

13. Byrne JA and Oldstone MBA. Biology of cloned cytotoxic T lymphocytes specific for lymphocytic choriomeningitis virus: clearance of virus in vivo. J Viol 1984; 51:682-6.

14. Chesbro B, Wehrly K. Studies on the role of the host immune response in recovery from friend virus leukemia II. Cell-mediated immunity. J Exp Med 1976; 143:85–99.

15. Plata F, Langlade-Demoyen P, Abastado JP, Berbar T and Kourilsky P. Retrovirus antigens recognized by cytolytic T lymphocytes activate tumor rejection in vivo. Cell 1987; 48:231.

16. Zinkernagel RM and Althage A. Antiviral protection by virus-immune cytotoxic T cells: infected target cells are lysed before infectious virus progeny is assembled. J Exp Med 1977; 145:644–51.

17. Quinnan GV, Kirmani N, Rook AH, Manishewitz JF, Jackson L, Moreschi G, Santos GW, Saral R, Burns WH. Cytotoxic T cells in cytomegalovirus infection. HLA-restricted T-lymphocyte and non-T-lymphocyte cytotoxic responses correlate with recovery from cytomegalovirus infection in bone marrow transplant recipients. N Engl J Med 1982; 307:6–13.

18. McMichael AJ, Gotch FM, Noble GR, Beare PAS. Cytotoxic T-cell immunity to influenza. N Engl J Med 1983; 309:13–7.

19. Medley GF, Anderson RF, Cox DR, Billard L. Incubation period of AIDS in patients infected via blood transfusion. Nature (London) 1987; 328:719–21.

20. Walker BD, Chakrabarti S, Moss B, Paradis TJ, Flynn T, Durno AG, Blumberg RS, Kaplan JC, Hirsch MS, Schooley RT. HIV-specific cytotoxic T lymphocytes in seropositive subjects. Nature (London) 1987; 328: 345–8.

21. Walker BD, Flexner C, Paradis TJ, Fuller TC, Hirsch MS, Schooley RT, Moss B. HIV-1 reverse transcriptase is a target for cytotoxic T lymphocytes in infected individuals. Science 1988; 240:64–6.

22. McMichael AJ, Michie CA, Gotch FM, Smith GL, Moss B. Recognition of influenza A virus nucleoprotein by human cytotoxic T lymphocytes. J Gen Virol 1986; 67:719–26.

23. Chakrabarti S, Robert Guroff M, Wong-Staal F, Gallo RC, Moss B. Expression of the HTLV–III envelope gene by a recombinant vaccinia virus. Nature (London) 1986; 320:535–7.

24. Lifson J, Feinberg MB, Reyes GR, Rabin L, Banapour B, Chakrabarti S, Moss B, Wong-Staal F, Steimer KS, Engelman EG. Induction of CD4-dependent cell fusion by the HTLV–III/LAV envelope glycoprotein. Nature (London) 1986; 323:725–8.

25. Flexner C, Broyles SS, Earl P, Chakrabarti S, Moss B. Characterization of human immunodeficiency virus *gag/pol* gene products expressed by recombinant vaccinia viruses. Virology 1988; 166:339–49.

26. Weinhold K, Matthews TJ, Ahearn PM, Langlois AJ, Lyerly HK, Tyler DS, Stine KC, Durach DT, Bolognesi DP. Cellular anti-gp120 cytolytic reactivities in HIV-1 seropositive individuals. Lancet 1988; 1:902–4.

27. Koenig S, Earl P, Powell D, Pantaleo G, Merli S, Moss B, Fauci AS. Group-specific, major histocompatibility complex class I-restricted cytotoxic responses to human immunodeficiency virus 1 (HIV-1) envelope proteins

by cloned peripheral blood T cells from an HIV-1 infected individual. Proc Natl Acad Sci USA 1988;85:8638–42.

28. Siliciano RF, Lawton T, Knall C, Karr RW, Berman P, Gregory T, Reinherz EL. Analysis of host-virus interaction in AIDS with anti-gp120 T cell clones: Effect of HIV sequence variation and a mechanism for CD4+ cell depletion. Cell 1988;54:561–75.

29. Plata F, Autran B, Martins LP, Wain-Hobson S, Raphael M, Maynard C, Denis M, Guillon JM, Debre P. AIDS-virus specific cytotoxic T lymphocytes in lung disorders. Nature (London) 1988;328:348–51.

30. Ennis FA, Wells MA, Butchko GM, Albrecht P. Evidence that cytotoxic T cells are part of this host's response to influenza pneumonia. J Exp Med 1978;148:1241–50.

31. Walker CM, Moody DJ, Stites DP, Levy JA. CD8+ lymphocytes can control HIV infection in vitro by suppressing virus replication. Science 1986;234:1536-6.

32. Kannagi M, Chalifoux LV, Lord C, Letvin NL. Suppression of simian immunodeficiency virus replication in vitro by CD8+ lymphocytes. J Immunol 1988;140:2237-42.

33. Laglade-Demoyen P, Michel F, Hoffenbach A, Vilmer E, Dadaglio G, Garcia-Pons F, Maynard C, Autran B, Wain-Hobson S, Plata F. Immune recognition of AIDS virus antigens by human and murine cytotoxic T lymphocytes. J Immunol 1988;141:1949.

34. Sethi KK, Naeher H, Stroehmann I. Phenotypic heterogeneity of cerebrospinal fluid-derived HIV-specific and HLA-restricted cytotoxic T cell clones. Nature (London) 1988;335:178–81.

35. Nixon DF, Townsend ARM, Elvin JG, Rizza CR, Gallway J, McMichael AJ. HIV-1 gag-specific cytotoxic T lymphocytes defined with recombinant vaccinia virus and synthetic peptides. Nature (London) 1988;336:484-7.

36. Townsend ARM, Rothbard J, Gotch FM, Bahadur G, Wraith D, McMichael AJ. The epitopes of influenza nucleoprotein recognized by cytotoxic T lymphocytes can be defined with short synthetic peptides. Cell 1986;44:959–68.

37. Koup RA, Sullivan JL, Levine PH, Brehler D, Mahr A, Mazzara G, McKenzie S, Panicali D. Detection of MHC class I restricted, HIV-specific cytotoxic T lymphocytes in the blood of infected hemophiliacs. Blood 1989;73:1909-14.

DEVELOPMENT OF VACCINE CANDIDATES

9

Biochemical and Immunologic Characterizations of HIV Envelope Glycoproteins Expressed by Recombinant Vaccinia Virus

Shiu-Lok Hu
Oncogen
Seattle, Washington

INTRODUCTION

Since the pioneering works of Panicali and Paoletti (1) and Moss et al. (2), vaccinia virus has been used extensively as a vector for the expression of various foreign genes. The advantages of using vaccinia virus as an expression vector are several. First, vaccinia virus infects a wide range of mammalian cells, offering a homologous system to study the expression and the processing of gene products of mammalian or mammalian virus origins. Second, infection with recombinant vaccinia virus is an efficient way to generate histocompatible targets cells for the study of cytotoxic T lymphocytes against specific viral antigens. Finally, recombinant vaccinia virus offers a promising approach to a new generation of vaccines. Immunization of animals with recombinant vaccinia viruses has resulted in protective immunity against a number of diseases and infections (for review, see Ref. 3), including simian AIDS caused by type D retroviruses (80).

Vaccinia virus has been used successfully for centuries as the vaccine against smallpox. It is heat-stable, dessication-tolerant, easy to produce and to administer. These properties have allowed the use of vaccinia virus for the global eradication of smallpox (4). These are relevant considerations for the development of vaccines against AIDS, since HIV infection has already become a worldwide health concern (5). Furthermore, use of recombinant vaccinia virus as a vaccine approach eliminates the risks associated with using whole HIV virions. These include theoretical risks of introducing retroviral genomes into otherwise healthy human beings, as well as realistic risks that may arise as a result of handling large quantities of HIV (6). It is, therefore, of interest to explore recombinant vaccinia virus as an approach to vaccines against AIDS.

Recombinant vaccinia viruses have been constructed (7-9) to express the envelope glycoproteins of HIV type 1 (HIV-1). In this article, I will summarize the biochemical and immunologic characterizations of these proteins and the preliminary results of the evaluation of these recombinants as potential AIDS vaccines.

BIOCHEMICAL CHARACTERIZATIONS OF HIV ENVELOPE GLYCOPROTEINS EXPRESSED BY RECOMBINANT VACCINIA VIRUSES

The envelope (*env*) gene of HIV-1 encodes for a polypeptide 856 amino acids in length (BRU or IIIB isolates). This polypeptides is heavily glycosylated and has an apparent molecular weight of 150-160 kD (gp150/160). Glycoprotein gp160 is proteolytically cleaved into an exterior glycoprotein of 110-120 kD (gp110/120) and a transmembrane glycoprotein of 41 kD (gp41) (10,11). Glycoprotein gp120 confers much of the T-lymphotropic properties of HIV because it contains the CD4 receptor binding site(s) (12-14). Together with gp41, it mediates syncytium formation in $CD4^+$ cells (15,16). The envelope glycoproteins have been the primary targets for HIV vaccine development to date.

We and others (7-9) have constructed recombinant vaccinia viruses expressing the envelope glycoproteins of HIV-1. These recombinants contain a chimeric gene consisting of the entire HIV-1 envelope-coding sequence inserted downstream form a vaccinia virus promoter (7.5K). This chimeric gene is inserted in the thymidine kinase gene of vaccinia virus. Upon infection of tissue cells, these recombinants direct the synthesis of three major glycoproteins immunoreactive with HIV-positive sera. They correspond to HIV-1 envelope glycoproteins gp160, gp120, and gp41. The processing and the localization of the recombinant-made glycoproteins appear to be similar to that of authentic HIV envelope glycoproteins. For example, recombinant gp160 is cleaved, presumably by host protease(s), into gp120 and gp41 (7,8; Fig. 1A), which are transported to the surface of recombinant-infected cells (8). Recombinant-made glycoprotein gp120 is released into infected cell culture medium (7,9; Fig. 1A), as has been observed for the HIV counterpart (17). In contrast, efficient cleavage of the precursor envelope glycoprotein is not observed for a chimeric gp160 expressed in a transformed mammalian cell line (18). The reason for this discrepancy has yet to be resolved.

Using vaccinia virus vectors, we have also expressed several mutant forms of the HIV envelope glycoproteins. Figure 1B describes some of these recombinants

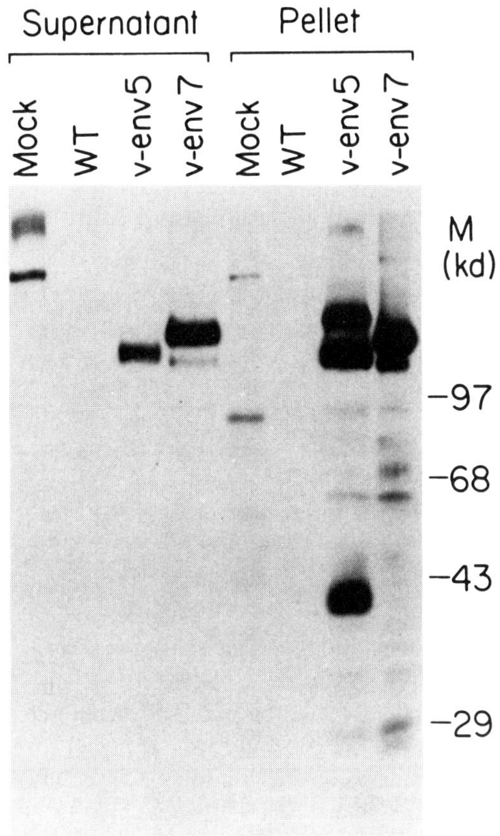

Figure 1A Radioimmunoprecipitation of recombinant-made HIV envelope glycoproteins by HIV-positive human serum. African green monkey kidney cells were infected with either vaccinia virus (WT), or recombinants containing HIV-1 *env* gene (v-env5 and v-env7). Immunoreactive proteins from infected cells (pellet) or from infected culture medium (supernatant) were resolved by SDS–PAGE.

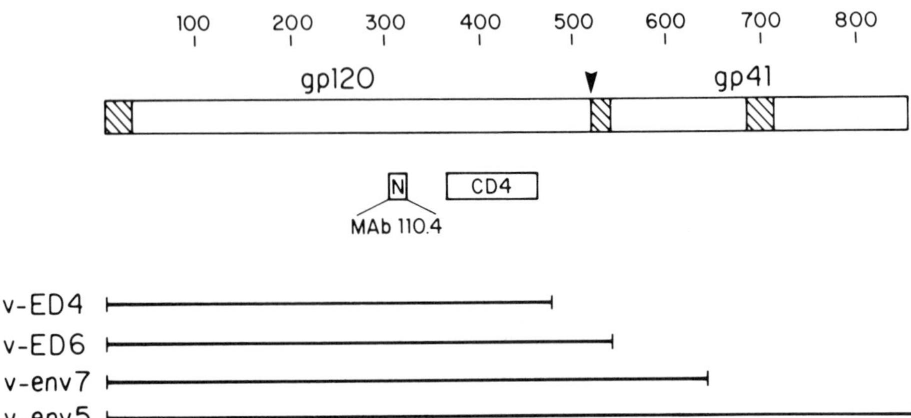

Figure 1B Envelope glycoproteins of HIV-1. Hatched areas indicate major hydrophobic regions. Locations of CD4-binding region (20,23) and the major neutralizing epitope (66–69) recognized by monoclonal antibody 110.4 (22,24) are as indicated. The following HIV *env*–specific amino acid sequences are expressed by vaccinia recombinant viruses: v-ED4, 1-467; v-ED6, 1-531; v-env7, 1-640; v-env5, 1-856. Numbering is based on HXB2 sequence compiled by Myers et al. (65).

that express a nested set of HIV *env*-related glycoproteins. These glycoproteins all share the same N-terminal sequence as HIV gp160, but have differently truncated carboxy-termini. These recombinants were used to study the sequence requirements for the membrane localization and the CD4-binding properties of HIV envelope glycoproteins.

Hydropathicity analysis of gp160 indicates the presence of three major hydrophobic regions. The N-terminal hydrophobic region is believed to be the signal sequence for the membrane localization of the glycoproteins. The role of the other two hydrophobic regions in gp41 is less clear. it has been suggested that both regions interact with lipid bilayers and serve as transmembrane anchor sequences for gp160 or gp41 (19). Alternatively, evidence exists indicating that only the C-terminal hydrophobic region serves as the anchor sequence (18,20) and that the other hydrophobic region at the N-terminus of gp41 facilitates membrane fusion (18,20-21). Result of our analysis supports the latter hypothesis. Recombinant v-env7 directs the synthesis of a 130 kD glycoprotein (amino acid number 1-640), which lacks the C-terminal hydrophobic region. In contrast to the full-length gp160, the truncated glycoprotein is efficiently secreted into infected cell medium (Fig. 1A) and is not present on infected cell surface (unpublished data). It should be noted that very little gp120 is processed from the truncated precursor, suggesting a possible requirement of membrane anchoring for the efficient cleavage of gp160.

Recombinant-made HIV gp120 (v-ED6, Fig. 1B) binds to CD4 receptors with similar affinity and specificity as authentic gp120 (22). This binding is drastically reduced when the C-terminal 44 amino acids of gp120 are removed, as in the case of the truncated gp120 produced by recombinant v-ED4 (22). This protein contains regions of gp120 at amino acid nos. 363, 419, and 426–437 previously identified by Kowalski et al. (20) and Lasky et al. (23) as essential for gp120–CD4 interactions. Our results indicate that the presence of these regions on gp120, although necessary, is not sufficient for its binding to CD4 receptor. This binding, however, is not affected by a neutralizing monoclonal antibody (mAb 110.4) that recognizes a major neutralization epitope (amino acid number 302–320) located within a highly variable region of gp120 (22,24; Fig. 1B). Neutralization of HIV infectivity by this and other similar antibodies (25) is therefore not likely to involve direct blocking of gp120–CD4 interactions, but rather through the inhibition of subsequent step(s) necessary for viral infection, such as the presumed associations between gp120 and gp41 (20) leading to the fusion of viral envelope and cell membrane and the formation of syncytium.

Recombinant vaccinia virus thus provides an altrernative system to study the biosynthesis and the biochemical properties of HIV envelope glycoproteins. Large quantities of HIV envelope glycoproteins can also be produced by recombinant vaccinia virus in a highly efficient expression system (25) and be used in the formulation of potential subunit vaccines against AIDS (26).

IMMUNOGENICITY STUDIES OF RECOMBINANT VACCINIA VIRUSES EXPRESSING HIV ENVELOPE GLYCOPROTEINS

Most of the work reported to date on the immunogenicity of vaccinia-HIV*env* recombinants has been done on recombinants that express the entire *env* gene. The ability of these recombinants to induce HIV-specific immune responses was first demonstrated in mice. Seroconversion was detected following a single inoculation of vaccinia-HIV*env* recombinant virus administered subcutaneously (7,9), or intraperitoneally (8). Most of these antibodies were directed to gp41 and gp160 as determined by immunoblot analysis (7,9), although some reactivity to gp120 could also be detected by immunoprecipitation analysis (8). Kieny et al. (9) observed that titers of HIV-specific antibodies generated by mice immunized with vaccinia-HIV*env* recombinant were low as compared to that of antivaccinia antibodies. This was attributed to the rapid loss of envelope antigens from the surface of recombinant-infected cells (9,27). Sera from recombinant-immunized mice generally contain no or very low titers (<1:20) of HIV-neutralizing activities (E. Kinney-Thomas and S.-L. Hu, unpublished results).

The immunogenicity of vaccinia-HIV*env* recombinant virus was also tested in several primate species. Contrary to the results obtained in mice, there is little or no HIV-specific antibody in macaques (*Macaca fascicularis*) following primary immunization with the recombinant virus (28). A second inoculation with the recombinant virus increased the titers of anti-HIV antibodies significantly (28). Low to moderate levels of HIV-neutralizing antibodies are also generated in *M. mulatta* (B. Moss, personal communication) and in *M. fascicularis* (E. Kinney-Thomas and S.-L. Hu, unpublished results) following repeated inoculations of the recombinant virus.

In addition to antibody responses, strong T-cell-mediated immunity to HIV was also elicited by immunization with the recombinant virus. This was first demonstrated by Zarling et al. (29), who showed that peripheral blood lymphocytes (PBL) from macaques immunized with vaccinia-HIV*env* recombinant virus proliferated and produced lymphokine interleukin-2 (IL-2) in response to stimulation by HIV antigens. In vivo, these IL-2-producing T-helper cells not only could promote B-cell differentiation for the production of antibodies against HIV, but also activate effector cells, such as cytotoxic T lymphocytes (CTL) and/or natural killer cells, to destroy HIV-infected cells.

The fact that HIV-specific cytotoxic T lymphocytes can indeed be induced by immunization with recombinant vaccinia-HIV*env* virus was first demonstrated in chimpanzees by Zarling et al. (30). PBLs from immunized chimpanzees showed strong proliferative response upon stimulation with HIV envelope antigens. Following expansion in the presence of envelope antigens, T-cell clones were established and were shown to be able to lyse autologous lymphoblastoid cell lines infected with recombinant vaccinia virus expressing HIV envelope antigens, but not those infected with parental vaccinia virus (30). These results demonstrate that the envelope glycoproteins of HIV not only can induce a CTL response in primates, but also can serve as a target for such a response. Unfortunately, no neutralizing antibody was detected in any of the immunized animals. Similar results were also reported by Girard and coworkers (4th International Conference on AIDS, 1988). They immunized chimpanzees with recombinant vaccinia virus expressing either HIV*env* alone, or together with IL-2. They then boosted the animals with inactivated HIV, or with formalin-fixed autologous cells infected with recombinant vaccinia-HIV*env* virus. No neutralizing antibody was observed. The lack of a strong neutralizing antibody response has also been observed in chimpanzees immunized with native or recombinant-produced HIV envelope antigens (31,32). The reason for these low responses is not yet understood.

Protective immunity has been observed in chimpanzees immunized with recombinant vaccinia virus expressing hepatitis B surface antigen, despite the fact that very little or no antibody was detected prior to challenge (33). Since immunization of chimpanzees with vaccinia-HIV*env* recombinant virus induced both HIV-specific antibodies (albeit nonneutralizing) and T-cell-mediated immunity (including CTL response), we sought to determine the effect of such immunization on subsequent challenge infection by HIV-1. Two experiments were performed. One involved six chimpanzees (two controls and four experimentals, see footnote to Table 1) challenged with a high dose of HIV (3×10^5 50% tissue culture infectious dose) and the other involved three animals (one control and two experimentals) challenged with a low dose of virus (100 $TCID_{50}$), all administered intravenously. Following the challenge, an anamnestic response was observed in all the vaccinia-HIV*env*-immunized animals, indicated by the immediate rise of HIV-specific antibody titers (Fig. 2). This early increase is specific for antibodies against envelope antigens (Fig. 3) and is correlated with the early appearance of HIV-neutralizing activities (34).Animals challenged with high doses of HIV showed seroconversion to core antigens between 4–6 weeks following infection, whereas those challenged with low doses did so between 8–10 weeks. There is no substantial difference between control and experimental animals in their antibody responses to core antigens, with the exception that one experimental animal (no. 72, Fig. 3) challenged with low dose of virus developed *gag*-specific antibody antigens 4–6 weeks earlier than the control animal. Viral antigenemia (p24) and viremia were detected in the sera of the two control animals infected with a high dose of HIV between 2–4 weeks following challenge (Table 1). This was not observed in the four experimental animals in the same group, nor in any of the three animals challenged with the low dose

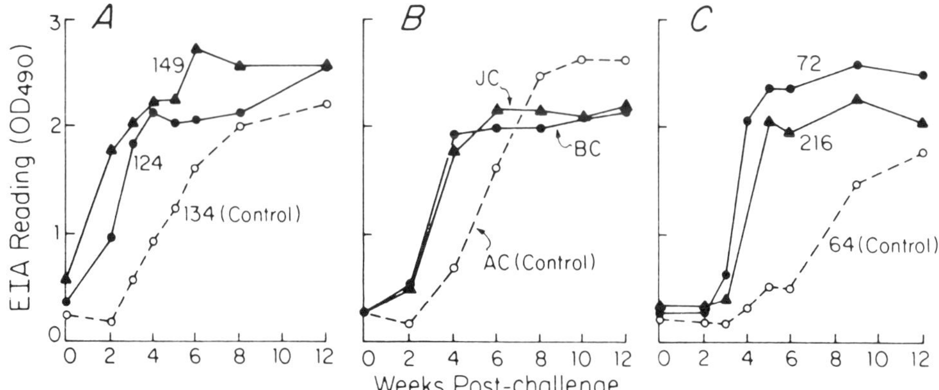

Figure 2 Seroconversion of HIV-infected chimpanzees. Serum samples were diluted 1:400, and HIV-specific antibodies were detected by enzyme-linked immunoassay (Genetic System, Corp.). Panels A, B, and C refer to three groups of animals used in this experiment. See footnote *a* of Table 1 for information on immunization and challenge.

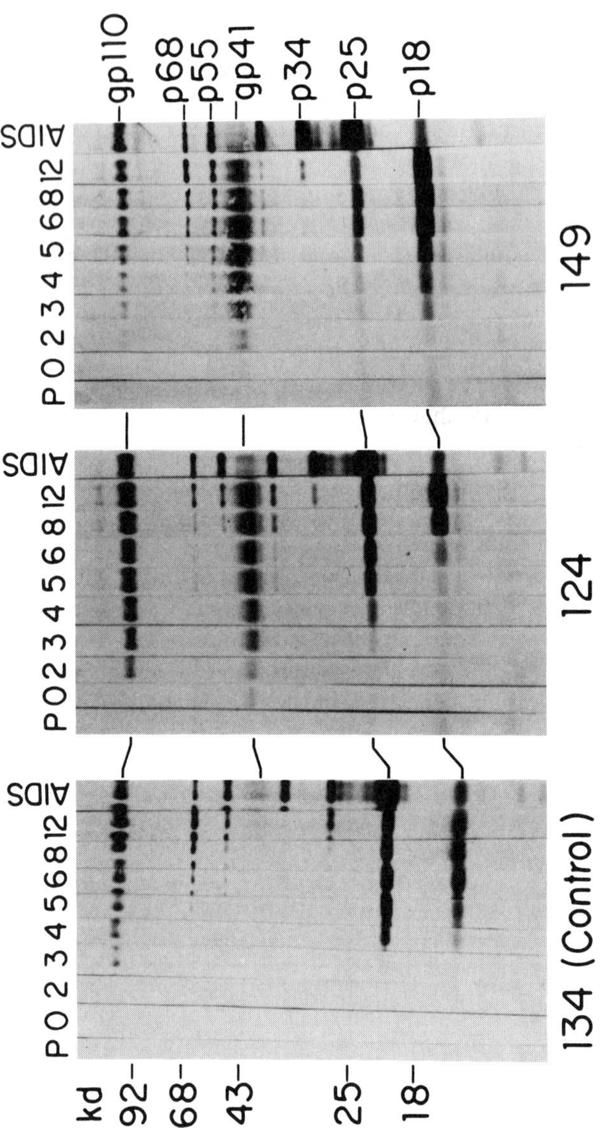

gp110
p68
p55
gp41
p34
p25
p18
AIDS
P O 2 3 4 5 6 8 12 A
149
AIDS
P O 2 3 4 5 6 8 12 A
124
AIDS
P O 2 3 4 5 6 8 12 A
134 (Control)
kd
92—
68—
43—
25—
18—
(A)

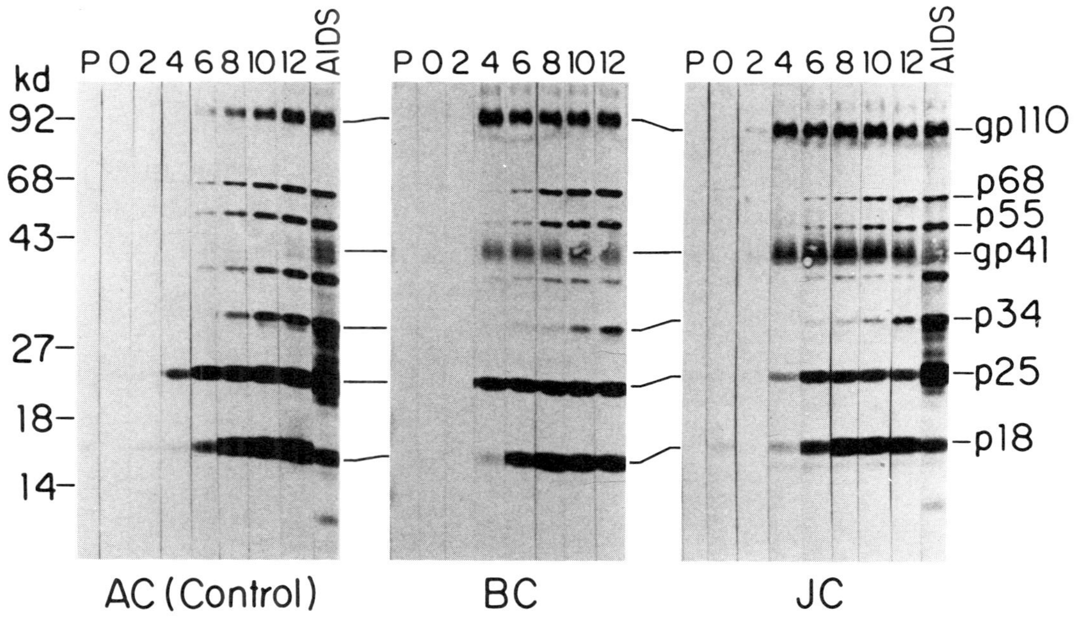

(B)

Figure 3 Western blot analysis of sera from HIV-infected chimpanzees. Serum samples were diluted 100-fold and tested for reactivity to purified HIV virion proteins by Western blot (Genetic Systems, Corp.) as previously described (34). See footnote a of Table 1 for information on immunization and challenge. P = prebleed; 0 = prechallenge; 2-12 = biweekly bleeds following challenge; AIDS = HIV-positive human serum. Panels A, B, and C refer to three groups of animals used in this experiment. Refer to Table 1 for information on immunization and challenge. Panel B is reproduced, with permission, from Hu et al. (34).

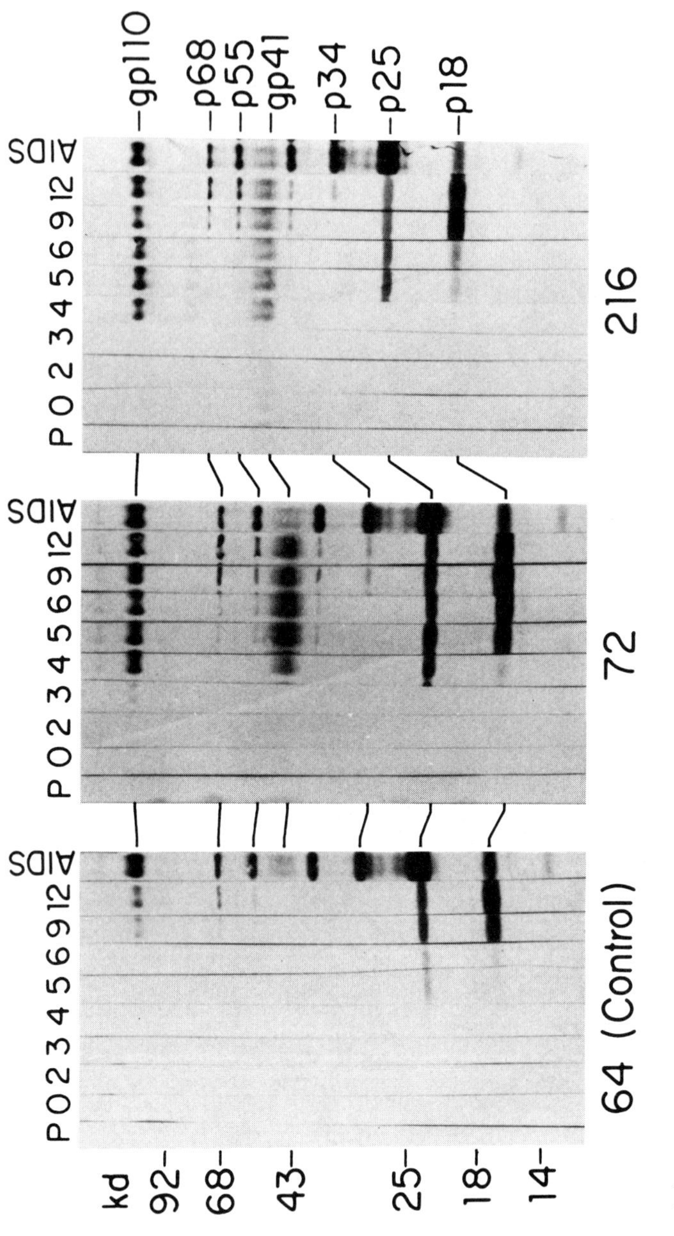

(C)

Figure 3 (Continued)

Table 1 Viral Antigenemia and Viremia in HIV-Infected Chimpanzees

Animal no.	Immunized with[a]	Challenge dose ($TCID_{50}$)	Weeks after challenge				
			0	2	3	4	$\geqslant 5$
134	v-HSVgD1NY	300,000	−	+[b]	++[c]	+	−
149	v-env5NY		−	−	−	−	−
124	v-env5NY		−	−	−	−	−
AC	v-HSVgD1WR	300,000	−	+	NT[d]	+	−
BC	v-env5WR		−	−	NT	−	−
JC	v-env5WR		−	−	NT	−	−
64	v-HSVgD1NY	100	−	−	−	−	−
72	v-env5NY		−	−	−	−	−
216	v-env5NY		−	−	−	−	−

[a]Control animals received recombinant vaccinia virus expressed glycoprotein D of herpes simplex virus type 1 (v-HSVgD1). Experimental animals received recombinant v-env5, which expresses the entire *env* gene of HIV. Suffixes NY and WR indicate, respectively, the parental virus as New York Board of Health or Western Reserve strains of vaccinia virus.
[b]+ = sera contain HIV core antigen (p24) by commercial tests (Genetic Systems Corp. or Abbott).
[c]Infectious virus (HIV-1) was detected in this serum sample by in vitro infectivity assays.
[d]Not tested.

of virus. However, all animals, both control and experimental, became persistently infected with HIV-1 as indicated by the presence of infectious virus following in vitro co-cultivation of PBLs from challenged animals with activated human PBLs (unpublished data). It therefore appears that although immunization with vaccinia-HIV*env* recombinant virus serves to potentiate HIV-specific antibody responses, the immunity generated is not sufficient to protect the animals from HIV-1 infection.

Whether immunization could have prevented the development of disease following HIV infection cannot be answered in the chimpanzee model, since HIV-infected chimpanzees do not develop clinical symptoms comparable to AIDS in humans. Alter et al. (35) reported the development of persistent lymphadenopathy in an animal transfused with large quantities of plasma from AIDS patients. It is of interest to note that in the chimpanzee challenge study described above (33), one of the two control animals challenged with a high dose of HIV-1 developed persistent lymphadenopathy similar to that observed in some HIV-infected humans. In contrast, none of the four immunized animals challenged with the same dose of HIV-1 showed any clinical symptoms. Based on these results, one could speculate that, although immunization did not prevent HIV infection, it might have affected the development of lymphadeno-pathy in these animals. Indeed, examples exist where immunization can effectively prevent disease, but not necessarily infection (36–38). Unfortunately, data cited above (33) do not warrant such conclusions, partly because of the lack of statistical significance and partly because of the limitations of the chimpanzee as a model for the study of human diseases caused by HIV infection.

Studies of human immune responses to HIV antigens have been largely limited to HIV-infected individuals. Several lines of evidence indicate that the immune responses of HIV-infected humans differ from that of experimentally infected chimpanzees (39–41). It is therefore of importance to study how humans respond to HIV antigens in the absence of HIV infection and to compare these responses to that observed in other animals species. Several ongoing clinical trials test the safety and immunogenicity of various recombinant-made and synthetic HIV antigens (7,9,42,43). Two of these studies focus on vaccinia-HIV*env* recombinants, one conducted by Zagury and his colleagues in France and in Zaire, and the other by Oncogen/Bristol-Myers in the United States.

Zagury et al. (44) reported that low titers of HIV-specific neutralizing antibodies as well as T-helper responses were obtained following a single immunization with vaccinia-HIV*env* recombinant virus. The neutralizing activity was largely against the homologous strain of HIV-1, whereas the T-cell response appeared to be more broadly reactive. Significant enhancement of immune responses was elicited by boosting first with paraformaldehyde-fixed autologous lymphocytes previously infected with vaccinia-HIV*env* recombiant virus, and then with gp160 made by recombinant vaccinia virus. Broadly reactive neutralizing antibodies and cell-mediated immunity, including CTL, helper T cells, immediate- and delayed-type hypersensitivity to gp160, were observed. Although there is no indication whether any of these immune responses would be protective against HIV infection, these results are certainly encouraging in that functional immune responses could be induced by immunization.

Although vaccinia virus itself has been used extensively, recombinant vaccinia-HIV*env* virus represents the first live recombinant virus tested in humans. There are many issues, both regulatory and scientific, that need to be addressed before this novel approach can be used as a realistic vaccine strategy. Toward this goal, we have initiated a Phase I clinical trial of vaccinia-HIV*env* recombinant virus under the approval of the Food and Drug Administration of the United States. The objective of this study is to evaluate parameters that affect the safety and the immunogenicity of such recombinant vaccinia virus in people with or without prior exposure to smallpox vaccine. Preliminary results indicate that there is no adverse effect due to immunization (L. Corey, personal communication). Immune responses are currently being evaluated.

FUTURE DIRECTIONS

In spite of the progress made in the study of HIV, major obstacles exist for the development of a safe and efficacious vaccine against AIDS. One of these difficulties lies in the poor understanding of immune markers indicative of protection against AIDS. For certain viral diseases, presence of neutralizing antibodies predicts protective immunity (45,46). Neutralizing antibodies have been detected in HIV-infected individuals (47,48). However, there is only weak correlation between the presence of such antibodies to lesser disease outcome (47-49). Initial attempts to demonstrate adoptive immunity by transfusing high-titered neutralizing human immunoglobulins to chimpanzees have failed to protect the animals against HIV infection (50). Other HIV-specific immune responses, such as antibody-dependent cellular cytotoxicity (ADCC) and cytolytic T lymphocytes (CTL), have also been detected in HIV-infected individuals (51-55). In other viral systems, these mechanisms play an important role in limiting viral infections by clearing virus-infected cells (56-58). Although it is not clear what role these immune mechansims would play in HIV infection, it is not unreasonable to assume that one of the operational goals of AIDS vaccine development is to elicit strong neutralizing antibodies, and helper T cell as well as CTL functions. Based on the work reviewed here (29,30,44), it is evident that, with appropriate regimen, immunization with recombinant vaccinia-HIV*env* virus could elicit all of these immune responses against HIV. Whether these responses are necessary and sufficient to protect against AIDS or HIV infection can only be answered in an appropriate test system.

Unfortunately, there is presently no suitable animal model to test vaccines against AIDS. Most studies to date utilize chimpanzees, which are scarce, costly, and do not develop AIDS as a result of HIV infection. In this regard, the chimpanzee model might be useful for identifying parameters that contribute to the development of AIDS in humans (39-41). But, as a system to test the efficacy of potential vaccines, chimpanzees are not ideal. Montagnier reported recently (4th International Conference on AIDS, 1988) that an AIDS-like disease can be induced in macaques following infection by HIV-2, which is similar to simian immunodeficiency virus (SIV) (59-61). If confirmed, macaques would be the system of choice to test vaccines against HIV-2. Alternatively, since SIV causes similar diseases in macaques as HIV does in humans (62), one could use SIV as a model to develop vaccines against SIV-induced AIDS in macaques and to establish immune markers that correlate with protection. The same approach will then be used to develop vaccines against HIV. Candidate vaccines that elicit immune responses comparable to those generated by successful SIV vaccines can then be tested for protection against HIV infection in chimpanzees and eventually for protection against AIDS in human. Recent demonstrations of HIV infection in rabbits (63) and in immunologically reconstituted mice (64) raise the possibility that these animal models could also be used for the testing of potential AIDS vaccines.

The extraordinarily high degree of genetic variability observed in HIV (65) poses a major challenge to the development of an AIDS vaccine. The envelope glycoproteins, which have been the primary targets for vaccine development, are also the least conserved antigens among various HIV isolates. The major neutralizing epitope of HIV-1 envelope glycoproteins has been localized in a highly variable region (66,67). Immunization with various proparations of envelope glycoproteins has generated neutralizing antibodies directed against predominantly the homologous strain of HIV (31,32,66-69). If these antibodies are shown to be protective against homologous HIV challenge, it is then possible to use mixtures of immunogens from various isolates to achieve a broader protection. In this regard, recombinant vaccinia virus may offer an advantage over other viral vectors (such as adenovirus) because of its large cloning capacity (25 kilobase pairs). Immunization with a single recombinant vaccinia virus expressing multiple foreign genes is able to elicit immune responses to each of these foreign antigens (70). However, for this "polyvalent vaccine" approach to be effective against HIV, one needs to identify the major serotypes and variants of HIV, the pattern of their cross-reactivity as well as the temporal and geographic variations of these variants. Since the answer to some of these questions may be difficult to obtain, it is important to explore immunization schemes that elicit cross-reactive immune responses to various HIV isolates (71,72). In this regard, one should consider not only envelope glycoproteins, but also other more conserved antigens (i.e., *gag, pol, nef*, etc.) as potential targets for recombinant vaccine developments.

A successful vaccine has to be both safe and efficacious. The safety of vaccinia virus has been well demonstrated in human populations. A small but definable risk has been associated with smallpox vaccination. Of the more common complications, the most severe form is generalized vaccinia in immunocompromised individuals (73). Being a live virus, vaccinia can also be accidentally transmitted (73). Therefore, the use of recombinant vaccinia virus as an approach to AIDS vaccine poses a unique dilemma, that is, if the vaccine is efficacious, it will be most needed in populations most likely to experience complications, i.e., those with high rates of HIV infction. Although these complications may not be as frequent as one might expect, generalized vaccinia after smallpox vaccination has been reported in a military recruit with HIV disease (74). It is therefore imperative that, if vaccinia-based vaccines are to be used, the immune status of prospective vaccinees should be prescreened, especially with regard to prior HIV infection. Second, precautions should be taken to minimize accidental infection of the vaccinees and their contacts. Third, further research should be directed at the development of a safe vector that can be used in immunocompromised individuals. Recent results indicate that vaccinia virus expressing IL-2 (75) may be useful as a vector for this purpose. Last, the potential complications due to the immune responses to HIV elicited by vaccination should also be considered. Immunoenhancement of viral infections has been documented (76). Although it remains controversial, evidence of immunoenhancement of HIV infection in vitro has been reported (77,78). It has also been suggested that the development of AIDS is related to autoimmune disorders triggered by immune responses to certain HIV antigens (see Ref. 79). So far, there has not been any untoward effect observed in people inoculated with any candidate AIDS vaccine, including recombinant vaccinia viruses. Further research, however, will be needed to confirm the long-term safety of these candidate vaccines. In this regard, an animal model, such as SIV infection of macaques, may be helpful to provide some insights.

SUMMARY

Vaccinia virus has been used as a vector to express the envelope glycoproteins of HIV. Recombinant-made envelope glycoproteins are correctly processed and are biologically active. Mutational analyses of the recombinant-made proteins allow us to define functional domains important to the cellular localization and the CD4-binding activity of HIV envelope glycoproteins. The potential of vaccinia-HIV*env* recombinants to serve as candidate vaccines against AIDS has been examined. Immunization with recombinant vaccinia-HIV*env* virus elicits HIV-specific immune responses, including neutralization antibodies, antibody-dependent cellular cytotoxicity, helper T-cell and cytotoxic T-lymphocyte functions. It is not clear at present if any of these immune responses could result in protection against AIDS. Proper animal models and extensive clinical trials will be needed before one could address such questions. Recombinant vaccinia virus offers several unique advantages as an approach to AIDS vaccine, although concern exists about its safety among populations with high HIV infections. Much more work is needed before the potential of such an approach can be realized.

ACKNOWLEDGMENTS

I wish to thank all my colleagues and collaborators whose names have been listed in the references cited below. This review would not have been possible without their work and contributions.

REFERENCES

1. Panicali D, Paoletti E. Construction of poxviruses as cloning vectors: Insertion of the thymidine kinase gene from herpes simplex virus into the DNA of infectious vaccinia virus. Proc Natl Acad Sci USA 1982; 79:4917–31.

2. Mackett M, Smith GL, Moss B. Vaccinia virus: A selectable eukaryotic cloning and expression vector. Proc Natl Acad Sci USA 1982; 79:7415–9.

3. Moss B, Flexner C. Vaccinia virus expression vectors. Ann Rev Immunol 1987; 5:305–24.

4. Henderson DA, Arita I. Utilization of vaccine in the global eradication of smallpox. In; Quinnan GV, ed. Vaccinia Viruses as Vectors for Vaccine Antigens. New York: Elsevier, 1985: 61–7.

5. Piot P, Plummer FA, Mhalu FS, Lamboray J-L, Chin J, Mann JM. AIDS: An international perspective. Science 1988; 239:573–9.

6. Weiss SH, Goedert JJ, Gartner S, Popovic M, Waters D, Markham P, di Marzo Veronese F, Gail MH, Barkley WE, Gibbons J, Gill FA, Leuther M, Shaw GM, Gallo RC, Blattner WA. Risk of human immunodeficiency virus (HIV-1) infection among laboratory workers. Science 1988; 239:68–71.

7. Hu S-L, Kosowski SG, Dalrymple J. Expression of AIDS virus envelope gene in recombinant vaccinia viruses. Nature (Lond.) 1986; 320:537–40.

8. Chakrabarti SM, Robert-Guroff M, Wong-Staal F, Gallo RC, Moss B. Expression of the HTLV–III envelope gene by a recombinant vaccinia virus. Nature (Lond.) 1986; 320:535–7.

9. Kieny MP, Rautmann G, Schmitt D, Dott K, Wain-Hobson S, Alizon M, Girard M, Chamaret S, Laurent A, Montagnier L, Lecocq J-P. AIDS virus env protein expressed from a recombinant vaccinia virus. Bio/Technology 1986; 4:790–5.

10. Robey WG, Safai B, Oroszlan S, Arthur LO, Gonda MA, Gallo RC, Fischinger PJ. Characterization of envelope and core structural gene products of HTLV–III with sera from AIDS patients. Science 1985; 228:593–5.

11. di Marzo Veronese F, De Vico AL, Copeland TD, Oroszlan S, Gallo RC, Sarngadharan MG. Characterization of gp41 as the transmembrane protein coded by the HTLV–III/LAV envelope gene. Science 1985; 229:1402–5.

12. Dalgleish A, Beverley PCL, Clapham PR, Crawford DH, Greaves MF, Weiss R. The CD4 (T4) antigen is an essential component of the receptor for the AIDS retrovirus. Nature (Lond.) 1984; 312:763–6.

13. Klatzmann D, Champagne E, Chamaret S, Gruest J, Guetard D, Hercend T, Gluckman JC, Montagnier L. T-lymphocyte T4 molecule behaves as the receptor for human retrovirus LAV. Nature (Lond.) 1984; 312:767–8.

14. McDougal JS, Kennedy MS, Sligh JM, Cort SP, Mawle A, Nicholson J. Binding of the HTLV–III/LAV to T4$^+$ T cells by a complex of the 110k viral protein and the T4 molecule. Science 1986; 231:382–6.

15. Lifson JD, Reyes GR, McGrath MS, Stein BS, Engleman EG. AIDS retrovirus induced cytopathology: giant cell formation and involvement of CD4 antigen. Science 1986; 232:1123–7.

16. Sodroski J, Goh WC, Rosen C, Campbell K, Haseltine WA. Role of the HTLV–III/LAV envelope in syncytium formation and cytopathicity. Nature (Lond.) 1986; 322:470-4.

17. Gelderblom HR, Reupke H, Pauli G. Loss of envelope antigens of HTLV-iii/LAV, a factor in AIDS pathogenesis? Lancet 1985; 2:1016-7.

18. Berman PW, Nunes WM, Haffar OK. Expression of membrane-associated and secreted variants of gp160 of human immunodeficiency virus type 1 in vitro and in continuous cell lines. J Virol 1988; 62:3135-42.

19. Modrow S, Hahn BH, Shaw GM, Gallo RC, Wong-Staal F, Wolf H. Computer-assisted analysis of envelope protein sequences of seven human immunodeficiency virus isolates: Prediction of antigenic epitopes in conserved and variable regions. J Virol 1987; 61:570-8.

20. Kowalski M, Potz J, Basiripour L, Dorman T, Goh WC, Terwilliger E, Dayton A, Rosen C, Haseltine W, Sodroski J. Functional regions of the envelope glycoprotein of the human immunodeficiency virus type 1. Science 1987; 237:1351-5.

21. Gallaher GR. Detection of a fusion peptide sequence in the transmembrane protein of human immunodeficiency virus. Cell 1987; 80:327-8.

22. Linsley PS, Ledbetter JA, Kinney-Thomas E, Hu S-L. Effects of anti-gp120 monoclonal antibodies on CD4 receptor binding by the env protein of HIV-1. J Virol 1988; 62:3695-702.

23. Lasky LA, Nakamura G, Smith DH, Fennie C, Shimasaki C, Patzer E, Berman PW, Gregory T, Capon DJ. Delineation of a region of the human immunodeficiency virus type 1 gp120 glycoprotein critical for interaction with the CD4 receptor. Cell 1987; 50:975-85.

24. Kinney-Thomas E, Weber JN, McClure J, Clapham PR, Singhal MC, Shriver MK, Weiss R. Neutralising monoclonal antibodies to the AIDS virus. AIDS 1988; 2:25-9.

25. Feurst TR, Earl PL, Moss B. Use of a hybrid vaccinia virus-T7 RNA polymerase system for expression of target genes. Mol Cell Biol 1987; 7:2538-44.

26. Barrett N, Mitterer A, Mundt W, Eibl J, Eibl M, Gallo RC, Moss B, Dorner F. Large scale production and purification of a vaccinia recombinant derived HIV-1 gp160 and analysis of its immunogenicity. AIDS Res Hum Retrov 1989; 5:159-71.

27. Kieny MP, Lathe R, Riviere Y, Dott K, Schmitt D, Girard M, Montagnier L, Lecocq J-P. Improved antigenicity of the HIV env protein by cleavage site removal. Protein Engineering 1988; 2:219-25.

28. Hu S-L, Morton W, Moran PA, McClure J, Kosowski SG, Zarling JM. Immune response to human immunodeficiency virus in macaques immunized with recombinant vaccinia virus. In: Chanock RM et al., eds. Modern approaches to new vaccines Cold Spring Harbor, NY: Cold Spring Harbor Laboratory, 1987: 231-5.

29. Zarling JM, Morton W, Moran PA, McClure J, Kosowski SG, Hu S-L. T-cell responses to human AIDS virus in macaques immunized with recombinant vaccinia viruses. Nature (Lond.) 1986; 323:344-6.

30. Zarling JC, Eichberg JW, Moran PA, McClure J, Sridhar P, Hu S-L. Proliferative and cytotoxic T cells to AIDS virus glycoproteins in chimpanzees immunized with a recombinant vaccinia virus expressing AIDS virus envelope glycoproteins. J Immunol 1987; 139:988-90.

31. Arthur LO, Pyle SW, Nara PL, Bess JW Jr, Gonda MA, Kelliher JC, Gilden RV, Robey WG, Bolognesi DP, Gallo RC, Fischinger PJ. Serological responses in chimpanzees inoculated with human immunodeficiency virus glycoprotein (gp120) subunit vaccine. Proc Natl Acad Sci USA 1987; 84:8583-7.

32. Berman PW, Groopman JE, Gregory T, Clapham PR, Weiss RA, Ferriani R, Riddle L, Shimasaki C, Lucas C, Lasky LA, Eichberg JW. Human immunodeficiency virus type 1 challenge of chimpanzees immunized with recombinant envelope glycoprotein gp120. Proc Natl Acad Sci USA 1988; 85: 5200-4.

33. Moss B, Smith GL, Gerin JL, Purcell RH. Live recombinant vaccinia virus protects chimpanzees against hepatitis B. Nature (Lond.) 1984 311:67-9.

34. Hu S-L, Fultz PN, McClure HM, Eichberg JW, Kinney-Thomas E, Zarling JM, Singhal MC, Kosowski SG, Swenson SG, Anderson DC, Todaro G. Effect of immunization with vaccinia-HIV *env* recombinant on HIV infection in chimpanzees. Nature (Lond.) 1987; 328:721-3.

35. Alter HJ, Masur H, Saxinger WC, Gallo RC, Macher AM, Lane HC, Fauci AS. Transmission of HTLV-III infection from human plasma to chimpanzees: an animal model for AIDS. Science 1984; 226:549-52.

36. Salk JE, Vaccination against paralytic poliomyelitis: performance and prospects. Am J Publ Health 1955; 45:575-96.

37. Olsen RG, Hoover EA, Schaller JP, Mathes LE, Wolff L. Abrogation of resistance to feline oncornavirus disease by immunization with killed feline leukemia virus. Cancer Research 1977; 37:2082-5.

38. Earl PL, Moss B, Morrison RP, Wehrly K, Nishio J, Chesebro B. T-lymphocyte priming and protection against Friend leukemia by vaccinia-retrovirus env gene recombinant. Science 1986; 234:728-31.

39. Wahren B, Morfeldt-Mansson L, Biberfeld G, Moberg L, Sonnerborg A, Ljungman P, Werner A, Kurth R, Gallo RC. Characteristics of the specific cell-mediated immune response in human immunodeficiency virus infection. J Virol 1987; 61:2017-23.

40. Eichberg JW, Zarling JM, Alter HJ, Levy JA, Berman PA, Gregory T, Lasky LA, McClure J, Cobb KE, Moran PA, Hu S-L, Kennedy RC, Chanh TC, Dreesman GR. T cell responses to human immunodeficiency virus (HIV) and its recombinant antigens in HIV infected chimpanzees. J Virol 1987; 61:3804-8.

41. Zarling JM, Eichberg JW, Moran PA, McClure J, Morton W, Alter H, Hu S-L. T-cell mediated immune responses to HIV in immunized and HIV-infected primates. In: Bolognesi D, ed. Human retroviruses, cancer, and AIDS: Approaches to prevention and therapy. New York: Alan R. Liss, Inc., 1988: 327-40.

42. Cochran MA, Ericson BL, Knell JD, Smith GE. Use of baculovirus recombinants as a general method for the production of subunit vaccines. In: Chanock RM et al., eds. Modern approaches to new vaccines Cold Spring Harbor, NY: Cold Spring Harbor Laboratory, 1987: 384-8.

43. Naylor PH, Naylor CW, Badamchian M, Wada S, Goldstein AL, Wang S-S, Sun DK, Thornton AH, Sarin PS. Human immunodeficiency virus contains an epitope immunoreactive with thymosin α_1 and the 30-amino acid synthetic p17 group-specific antigen peptide HGP-30. Proc Natl Acad Sci USA 1987; 84:2951-5.

44. Zagury D, Bernard J, Cheynier R, Desportes I, Leonard R, Fouchard M, Reveil B, Ittele D, Lurhuma Z, Mbayo K, Wane J, Salaun J-J, Goussard B, Dechazal L, Burny A, Nara P, Gallo RC. A group specific anamnestic immune reaction againt HIV-1 induced by a candidate vaccine against AIDS. Nature (Lond.) 1988; 332:728-1.

45. Essex M. Feline leukemia: A naturally occurring cancer of infectious origin. Epidemiol Rev 1982; 4:189-203.

46. Daniel MD, Letvin NL, Sehgal PK, Hunsmann G, Schmidt DK, King NW, Desrosiers, RC. Long-term persistent infection of macaque monkeys with the simian immunodeficiency virus. J Gen Virol 1987; 68:3183-9.

47. Weiss RA, Clapham PR, Chiengsong-Popov R, Dalgleish AG, Carne CA, Weller IVD, Tedder RS. Neutralization of human T lymphotropic virus type III by sera of AIDS and AIDS-risk patients. Nature (Lond.) 1985; 316:69-72.

48. Robert-Guroff M, Brown M, Gallo RC. HTLV-III-neutralizing antibodies in patients with AIDS and AIDS-related complex. Nature (Lond) 1985; 316:72-4.

49. Weber JN, Clapham PA, Weiss RA, Parker D, Roberts C, Duncan J, Weller I, Carne C, Tedder RS, Pinching AJ, Cheingsong-Popov R. Human immunodeficiency virus infection in two cohorts of homosexual men: neutralising sera of anti-gag antibody with prognosis. Lancet 1987; 1:119-21.

50. Prince AM, Horowitz B, Baker L, Shulman RW, Ralph H, Valinsky J, Cundell A, Brotman B, Boehle W, Rey F, Piet M, Reesink H, Tersmette M, Miedema F, Barbosa L, Memo G, Nastala CL, Allan JS, Lee DR, Eichberg JW. Failure of an HIV immune globulin to protect chimpanzees against experimental challenge with HIV. Proc Natl Acad Sci USA 1988; 85:6944-8.

51. Rook AH, Lane HC, Folks T, McCoy S, Alter H, Fauci AS. Sera from HTLV-III/LAV antibody-positive individuals mediate antibody-dependent cellular cytotoxicity against HTLV-III/LAV-infected T cells. J Immunol 1987; 138:1064-7.

52. Ljunggren K, Bottiger B, Biberfeld G, Karlson A, Fenyo E-M, Jondal M. Antibody-dependent cellular cytotoxicity-inducing antibodies against human immunodeficiency virus: Presence at different clinical stages. J Immunol 1987; 139:2263-7.

53. Walker BD, Chakrabarti S, Moss B, Paradis TJ, Flynn T, Durno AG, Blumberg RS, Kaplan JC, Hirsch MS, Schooley RT. HIV-specific cytotoxic

T lymphocytes in seropositive individuals. Nature (Lond.) 1987;328:345–58.

54. Walker BD, Flexner C, Paradis TJ, Fuller TC, Hirsch MS, Schooley RT, Moss B. HIV-1 reverse transcriptase is a target for cytotoxic T lymphocytes in infected individuals. Science 1988; 240:64–6.

55. Plata F, Autran B, Martins LP, Wain-Hobson S, Raphael M, Mayaud C, Denis M, Guillon J-M, Debre P. AIDS virus-specific cytotoxic T lymphocytes in lung disorders. Nature (Lond.) 1987; 328:348–51.

56. Shore SL, Cromeans TL, Romano TJ. Immune destruction of virus infected cells early in the infectious cycle. Nature (Lond.) 1976; 262:695–6.

57. Zinkernagel RM, Doherty PC. MHC restricted cytotoxic T cells: Studies on the biological role of polymorphic major transplantation antigens determining T cell restriction-specificity, function and responsiveness. Adv Immunol 1979; 27:51–63.

58. Britt WJ, Chesebro B. H-2D control of recovery from Friend virus leukemia: H-2D region influences the kinetics of the T lymphocyte response to Friend virus. J Exp Med 1983; 157:1739–45.

59. Clavel C, Guyader M, Guetard D, Salle M, Montagnier L, Alizon M. Molecular cloning and polymorphism of the human immune deficiency virus type 2. Nature (Lond.) 1986; 325:691–5.

60. Franchini G, Gurgo C, Guo H-G, Gallo RC, Collalti E, Fargnoli KA, Hall LF, Wong-Staal F, Reitz MS Jr. Sequence of simian immunodeficiency virus and its relationship to the human immunodeficiency viruses. Nature (Lond.) 1987; 328:539–43.

61. Chakrabarti L, Guyader M, Alizon M, Daniel MD, Desrosiers RC, Tiollais P, Sonigo P. Sequence of simian immunodeficiency virus from macaque and its relationship to other human and simian retroviruses. Nature (Lond.) 1987; 328:543–7.

62. Letvin NL, Daniel MD, Sehgal PK, Desrosiers RC, Hunt RD, Waldrom LM, MacKey JJ, Schmidt DK, Chalifoux LV, King NW. Induction of AIDS-like disease in macaque monkeys with T-cell tropic retrovirus STLV-III. Science 1985; 230:71–73.

63. Filice G, Cereda PM, Varnier OE. Infection of rabbits with human immunodeficiency virus. Nature (Lond) 1988; 335:366–9.

64. Namikawa R, Kaneshima H, Lieberman M, Weissman IL, McCune JM. Infection of the SCID-hu mouse by HIV-1. Science 1988; 242:1684–6.

65. Myers G, Josephs SF, Rabson AB, Smith TF, Wong-Staal F, (eds.) Human retroviruses and AIDS. Los Alamos-Los Alamos National Laboratory, 1988.

66. Palker TJ, Clark ME, Langlois AJ, Mathews TJ, Weinhold KJ, Randall RR, Bolognesi DP, Haynes BF. Type-specific neutralization of the human immunodeficiency virus with antibodies to env-encoded synthetic peptides. Proc Natl Acad Sci USA 1988; 85:1932–6.

67. Rusche JR, Javaherian K, McDanal C, Petro J, Lynn DL, Grimaila R, Langlois A, Gallo RC, Arthur LO, Fischinger PJ, Bolognesi DP, Putney SD, Mathews TJ. Antibodies that inhibit fusion of human immunodeficiency

virus-infected cells bind a 24-amino acid sequence of the viral envelope, gp120. Proc Natl Acad Sci USA 1988; 85:3198–202.

68. Mathews TJ, Langlois AJ, Bobey WG, Chang NT, Gallo RC, Fischinger PJ, Bolognesi DP. Restricted neutralization of divergent human T-lymphotropic virus type III isolates by antibodies to the major envelope glycoprotein. Proc Natl Acad Sci USA 1986; 83:9709–13.

69. Putney SD, Matthews TJ, Robey WG, Lynn DL, Robert-Guroff M, Mueller WT, Langlois AJ, Ghrayer J, Petteway SR Jr, Weinhold KJ, Fischinger PJ, Wong-Staal F, Gallo RC, Bolognesi DP. HTLV-III/LAV neutralizing antibodies to an E. coli produced fragment of the virus envelope. Science 1986; 234:1392–5.

70. Perkus ME, Piccini A, Lipinskas BR, Paoletti E. Recombinant vaccinia virus: Immunization against multiple pathogens. Science 1985; 229:981–4.

71. Ho DD, Kaplan JC, Rackausjas IE, Gurney ME. Second conserved domain of gp120 is important for HIV infectivity and antibody neutralization. Science 1988 239:1021–3.

72. Chanh TC, Dreesman GR, Kennedy RC. Neutralization of human immunodeficiency virus by a monoclonal anti-idiotype that mimics the viral receptor. Proc Natl Acad Sci USA 1987; 84:3891–5.

73. Arita I, Fenner F. Complications of smallpox vaccination. In: Quinnan GV, ed. Vaccinia viruses as vectors for vaccine antigens. New York: Elsevier, 1985.

74. Redfield RR, Wright DC, James WD, Jones TS, Brown C, Burke DS. Disseminated vaccinia in a military recruit with human immunodeficiency virus (HIV) disease. N Engl J Med 1987; 316:673–6.

75. Flexner C, Hugin A, Moss B. Attenuation of live recombinant vaccinia virus vactors by expression of human interleukin-2. In: Ginsberg H et al., eds. New chemical and genetic approaches to vaccination. Cold Spring Harbor, NY: Cold Spring Harbor Laboratory, 1988.

76. Porterfield JS. Antibody-dependent enhancement of viral infectivity. Adv Virus Res 1986; 31:335–55.

77. Robinson WE, Montefiori DC, Mitchell WM. Antibody-dependent enhancement of human immunodeficiency virus type 1 infection. Lancet 1988; 1:790–4.

78. Homsy J, Tateno M, Levy JA. Antibody-dependent enhancement of HIV infection. Lancet 1988; 1:1285–6.

79. Fauci AS. The human immunodeficiency virus: Infectivity and mechanisms of pathogenesis. Science 1988; 239:617–22.

80. Hu S-L, Zarling JM, Chinn J, Travis BM, Moran PA, Sias J, Kuller L, Morton WR, Heidecker G, Benveniste RE. Protection of macaques against simian AIDS by immunization with a recombinant vaccinia virus expressing the envelope glycoproteins of simian type-D retrovirus. Proc Natl Acad Sci USA 1989; 86:7213–7.

10

Large-Scale Production, Purification, and Immunologic Analysis of a Vaccinia Recombinant Derived HIV-1 gp160

Friedrich Dorner and Noel Barrett
Immuno AG
Vienna, Austria

Bernard Moss
National Institute of Allergy and Infectious Diseases
National Institutes of Health
Bethesda, Maryland

INTRODUCTION

The acquired immunodeficiency syndrome (AIDS) was first recognized in 1981 (1-3), and the etiologic agent associated with the disease was first isolated in 1983 (4) and identified as a retrovirus. The disease has spread rapidly in the intervening period so that an estimated 1-1.5 million people have been infected with the etiologic agent, the human immunodeficiency virus (HIV-1) in the United States alone (5). Initial surveillance studies in Central Africa suggest an annual incidence of AIDS of 550-1200 cases per million adults (6), and at least one case of the disease has been reported in 123 countries up to October 1987 (7). These data demonstrate the large-scale spread of the disease and demonstrate the urgent need for a vaccine against its etiologic agent.

Based on other retroviral models, such as murine, feline, bovine, and simian viruses, the obvious candidate for a vaccine to prevent primary infection is the envelope glycoprotein (8-13). Antibodies to this protein are also readily detectable in infected patients (14-16). The HIV-1 envelope protein is synthesized as a polyprotein precursor which is subsequently glycosylated within infected cells to give a glycoprotein with a mol. wt of 160 kDa (gp160), which is processed by proteolysis into a gp120 external glycoprotein and a gp41 transmembrane protein (14,16,17). It has been shown that the major envelope glycoprotein gp120 contains sites for binding to the receptor CD4 molecule on T4 cells (18–20), and it also contains sites which are recognized by neutralizing antibodies (17,21–23). There have also been reports that T-cell-mediated immune responses can be generated by immunization with gp120 (24) or a recombinant vaccinia virus coding for the HIV gp160 (25). However, as it has been reported that neutralizing epitopes are present on both the gp120 and gp41 proteins (26) and injection of chimpanzees with purified gp120 alone has failed to provide protection against infection with HIV-1 (52), we have decided to develop a candidate vaccine consisting of the full-length envelope glycoprotein.

HIV-1 envelope glycoproteins can be purified from virus or infected cells (21) but only in small amounts which make large-scale vaccine studies difficult. For this reason alternative approaches, which would allow production of larger quantities of a candidate vaccine, must be sought. A number of researchers have attempted to construct candidate vaccine which could be produced in larger quantities by cloning and expression of HIV proteins in bacterial (27), mammalian (23,28–30), and insect cell (31) systems. However systems which do not envisage protein expression in mammalian systems may result in production of proteins which are nonglycosylated or have glycosylation patterns different from that of the authentic virus-derived protein. This could result in alterations in the folding of the protein and the loss of conformational epitopes important in the induction of a specific humoral and cellular immune response.

For this reason we have attempted to develop a candidate vaccine using the full envelope glycoprotein in a eukaryotic expression vector. Vaccinia virus is a particularly useful vector in that recombinants can be readily constructed by integration of the foreign gene in a nonessential region of the vaccinia DNA and thus retain infectivity. When properly engineered the proteins are synthesized, processed, and transported to the membrane of infected cells. Although vaccinia virus infection leads to cell death, there is little lysis and the majority of cells remain intact, allowing easy extraction of the required protein from infected cells (32).

We have described a gp160 expression system based on coinfection of Vero cells with two recombinant vaccinia viruses (32), one of which contains the bacteriophage T7 RNA polymerase gene under control of a vaccinia promoter. The second recombinant contains the HIV-1 gp160 gene flanked by bacteriophage T7 promoter and termination sequences (32). We describe the large-scale production and purification of this protein from infected Vero cells. We have characterized it biochemically and have determined its immunogenicity in various animal models.

MATERIALS AND METHODS

Construction of Plasmids

Plasmids containing the HIV-1 gp160 and the T7 RNA polymerase have been previously described (32,33). Briefly, a 3.b kbp Sst I fragment containing the envelope gene (gp160) of HIV-I (HTLV-III$_B$) clone BH8 was inserted into M13mp18. In vitro mutagenesis generated on EcoRV site for ease of subcloning and a translation initiation codon with a eukaryotic consensus sequence. An additional EcoRV site was inserted following the termination codon of the gp160 gene. This fragment was then subcloned into an insertion recombinant plasmid via an endonuclease site. A plasmid containing the T7 RNA polymerase gene under the regulation of the vaccinia P7.5 promoter was constructed as follows. A 2.65 kbp DNA fragment, containing the entire T7 gene 1 coding region for T7 RNA polymerase, was excised with Bam H1 from plasmid pAR 1173 and inserted into the unique Bam H1 site of the plasmid pGS53.

Construction of Vaccinia Virus Recombinants

Recombinant viruses were prepared by infecting CV-1 cells with vaccinia virus (strain WR) and transfecting them with calcium phosphate precipitated plasmid DNA (34). The cells were harvested, and TK$^-$ recombinant viruses were isolated by plaque assay on thymidine kinase negative (TK$^-$) 143 cells (35) in the presence of BUdR and identified by DNA dot blot hybridization. Isolated virus was then plaque purified once more in TK$^-$ cells with BUdR selection, and virus stocks were prepared under nonselective conditions in Hela S3 cells.

Production of Recombinant Virus Stocks

High titer stocks of vaccinia recombinants were prepared by infecting Vero cells with 1 pfu virus/cell. After 2-3 days incubation at 37°C, the infected cells were shaken into the medium and pelleted by centrifugation at 5000 g for 20 min. The supernatant was poured off and stored at 4°C. The cells were then washed three times in PBS. A trypsin solution was then added to the cell suspension to give an end concentration of 0.025% trypsin. This suspension was then maintained at 37°C for 30 min with gentle stirring. The trypsinized cell suspension was then pooled with the medium supernatant and this was aliquoted and frozen at -80°C. This procedure increases the virus titer to approximately 10-fold that present in cell medium alone.

Large-Scale Cultivation of Vero Cells

A Vero cell inoculum was first prepared by passage of cells in plastic Roux and Roller bottles (Nunc) to produce sufficient cells to inoculate a 6-liter fermenter, which was then used as inoculum for a 40-liter vessel. A single ampule of Vero cells with a defined passage number was thawed from liquid nitrogen and passaged to produce 12 confluent Roller bottles. These cells were then trypsinized, resuspended in Medium 199 with 5% fetal calf serum, and mixed with a suspension of microcarriers (Cytodex 3, Pharmacia), which was then pumped into the fermenter to give a final concentration of 2×10^8 cells and 5 g microcarriers/liter. Medium was added at this stage to a volume of one third of the final working volume. The cells were allowed to adhere to the carriers for a 3-hour period during which the suspension was slowly stirred. After this period medium (DMEM with 5% FCS) was added to give the final working volume. When a cell number of 6-8×10^8/liter was achieved, continuous perfusion with DMEM with 5% FCS began. After a cell number of approximately 5×10^9/liter was achieved, the microcarriers were trypsinized and cells with microcarriers were pumped into a 40-liter fermenter, which contained 5 g/liter new microcarriers. After adsorption the fermenter was filled to a volume of 40 liters and cultivation proceeded as described above.

gp160 Production

When a cell density of 5×10^9/liter was achieved, the microcarriers were allowed to settle and the medium was pumped out. Five liters each of the two recombinants were pumped into the fermenter to give a moi of approximately 2 pfu of each recombinant per cell. After virus adsorption the fermenter were filled to a volume of 40 liters with medium 199 with 5% FCS. The fermenter was then perfused with 40 liters of the same medium over a 40-hr period. After this period approximately 80% of the cells were detached from the microcarriers, and they were pumped out with the medium. The remaining adhering cells were detached by washing with medium with rapid stirring, and they were pumped out and pooled with the first medium. Microcarriers were then removed by passage of this suspension through a 70 μm sieve. The cells were then pelleted by centrifugation in a Beckman JCF–Z continuous flow rotor at 16,000 g. The cell pellet, removed by scraping from the core, was weighed and frozen at $-80°C$ before processing for gp160 extraction and purification.

Purification

The thawed cell pellet for extraction of gp160 was resuspended in 10 volumes Tris-buffered saline (TBS) pH 7.4, with 1 mM $CuSO_4$, 0.5 mM $ZnCl_2$, and 0.1 mM PMSF. This was then passed through a Menten-Gaulin homogenizer at 1200 psi. The cell membrane resuspension was then pelleted at 25,000 g for 15 min. This pellet was then resuspended in 15 volumes of extraction buffer (50 mM Tris-HCl pH 8.3, 1% sodium deoxycholate, 1 mM $CuSO_4$, 0.5 mM $ZnCl_2$, 0.1 mM PMSF) and left at 25°C for 30 min. This suspension was then clarified by centrifugation at 100,000 g for 1 hr. The supernatant was then incubated for 16 hr with lentil-lectin sepharose. Fifty g wet gel were used per liter suspension. After adsorbtion of glycoproteins, the gel was washed with 50 mM Tris HCL pH 8.3, 0.25% deoxycholate with protease inhibitors. Bound proteins were then eluted with 5% methylglucoside in Tris buffer with 0.25% deoxycholate. The eluate was then diluted in TBS with 0.1% Tween-20. This was then incubated for 16 hr with sepharose-bound monoclonal antibody to HIV gp160. This was washed with TBS-Tween and TBS and then treated with 1000 units/liter DNAse and 50 units/liter RNAse in Tris-buffer pH 8.3, 1 mM $CaCl_2$, 1 mM $MgCl_2$. It was then washed with TBS, eluted with 3M KSCN, and dialyzed against TBS. The dialyzed eluate is adjusted to 1% Zwittergent and 5% Betain and adsorbed to a Mono Q matrix. This was then eluted with a KSCN gradient, and detergents were removed by a second lentil-lectin chromatography step. The glycoprotein was eluted with 5% methylglucoside as described above and dialyzed against TBS.

Neutralization Test

The test sera were diluted in twofold steps and incubated with 10^2 $TCID_{50}$ $HTLV-III_B$ or RF at 4°C for 2 hr. This was then added to 10^7 H9 cells in 1 ml medium. After adsorption for 1 hr, 9 ml of RPMI medium + 10% fetal calf serum and 2 μg Polybrene were added. The cultures were incubated at 37°C, and reverse transcriptase activity in the cell medium was determined 10 days postinfection. Neutralization titer was defined as the reciprocal of the serum dilution, which reduced the reverse transcriptase activity by greater than 90% compared to control cultures with preimmune serum.

Potency Test

The potency of the vaccine was determined by injecting mice with serial dilutions of gp160 alone or adjuvanted with different formulations. Groups of 10 mice were infected subcutaneously with 1 ml of fourfold dilutions of the test substance. A total of 50 mice were injected in each test. Forty-two days post immunization, each animal was bled by the retroorbital route. The different sera were diluted and examined for presence of HIV antibodies by ELISA determination (Sorin). All positive samples were recorded, and the effective dose 50 $(E.D._{50})$, i.e., the gp160 dose which results in seroconversion in 50% of immunized animals, was statistically determined by the method of Kaerber (36).

RESULTS

Enhanced Production of gp160 Using Double Infection System

The production of gp160 in infected mammalian cells was originally reported using a single vaccinia recombinant containing the HIV *env* gene under the direct control of a vaccinia promoter (28). The efficiency of HIV gp160 synthesis by the double infection system was compared with that of the single vaccinia recombinant (32). Cells were infected with equal amounts of the recombinant VTF-3, which contains the T7 polymerase gene under the control of the vaccinia P7.5 promoter, and with VPE-5, which contains the HIV *env* gene under the control of a T7 promoter. The synthesis of gp160 in these cells was compared with that in cells infected with the single VPE-7 recombinant under identical conditions to that of the double infection. Figure 1 illustrates an immunoblot analysis of extracts from recombinant infected CV-1 cells and HIV-1-infected H9 cells. Infection with both recombinant viruses results in expression of HIV proteins which comigrate with the authentic virus-derived gp160, gp120, and gp41 proteins. Densitometry of the bands corresponding to gp160 demonstrated that this protein was synthesized at a relative intensity ratio of 7.5:1 for the double infection and single vaccinia infection systems, respectively. This increased production with the double infection system was demonstrated in a number of different cell systems, including Vero cells.

Purification of Vaccinia-Derived gp160 from Vero Cells

The location of the recombinant gp160 in vaccinia-infected Vero cells was examined by immunofluorescence of unfixed cells. A monoclonal antibody specific for gp160 was used to stain cells 24 hr after infection, and this demonstrated that the gp160 was located on the surface of these cells. The tissue culture medium supernatant of such infected cells was concentrated and HIV-1 envelope proteins were purified from this material by immunoaffinity and lentil-lectin chromatography as described in Methods. No intact gp160 could be demonstrated in these supernatants although gp120 could be recovered (data not shown). This indicated that intact gp160 could be recovered only from the membranes of infected cells. A number of different treatments were examined for efficiency of gp160 extraction, and it was found that extraction with 1% deoxycholate resulted in the most efficient recovery of the protein (data not shown). This extraction process, as described in Methods, was then used for all further experiments, and the material was then purified by sequential lentil-lectin and immunoaffinity chromatography followed by ion exchange and a second lentil-lectin chromatography step (see Methods). The results of this multistep purification procedure are demonstrated in Figure 2. A single major band with MW 160 KD was detected by protein staining after this purification process.

Characterization of the Vaccinia-Derived Protein

The material purified as described above was subjected to SDS PAGE and then blotted onto nitrocellulose filters and incubated with monoclonal antibodies

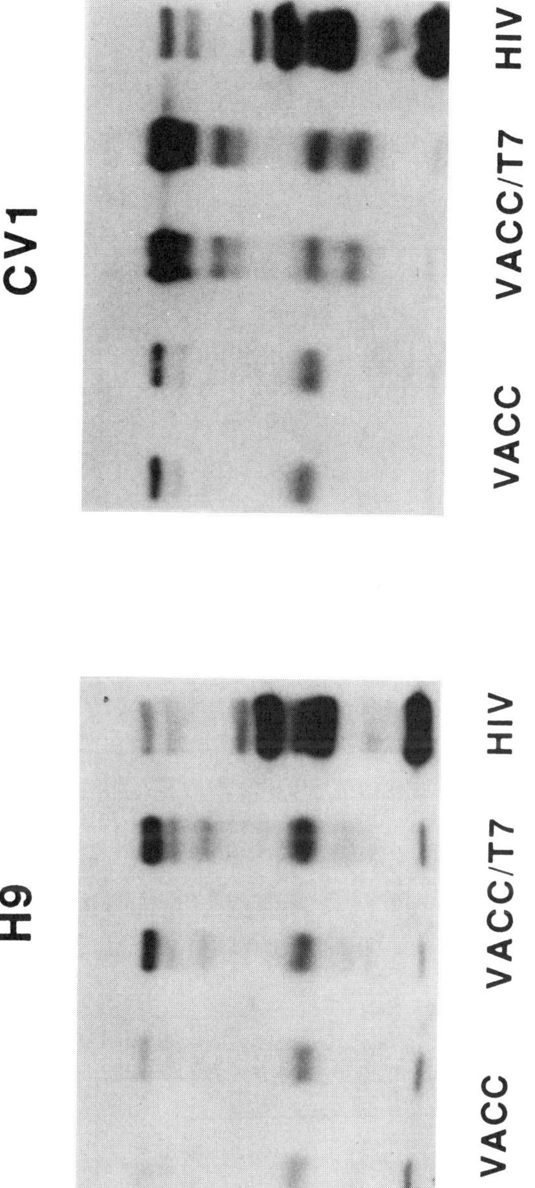

Figure 1 Polyacrylamide gel immunoblot of HIV-1 envelope proteins expressed in CV-1 cells by recombinant vaccinia virus VPE-7 (VACC) and by equal amounts of VTF7-3 and VPE-5 (VACC/T7) and in H9 cells by HIV-1. (Adapted from Ref. 31.)

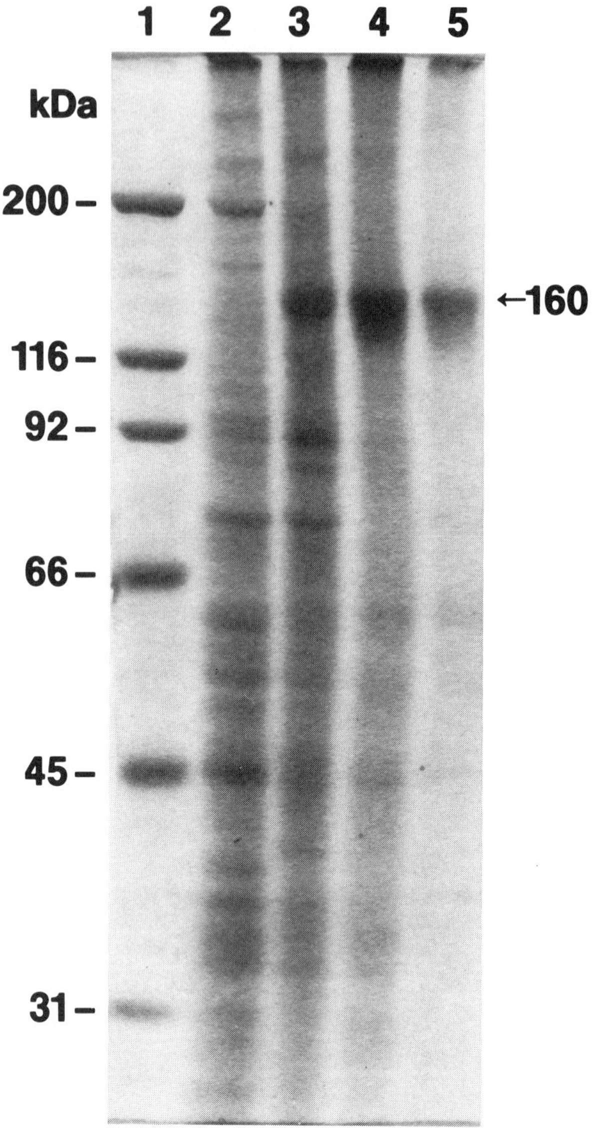

Figure 2 Polyacrylamide gel analysis of vaccinia recombinant-infected Vero cells after each purification step. The gel was stained with Coomassie blue. Lane 1, mol. wt. markers. Lane 2, deoxycholate extract. Lane 3, material eluted from lentil-lectin column. Lane 4, eluted from immuoaffinity column. Lane 5, eluted from second lentil-lectin column following ion exchange chromatography. (Adapted from Ref. 54.)

specific for HIV-1 gp120 and gp41. For comparison purposes a purified H9/HIV-1 preparation was also blotted onto nitrocellulose after SDS PAGE and was incubated with these monoclonals under identical conditions (Fig. 3). This immunoblot analysis demonstrated that both monoclonals against gp41 and gp120 reacted with the gp160 preparation purified from vaccinia-infected Vero cells, and this protein had a molecular weight identical to the gp160 present on the HIV-1 particle. No bands could be detected in the vaccinia-derived material equivalent to the gp120 and gp41, indicating that these breakdown products of the gp160 were not generated in the extraction and purification process from vaccinia-infected cells.

Morphological Analysis

We had earlier seen that attempts to analyze our gp160 preparations by PAGE under nondenaturing conditions were unsuccessful as the material did not enter the gel. This suggested that the gp160 may be present in a high molecular weight polymeric form. This hypothesis was also supported by our observations that hepatitis B Pre-S$_2$ antigen produced by a recombinant vaccinia virus in Vero cells was secreted from infected cells as a high molecular weight particle. We therefore carried out electron-microscopic analysis of the final purified material. Figure 4 illustrates that gp160 after final purification was present in a particulate form with a diameter in the range of 15–30 nm.

Determination of gp160 Yield from Infected Vero Cells

Routine production of gp160 was carried out in a 40-liter fermenter using 5 g of microcarriers per liter. This allowed us to achieve a cell density of approximately 5×10^9 cells/liter, i.e., a total cell number of 2×10^{11} cells. Infection with VPE-5 and VTF7-3 was carried out with a multiplicity of infection of 2 pfu of each recombinant per cell. Although it has been reported that a moi of 10 pfu per recombinant per cell is optimal (32), it was not practical to produce the large volume of virus required with such a high titer to obtain this multiplicity of infection. After infection with a moi of 2 pfu per recombinant per cell, the amount of gp160 recoverable from infected cells was measured over a period of 12–96 hr. Optimal yield of gp160 was obtained when the cells were harvested 40 hr postinfection. The yield of gp160 after each purification step was then determined. Table 1 describes the percentage yield after each step and demonstrates that a 10% yield of approximately 50 mg could be obtained from a single 40-liter fermenter under the conditions described in Methods.

Serologic Responses in Goats Immunized with Adjuvanted gp160

To determine the immunogenicity of our recombinant-derived gp160 and to obtain large amounts of HIV-specific antibodies, goats were injected with 50 μg

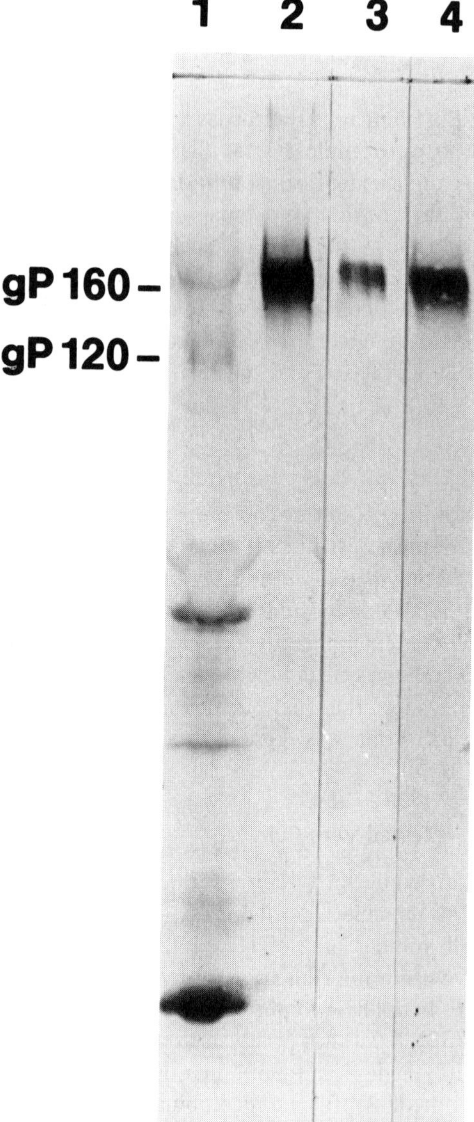

Figure 3 Immunoblot analysis of purified gp160. Samples were subjected to polyacrylamide gel electrophoresis, transferred to nitrocellulose, and probed with human antiserum or monoclonal antibodies. Lane 1, HIV-1 preparation from infected H9 cells probed with human HIV-1 antiserum. Lane 2, purified gp160 probed with the same antiserum. Lane 3, purified gp160 probed with a gp120-specific monoclonal. Lane 4, purified gp160 probed with a gp41-specific monoclonal. (Adapted from Ref. 54.)

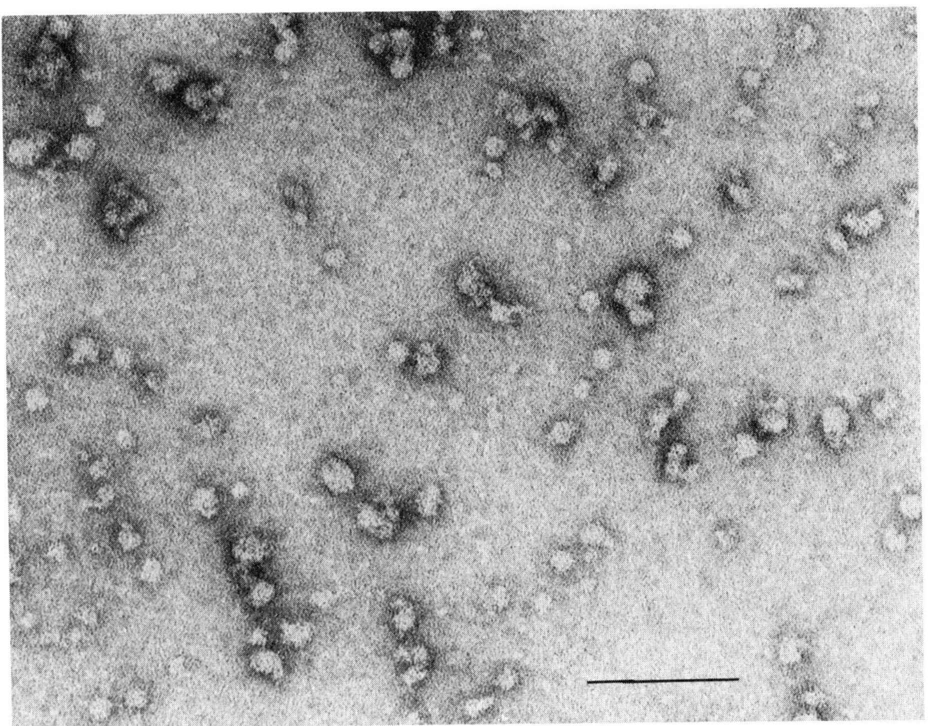

Figure 4 Electron micrograph of purified gp160 (bar = 100 nm). (Adapted from Ref. 54.)

gp160 per dose adjuvanted with 0.2% Al(OH)₃ or with complete Freund's adjuvant. Booster injections of 50 μg were given at regular intervals adjuvanted with 0.2% Al(OH)₃ or incomplete Freund's adjuvant, respectively. Specific gp160 antibodies were measured by standard ELISA techniques using a commercial whole virus kit (Sorin) and with plates coated with highly purified vaccinia-derived gp160. The goats immunized with gp160 in complete Freund's adjuvant showed an early serologic response to the first immunization and specific antibody levels as demonstrated by binding to gp160-coated plates continued to increase until after the eighth booster (Fig. 5). Maximum titer obtained for this goat was 1:102,400 in the gp160 ELISA and 1:12,800 in the Sorin test. In contrast the goats immunized with gp160 in alum demonstrated a much weaker antibody response with a maximum titer of 1:400 being obtained.

Determination of Neutralizing Antibody Activity

The virus neutralization capacity of selected sera from two goats immunized with gp160 and Freund's adjuvant was tested as described in Methods. Both

Table 1 Calculation of gp160 Recovery from a 40-Liter Fermenter After Each Purification Step

	Volume (ml)	Protein (mg)	gp160 ELISA[a] (mg)	μg gp160/ 10^8 cells	%
DOC extraction	4,500	22,600	450	225	100
1° L–L-eluate	250	500	300	150	67
HIV–IgG eluate	200	100	150	75	30
IEX eluate	50	–	–	–	–
2° L–L-eluate	100	30	50	25	11

[a]Determined using a highly purified gp120 standard obtained from HIV-1-infected H9 cells.
Source: Adapted from Ref. 54.

these animals had high binding antibody titers as determined by ELISA but failed to neutralize 10^2 TCID$_{50}$ even after a total of three immunizations (Table 2). However, further boostering resulted in HTLV–IIIB neutralizing antibodies first appearing in both animals 14 weeks after initial immunization. No neutralizing activity directed against the RF strain could, however, be detected at this stage. Antibodies capable of neutralizing the RF strain first appeared 25 weeks after initial immunization and after seven injections. In comparison two human sera which had high titer gp160-specific antibodies had neutralizing titers of 1:320 against III$_B$ and 1:160 and 1:80 against RF.

Potency Determination in Mice Using Different Adjuvant Formulations

The data presented in Figure 5 illustrate the importance of adjuvants in presentation of an antigen to the immune system. As the ultimate aim of this study was to develop a vaccine for human use and Freund's adjuvant is not suitable for this purpose, we looked at the efficacy of a number of other antigen presentation systems. We determined the potency of gp160 in alum, Freund's adjuvant, ISCOMS, and deoxycholate with alum. The ED$_{50}$ of these different preparations was determined in mice as described in Methods. Table 3 demonstrates that the most immunogenic preparation was gp160 in 0.2% Al(OH)$_3$ and 0.25% deoxycholate with values of 90, 120, and 210 ng/ml in the three tests carried out.

DISCUSSION

The development of a vaccine which will provide protection against primary HIV infection was the object of this study. An HIV candidate vaccine must be safe, must be available in large quantities, and must induce an immune response which will preferentially prevent virus infection or at least prevent development of disease. The full-length HIV envelope protein gp160 has been chosen as the best candidate for such a vaccine. It is not possible to use an inactivated whole virus vaccine to immunize humans as this virus contains a reverse transcriptase which if not fully inactivated could possibly cause the integration of proviral DNA in the host cell DNA. It is also difficult to envisage the use of virion-derived envelope glycoprotein as only very small amounts can be purified from the virion or from HIV-infected cells (21).

For this reason we have attempted to develop a candidate vaccine using the full-length envelope glycoprotein expressed in vaccinia virus–infected Vero cells. Such vaccinia recombinants had previously been shown to be successful in inducing protective immune responses against the retrovirus Friend leukemia virus

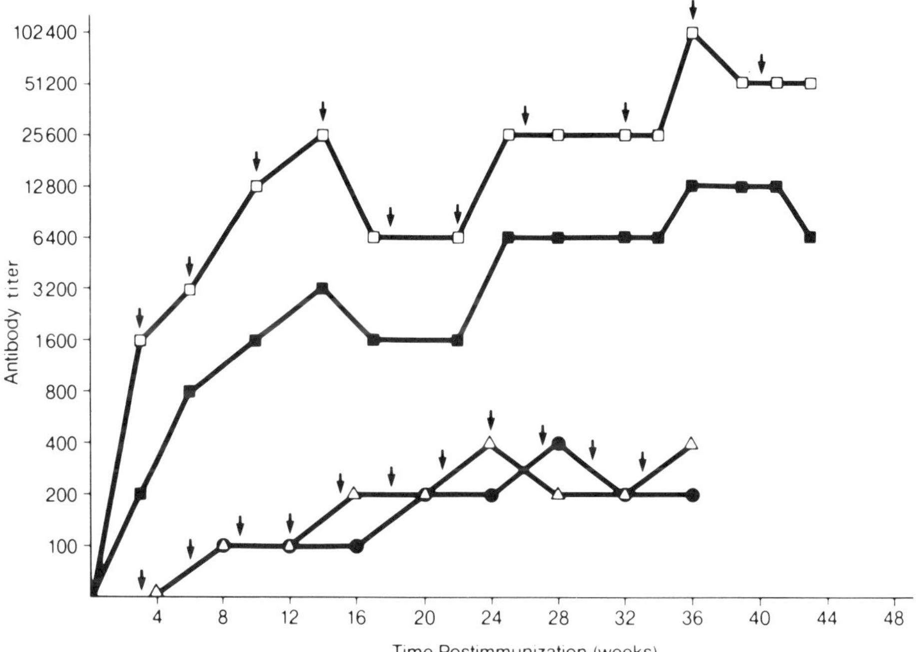

Figure 5 Binding antibody titers in goats injected with gp160. (□——□) Immunized using Freund's adjuvant, antibody titer measured with gp160-coated plates. (■——■) Immunized using Freund's adjuvant, antibody titer measured with Sorin kit. (△——△) Immunized using Al (OH)$_3$ as adjuvant, antibody titer measured with gp160-coated plates. (●——●) Immunized using Al (OH)$_3$ as adjuvant, antibody titer measured with Sorin kit. (Adapted from Ref. 54.)

Table 2 Neutralizing Activity of Human- and gp160-Immunized Goat Sera against HIV-1 (III$_B$) and RF

Serum	ELISA titer (GP160-specified	Time postimmunization (weeks)	Immunizations (no.)	Neutralizing titer[a]	
				III$_B$	RF
Human 1	512,000	—	—	320	160
Human 2	256,000	—	—	320	80
Goat 85	12,800	10	3	<5	<5
Goat 85	25,600	14	4	20	<5
Goat 85	25,600	25	7	40	10
Goat 85	102,400	36	9	80	20
Goat 4	6,400	10	3	<5	<5
Goat 4	25,600	14	4	20	<5
Goat 4	102,400	25	7	40	10
Goat 4	102,400	36	9	40	10

[a]Neutralization was determined by evaluation of reverse transcriptase activity in supernatants of H9 cells cultured for 10 days in the presence of 10^2 TCID$_{50}$ HIV-1. Values are the inverse of antiserum dilutions that inhibited reverse transcriptase activity $\geqslant$90%.
Source: Adapted from Ref. 54.

Table 3 Determination of the Potency of a gp160 Vaccine in Mice with Different Adjuvant Formulations

Vaccine formulation	Maximum dose (μg)	Number of seroconverting animals[a]	ED_{50} (μg)	Max. titer anti-gp160[b]
gp160 (plain)	40	8	28.3	10
gp160 (ISCOM)	20	9	1.52	100
gp160 + CFA	10	15	2.29	100
gp160 + 0.2% Al (OH)$_3$	10	4	>10	100
gp160 + 0.25% DOC + 0.2% Al (OH)$_3$	5	28	0.21	500
gp160 + 0.25% DOC + 0.2% Al (OH)$_3$	5	32	0.12	100
gp160 + 0.25% DOC + 0.2% Al (OH)$_3$	5	34	0.09	1000

[a]A total of 50 animals were injected in each test.
[b]Antibody titer was determined using Sorin ELISA kit.
Source: Adapted from Ref. 54.

(37), and against a wide variety of other viral diseases (38-44), and expression in infected Vero cells allows large-scale production of the desired protein.

The production of vaccinia recombinants expressing HIV-I gp160 has been reported by a number of groups (28,29,30). We have described here the use of a double infection system using one recombinant which codes for the bacterio-phage T7 polymerase and a second which codes for gp160 under the control of a T7 promoter (32). This resulted in an eightfold increase in gp160 production compared to the standard single recombinant system with gp160 under the control of a vaccinia promoter (see Fig. 1).

Vaccinia virus recombinants may be used in two ways in developing a vaccine. One method is to use the whole recombinant virus itself as an immunogen, i.e., as a live vaccine. This has been done successfully with recombinants expressing the hepatitis B surface antigen, and immunization with such a recombinant has resulted in protection of chimpanzees against challenge with live virus (40). However, chimpanzees immunized with vaccinia recombinants expressing the HIV-1 gp160 were not protected against challenge with various doses of HIV-1 (45). This may be due to the fact that it is not optimal to administer a booster injection without a long interval between injections as the replicating virus results in a strong protective response against further vaccinia virus infections. For this reason we have decided to develop a candidate vaccine by purification of the gp160 from infected mammalian cell cultures. The multistep purification procedure described here results in isolation of a highly purified protein (see Fig. 2), which is identical in molecular weight and its reaction with specific HIV monoclonal antibodies to the virus-derived protein (see Fig. 3). E.M. analysis of the final purified product also demonstrated that it was organized as a particle of approx. 15-30 nm diameter (see Fig. 4). This may be important as regards the immunogenicity of the protein as the arrangement of a protein in such a particle or as an ISCOM preparation generally leads to increased immunogenicity (52).

This highly purified protein may be produced in large amounts from Vero cells cultivated on microcarriers in fermenters. This is presently being produced in 40-liter capacity fermenters, as this provides sufficient material for experimen-tal purposes. However, it is technologically possible to develop fermenters with capacities up to 1000 liters, which would enable the large-scale production of a vaccine for human use.

The initial serologic analysis of this particulate gp160 demonstrated that the adjuvantation of this material was critical to eliciting a significant immune response. Adjuvantation with alum, which is the standard preparation used for human vaccines, resulted in a weak humoral immune response after injection into goats with a maximum titer of 400 being obtained. However the use of Freund's adjuvant in association with gp160 drastically improved the response and led to development of extremely high antibody titers as measured with two

ELISA systems. These antibodies were also capable of neutralizing HIV infectivity in vitro with type-specific antibodies first appearing 14 weeks after initial immunization. Antibodies capable of neutralizing the widely divergent RF strain of HIV first appeared 25 weeks after initial immunization and after six booster injections (see Table 2). This is in agreement with data from the murine leukemia system where immunization of animals with an envelope gp70 from a single species first gave rise to a type-specific neutralizing antibody. With additional immunization a broadly neutralizing antibody developed so that a late serum could neutralize a variety of virus types (46). In addition a recent report on the injection of vaccinia-derived gp160 into humans (47) describes the development of a high-titer group-specific neutralization approximately 100 days after initial injections. However, this is not in agreement with data published on the Baculovirus-derived gp160. Sera derived from animals immunized with gp160 purified from insect cells infected with recombinant Baculovirus had type-specific but not group-specific neutralizing activity (31). Repeated booster injections with this material resulted in no change in the neutralization pattern in contrast to our data. This may be due to the fact that the glycosylation in insect cells is different from that of mammalian cells. In addition this material is extracted by SDS treatment, which may lead to the loss of conformational epitopes important for induction of group specific neutralization. However, it has also been reported that a nonglycosylated *E. coli*-derived HIV protein representing the transmembrane gp41 was able to elicit low-titer group-specific neutralizing activity (24). This data suggests that glycosylation of the envelope proteins may not be important for eliciting group-specific antibodies.

Although the role of glycosylation is still not clear, it is evident from our data that the manner of presentation of antigen to the immune system by adjuvantation is crticial to the development of a strong humoral immune response (see Figs. 4,5). As Freund's adjuvant may not be used in humans, we looked at a number of possible adjuvant formulations which could be suitable for a human vaccine. Potency tests in mice demonstrated that the combination of sodium deoxycholate and alum resulted in a greatly increased immunogenicity of gp160 when tested in mice. Safety studies in a number of animal models have indicated that this formulation may be suitable for human use (48,49). Experiments are in progress in goats and other animal models to determine whether group-specific neutralizing antibodies can also be elicted with this adjuvant formulation. We are also looking at the efficiency of the cellular immune response to various gp160 vaccine preparations, and this data will allow us to begin protection studies in chimpanzees, which are the ultimate test of the efficacy of a candidate vaccine before immunizing humans. This will also allow us to examine the possibility of the development of an autoimmunosuppressive reaction following immunization. This has been reported to be a possibility as a result of molecular mimicry involving gp160, CD4 molecules, antibodies, and CD4-acceptor sites (50). It has also been reported that components of serum in HIV-1-infected or immunized individuals may enhance viral infection and mask neutralizing antibody activity (51). This hypothesis must be examined by virus challenge of gp160-immunized chimpanzees before beginning human trials.

ACKNOWLEDGMENTS

We thank Drs. T. Fuerst and P. Earl, NIAID, for seed stocks of recombinant vaccinia viruses; Dr. D. P. Bolognesi, Duke University Medical Center for supplying HIV-1-derived gp160; Dr. U. Sleytr, University of Vienna, for electron microscopy; Ms. Sieglinde Szabo and Ms. Ulrike Zapletal for excellent secretarial assistance.

REFERENCES

1. Gottlieb MS, Schroff R, Schanker HM, Weisman JD, Fan PT, Wolf RA, Saxon A. Pneumocystis carinii pneumonia and mucosal candidiasis in previously healthy homosexual men. N Engl J Med 1981; 305:1425–31.
2. Masur H, Michelis MA, Greene JB, Onorato I, Vande Stouwe RA, Holzman RS, Wormser G, Brettman L, Lange M, Murray WH, Cunningham-Rundles S. An outbreak of community-acquired Pneumocystis carinii pneumonia. N Engl J Med 1981; 305:1431–8.
3. Siegal FP, Lopez C, Hammer GS, Brown AE, Kornfeld SJ, Gold J, Hassett J, Hirschman SZ, Cunningham-Rundles C, Adelsberg BR, Parham DM, Siegal M, Cunningham-Rundles S, Armstrong D. Severe acquired immunodeficiency in male homosexuals manifested by chronic penianal ulcerative herpes simplex lesions. N Engl J Med 1981; 305:1439–44.
4. Barré-Sinoussi F, Chermann JC, Rey F, Nugeyre MT, Charmaret S, Gruest J, Dauguet C, Axer-Blin C, Vézinet-Brun F, Rouzioux C, Rozenbaum W, Montagnier L. Isolation of a T-lymphotropic retrovirus from a patient at risk for acquired immunodeficiency syndrome. Science 1983; 220:868–71.
5. May RM, Anderson RM. Transmission dynamics of HIV infection. Nature 1987; 326:137–42.
6. Quinn TC, Mann JM, Curran JW, Piot P. AIDS in Africa: An epidemiologic paradigm. Science 1986; 234:955–63.
7. World Health Organization (WHO). Wkly Epidemiol Rec 1987; 62:301.
8. Hunsmann G, Moenning V, Schafer W. Properties of mouse leukemia viruses. IX. Active and passive immunization of mice against Friend leukemia with isolated viral gp71 glycoprotein and its corresponding antiserum. Virology 1975; 66:7–9.
9. Hunsmann G, Schneider J, Schulz A. Immunoprevention of Friend virus induced erythroleukemia by vaccination with viral envelope glycoprotein complexes. Virology 1981; 113:602–12.

10. Hunsmann G, Pedersen NC, Theilen GH, Bayer H. Active immunization with feline leukemia virus envelope glycoprotein suppresses growth of virus-induced feline sarcoma. Med Microbiol Immunol 1983; 171:223–41.

11. Lewis MG, Mathes LE, Olson RG. Protection against Feline leukemia by vaccination with a subunit vaccine. Infect Immun 1981; 34:888–94.

12. Osterhaus A, Weijer K, Uytedehagg F, Jarrett O, Sundquist B, Morein B. Induction of protective immune response in cats by vaccination with feline leukemia virus iscom. J Immunol 1985; 135:591–6.

13. Fischinger PJ, Schafer W, Bolognesi DP. Neutralization of homologous and heterologous oncornaviruses by antisera against the p15(E) and gp71 polypeptides of Friend murine leukemia virus. Virology 1976; 71:169–84.

14. Allan JS, Coliga JE, Barin F, McLance MF, Sodroski JG, Rosen CA, Haseltine WA, Lee TH, Essex M. Major glycoprotein antigens that induce antibodies in AIDS patients are encoded by HTLV–III. Science 1985; 228:1091–3.

15. Barin F, McLane MF, Allan JS, Lee TH, Groopman JE, Essex M. Virus envelope protein of HTLV-III represents major target antigen for antibodies in AIDS patients. Science 1985; 228:1094–6.

16. Veronese FD, DeVico AL, Copeland TD, Oroszlan S, Gallo RC, Sarngadharan MG. Characterization of highly immunogenic p66/p51 as the reverse transcriptase of HTLV–III/LAV. Science 1985; 229:1402–5.

17. Robey WG, Safai B, Oroszlan S, Arthur LO, Gonda MA, Gallo RC, Fischinger PJ. Characterization of envelope and core structural gene products of HTLV–III with sera from AIDS patients. Science 1985; 228:593–5.

18. Dalgleish AG, Beverley PCL, Clapham PR, Crawford DH, Greaves MF, Weiss RA. The CD4 (T4) antigen is an essential component of the receptor of the AIDS retrovirus. Nature (London) 1984; 312:763–8.

19. Klatzmann D, Champagne E, Chamaret S, Gruest J, Guetard D, Hercend T, Cluckman J-C, Montagnier L. T-lymphocyte T4 molecule behaves as the receptor for human retrovirus LAV. Nature (London) 1984; 312:767–70.

20. McDougal JS, Kennedy MS, Sligh JM, Cort SP, Mawle A, Nicholson JKA. Binding of HTLV–III/LAV to T4$^+$ T cells by a complex of the 110K viral protein and the T4 molecule. Science 1985; 231:382–5.

21. Robey WG, Arthur LO, Matthews TJ, Langlois A, Copeland TD, Lerche NW, Oroszlan S, Bolognesi DP, Gilden RV, Fischinger PJ. Prospect for prevention of human immunodeficiency virus infection: Purified 120-kDa envelope glycoprotein induces neutralizing antibody. Proc Natl Acad Sci USA 1986; 83:7023–7.

22. Matthews TM, Langlois A, Robey WG, Chang NT, Gallo RC, Fischinger PJ, Bolognesi DP. Restricted neutralization of divergent HTLV–III LAV isolates by antibodies of the major envelope glycoprotein. Proc Natl Acad Sci USA 1986; 83:9709–13.

23. Lasky LA, Groopman JE, Fennie CW, Benz PM, Capon DJ, Dowbenko DJ, Nakamura GR, Nunes WM, Renz ME, Berman PW. Neutralization of the AIDS retrovirus by antibodies to a recombinant envelope glycoprotein. Science 1986; 233:209–12.

24. Krohn K, Robey WG, Putney S, Arthur L, Nara P, Fischinger P, Gallo RC, Wong-Staal F, Ranki A. Specific cellular immune response and neutralizing antibodies in goats immunized with native or recombinant envelope proteins derived from human T-lymphotropic virus type III$_B$ and in human immunodeficiency virus-infected men. Proc Natl Acad Sci USA 1987; 84: 4994-8.

25. Zarling JM, Morton W, Moran PA, McClure J, Kosowski SG, Hu S-L. T-cell responses to human AIDS virus in macaques immunized with recombinant vaccinia viruses. Nature 1986; 323:344.

26. Chanh TC, Dreesman GR, Kanda P, Linette GP, Sparrow JT, Ho DD, Kennedy RC. Induction of anti-HIV neutralizing antibodies by synthetic peptides. The EMBO Journal 1986; 5:3065-71.

27. Putney SD, Matthews TJ, Robey WG, Lynn DL, Robert-Guroff M, Mueller WT, Langlois AJ, Ghrayeb J, Petteway SR, Weinhold KJ, Fischinger PJ, Wong-Staal F, Gallo RC, Bolognesi DP. HTLV-III/LAV Neutralizing antibodies to an *E. coli* produced fragment of the virus envelope. Science 1986; 234:1392-5.

28. Chakrabarti S, Robert-Guroff M, Wong-Staal F, Gallo RC, Moss B. Expression of the HTLV-III envelope gene by a' recombinant vaccinia virus. Nature 1986; 320:535-7.

29. Hu S-L, Kosowski SG, Dalrymple JM. Expression of AIDS virus envelope gene in recombinant vaccinia viruses. Nature 1986; 320:537-40.

30. Kieny MP, Rautmann G, Schmitt D, Dott K, Wain-Hobson S, Alizon M, Girard M, Chamaret S, Laurent A, Montagnier L, Lecocq J-P. AIDS virus ENV protein expressed from a recombinant vaccinia virus. Biotechnology 1986; 4:790-5.

31. Rusche JR, Lynn DL, Robert-Guroff M, Langlois AJ, Liverly HK, Carson H, Krohn K, Ranki A, Gallo RC, Bolognesi DP, Putney SD, Matthews TJ. Humoral immune response to the entire human immunodeficiency virus envelope glycoprotein made in insect cells. Proc Natl Acad Sci USA 1987; 84:6924-8.

32. Fuerst TR, Earl PL, Moss B. Use of a hybrid vaccinia virus-T7 RNA polymerase system for expression of target genes. Molecular and Cellular Biology 1987; 7:2538-44.

33. Fuerst TR, Niles EG, Studier FW, Moss B. Eukaryotic transient-expression system based on recombinant vaccinia virus that synthesizes bacteriophage T7 RNA polymerase. Proc Natl Acad Sci USA 1986; 83:8122-6.

34. Mackett M, Smith GL, Moss B. General method for the production and selection of infectious vaccinia virus recombinants expressing foreign genes. J Virol 1984; 49:857-64.

35. Rhim JS,Cho HY, Huebner RJ. Non-producer human cells induced by murine sarcoma virus. Int J Cancer 1975; 15:23-9.

36. Kaerber G. Beitrag zur kollektiven Behandlung pharmakologischer Reihenversuche. Arch Exp Pathol Pharmakol 1981; 162:480-3.

37. Earl PL, Moss B, Morrison RP, Wehrly K, Nishio J, Chesebro B. T-lymphocyte priming and protection against Friend leukemia by vaccinia-retrovirus *env* gene recombinant. Science 1986; 234:728-31.

38. Smith GL, Murphy BR, Moss B. Construction and characterization of an infectious vaccinia virus recombinant that expresses the influenza hemagglutinin gene and induces resistance to influenza virus infection in hamsters. Proc Natl Acad Sci USA 1983; 80:7155-9.

39. Wiktor TF, MacFarlan RI, Reagan KJ, Dietzschold B, Curtis PJ, Wunner WH, Kieny M-P, Lathe R, Lecocq, J-P, Hockett M, Moss B, Koprowski H. Protection from rabies by a vaccinia virus recombinant containing the rabies virus glycoprotein gene. Proc Natl Acad Sci USA 1984; 81:7194-8.

40. Moss B, Smith GL, Gorin JL, Purcell RH. Live recombinant vaccinia virus protects chimpanzees against hepatitis B. Nature 1984; 311:67-9.

41. Mackett M, Yilma T, Rose JK, Moss B. Expression of VSV genes and protective immunization of mice and cattle. Science 1985; 227:433-5.

42. Mackett M, Arrand JR. Recombinant vaccinia virus induces neutralizing antibodies in rabbits against Epstein-Barr virus membrane antigen gp 340. The EMBO Journal 1985; 4:3229-34.

43. Elango N, Prince GA, Murphy BR, Venkatesan S, Chanock RM, Moss B. Resistance to human respiratory syncytial virus (RSV) infection induced by immunization of cotton rats with a recombinant vaccinia virus expressing the RSV G glycoprotein.Proc Natl Acad Sci USA 1986; 83:1906-10.

44. Zarling JM, Moran PA, Lasky LA, Moss B. Herpes simplex virus (HSV)-specific human T-cell clones recognize HSV glycoprotein D expressed by a recombinant vaccinia virus. J Virol 1986; 59:506-9.

45. Hu S-L, Fultz PN, McClure HM, Eichberg JW, Thomas EK, Zarling J, Singhal MC, Kosowski SG, Swenson RB, Anderson DC, Todaro G. Effect of immunization with a vaccinia-HIV *env* recombinant on HIV infection of chimpanzees. Nature 1987; 328:721-3.

46. Schäfer W, Bolognesi DD. Relationships between viral structural and cell-surface antigens and their possible significance in immunological defense mechanisms. In Hanna MA Jr, Rapp F., ed. Contemporary topics in immunobiology, Vol. 6. New York: Plenum, 1977:127-67.

47. Zagury D, Bernard J, Cheynier R, Desportes I, Leonard R, Fouchard M, Reveil B, Ittele D, Lurhuma Z, Mbayo K, Wane J, Salaun J-J, Goussard B, Dechazal L, Burny A, Nara P, Gallo RC. A group specific anamnestic immune reaction against HIV-1 induced by a candidate vaccine against AIDS. Nature 1988; 332:728-31.

48. Nagy LK. The effect of deoxycholate on cholera vaccine. Progr Immunobiol Standard 1972; 5:341-7.

49. Mussgay M, Weiland E. Preparation of inactivated vaccines against alpha-viruses using semliki forest virus—white mouse as a model. I. Inactivation experiments and evaluation of double inactivated subunit vaccines. Intervirology 1973; 1:259-68.

50. Martinez-A C, De La Hera A, Alonso JM, Marcos MAR, Marquez C, Toribio ML, Coutinho A. Immunological consequencing of HIV infection: Advantage of being low responder casts doubts on vaccine development. Lancet 1988; 1:454–7.
51. Robinson WE, Montefiori DC, Mitchell WM. Antibody-dependent enhancement of human immunodeficiency virus type 1 infection. Lancet 1988; 1:790–4.
52. Berman PW, Groopman JE, Gregory T, Clapham PR, Weiss RW, Ferriani R, Riddle L, Shimasaki C, Lucas C, Lasky LA, Eichberg JW. Human immunodeficiency virus type 1 challenge of chimpanzees immunized with recombinant envelope glycoprotein gp 120. Proc Natl Acad Sci USA 1988; 85: 5200–4.
53. Morein B, Sundquist B, Höglund S, Dalsgaard K, Osterhaus A. Iscom, a novel structure for antigenic presentation of membrane proteins from enveloped viruses. Nature 1984; 308:457–4.
54. Barrett N, Mitterer A, Mundt W, Eibl J, Eibl M, Gallo RC, Moss B, Dorner F. Large-scale production and purification of a vaccinia recombinant-derived HIV-1 gp160 and analysis of its immunogenicity. AIDS Res Human Retroviruses 1989; 5:159–71.

11

CD4-gp120 Interaction
Idiotype Mimicry as Putative Vaccines and Therapeutics Against HIV Infection

Ronald C. Kennedy and Tran C. Chanh
Southwest Foundation for Biomedical Research
San Antonio, Texas

Vernon C. Maino and Noel L. Warner
Becton Dickinson Monoclonal Center
Mountain View, California

Wayne C. Koff
National Institute of Allergy and Infectious Diseases
National Institutes of Health
Bethesda, Maryland

INTRODUCTION

The network theory of immune regulation was first proposed by Jerne (1) to explain how idiotype–anti-idiotype interactions may be involved in regulating the immune response to an antigen. An idiotype (Id) defines the variable (V) region of the antibody molecule and often serves as a V region phenotypic marker. Because the V region of the antibody molecule also contains the antigen-binding region, the area of the antibody molecule also contains the antigen-binding region, the area of the antibody that makes contact with the antigen has been referred to as the paratope. It becomes important to remember that even within a single antibody molecule, different areas within the V region are capable of combining with different antigenic determinants. Thus, antigen binding to the antibody requries sufficient complementarity between the antigen and the antibody molecule to generate the attractive forces necessary for this interaction to occur. This complementarity or fitting of structural conformations plays a dual role in both antigen-binding to an antibody molecule and antigen mimicry by potential antiantibodies that recognize the conformation or 3-D structure expressed by the V region of an antibody molecule.

In early studies, antisera were generated against homologous immunoglobulins, such as myeloma or Bence Jones proteins. After the appropriate absorptions, these antisera reacted only with the myeloma proteins used as the immunogen and not with other myelomas or conventional antibodies. Only in rare instances were exceptions to this antigenic individuality noted in early studies. The first reports of antigenic individuality were based on studies with human myeloma proteins (2,3) and extended to a series of conventional antibodies in humans (4) and rabbits (5). In each of these instances, the antisera generated against either the myeloma proteins or conventional antibodies recognized only the immunizing immunoglobulin preparation. Cross-reactions with other myeloma proteins or antibodies were not detected. Thus, each antiserum detected unique or private determinants present on the V region of the antibody molecule used to immunize an appropriate host. The term Id was originally proposed by Oudin and Michael (6) to designate determinants unique to a small set of antibody molecules. An additional term was coined for the immunogenic potential of individual areas or determinants expressed on the surface of the antigen-binding region that encompasses a single antibody molecule and is referred to as the idiotope. Idiotope by definition implies monoclonality, and the unique collection of idiotopes present on each antibody molecule is referred to as an Id. The Id is often defined serologically by generating anti-idiotypic antiserum (anti-Id or Ab-2), whereby the Id can behave as an antigen and induce the production of antibodies against itself. It is noteworthy that the paratope may or may not be the same site as that recognized by the anti-Id. Therefore, the idiotope and paratope may represent distinct sites within the V region of an antibody molecule, the paratope being the area that binds antigen and the idiotope being a site that binds the anti-Id.

The early studies described above defined Id as predominantly private or unique Id determinants. However, shared Id that were common to more than one antibody preparation and that were found in numerous individuals within a given species have been termed by different investigators as public, shared, cross-reactive, or IdX determinants (for a review see reference 7). Shared Ids have been observed in a wide variety of species with antibodies generated to numerous antigens. The detection of a shared Id on antibodies of a given specificity expressed within one inbred strain of mice and not expressed in another have been used as V region phenotypic markers (reviewed in Ref. 8). In later sections, we will further discuss the detection of shared Ids and how serologic characteristics have been used in an attempt to classify anti-Id. Specific classes of anti-Id may be involved in developing potential anti-Id based vaccine strategies against numerous infectious organisms.

Anti-Id Modulation and Id Networks

Numerous studies have documented the manipulation of the immune response by injection of anti-Id. In particular, antigen exposure following injections of the anti-Id resulted in either suppression of Id positive, antigen-binding molecules or increased Id expression and antigen-binding activity (reviewed in Ref. 9). The generation of auto anti-Id (reviewed in Ref. 10) provided further evidence that immune regulation involves a series of Id networks. The characterization of anti-anti-Id (Ab-3) revealed that in some instances these antibodies were not able to bind the antigen used in the induction of the Id-expressing Ab-1 preparation. However, with the framework of Jerne's initial network proposal, Ab-3 can be produced with specificity to bind the original antigen by mimicking the Ab-1. Thus, the Ab-3 has a structure or a confromational fit that allows it to bind the Id expressed on the surface of the Ab-2. Alternatively, the Id of the Ab-1 has a structural conformation which allows the Ab-2 favorable attractive forces for binding. Thus, the conformation of the Ab-3 should represent the mirror or internal image of the original Id of the Ab-1 and have the capacity to bind antigen. Several kinds of Ab-3 molecules can be produced that differ in their abilities to bind the original antigen and Id expression (reviewed in Ref. 11).

SEROLOGIC CLASSIFICATION OF ANTI–ID

Anti-Id reagents have been serologically classified according to their specificity and recognition of Id (12). This classification has been modified to be consistent with alternative serologic specificities that have been recognized as it relates to the Id–anti-Id reactivity (13). Those anti-Ids or Ab-2 which recognize determinants distinct from the antigen-binding site of the Ab-1 and can bind the Ab-1 at the same time that the Ab-1 binds its antigen are designated as Ab-2 alpha. Antigen-inhibitable Ids have been divided into Ab-2 beta and Ab-2 gamma subclasses. Those anti-Ids that display the biological functions of the antigen recognized by the Ab-1 are called Ab-2 beta or the internal image class of anti-Id. It is these types of anti-Ids which were initially proposed by Nisonoff and Lamoyi in 1981 (14) as potentially applicable to vaccine development. An Ab-2 gamma recognizes Id within the antigen-binding site of the Ab-1, but no biological mimicry of the antigen exists. This classification scheme is not without pitfalls. It is possible that an Ab-2 alpha could induce an antigen-binding site conformation change and thereby inhibit the antigen-binding to Ab-1 as the result of recognizing noncombining site-related V region determinants. Affinity of the Ab-1 and Ab-2 for each other as well as antigen for Ab-1 may also play an important role as it relates to attempted serologic classification of the anti-Id (15). The most attention for anti-Id–based vaccines has been placed on Ab-2 beta subclass of anti-Id which can exhibit serologic characteristics of molecular mimicry. This mimicry is associated with an antigen of an infectious agent. However, recent studies have implicated other classes of Ab-2 for immune modulation or as putative vaccines or therapeutic agents (16,17). A large number of studies have implicated anti-Ids as potential vaccines for a variety of infectious agents and for tumors (reviewed in Refs. 18-20). The first situation whereby an anti-Id had potential as a vaccine for an infectious agent involved the Trypanosoma parasite (21). Studies following this initial report on the potential use of anti-Id–based vaccine strategies included hepatitis B virus and the rabies virus system (22-24). Other systems, whereby anti-Ids have been implicated as putative vaccines against infectious viral agents, are summarized in Table 1. It is of interest that certain Ab-2 subclasses of anti-Id appear genetically restricted in their ability to induce an antiantigen immune response. Such an instance of IgCh genetic restriction was reported in the Trypanosoma system (25). In this study, the ability to induce a murine Ab-3 which recognized Trypanosoma was shown to be dependent and linked to the expression of the proper IgCh genes. Such genetic restriction placed doubt on the use of anti-Id–based vaccines in outbred populations. However, further characterization of the anti-Id utilized in the Trypanosoma system indicated that the anti-Id preparation failed to exhibit any Ab-2 beta activity. Other studies have shown that anti-Id of the Ab-2 beta subclass are not genetically restricted and will induce Ab-3 response with antigen-binding activity across species barriers (26).

POSSIBLE ADVANTAGES OF ANTI–IDIOTYPE–BASED VACCINES

There are several reasons to suggest that an anti-Id–based vaccine represents a viable as well as a preferred alternative to conventional vaccines in specific situations. The first advantage would be in instances where there is difficulty in obtaining adequate amounts of antigen. This would occur when the organism producing the infectious disease is difficult to obtain or when in vitro tissue culture systems for growth of the organism is not available. Examples of this include the infectious agents of leprosy and those of many protozoal diseases. Two other possible advantages are that anti-Ids are not infectious and may therefore be extremely useful when a conventional attentuated vaccine has a high propensity for reverting to a virulent form or when killed viral vaccines could potentially contain contaminating products injurious to the nonimmune host. A fourth advantage would occur when immunity to a single epitope on an infectious agent is adequate for inducing protection. Some infectious agents contain antigenic determinants in common with host tissue or body components leading to the development of a cross-reactive autoimmune response. An anti-Id vaccine

Table 1 Systems Where Published Studies on Anti-Id Have Been Described Which Induce Immune Response Against Viral Antigens Associated with Infectious Organisms

Viral system	Disease	Reference
Cytomegalovirus	Latent disease	86
Coxsackievirus	Myocarditis	87
Feline leukemia virus	Immunodeficiency diseases	11
Heptatitis B virus	Serum hepatitis	22
		88
		89
		16
Human immunodeficiency virus	AIDS	71
		81
Herpes simplex virus	Encephalitis, latent disease	31
		91
		92
		93
Influenza virus	Influenza	94
Mouse mammary tumor virus	Murine tumors	95
Newcastle disease virus	Newcastle disease	96
Poliovirus	Poliomyelitis	97
Rabies virus	Rabies	23
		32
Reovirus	Encephalitis	98
Sendai virus	Systemic infection	99
		100
SV40	Murine tumors	101

could theoretically induce immunity to a single epitope and bypass a possible autoimmune outcome. The ability of an anti-Id to mimic a nonproteinaceous antigen leads to a fifth possible advantage. Studies have implicated this potential based on the capsular polysaccharides of pathogenic bacteria (27,28). Alternatively, an anti-Id that mimics the capsular polysaccharide of pathogenic bacteria may be useful in neonates who normally do not develop an immune response until late in ontogeny (27). The polysaccharide structure or conformation can be mimicked by antibody molecule, which is protein in nature, thereby utilizing the potential application of anti-idiotypes as vaccines in nonresponding neonates

(27,29,30). Therefore, a sixth possible application would then be to circumvent the potential nonresponsiveness to certain kinds of antigens in neonates. A seventh advantage consists of the ability of the anti-Id to modulate an immune response. One can select those idiotopes from which the most desirable immune response would result. It may be possible to enhance or prime the production of those specific antibodies utilizing anti-Id immunization prior to antigenic challenge (22,31,32). The ability of anti-Id to prime the immune response to a subsequent immunization with a viral antigen has been reported for hepatitis B surface antigen (HBsAg) and rabies virus glycoprotein. Another possible advantage of anti-Id–based vaccine occurs when the organism exhibits a high degree of genomic diversity. Anti-Ids can be used to induce an immune response to conformational determinants, such as sites of interaction with cell surface receptors that may be share by strains or different isolates of the organism. The latter advantage of anti-Id is the theoretical conception for the use of anti-Id–based vaccine strategies against human immunodeficiency virus (HIV). The ninth advantage would be the induction of immunity against toxins in which the toxic nature of the compound precludes its use for immunization. The potential advantages of anti-Id vaccine strategies are summarized in Table 2.

IDIOTYPE NETWORKS IN HBV INFECTION

Our interest in anti-Id–based vaccines resulted from studies involving the in vivo modulation effects of an anti-Id preparation that exhibited serologic mimicry of HBsAg (for a review see Ref. 33). Immunization of mice with anti-Id prior to HBsAg injection resulted in an increased number of spleen cells secreting IgM anti-HBs (22). Spleen cells also were induced to secrete anti-HBs by the administration of anti-Id without antigen exposure. Serologic analysis showed that anti-Id given in saline induced primarily an IgM anti-HBs response, whereas alum-precipitated anti-Id produced an IgG anti-HBs response when administered prior to HBsAg (23). Direct binding and inhibition studies demonstrated that the anti-Id–induced anti-HBs recognized the group-specific *a* determinant of HBsAg (34). The Id expressed by the anti-HBs Ab-3 population was shared with anti-HBs Ab-1 preparations produced in humans naturally infected with human hepatitis B virus (HBV). Since previous studies by others had shown that antibodies to the *a* determinant confer protection from HBV infection, our studies suggested the potential use of anti-Id as a vaccine or vaccine primer for HBV infection. To further evaluate this possibility, we immunized mice with anti-Id in conjunction with a cyclic synthetic peptide analogous to an HBsAg *a* determinant (31). Anti-HBs titers comparable to HBsAg immunization alone were produced in BALB/c mice. In addition, high anti-HBs titers were obtained by injecting HBsAg following anti-Id priming.

Table 2 Potential Advantages of Anti-Idiotypic Antibody–Based Vaccine Strategies

1. Difficulty in obtaining adequate amounts of the organism in question (not easy to produce adequate amounts of the protective antigen, i.e., leprosy).

2. Attenuated vaccine has a propensity for reverting to a virulent form (unlikely, but a possibility).

3. Killed vaccine contains contaminating products that may induce a deleterious immune response (polio vaccine and SV40).

4. Immunity to a single epitope is adequate for inducing protection (infectious agent contains antigens cross-reactive with host tissue antigens) (vaccine for dental caries).

5. Mimic nonproteinaceous antigens (carbohydrates, polysaccharides, glycolipids).

6. Potential use in neonates who do not respond to conventional polysaccharide-based capsular vaccines of bacteria.

7. Use an anti-Id for priming the immune response to an infectious agent (immune selection for a specific antieptiopic response or idiotopic expression).

8. Organism exhibits a high degree of genomic diversity, yet exhibits conserved receptor tropism (HIV).

9. Use for mimicking toxins or substances toxic in vivo.

The next step was to test our anti-Id preparation in chimpanzees, the relevant animals model for HBV infection. Two chimpanzees were immunized with the rabbit anti-Id, while two control animals were either untreated or were given a nonimmune rabbit antibody preparation. Four injections of the anti-Id preparation elicited an anti-HBs Ab-3 response with specificity for the anti-Id (35). All four chimpanzees were challenged with infectious HBV. Both control chimpanzees developed clinical and serologic characteristics consistent with an active HBV infection, whereas the two anti-Id-treated chimpanzees were protected from infection. These results indicated that anti-Id preparations might represent candidates for vaccines against human diseases. Recent studies have indicated that anti-Id immunized chimpanzees have anti-HB levels indicative of protective immunity 3 years following the infectious challenge. In addition, peripheral blood lymphocytes (PBL) from the anti-Id–immunized chimpanzees exhibited HBsAg-specific in vitro proliferation. Thus, the anti-Id appeared to induce both B- and T-cell immunity in chimpanzees (Kennedy and Eichberg, unpublished observation). Based on the above studies, we decided that Id-based vaccine strategies may represent an alternative vaccine candidate for controlling human immunodeficiency virus (HIV) infection.

CONSIDERATIONS WHEN DEVELOPING A VACCINE FOR HIV

An important consideration when designing vaccine strategies for HIV is the fact that there exists among different isolates a high degree of genetic polymorphism, especially within gp120. This hypervariability within the envelope gene is highly reminiscent of the situation with other lentiviruses. In addition, studies have indicated that the humoral immune response induced to purified HIV envelope proteins in experimental animals exhibits predominantly type-specific in vitro neutralizing antibody activity. Such antibody fails to neutralize genetically divergent isolates of HIV. An effective vaccine should contain all potential group-common neutralizing epitopes without including the potentially divergent hyper-variable regions of the virus. In addition, HIV infection may be conferred by either cell-free or cell-associated virus. A vaccine candidate should be able to induce cell-mediated immunity along with antibodies that mediate antibody-dependent cell-mediated cytotoxicity (ADCC), which may play a role in the destruction of infected cells prior to transmission of the virus (reviewed in Ref. 36). HIV may become latently infected in cells and may avoid the immune system by remaining dormant within cells for a period of time. This adds an additional constraint when perceiving strategies for developing a vaccine against HIV. One must also be aware of the possibility of viral enhancement, whereby an immune response may be produced against the virus, which enhances its infectivity by promoting the uptake in Fc-bearing lymphoid cells such as mono-cytes and macrophages. The above constraints and considerations for developing an HIV-based vaccine strategy do not appear to reside within vaccine strategies that have been successful relative to other infectious viral agents. Therefore, new kinds of approaches and strategies such as the anti-Id–based vaccine concepts should be examined for their potential usefulness in controlling HIV infection.

CD4–HIV gp120 INTERACTION

The biochemical and molecular characterization of the human CD4 and murine L3T4 molecules has suggested that these molecules are members of the immuno-globulin supergene family (37,38). The nucleotide and predicted amino acid sequences of CD4 indicate that the CD4 molecule possesses a 23 amino acid leader sequence which is followed by a V-like region. This V region with the amino terminal portion of CD4 exhibits 32% homology to the immunoglobulin light chain and contains one intrachain disulfide bond (cysteine residues at positions 16 and 84). The CD4 molecule also appears to exhibit a joining (J)-like region, which displays both sequence homology to the immunoglobulin J- and T-cell receptor (TCR) regions. There exists a third extracellular domain, which appears to be unrelated to any known protein and exhibits two potential glycosylation sites containing the sequence (Asn-Leu-Thr) which will allow for potential N-link glycosylation. The CD4 molecule also exhibits a transmembrane portion which contains approximately 50% homology to the class II major histocompatability complex (MHC) beta chain and a highly charged cytoplasmic region of approximately 40 amino acids. The molecular biochemical and functional characteristics of the murine L3T4 shares significant homology with the human CD4. It is not unreasonable to speculate that based on structural similarities of CD4 to immunoglobulin, the CD4 structure may be involved in cell–cell interactions. The extracellular sequence of the CD4 molecule includes six cysteine residues at amino acid positions 16, 84, 130, 159, 302, and 345. These cysteines may represent potential sites for intrachain disulfide bond formation. Such loop structures are reminiscent of the immunoglobulin-like domains. In the murine L3T4 molecule, analogous cysteine residues have been shown to form three disulfide bridges which exist between adjacent pairs of cysteine residues (39). The possibility exists that similar linkages may occur in humans. Thus, the CD4 molecule appears to exhibit four immunoglobulin-related domains (40,41).

The CD4 molecule is a T-cell membrane glycoprotein that has been implicated in mediating the T-cell-target cell interaction by recognizing the MHC class II antigens (42–49) (see Fig. 1). It is preferentially expressed on the surface of the T-helper inducer/subset of lymphocytes (50). It has been proposed that the CD4 molecule binds monomorphic epitopes of MHC class II molecules in order to enhance the avidity of the T-cell antigen-specific recognition (51–53). Several groups of investigators have shown convincing evidence that CD4 glycoprotein serves as a receptor for HIV binding (54–58). A panel of approximately 25 monoclonal anti-CD4 antibodies were tested for the ability to block HIV binding to target cells and to compete with each other for binding to CD4. The results suggested that the HIV binding site on CD4 is a relatively large site because antibodies from two noncompeting groups can inhibit HIV binding extremely efficiently (59). This suggests that the binding site on CD4 may contain distinct epitopes which are essential in promoting HIV binding.

Recent studies utilizing synthetic peptide analogues to amino acid sequences of human CD4 and human CD4-murine L3T4 chimeric molecules, along with point mutations affecting the primary amino acid sequence of the CD4 molecule, indicate that the amino terminal portion of CD4 is inovlved in binding gp120 (60-62). These authors also conclude that monoclonal anti-CD4 preparations which inhibit the CD4–gp120 interaction map to both the first and second immunoglobulin-like domains. These domains contain intrachain disulfide bonds formed by cysteine residues 16 to 84 and 130 to 159, respectively, on the CD4 molecule. It remains to be determined whether two distinct sites are involved in the CD4 binding to gp120 or whether blocking monoclonal antibodies which recognize a carboxyl CD4 site (carboxyl of residues 1 to 83)

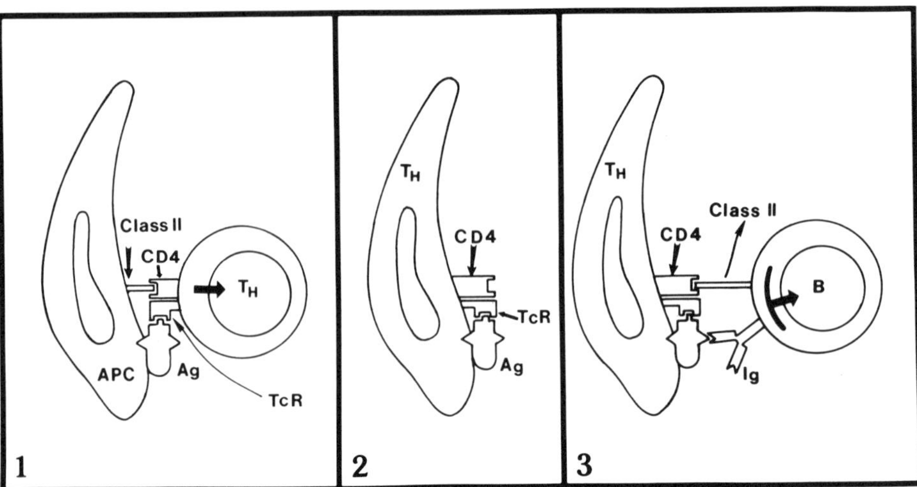

Figure 1 The potential interaction between monomorphic MHC class II determinants and the CD4 molecule as it relates to the induction of an immune response is depicted. In panel 1, an antigen-presenting cell (APC) presents antigen (Ag) with specificity for the TcR to a T_H cell. This interaction may require an additional interaction between class II on the APC and CD4 on the T_H cell. In panel 2, the T_H cell exhibits Ag bound to the TcR. In panel 3, the T_H cell presents Ag with specificity for the immunoglobulin (Ig) receptor to a B cell. Again, this interaction may require an interaction between class II and CD4 for proper presentation of the Ag to the Ig receptor. Thus, class II and gp120 may both represent ligands of the CD4 receptor molecule.

induce a conformational change that affects the CD4–gp120 reaction. Other investigators have mapped the gp120 binding site to the two amino terminal domains of CD4 (63–65). Reports have also demonstrated that soluble CD4 protein can abrogate HIV infectivity (65–69). The important finding in these reports is that the soluble CD4 protein did not induce in vitro immunosuppression which presumably occurs by inhibition by specific class II-T cell interactions (68).

There appear to be two possible approaches when one considers anti-Id–based vaccine and therapeutic strategies for HIV (Fig. 2). The first approach for a vaccine would be to mimic the envelope glycoprotein gp120 and use an anti-Id to induce an Ab-3 response which had anti-HIV gp120 binding activity. An alternative approach for developing an Id-based vaccine would use antibodies that recognize the CD4 molecule and generate an anti-Id whereby the anti-Id would mimic CD4 and bind HIV. In the first instance the Ab-2 would be the vaccine and the resulting immune response would be an Ab-3 with HIV-binding capacity. In the latter case, the Ab-1 or anti-CD4 would represent the vaccine preparation; the resulting immune response would be an Ab-2 which mimics CD4 and exhibits anti-HIV activity. Using anti-Id to either mimic specific epitopes of gp120 or the CD4 molecule may represent a means by which one can circumvent the problem associated with the high degree of polymorphism in gp120 of HIV. These two possibilities based on putative anti-Id vaccines for HIV will be discussed below. For an Id-based therapeutic approach, an Ab-1 or Ab-3 with group-common neutralizing anti-HIV activity could be passively administered similar to an immune gamma globulin preparation. Alternatively, an anti-Id with serologic mimicry of CD4 could be administered passively, such that a monoclonal antibody serves to bind HIV and HIV-infected cells in vivo similar to studies proposed with soluble CD4. The advantage of a monoclonal anti-Id that mimics CD4 over soluble CD4 is that the antibody preparation will have a longer half-life in vivo. Thus, this preparation would be more cost-effective as a therapeutic agent when compared to recombinant soluble CD4. Thus, two different

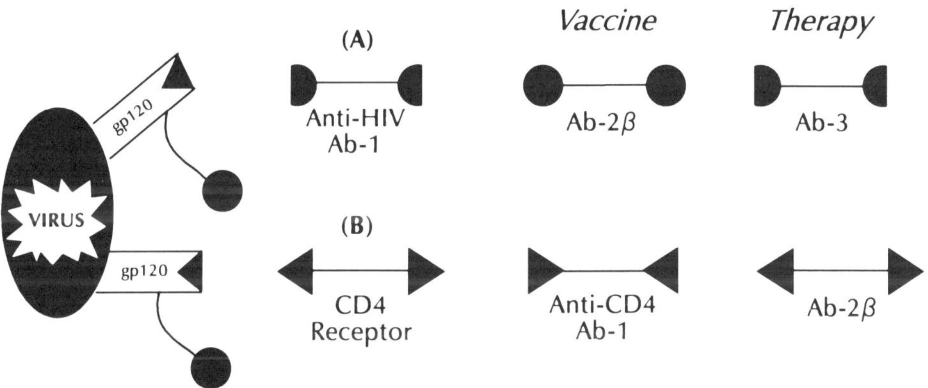

Figure 2 Two potential Id-based strategies for developing vaccines and therapeutics to control HIV infection. In panel A, an anti-Id (Ab-2 beta) mimics a determinant of gp120. The Ab-2 beta is generated against a group-specific neutralizing Ab-1 preparation which recognizes this epitope and the anti-Id is the vaccine. This Ab-2 beta induces an Ab-3 response which mimics the Ab-1. The Ab-3 binds gp120 and neutralizes HIV infectivity by reacting with this gp120 epitope. Both the Ab-1 and Ab-3 preparations exhibit anti-gp120 activity and may be useful as therapeutic agents. In panel B, the anti-CD4 (Ab-1) is the vaccine and induces an anti-Id (Ab-2 beta) that structurally mimics CD4 and binds gp120. A monoclonal Ab-2 beta will mimic CD4 and could represent a therapeutic agent.

Id-based strategies exist when one considers these approaches as putative vaccines and/or therapeutics for HIV.

STUDIES ON IDIOTYPE-BASED STRATEGIES FOR HIV

We and others reasoned that an Ab-2 beta anti-Id response generated against anti-CD4 antibodies (Ab-1) recognizing HIV blocking determinants on the CD4 molecule could mimic CD4 and bind to the HIV envelope glycoprotein (70,71). One could anticipate that the interaction of the anti-Id binding to gp120 could inhibit HIV binding to CD4 on target cells resulting in viral inactivation. In this context, a number of investigators have recently reported the isolation of monoclonal anti-Id that exhibited properties consistent with Ab-2 beta reactivity and recognition of HIV (71-74). Our laboratory reported the isolation of an IgM mouse monoclonal anti-Id against anti-Leu3a that demonstrated reactivity for gp120 by Western blot analysis and exhibited HIV neutralizing activity in vitro (71). In addition, two other laboratories have recently reported the generation of murine monoclonal anti-Id which were raised against anti-CD4 monoclonal antibodies that blocked the HIV infection of T-cell lines (72-74). These monoclonal anti-Id appeared to mimic CD4 in that they had the capacity to neutralize HIV infectivity in vitro and/or bind antigens associated with gp120 in Western blot analysis. One of these reagents also demonstrated complement-dependent cytolysis of HIV-infected cells by the monoclonal anti-Id in the presence of rabbit antimouse reagent (74). It was reported that this monoclonal anti-Id exhibited the capacity to neutralize divergent HIV-1 strains including Haitian and African isolates. In collaboration with A. Dalgliesh (75), our laboratory has immunized BALB/c mice with anti-Leu3a. A polyclonal anti-Id was induced that exhibited in vitro neutralizing activity against divergent HIV-1 isolates as well as a strain of HIV-2. Thus, the anti-Id reported in this study effectively inhibited syncytium formation utilizing HIV isolates HTLV–IIIB, ARV-2, RF, MN, and HIV-2$_{Rod}$ (75). These data indicate that an anti-Id response can mimic a conformational epitope on CD4 which binds HIV-1 and HIV-2 at sites where gp120 interacts with the CD4 receptor. Reports of a polyclonal anti-Id response which recognizes gp120 associated with HIV has also been reported by other investigators who have utilized blocking anti-CD4 preparations to immunize mice (76).

Our laboratories have been examining the potential use of mouse monoclonal anti-CD4 preparations for inducing HIV gp120 specific immune responses in nonhuman primate species. In our initial experiments, we immunized baboons with a combination of OKT4A and anti-Leu3a, two murine monoclonal anti-CD4 preparations that block gp120 binding to CD4, intramuscularly as an alum precipitate. Following multiple immunizations, an antibody response was detected in the baboons that recognized HIV envelope glycoproteins by western blot analysis (77). A weak antibody response was observed in the baboon antisera that recognized SIV gp120 (78). This study suggested that an anti-Id response induced in baboons to anti-CD4 immunization may serologically mimic CD4 and bind a cross-reactive epitope on HIV and SIV gp120. We have recently extended these studies and have immunized additional baboons with several other mouse monoclonal anti-CD4 antibodies (including anti-Leu3a), either individually or as a cocktail preparation, and characterized the anti-Id responses. Depending on the monoclonal anti-CD4 preparation(s) used for immunization, the baboon anti-Id responses in certain instances detected either private or cross-reactive anti-CD4 Ids. The baboons that received cocktail monoclonal anti-CD4 preparations demonstrated a broadening of the cross-reactive Id response. The anti-Id response appeared to recognize a combining site-related Id based on inhibition of the CD4-monoclonal anti-CD4 reaction. Utilizing Western blot anlaysis, a weak and variable anti-HIV gp120 response was detected in some of the baboons immunized with the monoclonal anti-CD4 preparations. Some cross-reactivity with SIV gp120 was also observed. The detection of an anti-HIV gp120 response did not correlate with anti-Id titer, detection of a cross-reactive Id, or recognition of the anti-CD4 combining site by the anti-Id. Studies have suggested that intravenous immunization of mice with monoclonal anti-L3T4 (L3T4 is the murine CD4 analogue) induced long-term immunosuppression (79,80). To date no indication of anti-CD4-induced immunosuppression has been observed in any of the anti-CD4 immunized baboons as determined by mitogen-induced in vitro proliferation.

In addition, we also immunized rhesus monkeys with monoclonal anti-CD4 preparations. The anti-Id response obtained in rhesus monkeys was serologically similar when compared to that induced in baboons. An anti-SIV gp120 response was observed in some of the rhesus monkeys following multiple intramuscular immunizations with the anti-CD4 preparations.

Studies by one of our collaborators have used anti-Leu3a to immunize HIV-infected individuals to assess the safety and therapeutic potential of anti-Leu3a treatment in infected humans (A. G. Dalgleish, personal communication). It should be noted that although these monoclonal and polyclonal anti-Id antibodies are interesting with respect to the suggested HIV reactivities, the neutralizing and binding activities of these antibodies occurred at significantly high concentrations and therefore suggest that the affinities of the purported HIV reactivities of these antibodies are very low. The inability thus far to generate high-affinity HIV-reactive anti-Id antibodies may be significant in the development of a useful vaccine for HIV. Therefore, it is believed that the development of high-affinity HIV-reactive anti-Id responses represents one of the most critical challenges in the effort to establish a protective anti-Id response. Our laboratories have mapped monoclonal anti-CD4 antibodies that inhibit binding of HIV-1 to CD4-positive T-cells and inhibit syncytia formation by HIV-1 and

SIV to several distinct epitopes expressed on the CD4 molecule. As a part of our strategy for testing as an Id-based vaccine in primates, it is our intention to prepare a cocktail of different monoclonal anti-CD4 antibodies representing distinct CD4 epitope reactivities that block both HIV-1 and SIV syncytia formation. In addition, we are evaluating the role of adjuvants and synthetic peptides derived from idiotypic sequences of Ab-1 antibodies in the enhancement of idiotypic immunogenicity. We are also examining the use of anti-Id to anti-CD4 to induce an Ab-3 response that binds CD4 and prevents in vitro infection by cell-associated virus.

Our laboratories have also been interested in using anti-Id to mimic the envelope glycoprotein of HIV. We have generated a specific rabbit anti-Id that recognizes chimpanzee antibodies directed against gp41, which is associated with a synthetic gp41 peptide (81). This synthetic peptide defines a group-common HIV-1-neutralizing epitope which was associated with an immune response induced in both mice and rabbits (82,83). The antibody response to the peptide in chimpanzees recognized both gp160 and gp41 by radioimmunoprecipitation and Western blots, however, it failed to neutralize HIV infectivity in vitro. This chimpanzee antibody preparation was affinity purified on synthetic peptide-containing, immunoadsorbent columns and used to immunize rabbits. The anti-Id response, based on serologic classification, appeared to represent a noninternal image, anti-Id, or an Ab-2 alpha. The chimpanzee Id-rabbit anti-Id reaction could not be inhibited by either recombinant gp160 or the synthetic gp41 peptide. Immunization of BALB/c mice with the polyclonal anti-Id induced an antipeptide response which bound gp41 by Western blots. The Id expressed in the anti-gp41 response in mice is not normally detected in the murine gp160 immune response to the synthetic peptide. This study suggested that this anti-Id may activate normally silent or dormant clones. Recent studies by our laboratories have suggested that a monoclonal anti-Id of the Ab-2 alpha class can similarly induce an antigen-positive, Id-positive response in BALB/c mice whereby the Id which was expressed by anti-Id immunization was normally silent or dormant. Further studies with the monoclonal anti-Id indicated that immunization across species barriers, such as rabbits, induced an antigen-negative, Id-positive response (84). It appears that this class of anti-Id can induce an immune response, be it antigen-positive or antigen-negative, that expresses an Id not normally detected during the course of the immune response to the nominal antigen. Perhaps the use of anti-Id to prime or induce an immune response with serologic characteristics associated with the Ab-1 may be important in activating clones of cells that do not normally respond during the immune response to the nominal antigen. Thus, anti-Id can be used not only to mimic a given antigen, but also to induce normally silent or dormant clones of cells to express immunologic specificities that would not be induced in instances whereby the host was immunized with the nominal antigen. It appears that both classes of anti-Ids, namely the internal image and noninternal image, may be useful in expanding the immune response to a given infectious agent. The role of the latter class of anti-Id, as it relates to HIV-based vaccines and possible immunotherapy remains to be determined.

An anti-Id has been produced against an immunoglobulin fraction of sera from asymptomatic humans that exhibited antisyncytial activity (85). This polyclonal anti-Id preferentially inhibited the ability of the polyclonal human Ab-1 to immunoprecipitate gp160, but not gp120. This anti-Id appears to identify a surface molecule unique to both CD4-positive and CD4-negative human T-cell lines, but not present on murine T-cell lines. The authors conclude that this anti-Id may identify an ancillary molecule on human T cells important in HIV–T-cell interactions. Therefore, anti-Ids appear to have potential, as both vaccines and as reagents to identify virus–cell receptor interactions. Together, these recent studies implicate anti-Ids as reagents that can interfere with the HIV gp120–CD4 interaction and could be useful in identifying other molecules involved in HIV infectivity of T cells.

CONCLUDING REMARKS

Since the initial postulate of Jerne that the immune response to an antigen is regulated by a series of Id–anti-Id reactions, numerous studies have demonstrated that anti-Id reagents may regulate the immune response to a wide variety of antigens, including those associated with infectious agents such as HIV. Although the data is still not conclusive that Id networks may be involved in HIV infection and/or pathogenesis, based on the present studies and studies of other vaccine candidates, it is not unreasonable to speculate that Id-based reagents may have a role as putative vaccines and/or therapeutic agents in controlling HIV infection. An example of a putative Id cascade and the generation of Ab-1, Ab-2, and Ab-3 populations based on exposure to HIV is depicted in Figure 3. Several of the Ab-2 populations have the capacity of inducing an Ab-3 response that binds HIV. The Ab-2 can also induce selected Id expression on the Ab-3 molecules. Since the Id is a serologic representative and phenotypic marker of the V region and a given V region is encoded by germ line genes, the induction of an Ab-3 response with anti-HIV activity can potentially be preprogrammed for Id expression by the activation of a particular V-region germ line gene product. Certainly, somatic mutation and recombination events which occur during V_D, V_J, and V_H or V_J and V_L joining also play a role in the Id repertoire. However, current vaccine strategies that immunize with HIV antigens have very little control over what V-region products will be expressed. The host and the immune system determine what HIV-specific immunity will result from HIV antigen stimulation. The possible use and an advantage of anti-Id strategies is the potential preprogramming of the V-region repertoire based on Id

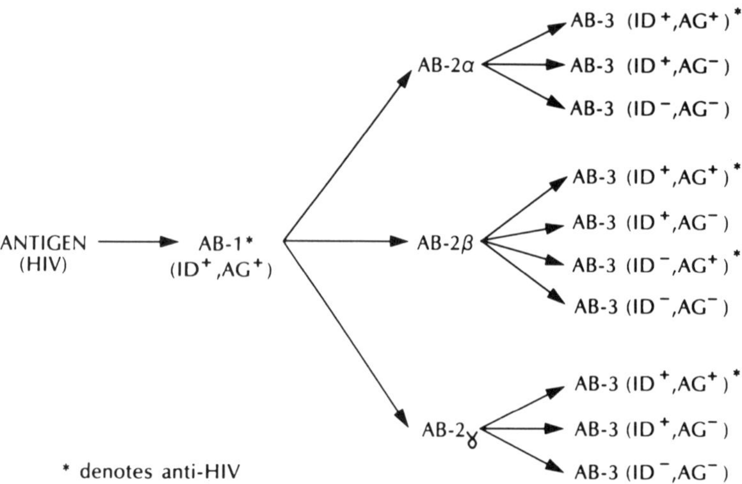

Figure 3 An example of how an idiotype cascade resulting from HIV infection may be used to generate anti-Id (Ab-2) reagents that will induce various Ab-3 subpopulations. Each anti-Id subclass can induce an Ab-3 population that will bind HIV and express an Id shared by the Ab-1 (ID$^+$, AG$^+$). In addition, other Ab-3 populations can be produced which may or may not express a similar Id specificity shared by the Ab-1 and will not bind HIV. The Ab-2 beta subclass can also induce a subpopulation of Ab-3 that will bind HIV and not express the Id of the Ab-1 (ID$^-$, AG$^-$). Alternatively, the induction of an auto-anti-Id response resulting from HIV infection that mimics gp120 could bind CD4. This may result in immunosuppression and CD4 cell depletion because of the auto-anti-Id (Ab-2 beta) binding CD4 on the surface of lymphocytes. Whether or not manipulation of an Id cascade in HIV will be beneficial or detrimental to resolution of infection remains to be determined.

expression prior to HIV antigen stimulation. Thus, if protective immunity requires an anti-HIV response that expresses a given Id (namely, Id^a), and HIV immunization or infection induces an anti-HIV response which expresses a different Id (namely, Id^b), which does not confer protection, then current vaccine strategies using HIV antigens will not be useful. An anti-Id immunization with a reagent that exhibits specificity for Id^a can potentially preprogram the Id selection such that HIV immunization or infection following anti-Id exposure should result in a anti-HIV response where Id^a predominates over Id^b.

Anti-Id and its potential as vaccine strategies have been looked on by other investigators as the most esoteric approach in developing a putative vaccine for HIV. However, based on the failure of the other approaches as they relate to inducing a protective immune response to HIV in relevant animal models, one must not rule out the possibility that Id-based vaccine strategies may have advantages and usefulness in this type of infection. It is also not clear what role vaccines and/or therapies will play as they relate to latent infections. If one could maintain a given Id network at a level which prevents the induction of a latently infected cell to viral replication and active infection, then this may represent a means by which successful therapeutic strategies could be developed. This may be possible not only for HIV, but also for other latent infections. The possibility of using Id-based vaccine strategies and anti-Id immunogens to control HIV infection in concert with other strategies has been described above. This may represent a possibility as it relates to modulating the immune response to HIV. Indeed, anti-Id priming of in vivo immune responses has been reported for HBsAg and rabies virus (22,31,32). It was our purpose in this review to define in very real terms what Id are, historically how they were derived, and their potential use in combating AIDS, either as vaccines or therapeutics.

ACKNOWLEDGMENTS

This work was supported by National Cooperative Vaccine Development Grant AI 26462 from the National Institute of Health.

REFERENCES

1. Jerne NK. Towards a network theory of the immune system. Ann Immunol (Paris); 1974; 125C:373–89.
2. Lohss F, Weiler E, Hillman G. Myolom-plasma-proteine. III. Mitteilung zur Immunochemie der -myleom- proteine. Z Naturforsch 1953; 8B:625–31.
3. Slater RJ, Ward SM, Kunkel HG. Immunological relationships among the myeloma proteins. J Exp Med 1955; 101:85–108.
4. Kunkel HG, Mannik M, Williams RC. Individual antigenic specificity of isolated antibodies. Science 1963; 140:1218–9.
5. Oudin J, Michael M. Une nouvelle forme d'allotypie des globulines du serum de Lapin, apparemment liee a loa fonction et a la specificite anticorps. CR Acad Sci (Paris) 1963; 257:805–8.
6. Oudin J, Michael M. Idiotypy of rabbit antibodies. I. Comparison of idiotypy of antibodies against Salmonella typhi with that of antibodies against other bacteria in the same rabbits, or of antibodies against Salmonella. J Exp Med 1969; 138:595–617.
7. Weigert M, Potter M. Antibody variable-region genetics: Summary and abstracts of the Homogeneous Immunoglobulin Workshop VII. Immunogenetics 1977; 4:401–35.
8. MaKela O, Karjalainen K. Inherited immunoglobulin idiotypes of the mouse. Immunol Rev 1977; 34:119–38.

9. Bona CA. (ed) Biological applications of anti-idiotypes, Vol II. Boca Raton, Fl.: CRC Press, 1988.

10. Rodkey LS. Autoregulation of immune responses via idiotype network interactions. Microbiol Rev 1980; 44:631–59.

11. Uytdehaag FGCM, Bunschoten H, Weijer K, Osterhaus ADME. From Jenner to Jerne: Towards idiotype vaccines. Immunol Rev 1986; 90:93–113.

12. Jerne NK, Roland J, Cazenave P-A. Recurrent idiotopes and internal images. EMBO J 1982; 1:243–7.

13. Bona C, Kohler H. Anti-idiotypic antibodies and internal images. In J. C. Venter, C. M. Fraser, and J. Linstrom, ed. Monoclonal and anti-idiotypic antibodies: Probes for receptor structure and function. New York: Alan R. Liss, 1984: 141–9.

14. Nisonoff A, Lamoyi E. Implications of the presence of an internal image of the antigen in anti-idotypic antibodies: Possible application to vaccine production. Clin Immunol Immunopathol 1981; 21:397–406.

15. Stevens FJ, Jwo J, Caperos W, Kohler H, Schiffer M. Relationships between liquid- and solid-phase antibody association characteristics: Implications for the use of competitive ELISA techniques to map the spatial location of idiotopes. J Immunol 1986; 137:1937–44.

16. Schick MR, Dreesman GR, Kennedy RC. Induction of an antihepatitis B surface antigen response in mice by noninternal image (Ab2 alpha) anti-idiotypic antibodies. J Immunol 1987; 138:3419–25.

17. Huang J-H, Ward RE, Kohler H. Idiotope antigens (Ab2 alpha and Ab2 beta) can induce in vitro B cell proliferation and antibody production. J Immunol 1986; 137:770–6.

18. Dreesman GR, Kennedy RC. Anti-idiotypic antibodies: Implications of internal image-based vaccines for infectious diseases. J Infect Dis 1985; 151:761–5.

19. Hiernaux JR. Idiotypic vaccines and infectious diseases. Infect Immun 1988; 56:1407–13.

20. Kennedy RC, Zhou E-M, Lanford RE, Chanh TC, Bona CA. Possible role of anti-idiotypic antibodies in the induction of tumor immunity. J Clin Invest 1987; 80:1217–24.

21. Sacks DL, Esser KM, Sher A. Immunization of mice against African trypanosomiasis using anti-idiotypic antibodies. J Exp Med 1982; 155:1108–19.

22. Kennedy RC, Adler-Storthz K, Henkel RD, Sanchez Y, Melnick JL, Dreesman GR. Immune response to hepatitis B surface antigen: Enhancement by prior injection of antibodies to the idiotype. Science 1983; 221:853–55.

23. Reagan KJ, Wunner WH, Wiktor TJ, Koprowski H. Anti-idiotypic antibodies induce neutralizing antibodies to rabies virus glycoprotein. J Virol 1983; 48:660–6.

24. Kennedy RC, Dreesman GR. Enhancement of the immune response to hepatitis B surface antigen. In vivo administration of anti-idiotypes induces anti-HBs that expresses a similar idiotype. J Exp Med 1984; 159:655–65.

25. Sacks DL, Sher A. Evidence that anti-idiotype induced immunity to experimental African trypanosomiasis is genetically restricted and requires recognition of combining site-related idiotopes. J Immunol 1983; 131: 1511-5.

26. Kennedy RC, Eichberg JW, Dreesman GR. Lack of genetic restriction by a potential anti-idiotype vaccine for type B viral hepatitis. Virology 1986; 148:369-74.

27. Stein KE, Soderstrom T. Neonatal administration of idiotype or anti-idiotype primes for protection against *Escherichia coli* K 13 infection in mice. J Exp Med 1984; 160:1001-11.

28. Esternink MAJ, Campagnari AA, Wirth MA, Apicella MA. Development and characterization of an anti-idiotype antibody to the capsular polysaccharide of *Neisseria meningitidis* serogroup C. Infect Immun 1988; 56:1120-7.

29. McNamara MK, Ward RE, Kohler H. Monoclonal idiotope vaccine against *Streptococcus pneumoniae* infection. Science 1984; 226:1325-6.

30. McNamara MK, Ward RE, Huang J-H, Kohler, H. Idiotope vaccine against *Streptococcus pneumoniae*. A precursor study. J Immunol 1987; 139: 2775-80.

31. Kennedy RC, Sparrow JT, Sanchez Y, Melnick JL, Dreesman GR. Enhancement of viral hepatitis B antibody (anti-HBs) response to a synthetic cyclic peptide by priming with anti-idiotype antibodies. Virology 1984; 136:247-52.

32. Reagan KJ. Modulation of immunity to rabies virus induced by anti-idiotypic antibodies. Curr Top Microbiol Immunol 1985; 119:15-30.

33. Kennedy RC. Idiotype networks in hepatitis B virus infection. Curr Top Microbiol Immunol 1985; 119:1-19.

34. Kennedy RC, Melnick JL, Dreesman GR. Antibody to hepatitis B virus induced by injecting antibodies to the idiotype. Science 1984; 223:930-1.

35. Kennedy RC, Eichberg JW, Lanford RE, Dreesman GR. Anti-idiotypic antibody vaccine for type B viral hepatitis in chimpanzees. Science 1986; 232:220-3.

36. Koff WC, Hoth DF. Development and testing of AIDS vaccines. Science 1988; 241:426-32.

37. Maddon PJ, Littman DR, Godfrey M, Maddon DE, Chess L, Axel R. The isolation and nucleotide sequence of a DNA encoding the T-cell surface protein T4: a new member of the immunoglobulin gene family. Cell 1985; 42:93-104.

38. Maddon PJ, Molineaux SM, Maddon DE, Zimmerman KA, Godfrey M, Alt FW, Chess L, Axel R. Structure and expression of the human and mouse T4 genes. Proc Natl Acad Sci USA 1987; 84:9155-9.

39. Classon BJ, Tsagaratos J, McKenzie IFC, Walker ID. Partial primary structure of the T4 antigens of mouse and sheep: Assignment of intrachian disulfide bonds. Proc Natl Acad Sci USA 1986; 83:4499-503.

40. Clark SJ, Jefferies WA, Barclay AN, Gagnon J, Williams AF. Peptide and nucleotide sequences of rat CD4 (W3/25) antigen: Evidence for derivation

from a structure with four immunoglobulin-related domains. Proc Natl Acad Sci USA 1987; 84:1649–53.

41. Littman DR, GEttner SN. Unusual intron in the immunoglobulin domain of the newly isolated murine CD4 (L3T4) gene. Nature 1987; 325:453–5.

42. Swain SL. T cell subsets and the recognition of MHC Class. Immunol Rev 1983; 74:129–42.

43. Krensky AM, Reiss CS, Mier JW, Strominger JL, Burakoff SJ. Long-term human cytolytic T-cell lines allospecific for HLA–DR6 antigen are OKT4[+]. Proc Natl Acad Sci USA 1982; 79:2365–9.

44. Spits H, Borst J, Terhorst C, de Vries JE. The role of T cell differentiation markers in antigen-specific and lectin-dependent cellular cytotoxicity mediated by T8[+] and T4[+] human cytotoxic T cell clones directed at class I and class II MHC antigens. J Immunol 1982; 129:1563–9.

45. Neuer SC, Schlossman SF, Reinherz EL. Clonal analysis of human cytotoxic T lymphocytes: T4[+] and T8[+] effector T cells recognize products of different major histocompatibility complex regions. Proc Natl Acad Sci USA 1982; 79:4395–9.

46. Wilde DB, Marrack P, Kappler J, Dialynas DP, Fitch FW. Evidence implicating L3T4 in class II MHC antigen reactivity: monoclonal antibody GK1.5 (anti-L3T4a) blocks class II MHC antigen-specific proliferation, release of lymphokines, and binding by cloned murine helper T lymphocyte lines. J Immunol 1983; 131:2178–83.

47. Swain SL, Dialynas DP, Fitch FW, English M. Monoclonal antibody to L3T4 blocks the function of T cells specific for class 2 major histocompatibility complex antigens. J Immunol 1984; 132:1118–23.

48. Gay D, Maddon P, Sekaly R, Talle MA, Godfrey M, Long E, Goldstein G, Chess L, Axel R, Kappler J, Marrack P. Functional interaction between human T-cell protein C4 and the major histocompatibility complex HLA–DR antigen. Nature 1987; 328:626–9.

49. Doyle C, Strominger JL. Interaction between CD4 and class II MHC molecules mediates cell adhesion. Nature 1987; 330:256–9.

50. Reinherz EL, Schlossman SR. The differentiation of function of human T lymphocytes. Cell 1980; 19:821–7.

51. Dialynas DP, Quan ZS, Wall KA, Pierres A, Quintans J, Loken MR, Pierres M, Fitch FW. Characterization of the murine T cell surface molecule, designated L3T4, identified by monoclonal antibody GK1.5: Similarity of L3T4 to the human Leu-3/T4 molecule. J Immunol 1983; 131:2445–51.

52. Marrack P, Endres R, Shimonkevitz R, Zlotnik A, Dialynas D, Fitch F, Kappler J. The major histocompatibility complex-restricted antigen receptor on T-cells. II. Role of the L3T4 product. J Exp Med 1983; 158:1077–91.

53. Shaw S, Goldstein G, Springer TA, Biddison WE. Susceptibility of cytotoxic T lymphocyte (CTL) clones to inhibition by anti-T3 and anti-T4 (but not anti-LFA-1) monoclonal antibodies varies with the "avidity" of CTL-target interaction. J Immunol 1985; 134:3019–26.

54. Klatzmann D, Barré-Sinoussi F, Nugeyre MT, Dauguet C, Vilmer E, Griscelli C, Brun-Vezinet F, Rouzioux C, Gluckman JC, Chermann J-C, Montagnier L. Selective tropism of lymphadenopathy associated virus (LAV) for helper-inducer T lymphocytes. Science 1984; 225:59–63.
55. Dalgleish AG, Beverley PCL, Clapham PR, Crawford DH, Greaves MF, Weiss RA. The CD4 (T4) antigen is an essential component of the receptor for the AIDS retrovirus. Nature 1984; 312:763–7.
56. McDougal JS, Mawle A, Cort, SP, Nicholson JKA, Cross GD, Scheppler-Campbell JA, Hicks D, Sligh J. Cellular tropism of the human retrovirus HTLV–III/LAV. I. Role of T cell activation and expression of the T4 antigen. J Immunol 1985; 135:3151–62.
57. McDougal JS, Kennedy MS, Sligh JM, Cort SP, Mawle A, Nicholson JKA. Binding of HTLV–III/LAV to T4$^+$ T cells by a complex of the 110K viral protein and the T4 molecule. Science 1986; 231:382–5.
58. Maddon PJ, Dalgleish AG, McDougal JS, Clapham PR, Weiss RA, Axel R. The T4 gene encodes the AIDS virus receptor and is expressed in the immune system and the brain. Cell 1986; 47:333–48.
59. Sattentau QJ, Dalgleish AG, Weiss RA, Beverley PCL. Epitopes of the CD4 antigen and HIV Infection. Science 1986; 234:1120–3.
60. Jameson BA, Rao PE, Kong LI, Hahn BH, Shaw GM, Hood LE, Kent SBH. Location and chemical synthesis of a binding site for HIV-1 on the CD4 protein. Science 1988; 240:1335–9.
61. Landau NR, Warton M, Littman DR. The envelope glycoprotein of the human immunodeficiency virus binds to the immunoglobulin-like domain of CD4. Nature 1988; 334:59–162.
62. Peterson A, Seed B. Genetic analysis of monoclonal antibody and HIV binding sites on the human lymphocyte antigen CD4. Cell 1988; 54:65–72.
63. Berger EA, Fuerst TR, Moss B. A soluble recombinant polypeptide comprising the amino-terminal half of the extracellular region of the CD4 molecule contains an active binding site for human immunodeficiency virus. Proc Natl Acad Sci USA 1988; 85:2357–61.
64. Richardson NE, Brown NR, Hussey RE, Vaid A, Matthews TJ, Bolognesi DP, Reinherz EL. Binding site for human immunodeficiency virus coat protein gp120 is located in the NH_2-terminal region of T4 (CD4) and requires the intact variable-region-like domain. Proc Natl Acad Sci USA 1988; 85:6102–6.
65. Traunecker A, Luke W, Karjalainen K. Soluble CD4 molecules neutralize human immunodeficiency virus type 1. Nature 1988; 331:84–6.
66. Smith DH, Byrn RA, Marsters SA, Gregory T, Groopman JE, Capon DJ. Blocking of HIV-1 infectivity by a soluble, secreted form of the CD4 antigen. Science 1987; 238:1704–7.
67. Fisher RA, Bertonis JM, Meier W, Johnson VA, Costopoulos DS, Liu T, Tizard R, Walker BD, Hirsch MS, Schooley RT, Flavell RA. HIV infection is blocked in vitro by recombinant soluble CD4. Nature 1988; 331: 76–8.

68. Hussey RE, Richardson NE, Kowalski M, Brown NR, Chang H-C, Siliciano RF, Dorfman T, Walker B, Sodroski J, Reinherz EL. A soluble CD4 protein selectively inhibits HIV replication and syncytium formation. Nature 1988; 331:78–81.

69. Deen KC, McDougal JS, Inacker R, Folena-Wasserman G, Arthos J. Rosenberg J, Maddon PJ, Axel R, Sweet RW. A soluble form of CD4 (T4) protein inhibits AIDS virus infection. Nature 1988; 331:82–4.

70. McDougal JS, Nicholson JKA, Cross GD, Cort SP, Kennedy, MS, Mawle AC. Binding of the human retrovirus HTLV-III/LAV/ARV/HIV to the CD4 (T4) molecule: Conformation dependence, epitope mapping, antibody inhibition and potential for idiotypic mimicry. J Immunol 1986; 137: 2937–44.

71. Chanh TC, Dreesman GR, Kennedy RC. Monoclonal anti-idiotypic antibody mimics to CD4 receptor and bind human immunodeficiency virus. Proc Natl Acad Sci USA 1987; 84:3891–5.

72. Rieber EP, Chen H, Federle C, Riethmuller G. Characterization of soluble serumfactor(s) which suppress Ig E-synthesis in vitro. Immunobiology 1987; 4:175.

73. Rieber EP, Chen H, Federle C, Riethmuller G. Monoclonal anti-CD4-idiotype antibody recognizing the HIV-envelop GP120. International Conference on Aids, 4th, Stockholm, Sweden, 1988, Book I, Final Program, Abstracts. p. 242(3089).

74. Ohno T, Nakamura M, Kamada M, Watanabe M, Kohno Y, Kobayashi M. Complement dependent cytolysis of HIV infected cells with anti-idiotype monoclonal antibodies against the CD4 molecule. International Conference on Aids, 4th, Stockholm, Sweden, 1988, Book 1, Final Program, Abstracts. p. 216(2211).

75. Dalgleish AG, Thomson BJ, Chanh TC, Malkovsky M, Kennedy RC. Neutralization of HIV isolates by anti-idiotypic antibodies which mimic the T4 (CD4) epitope: A potential AIDS vaccine. Lancet 1987; 2:1047–50.

76. Sattentau QJ, Weber JN, Weiss RA, Beverley PCL. Antisera to Leu3a with anti-idiotypic activity react with gp110/130 of HIV-1 and LAV-2. International Conference on Acquired Immunodeficiency Syndrome (AIDS)., Washington D.C., 1987, Abstracts. p. 160(TH.9.4).

77. Chanh TC Alderette BE, Zhou E-M, Kennedy RC. Anti-idiotypic antibodies against OKT4A bind to human immunodeficiency virus. Fed Proc 1987; 46:1352(6041) (Abstract).

78. Kennedy RC, Allan JS, Zhou, E-M, Buck DW, Warner NL, Maino VC, Chanh TC, et al. Strategies to develop idiotype-based vaccines for HIV. International Conference on Aids, 4th, Stockholm, Sweden, 1988, Book 1, Final Program, Abstracts, p. 217(2213).

79. Strober S. Approaches to human immune tolerance. Immunol. Today 1986; 7:153–155.

80. Benjamin RJ, Waldman H. Induction of tolerance by monoclonal antibody therapy. Nature 1986; 320:449–51.

81. Zhou E-M, Chanh TC, Dreesman GR, Kanda P, Kennedy RC. Immune response to human immunodeficiency virus. In vivo administration of anti-idiotype induces an anti-gp160 response specific for a synthetic peptide. J Immunol 1987; 139:2950-6.

82. Chanh TC, Dreesman GR, Kanda P, Linette GP, Sparrow JT, Ho DD, Kennedy RC. Induction of anti-HIV neutralizing antibodies by synthetic peptides. EMBO J 1986; 5:3065-71.

83. Dalgleish AG, Chanh TC, Kennedy RC, Kanda P, Clapham PR, Weiss RA. Neutralization of diverse HIV-1 strains by monoclonal antibodies raised against a gp41 synthetic peptide. Virology 1988; 165:209-15.

84. Zhou E-M, Lohman KL, Kennedy RC. Administration of noninternal image anti-idiotypic antibodies induces idiotype restricted response specific for human immunodeficiency virus envelope glycoprotein epitopes. Virology, in press.

85. Weiner DB, Williams WV, Hoxie JA, Greene MI. Identification of ancillary molecules on human T cells important in HIV-1 T cell interactions. International Conference on Aids, 4th, Stockholm, Sweden, 1988, Book 2, Program and Abstracts p. 120(2577).

86. Keay S, Rasmussen L, Merigan TC. Syngeneic monoclonal anti-idiotype antibodies that bear the internal image of a human cytomegalovirus neutralization epitope. J Immunol 1988; 140:944-948.

87. Paque RE, Miller R. Modulation of murine Coxsackievirus-induced myocarditis utilizing anti-idiotypes. Viral Immunol 1987; 1:207-224.

88. Thanavala YM, Brown SE, Howard CR, Roitt IM, Steward MW. A surrogate hepatitis B virus antigenic epitope represented by a synthetic peptide and an internal image antiidiotype antibody. J Exp Med 1986; 164:227-236.

89. Colucci G, Beazer Y, Waksal S. Interactions between HBV and polymeric human serum albumin. II. Development of syngeneic monoclonal anti-anti-idiotypes which mimic hepatitis B surface antigen in the induction of immune responsiveness. Eur J Immunol 1987; 17:371-374.

90. Kennedy RC, Adler-Storthz K, Burns JW, Henkel RD, Dreesman GR. Antiidiotype modulation of herpes simplex virus infection leading to increased pathogenicity. J Virol 1984; 50:941-953.

91. Gell PGH, Moss PAH. Production of cell-mediated immune response to herpes simplex virus by immunization with anti-idiotypic heteroantisera. J Gen Virol 1985; 66:1801-1804.

92. Lathey JL, Courtney RJ, Rouse BT. Production, binding characteristics, and immunogenicity of heterologous anti-idiotypic antibody to herpes simplex virus glycoprotein C. Viral Immunol 1987; 1:13-24.

93. Lathey J, Martin S, Rouse B. Suppression of delayed type hypersensitivity to herpes simplex virus type I following immunization with anti-idiotypic antibody: an example of split tolerance. J Gen Virol 1987; 68:1092-1102.

94. Mayer R, Ioannides C, Moran T, Johansson B, Bona C. Effect of syngeneic anti-idiotypic antibody on influenza virus neuraminidase antibody response. Viral Immunol 1987; 1:121-134.

95. Raychaudhuri S, Saeki Y, Chen J-J, Kohler H. Tumor-specific idiotype vaccines. III. Induction of T helper cells by anti-idiotype and tumor cells. J Immunol 1987; 139:2096–2102.
96. Tanaka M, Sasaki N, Seto A. Induction of antibodies against Newcastle Disease Virus with syngeneic anti-idiotype antibodies in mice. Microbiol Immunol 1986; 30:323–331.
97. Uytdehaag FGCM, Osterhaus ADME. Induction of neutralizing antibody in mice against poliovirus type II with monolonal anti-idiotypic antibody. J Immunol 1985; 134:1225–1229.
98. Sharpe AH, Gaulton GN, McDade KK, Fields BN, Greene MI. Syngeneic monoclonal antiidiotype can induces cellular immunity to reovirus. J Exp Med 1984; 160:1195–1205.
99. Ertl HCJ, Finberg RW. Sendai virus-specific T-cell clones; Induction of cytolytic T cells by an anti-idiotypic antibody directed against a helper T-cell clone. Proc Natl Acad Sci USA 1984; 81:2850–2854.
100. Ertl HCJ, Homans E, Tournas S, Finberg RW. Sendai virus-specific T cell clones. V. Induciton of a virus-specific response by antiidiotypic antibodies directed against a T helper cell clone. J Exp Med 1984; 159:1778–1783.
101. Kennedy R, Dreesman G, Butel J, Lanford R. Suppression of in vivo tumor formation induced by simian virus 40-transformed cells in mice receiving antiidiotypic antibodies. J Exp Med 1985; 161:1432–1449.

12

Prophylactic and Therapeutic Immunization Against AIDS
Theoretical Considerations Underlying a
Modified Noninfectious Whole Virus Approach

Jonas Salk with Merril J. Gersten
The Salk Institute for Biological Studies
San Diego, California

In designing strategies to prevent either HIV infection or disease, consideration must be given to the intrinsic properties of the causative virus that may render ineffective measures useful in dealing with simpler viruses. Among these are 1) the ability of HIV to enter CD4 cells and macrophages directly, 2) its efficient cell-to-cell transfer, and 3) its ability to integrate into host DNA to persist indefinitely. Moreover, persistent HIV infection induces immunopathic (host-originated), in addition to cytopathic (virus-originated) pathology. In view of these considerations, it has been suggested that prevention of disease may be more readily achievable than prevention of infection (1). Nevertheless, even though transient, inapparent infection at the cellular level may not be prevented, it may be possible, through appropriate immunologic (pre) conditioning, to prevent the *establishment* of persistent systemic infection, as reflected in positive viral cultures and an immune response. Both the long latent period before the onset of AIDS and anecdotal reports of virus clearing in previously infected humans and observations in chimpanzees (2) suggest that immunoprotective factors are elicited by the virus that limit, and may even eliminate, HIV infection by mechanisms still to be clarified. It is likely that cellular immune mechanisms, and cytotoxic T cells in particular, are involved in such phenomena.

Seen in this perspective, post-HIV infection events may be modulated through immunologic intervention either by 1) prepriming the immune system, by active immunization of HIV seronegatives, to respond anamnestically to subsequent HIV exposure, to prevent establishment of infection and/or disease, or 2) through active and/or passive immunization of HIV seropositives, to prevent, arrest, or reverse the development of disease, by limiting already established HIV infection (3).

These hypotheses are testable using an HIV immunogen comprised of native HIV molecules present in a purified and concentrated preparation of tissue-culture adapted HIV which is 1) treated to destroy infectivity, 2) depleted of the outer envelope glycoprotein, gp120, and 3) incorporated into a suitable, potent immunologic adjuvant. The purpose is to induce a broad spectrum of immune response, both cellular and humoral, which will include such immunologic specificities and modalities as may be necessary for preventing HIV infection and/or disease.

IMMUNOGEN PREPARATION AND COMPOSITION

Of primary importance in developing a noninfectious virus preparation for human immunization, and especially a retrovirus, is the question of the reliability of the inactivation process. For this reason use of mutliple procedures that are individually effective in destroying HIV infectivity are preferred in that they provide a wide margin of effectiveness and therefore of safety. As an example, β-propriolactone and gamma-radiation are being employed sequentially for the inactivation of a gp120-depleted virion.

The use of a gp120-depleted immunogen for these purposes is based, in part, on the difficulty of retaining this protein on the virion in the course of virus purification and concentration. Moreover, the persistence of antienvelope protein antibody, after other anti-HIV antibodies are lost, suggests the possibility that such antibody may be protective of the virus rather than the host. Such a gp120 immunogen, if used for prophylactic immunization, has the advantage of making it possible to distinguish an individual who became seropositive as a result of immunization from one in whom seropositivity was induced by infection. An envelope-depleted preparation also avoids any question regarding the possible role of (vaccine-induced) anti-gp120 antibody in facilitating viral spread through virus enhancement (1,4), or in contributing to immunopathogenesis (5,6). Such a gp120-depleted immunogen otherwise contains a wide range of other viral antigens, as is revealed by Gibbs et al. (2) in a comparison of the antibody response induced in a vaccinated seronegative chimpanzee (A-36) with that seen in animals that became seropositive as a result of infection (A-3 and A-86C) (Fig. 1). Included in such a preparation are antigens associated with the induction of ADCC (7), neutralizing (8), proliferative (9), and cytotoxic T-cell (10,11) effects, the functional significance of each of which for immunity to infection and/or disease remains to be established.

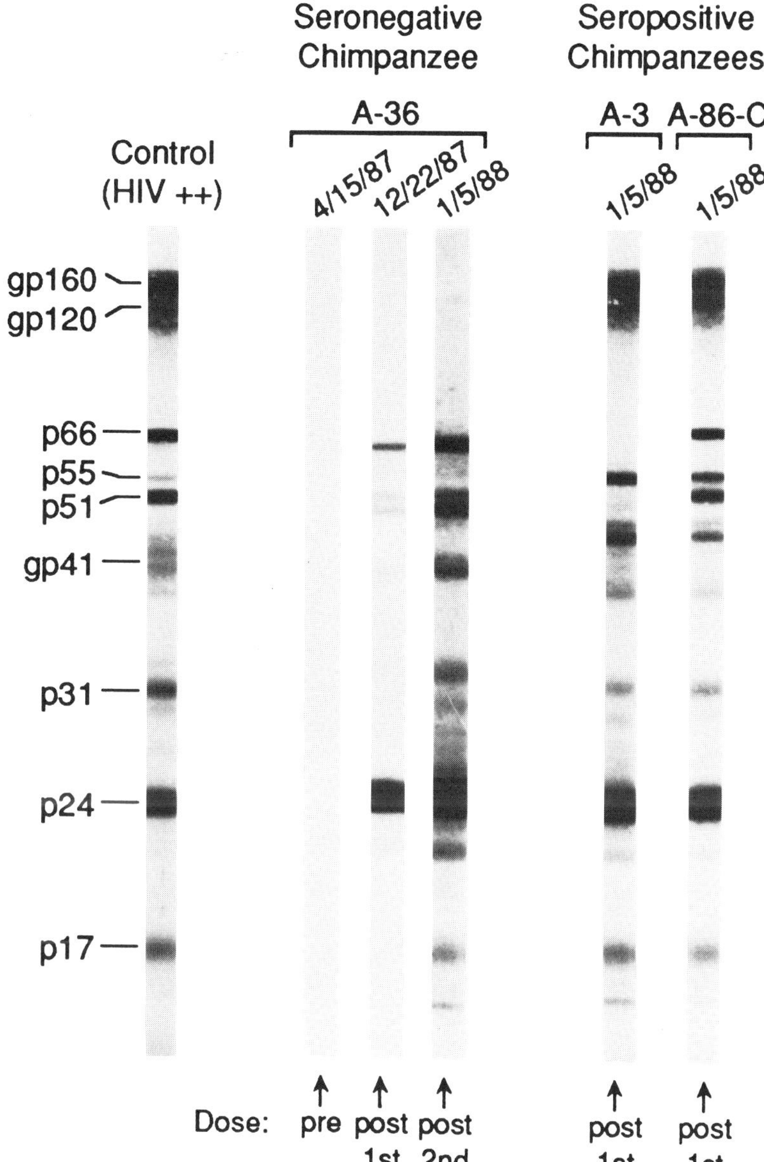

Figure 1 Western blot of sera from chimpanzees immunized with the envelope-depleted inactivated HIV immunogen in IFA. Dates of immunization: *A-36*–4/15/87 and 12/22/87; *A-3*–6:12/87; *A-86-C*–4/15/87. HIV positive control (lane 1), chimpanzee A-36 (lanes 2–4), and chimpanzees A-3 and A-86-c (lanes 5 and 6). (From Ref. 2.)

STUDIES IN ANIMALS

Dose-response studies carried out in rabbits by Peters et al. (12) have shown the effectiveness of such a noninfectious immunogen in inducing a broad anti-HIV antibody response exclusive of anti-gp160/120. The anti-p24 response observed in rabbits given two doses, administered one month apart, of 1–100 μg of virus antigen emulsified in IFA is presented in Figure 2. Comparable doses of immunogen administered in alum induced significantly lower responses (Fig. 2). Moreover, in contrast to the prompt and sustained responses induced by virus emulsified in IFA, those induced by the alum preparation did not appear until after the second dose and were less well sustained.

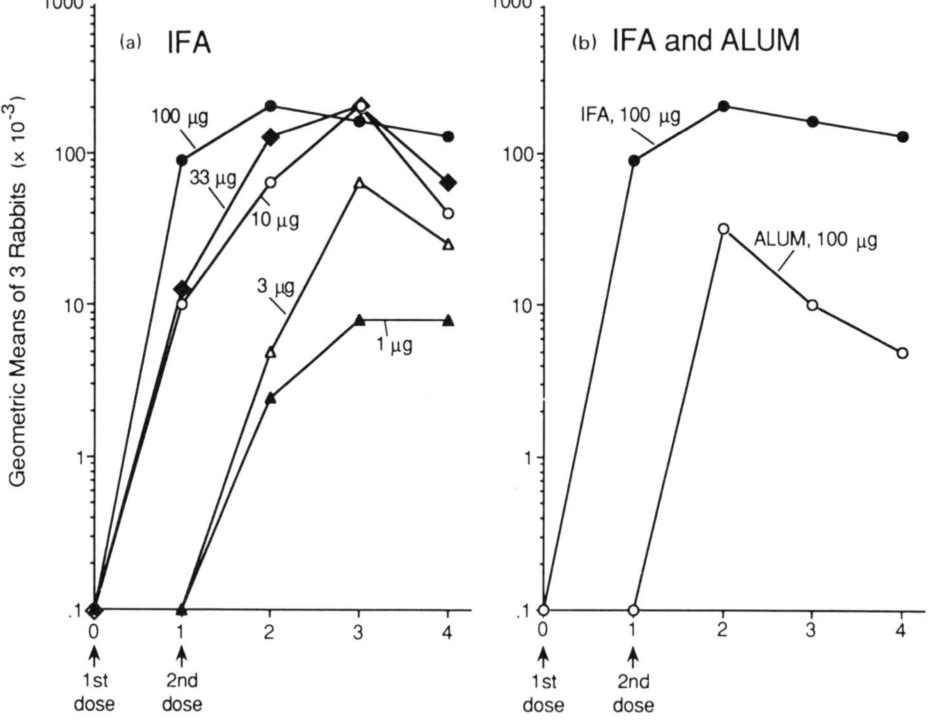

Figure 2 Anti-p24 response of rabbits inoculated twice with (a) different doses (1–100 μg) of the inactivated HIV immunogen in IFA; (b) 100 μg of the inactivated HIV immunogen in IFA or alum. In all cases, the two doses were administered one month apart. The points plotted represent the geometric mean titer for groups of three animals. For the purpose of calculating the geometric mean, titers of less than 2000 were assigned a value of 1000. (From Ref. 12.)

Studies of the immune response to the immunogen, emulsified in IFA, have been carried out in chimpanzees by Gibbs et al. (2). The preparation employed was administered to two previously infected seropositive chimpanzees (A-3 and A-86C) and one seronegative (A-36) animal. A secondary-type response developed after a single dose in the two seropositive chimpanzees, and primary- and secondary-type responses occurred after a first and second dose, respectively, in the seronegative animal. These animals, as well as a naive control animal (A-189a), were subsequently challenged with 40 chimpanzee infectious doses of HIV-1 by the intravenous route. Table 1 shows the patterns of anti-p24 response and of virus recovery in each chimpanzee following viral challenge, and Table 2 presents a summary of the inferences drawn from the experimental results. Hereafter the chimpanzees are referred to in terms of the *pattern* of immunologic and virologic response manifested after challenge, to emphasize that postinfection events are significantly affected by preinfection immunologic experience.

At the time of challenge, pattern A chimpanzees were negative for virus as assessed by co-cultivation of their PBL with virus-susceptible indicator cells. Although pattern A and B chimpanzees had similar prechallenge anti-p24 levels (Table 1), the pattern B animal, like the control, became detectably infected (PBL co-culture positive), whereas the pattern A animals did not. The difference in infectability between patterns A and B is reflected in the anamnestic humoral response manifested by the pattern B chimpanzee following virus challenge, and the absence of any humoral response in the pattern A animals. Although patterns A and B differed significantly in that anti-gp120 antibody was absent in pattern B, it is unlikely that this could account for the observed differences in the course of infection, since anti-gp120 seems to be associated neither with in vivo protection against infection (13), nor in vivo elimination of virus. One may infer, therefore, that the critical difference between patterns A and B may be associated with the degree of HIV cellular immunity present in each. This presumes that a sufficient cellular immunity developed in the pattern A chimpanzees, as a result of their primary HIV infection, which reduced their burden of virus-infected cells below the level of detectability, and also protected them against subsequent reinfection. This interpretation raises the possibility that with a suitably formulated noninfectious immunogen it may be possible, in humans, to induce a sufficient degree of HIV cellular (and humoral) immunity to simulate the immunologic status of the pattern A chimpanzees, thereby enabling the individual to resist the establishment of HIV infection, and possibly to reverse this process if HIV infection is already established.

STUDIES IN SEROPOSITIVE SUBJECTS

In view of the humoral immune response patterns observed in seropositive chimpanzees, and the absence of toxicity, Levine et al. (14) initiated exploratory

Table 1 Comparison of Serologic and Virologic Response Patterns in Chimpanzees Post-HIV Challenge

	Anti p24 $(\times 10^{-3})$				HIV culture (PBL)			
Chimpanzee #:	A86c	A3	A36	A189a	A86c	A3	A36	A189a
Status at immunization:	pos.	pos.	neg.	neg.	neg.[a]	neg.[a]	neg.	neg.
Immunization:	yes	yes	yes	no	yes	yes	yes	no
Weeks postchallenge								
0	8	32	16	0	−	−	−	−
1	16	32	16	0				
2	64	32	32	0	−	−	+	+
3	32	32	32	0				
4	16	16	64	0				
5	16	64	256	2	−	−	+	+
6	16	32	256	4	−	−	+	+
7	16	64	256	4				
8	16	64	256	8	−	−	+	+
9	16	64	256	8	−	−	+	+
10	4	64	256	4	−	−	+	+
12	16	64	256	NT	−	−	+	+
14	16	64	256	2	−	−	−	+
18	16	64	256	1				
Response pattern:	A	A	B	C	A	A	B	C

[a]Previously virus culture positive.

Table 2 Hypothesized Correlation Between Preexposure HIV Immunity
Patterns and Clinical Consequences of Exposure to HIV in Humans

	Preexposure Immunity		Postexposure Clinical consequences	
Patterns	CMI	HI	Infection	Disease
A	+	+	−	−
B	−	+	+	?
C	−	−	+	+

toxicity and immunogenicity studies in virus culture–positive HIV serpositive
individuals with persistent generalized lymphadenopathy. No toxic or other
adverse effects were observed in 9 subjects initially inoculated IM with the
immunogen in IFA, or in 10 subjects initially inoculated ID with the immunogen
in saline. In both groups a second dose was given via the reciprocal route. The
clear anamnestic response observed in the seropositive chimpanzees by Gibbs et
al. (2) was not observed in the seropositive humans. This difference is not fully
explained, but may be related to the fact that the seropositive humans were
positive for HIV, as revealed by PBL cultures, in contrast to the seropositive
chimpanzees that appeared to be free of infectious virus at the time of immunization. Conceivably, immune suppression resulting from the presence of HIV
infection, as well as the presence of already maximal responses due to continuing
viral antigenic stimulation, could account for the lack of response in the seropositive humans.

Even though anamnestic humoral responses were not observed in the seropositive human subjects, there seems to have been an effect on some components of the cellular immune system, since DTH responsiveness to nonspecific
antigens developed in some who were initially anergic and increased in others.
Furthermore, CD4 cell levels, as compared to historical control data from these
same individuals, tended to be stably maintained during the course of a year
postimmunization. An additional 27 matched treated and control pairs are being
followed by Levine et al. (14) to see if observations in this group of 54 individuals confirm any of the trends observed in the uncontrolled studies in 19
subjects referred to above.

The results of recently reported studies of passive immunization by Jackson
et al. (15) and by Karpas et al. (16) warrant confirmation and amplification. In
view of the significance of antibodies to nonenvelope antigens in mediating the
reported beneficial effects in subjects with advancing disease (15), future studies

of passive immunization may be facilitated by the availability of hyperimmune IgG prepared from the plasma of HIV seronegatives immunized with an inactivated, gp120-depleted, HIV immunogen administered in a potent immunologic adjuvant (Fig. 2).

PERSPECTIVE

The foregoing suggests that a multiple-strategy approach needs to be explored to study the prospects for immunization against HIV infection and/or disease, as set forth in Figure 3. Such an approach should include attempts at both therapeutic immunization of symptomatic and asymptomatic seropositives, as well as prophylactic immunization of at-risk seronegatives. Active immunization should be studied, not only in seronegatives but also in seropositives sufficiently immunocompetent to mount an immune response. For more severely immunocompromised seropositives, passive immunization needs to be explored using HIV-IgG. The latter might be prepared by immunizing low-risk seronegatives with the envelope-depleted noninfectious immunogen. For treating newborns of HIV-infected mothers, passive combined with active immunization would be appropriate.

In terms of pathogenesis and pathology, the HIV-infected individuals referred to in Figure 3 bear similarities not only to individuals harboring a latent virus,

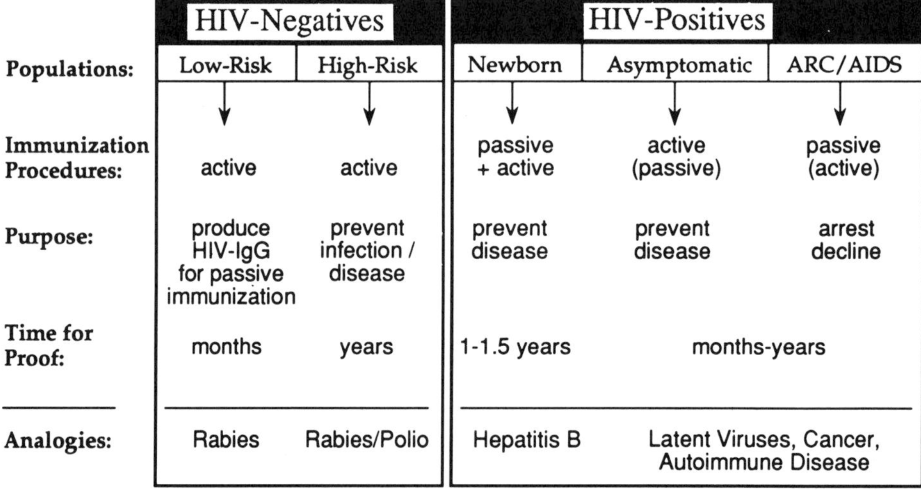

Figure 3 A multistrategy approach to the prevention and treatment of AIDS using a noninfectious HIV immunogen.

but also to those with cancer and autoimmune diseases. They are cancer-like in that the primary unit of pathology seems to be an infected *cell*; they are auto-immune-like in that a significant degree of CD-4 cell functional impairment and destruction appears to be the result of immunopathic mechanisms directed, in part, at viral antigens on the surface of uninfected cells. Accordingly, the strategies here proposed include an exploration of approaches to curb or eliminate virus-expressing cells, and the associated antigenemia, as well as an investigation of means for preventing the establishment and spread of HIV-infected cells in the host. For these purposes, amplification of the cellular arm of the HIV immune response is of particular importance; and the anticipated benefit is prolongation or restoration of the asymptomatic state in HIV-infected individuals, whether or not they are able to revert to an infection-free status.

The objective of these suggestions is thus to alter both the perception and the reality of a diagnosis of HIV infection from that of a death sentence to that of an infection with which one can live, similar to other chronic, latent viral infections, such as HSV, CMV, and EBV. In this way, infected individuals might be able to maintain quiescent infections through the maintenance of cellular and humoral immune effectors, and, under exceptional circumstances, might eliminate virus completely.

As implied in Figure 3, exploratory testing of the usefulness of these approaches needs to be conducted in human subjects, in part, because no fully appropriate animal model for the HIV-infected human exists. In chimpanzees HIV appears not to cause disease in the time-span observed thus far; and the SIV-rhesus model exhibits a more rapid course, due to its predominantly viral-induced cytopathology, than does HIV in humans. Thus, SIV-induced disease and death may occur within several months of infection, and often in the absence of a detectable immune response (17). Conversely, HIV-related CD4 cell destruction in humans occurs slowly, and only after the appearance of virus-specific antibody. In humans, immunopathic mechanisms thus appear to contribute more significantly to the pathogenesis of AIDS (5,6,18). This aspect of pathogenesis, together with the prolonged asymptomatic phase, distinguishes HIV infection of humans from SIV infection of rhesus monkeys, and provides the rationale for considering immunologic interventions that may halt or reverse progress of HIV infection to the stage of symptomatic disease.

The strategy here proposed for the study of prophylactic and therapeutic interventions for the control of HIV infection is but one of many that are under investigation. The approaches suggested in Figure 3 can be explored with knowledge and technology that we now possess. If any show promise, then more effective and more specific means could be developed based on the insights and experience gained in the course of using a noninfectious immunogen such as here proposed. Nevertheless, the therapeutic and prophylactic probes presently available may now be used to test their capacity to activate, alter, or preselect cellular and humoral immune response patterns to HIV. By observing the alterations in immune response patterns so induced, and correlating these with clinical and virologic consequences, it may be possible to gain insights as to which of the immunologic responses to HIV are critical to the control of HIV infection and AIDS.

NOTE ADDED IN PROOF

Continued monitoring of the HIV-challenged chimpanzees has revealed continued negative HIV cultures in A3 and A86c, continued positive cultures in A189a, and a sustained conversion to culture negativity in A36, beginning at 7 months. Further observations made in the human subjects have suggested that the presence of *HIV-specific* DTH, unrelated to the presence or absence of nonspecific DTH, plays a significant role in retarding the rate of progression of the HIV infection.

ACKNOWLEDGMENTS

The chimpanzee studies referred to in this paper have been carried out in collaboration with C. J. Gibbs of the National Institutes of Health. The human studies were conducted in collaboration with B. E. Henderson and A. Levine at the University of Southern California School of Medicine. Antibody and viral culture determinations were carried out in collaboration with D. J. Carlo, F. Jensen, and R. Peters of the Immune Response Corp. The assistance of Ami Koide in the preparation of the manuscript is greatly appreciated.

REFERENCES

1. Ada GL Prospects for HIV vaccines. J Acq Imm Def Syndr 1988; 1:295–303.
2. Gibbs CJ, Peters R, Gravell M, Johnson B, Jensen FC, Carlo DJ, Salk J. HIV immunization and challenge of HIV seropositive and seronegative chimpanzees. Submitted, 1989.
3. Salk J. Prospects for the control of AIDS by immunizing seropositive individuals. Nature 1987; 327:473–6.
4. Porterfield JS. Antibody-dependent enhancement of viral infectivity. Adv Virus Res 1986; 31:335–55.
5. Martinez-A, C, De La Hera A, Alonzo JM, Marcos MAR, Marquez C, Toribio ML, Coutinho A. Immunological consequences of HIV infection: advantage of being low responder casts doubt on vaccine development. Lancet 1988; 1:454–7.

6. Ziegler JL, Stites DP. Hypothesis: AIDS is an autoimmune disease directed at the immune system and triggered by a lymphotropic retrovirus. Clin Immunol Immunopathol 1986; 41:305-13.

7. Rook AH, Lane HC, Folks T, McCoy S, Alter H, Fauci AS. Sera from HTLV-III/LAV antibody positive individuals mediates antibody-dependent cellular cytotoxicity against HTLV-III/LAV-infected T cells. J Immunol 1987; 138:1064-7.

8. Ranki A, Weiss SH, Valle SL, Antonen J, Krohin KJE. Neutralizing antibodies in HIV (HTLV-III) infection: Correlation with clinical outcome and antibody response against different viral proteins. Clin Exp Immunol 1987; 69:231-9.

9. Wahren B, Morfeldt-Maansson L, Biberfeld G, Moberg L, Sonnenborg A, Liungman P, Werner A, Kurth R, Gallo R, Bolognesi D. Characteristics of the specific cell-mediated immune response in human immunodeficiency virus infection. J Virol 1987; 61:2017-23.

10. Walker BD, Chakrabati S, Moss B, Paradis TJ, Flynn T, Durno AG, Blumberg RS, Kaplan JC, Hirsch MS, Schooley RT. HIV-specific cytotoxic T lymphocytes in seropositive individuals. Nature 1987; 328:345-8.

11. Walker BD, Flexner C, Paradis TJ, Fuller TC, Hirsch MS, Schooley RT, Moss B. HIV-1 reverse transcriptase is a target for cytotoxic T lymphocytes in infected individuals. Science 1988; 240:64-6.

12. Peters RE, Jensen FC, Carlo DJ, Salk J. Dose response studies in rabbits of an envelope-depleted non-infectious HIV immunogen combined with different immunological adjuvants. In preparation, 1989.

13. Berman PW, Groopman JE, Gregory T, Clapham PR, Weiss RA, Ferriani R, Riddle L, Shimasaki C, Lucas C, Lasky LA, Eichberg JW. Human immunodeficiency virus type 1 challenge of chimpanzees immunized with recombinant envelope glycoprotein gp120. Proc Natl Acad Sci USA 1988; 85:5200-4.

14. Levine A, Henderson BE, Groshan S, Carlo D, Shepard HW, Salk J, et al. Immunization with inactivated, envelope-depleted HIV immunogen in HIV infected men with ARC: Preliminary report of exploratory studies in progress. In preparation, 1989.

15. Jackson GG, Rubenis M, Knigge M, Perkins JT, Paul DA, Despotes JC, Spencer P. Passive immunoneutralization of human immunodeficiency virus in patients with advanced AIDS. Lancet 1988; 2:647-52.

16. Karpas A, Hill F, Youle M, Cullen V, Gray J, Byron N, Hayhoe F, Tenant-Flowers M, Howard L, Gilgen D, Oates JK, Hawkins D, Gazzard B. Effects of passive immunization in patients with the acquired immunodeficiency syndrome-related complex and acquired immunodeficiency syndrome. Proc Natl Acad Sci USA 1988; 85:9234-7.

17. Gardner MB, Jennings M, Carlson JR, Lerche N, McGraw T, Luciw P, Marx P., Pedersen N. Post-exposure immunotherapy of simian immunodeficiency (SIV) infected rhesus with an SIV immunogen. J Med Primatol 1989; 18:321-8.

18. Shearer GM. AIDS: An autoimmune pathologic model for the destruction of a subset of helper T lymphocytes. Mt Sinai J Med 1986; 53:609-15.

ANIMAL MODELS FOR VACCINE DEVELOPMENT AND EFFICACY STUDIES

13

Equine Infectious Anemia Virus
A Natural Model for the Immunologic Management of Lentivirus Infections

Ronald C. Montelaro, Charles J. Issel, and Susan L. Payne
Louisiana State University
Baton Rouge, Louisiana

Keith Rushlow
Battelle Memorial Institute
Columbus, Ohio

INTRODUCTION

Animal lentiviruses provide important model systems for studying mechanisms of viral replication and pathogenesis and for developing and evaluating strategies for AIDS vaccines. Equine infectious anemia (EIA), which was one of the first diseases to be assigned a viral ("filterable") etiology in 1904 (1), offers a uniquely dynamic lentivirus infection in which to examine the nature and role of antigenic variation during persistent infections. Moreover, EIA is the only lentivirus system in which the infected animal routinely brings viral replication under immunologic control, despite rapid and varied changes in the antigens of the infecting equine infectious anemia virus (EIAV). Thus, an elucidation of the specific immune responses that affect control of virus replication should provide important information on the immune status to be achieved by candidate vaccines.

During the past several years we have developed an experimental infection model system in which Shetland ponies inoculated with a standard EIAV strain develop recurrent cycles of viremia and illness characteristic of chronic EIA (2). We have also analyzed in detail the antigens of EIAV and the variation that occurs in these antigens during persistent infections (3–10). Most recently we have begun a characterization of the virus-specific immune responses and the manner in which they change in response to antigenic variations in the virus. The results of these studies indicate that the recurrent nature of EIA can be attributed to the sequential evolution of EIAV variants that temporarily circumvent established host immune responses. After exposure to a sufficient number of variants, however, the immune responses apparently "mature" to a state capable of suppressing any further significant virus replication.

The purpose of this review is to summarize the salient features of the EIAV system and to relate these properties to the development of vaccines against the human immunodeficiency virus (HIV).

CLINICAL ASPECTS OF EIA

The clinical responses of horses following natural or experimental infections by EIAV can be divided into characteristic stages (Fig. 1). Acute EIA, characterized by fever and hemorrhages, is typically associated with the first exposure to virus

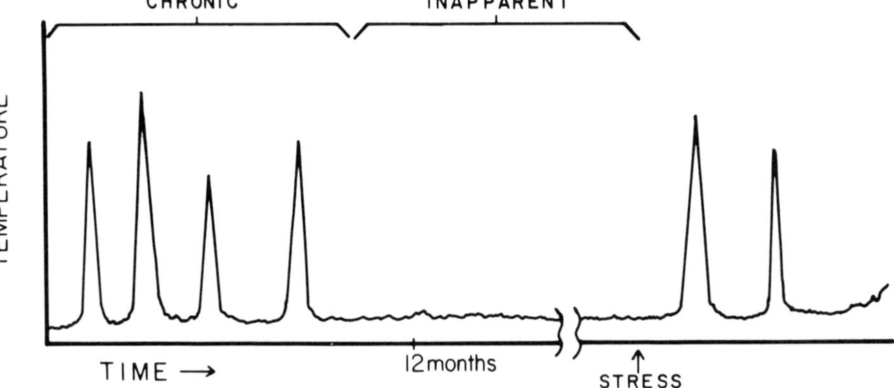

Figure 1   Schematic representation of the clinical response of a horse after infection by EIAV. Clinial episodes of EIA are represented by peaks of fever above normal animal temperatures. The chronic form of disease is characterized by recurrent clinical episodes which occur at unpredictable intervals during the first year after infection. At this time animals usually no longer display any obvious clinical signs, although recrudescence of disease can be induced years later by stress or the administration of immunosuppressants. The clinical response of animals is variable and depends, in part, on host resistance factors, virus virulence factors, and environmental factors (e.g., weather, work, hauling, etc.).

and appears to correlate with massive virus replication in and destruction of macrophages. The more classical symptoms of EIA (anemia, weight loss, edema, leukopenia, etc.) are observed later during recurring cycles of viremia and illness which appear at irregular intervals separated by weeks or months. This stage of disease is called chronic EIA. The frequency and severity of disease episodes decline with time and the chronic stage of disease usually ends within the first year after infection and an average of 6-8 clinical episodes. The exact progression of disease, however, depends on the infecting strain of EIAV and characteristics of the individual animal and its environment (general health, work load, etc.). For example, some infections may result in extensive encephalopathy, while others may show no manifestations of this pathology.

During disease episodes, viremia levels can range from 10^2-10^4 TCID$_{50}$ allowing easy recovery of virus from plasma incubated on cultured cells (2). In contrast, plasma viremia levels are typically negligible during afebrile periods. It has been clearly demonstrated that EIA can be transmitted by whole blood transfer to naive animals from infected animals displaying the chronic stage of disease. These blood transfers can be mediated by man (hypodermic needles, scalpels, etc.) or by insect vectors (11-13). In fact, transmission has been accomplished by allowing a single horse fly (*Tabanus fuscicostatus*) to take a partial blood meal on an infected pony during an acute clinical period and immediately finish its meal on a naive pony. The transfer of blood by this species has been estimated at 6 nl, and efficient transmission of EIAV from donors with plasma viremias of 10^6 horse ID$_{50}$ per ml has been reported with this horse fly species. Mosquitoes or other biting insects are less efficient in transmitting EIAV between animals.

Following the chronic stage of disease, most infected horses enter an inapparent stage during which there is an absence of any clinical symptoms or detectable levels of plasma viremia. The animal continues to harbor EIAV, however, as evidenced by the fact that disease can be efficiently transmitted by experimental transfer of whole blood (250 ml) from inapparently infected to naive horses. In addition, it has been demonstrated that recrudescence of chronic EIA can be induced in some inapparently infected horses by administration of immunosuppressants (e.g., dexamethasone) or by stress, even in certain animals that have been free of febrile episodes for years (14). This ability to induce chronic EIA in inapparent carriers suggests an active immunologic management of virus replication that can be overcome by suppressing or stressing the immune system.

The target cell of EIAV appears to be cells of the monocyte/macrophage lineage; there is no detectable infection of lymphocytes, nor is there apparent immunosuppression. In these regards, EIAV resembles visna virus and caprine arthritis encephalitis virus (CAEV) and differs from the human and simian (SIV) immunodeficiency viruses. Like HIV and SIV, however, EIAV infections manifest clear stages of apparent and inapparent infection, unlike visna virus and CAEV, which both induce slow, progressively degenerative clinical manifestations. In the case of HIV, the latent or inapparent period is the initial stage of infection, while in EIAV the inapparent period is observed during the final stage of infection.

Thus, the periodic nature of EIAV offers a uniquely dynamic model for examining lentivirus persistence in the presence of apparently competent host immune responses. In addition, EIAV-infected horses represent the only lentivirus system in which the infected animal routinely establishes control of viral replication, presumably resulting from cumulative immune responses produced against a series of virus variants generated during the first year postinfection. An elucidation of the immune factors which affect control of EIAV replication, even in the face of rapid and extensive antigenic variations of the infecting virus, should provide important insights into potential strategies for lentivirus vaccine development.

EIAV ANTIGENS

General Properties of Virion Proteins

EIAV is assigned to the lentivirus subfamily of retroviruses based on characteristic similarities in morphology, serologic relatedness, genetic organization and sequence homologies, and the role of monocytes/macrophage as target cells. The EIAV genome has been completely sequenced (15–17) revealing a genomic organization of EIAV that is similar to HIV in that the RNA encodes three primary genes, *gag, pol*, and *env* (Fig. 2). The *gag* and *pol* genes overlap, while the *env* gene is nonoverlapping. The genome also contains three short open reading frames (orfs), S1 and S2, located in the intergenic region between *pol* and *env*, and S3, located within the 3' coding region of the *env* gene. These orfs appear to mediate transactivation, although gene products have not yet been identified (18,19). The *gag* gene encodes four structural proteins in the order 5'-p15-p26-p11-p9-3', while the *env* gene encodes two glycoproteins in the order 5'-gp90-gp45-3'. The *pol* gene product is uncharacterized.

We have recently developed HPLC procedures which accomplish the purification of all EIAV *gag* and *env* proteins from purified virus in a single step (20). The availability of purified proteins has permitted a detailed cataloging of protein biochemical properties, including molecular weights, stoichiometry, amino acid compositions and sequences, isoelectric points, and patterns of modification (glycosylation, phosphorylation, fatty acylation, etc.) (3,4,26).

A schematic model depicting the structural organization of EIAV proteins is presented in Figure 3. The virus, which is about 100 nm in diameter, contains an oblong core characteristic of lentiviruses contained within the lipid envelope of

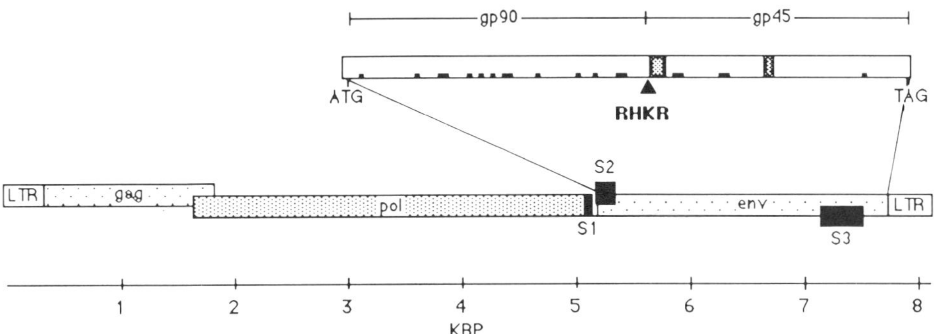

Figure 2 Genomic organization of EIAV (15,16). Structural features include overlapping *gag* and *pol* genes and a nonoverlapping *env* gene. Three short open reading frames (S1, S2, and S3) were identified by nucleotide sequence analysis. The *env* gene is expanded to show the basic peptide cleavage site (RHKR) used to generate mature gp90 and gp45. Hydrophobic regions in gp45 are shown as shaded boxes. Potential N-linked glycosylation sites are shown as boxes (15,16).

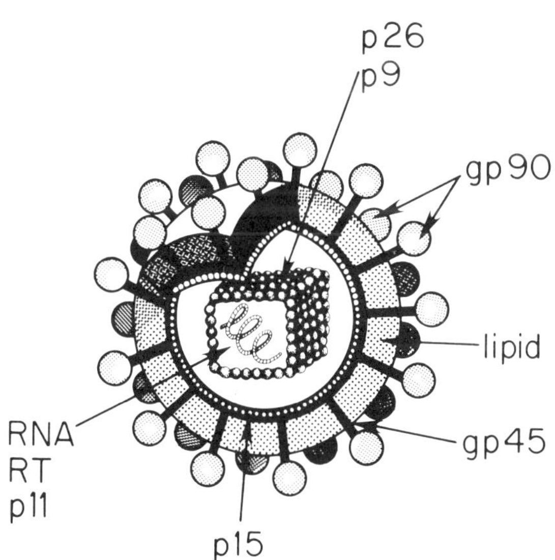

Figure 3 Structural model for the EIAV virion based on Refs. 3 and 4. RT - reverse transcriptase.

the virion. The envelope of the virus contains several hundred copies each of two distinct glycoproteins, gp90 and gp45. The gp90 component is highly glycosylated and is loosely associated with the virus particle; it can be efficiently retained if virus is purified on glycerol gradients, but is stipped from the virion if sucrose gradients are employed. In contrast, the gp45 is a slightly glycosylated and very hydrophobic protein which apparently spans the lipid bilayer of the viral envelope. EIAV gp90 and gp45 contain approximately equal numbers of amino acid residues; the apparent difference in molecular weight is attributable to the degree of glycosylation. The final envelope component is p15, a fatty acylated protein which forms a continuous matrix immediately beneath the lipid bilayer. There are approximately 3000 copies of p15 per virus particle, representing just enough protein to form a continuous monolayer beneath the lipid. The p15 component may be slightly phosphorylated (4).

The internal core of EIAV contains several thousand copies each of the other *gag* proteins (p26, p11, and p9). EIAV p26, the most abundant structural protein, is the primary constituent of the core shell and is the antigen employed in commercial diagnostic tests for virus-specific antibody in horses. The other core shell component appears to be the acidic protein p9. The p11 protein is highly basic and tightly associated with the RNA genome of the virus, along with 5-10 copies of reverse transcriptase, forming the ribonucleoprotein complex enclosed within the core shell.

The *gag* proteins of EIAV display significant sequence homologies with the corresponding proteins of HIV (15) and limited serologic cross-reactivities have been reported for the major core proteins of these viruses (HIV p24 and EIAV p26) (21,22). The *env* proteins of EIAV and HIV share remarkable similarities in structural features, but only very limited sequence homology (16,17). It has been reported that sera from EIAV-infected horses react strongly with HIV gp120 in radioimmunoprecipitation assays (23), however, this reactivity appears to be mediated by carbohydrate, rather than peptide, moieties of gp120 (24).

Protein Antigenicity

A variety of immunoassays indicate that the predominant antibody responses in EIAV-infected horses are directed against gp90 and gp45, with only minor antibody populations against the core proteins p26 and p 15 (5,25). The nature and kinetics of antigen-specific immune responses are discussed below. In this section, details of the molecular nature of these antigens are described.

The antigenic reactivity of EIAV gp90 has been analyzed, and the results indicate that the antibody contained in immune serum from persistently infected horses is directed predominantly against the peptide portions of gp90; only a minor antibody reactivity is detectable with the oligosaccharide components of the molecule (26). Moreover, the antibodies appear to be overwhelmingly specific for linear, rather than conformational epitopes, as the levels of antibody binding are not significantly affected by treatment of gp90 with detergents, salt, or reducing agents that modify protein conformation. In this regard, EIAV gp90 apparently differs from HIV gp120, whose reactivity with immune sera can be significantly influenced by the conformational state of the antigen.

A panel of monoclonal antibodies has been generated and used to identify the epitopes of the EIAV glycoproteins (10,27). The results of these studies reveal six antibody-binding sites (90A-F), which appear to define four gp90 epitopes designated 90A, 90B/F, 90C/D, and 90E). Two of these epitopes, C/D and E, are involved in virus neutralization by monoclonal antibodies. Two nonoverlapping and nonneutralizing epitopes (45A and 45B) are recognized by a limited panel of monoclonal antibodies specific for gp45. As observed with the antibodies contained in immune sera, the binding of monoclonal antibodies does not appear to depend significantly on protein conformation as binding efficiencies are not altered by changing detergent, salt, or reducing conditions. Competitive binding studies between the monoclonal antibodies and polyclonal immune sera from EIAV-infected horses demonstrate that the antigenic sites defined by the monoclonal antibodies are also recognized by equine antibodies produced during persistent infections. As noted below, however, it appears that the equine antibodies recognize additional sites on gp90 not identified by our panel of monoclonal antibodies.

To further localize the antibody-binding sites of gp90 and gp45, we have assayed the antigenicity of selected segments of EIAV glycoproteins expressed in *E. coli* using plasmids under the control of the *trp* operon (28). The *env* gene regions cloned and used for antigen production in *E. coli* are detailed in Figure 4, and the reactivity pattern of each recombinant antigen with the panel of monoclonal antibodies is summarized in Table 1. The results of these studies (summarized in Fig. 4, panel B) indicate that epitope 90A is localized to the amino terminal of gp90, while epitopes 90B, C, D, and F localize to the middle one third of the glycoprotein; epitope 90E has yet to be localized to a specific peptide region. These results then are in excellent agreement with the results of competitive ELISA assays that indicated a tight clustering of 90B, C, D, and F antibody-binding sites (27). One of the two identified gp45 epitopes, 45B, was localized to the amino terminal end of gp45 in a region bounded on either side by hydrophobic stretches of amino acid residues (Fig. 4, panel B); epitope 45A has not been localized yet. Thus, in agreement with the data cited above, the binding of antibodies to specific *E. coli* recombinant proteins indicates that epitopes 90A, 90B, 90C, 90D, 90F, and 45B represent continuous, carbohydrate-independent epitopes. Synthetic peptide methodologies are currently being used to refine further the localization of epitopes to specific amino acid sequences of EIAV glycoproteins.

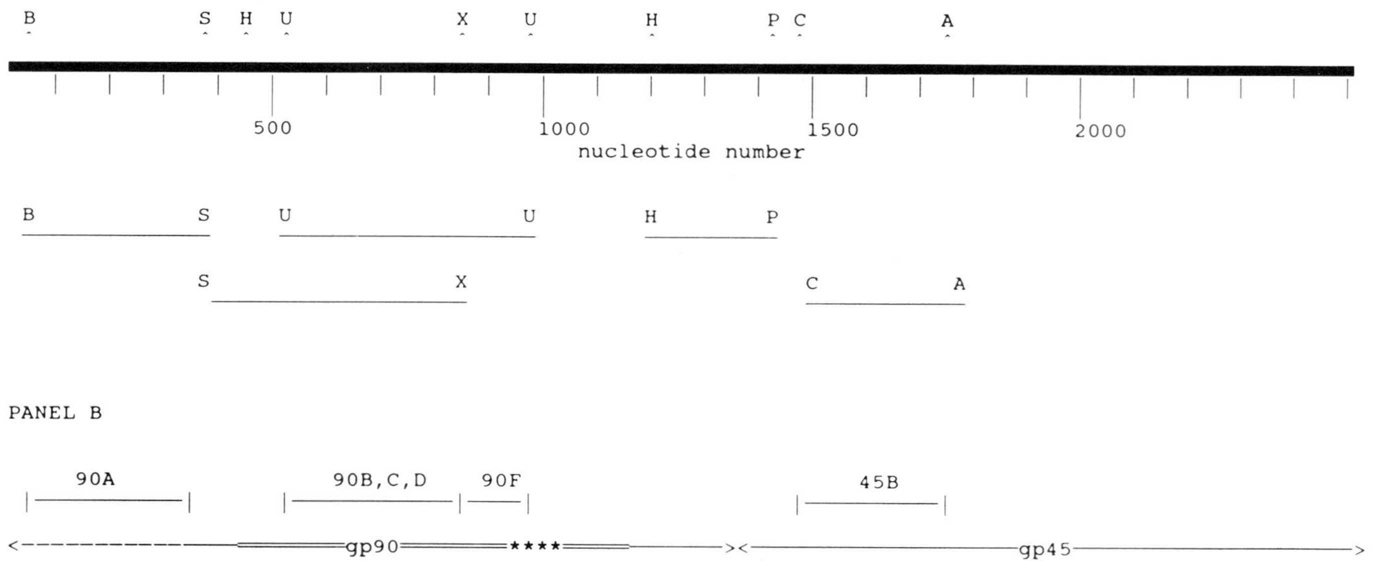

Figure 4 Panel A. Restriction enzyme map of the EIAV *env* gene showing DNA fragments cloned into *E. coli* expression vectors. A, AluI; B, BamHI; C, ScaI; H, HindIII; P, HpaI; U, Sau3A; X, XbaI. Panel B. Linear representation of the envelope glycoproteins gp90 and gp45 showing localization of epitopes based on the reactivity of a panel of monoclonal antibodies to expressed *env* gene fragments. The variable and hypervariable regions of gp90 (as predicted by DNA sequence analysis) are indicated by double lines and stars, respectively.

The recombinant peptide antigens described above were also assayed for reactivity against a panel of sera from horses naturally infected with unknown strains of EIAV and from ponies experimentally infected with prototype-derived EIAV strains (28). The representative data presented in Table 1 indicate that most of the glycoprotein expressions are reactive with at least some of the reference sera. Certain proteins e.g., the carboxy terminus of gp90 (HindIII-HpaI) and the gp45 Sca-Alu fragment, are recognized strongly by all test sera. The other proteins are recognized only by certain sera. These variations in range of reactivity appear to correlate with the "conserved" and "variable" glycoprotein regions previously deduced by comparative nucleic acid sequences of related EIAV isolates (9), as discussed below. The data also confirm that continuous, oligo-saccharide-independent peptide epitopes are immunogenic during persistent infections in horses, as well as in inoculated mice. However, the reactivity of the HindIII-HpaI fragment, representing the carboxy terminus of gp90, with all of the horse immune sera indicates an immunogenic region of this glycoprotein not defined by the existing panel of monoclonal antibodies.

Antigenic Variation

The unique periodic nature of chronic EIA can evidently be attributed to the sequential evolution of antigenic variants of EIAV that temporarily escape established humoral and cellular immune responses (Fig. 5). The initial evidence for EIAV antigenic variation is based on comparative neutralization assays employing virus isolates and immune sera recovered from chronically infected horses during various stages of disease. For example, Kono et al. (29) demonstrated over 15 years ago that, in general, sera from infected horses were capable of neutralizing virus isolated prior to the time of serum collection, but had no effect on the infectivity of virus isolates recovered at intervals after the serum time point. Ironically, this pioneering work by Kono, which first indicated a role of antigenic variation in retrovirus persistence, was widely accepted by veterinarians and largely unknown among retrovirologists! Although the actual role of neutralizing antibodies in controlling EIAV replication is questionable (see below), the role of antigenic variation in maintaining persistence appears to be well established. More recently a detailed characterization of EIAV antigenic variation has been made possible by the development of an animal model system in which Shetland ponies, inoculated with a standard strain of EIAV, reproducibly develop chronic EIA during which EIAV isolates can be efficiently recovered during sequential cycles of disease (21). A panel of over 20 of these virus isolates has been characterized by a variety of immunologic and biochemical procedures to ascertain the nature of antigenic variation in EIAV (5-10).

The major conclusions of this survey can be demonstrated by examining the properties of a panel of 13 virus isolates recovered during febrile episodes in

Table 1 Reactivity of Monoclonal Antibodies and Horse Immune Sera to Expressed Regions of EIAV gp90 and gp45 in Western Blot Assays

mAb/epitope	Antigen[a]						
	gp90	gp45	Bam/Sma	Sma/Xba	Sau3A	Hind/Hpa	Sca/Alu
86 90A	+[b]	–	+	–	–	–	–
87 90B	+	–	–	+	+	–	–
98 90C	+	–	–	+	+	–	–
115 90D	+	–	–	+	+	–	–
128 90E	–	–	–	–	–	–	–
71 90F	+	–	–	–	+	–	–
105 45A	–	+	–	–	–	–	–
90 45B	–	+	–	–	–	–	+

Animal	Nature of infection							
82	E[c]	+	+	−	+	+	+	+
96	E	+	+	−	+	+	+	+
127	E	+	+	+	+	+	+	+
727	E	+	+	(+)	(+)	+	+	+
6	N	+	+	−	−	+	+	+
7	N	+	+	−	−	+	+	+
8	N	+	+	−	−	−	+	+
10	N	+	+	−	−	−	+	+
11	N	+	+	−	−	−	+	+
12	N	+	+	−	+	(+)	+	+
13	N	+	+	−	−	−	+	+
14	N	+	+	−	−	−	+	+
15	N	+	+	+	(+)	−	+	+
16	N	+	+	−	−	−	+	+
17	N	(+)	−	−	−	−	+	+
19	N	+	+	−	−	−	+	+
20	N	+	+	−	−	−	+	+

[a]Antigens tested are HPLC-purifed gp90 and gp45 and various recombinant peptide expression depicted in Figure 3.

[b]+, (+), and − designate positive, weak positive, and negative results, respectively in Western blot analyses.

[c]E = experimental infection with prototype virus or strains derived by backpassage of prototype virus; N = natural infection with unknown strains of EIAV. All test sera were shown to be positive in the standard reference immunoassay employing agar gel immunodiffusion procedures (37).

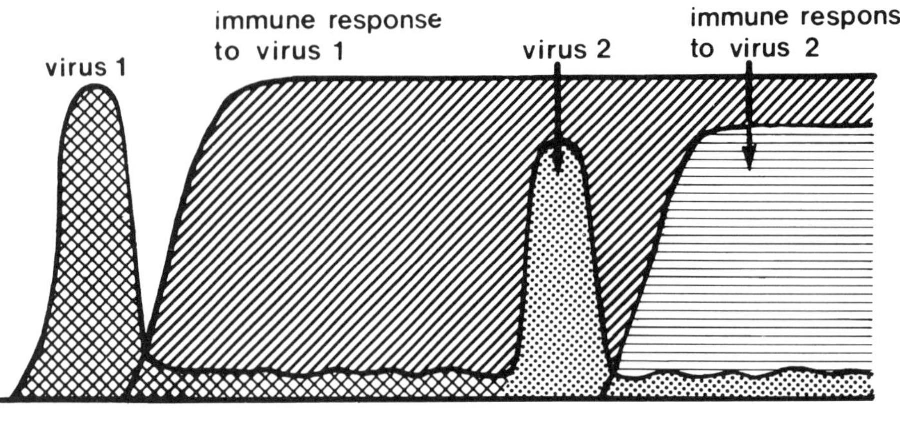

Figure 5 Model for the recurrent episodes of EIA during the chronic stage of disease. The infecting virus replicates in the horse producing a viremia and associated clinical signs of EIA. This viremia is brought under control by immune responses from the infected animal, and clinical manifestations of the disease disappear. However, mutations occurring during the replication of the infecting virus produce novel antigenic stains of virus which are able to circumvent host immune responses, resulting in a subsequent viremia and recurrence of disease. This process can repeat itself.

three experimentally infected ponies (Table 2). Each virus isolate was initially examined in homologous neutralization assays using serum samples collected during sequential afebrile periods in the respective infected ponies. The results of these assays reveal several important properties of persistent EIAV infections. First, within each group of virus isolates from a single pony it can be demonstrated that each virus isolate can only be inactivated by serum samples taken *after* the clinical episode of origin; none of the virus isolates can be neutralized by serum samples taken *prior* to the disease cycle of origin. Second, cross-neutralization assays indicate that each virus isolate is antigenically distinct, although an occasional low level of cross-reactivity can be detected in the neutralization assays. The antigenic uniqueness of most isolates can also be demonstrated by assaying the reactivity of each virus isolate in Western blots using a panel of monoclonal antibodies specific for gp90 and gp 45, respectively (Table 2). These binding data demonstrate variation at individual eptiopes defined by the panel of monoclonal antibodies based on binding assays. However it should also be noted that variation of EIAV can result in altered glycoprotein structures that continue to bind a neutralizing monoclonal antibody, but which are no longer neutralized as a result of antibody binding (10). Thus, structural variations may also result in changes in function, without complete abrogation of the antibody binding properties of the glycoprotein.

These antigenic analyses indicate that a distinct antigenic variant is associated with each febrile episode in an experimentally infected animal and that the evolution of a new predominant strain of virus can take as little as 2 weeks or as long as several months. There is no detectable common pattern of variant evolution in the parallel infections in different ponies. Thus, EIAV antigenic variation differs from that observed in visna virus (30,31), in that the former is evidently more rapid and more random.

The biochemical nature of antigenic variation among the panel of EIAV isolates has been examined by peptide and glycopeptide mapping procedures to compare viral proteins and by oligonucleotide fingerprint analysis to compare genomic RNA (5-10). The peptide/glycopeptide variations are specific for the viral envelope glycoproteins (gp90 and gp45); no structural alterations are observed among the internal viral proteins of the respective virus isolates. The combination of peptide and glycopeptide mapping indicates that each of the 13

Table 2 Properties of 13 Virus Isolates Recovered During Febrile Episodes in Three Experimentally Infected Ponies

EIAV isolates	Isolation day postinoculation	Epitopes gp90	gp45
Pony 91			
P3.1–1	12	ABCD	A
P3.1–2	32	ABCDE	A
P3.1–3	58	ABF	A
P3.1–4	198	AE	A
Pony 127			
P3.2–1	13	AD	AB
P3.2–2	41	ABCD	AB
P3.2–3	99	ABCDF	AB
P3.2–4	137	AE	AB
P3.2–5	158	AE	AB
Pony 135			
P3.3–1	16	ACD	A
P3.3–2	46	ABCDF	AB
P3.3–3	75	ABCDF	AB
P3.3–4	107	A	AB

virus isolates contain structurally unique gp90 and gp45 components, as no two maps were identical in pairwise comparisons. Moreover, analysis of the variant peptides detected among sequential virus isolates from each pony reveals that peptide alterations appearing in one isolate are not necessarily retained in the next or successive variants in that pony. Similarly, the oligonucleotide fingerprints differentiate among all of the virus isolates and once again demonstrate a noncumulative pattern of variation among sequential isolates. Pairwise comparisons of oligonucleotide fingerprints typically identify three to four variant oligonucleotides out of a total of over 50 oligonucleotides resolved for each genomic RNA. The degree of protein and genomic variation detected by these procedures suggests that the antigenic variation observed in EIAV is the result of random point mutations in the viral RNA, some of which result in altered glycoprotein amino acid sequences. Alterations in peptide maps and oligonucleotide fingerprints have not been detected during passage of the virus isolates in tissue culture, indicating the importance of immune selection in generating variants in horses. In these aspects, EIAV antigenic variation closely resembles variation in visna virus (30,31). However, the apparently noncumulative and completely random nature of EIAV variation is in marked contrast to the cumulative, common patterns of variation described for visna virus.

To directly relate the observed antigenic and structural variations to nucleotide sequence variation in EIAV, the *env* gene sequences of four virus isolates obtained from pony 91 were determined and compared (9). Figure 6 schematically depicts the patterns of sequence variation observed in the *env* genes of these isolates. All but one difference in nucleotide sequence among the four virus isolates resulted from single base substitutions; a single three-base insertion was observed in isolate P3.2-5. Overall, the nucleotide divergence between any pair of virus isolates ranges from 16 to 37 bases of a total fo 2583 bases in the *env* gene. Approximately 75% of all nucleotide substitutions result in amino acid replacements, and amino acid divergence ranges from 11 to 29 residues out of 860 total. In light of the extent of variation observed in peptide mapping, the relatively low level of nucleotide (0.6-1.4%) and amino acid (1.3-3.4%) divergence is somewhat surprising. However, the majority of all amino acid substitutions are nonconservative, predicting probable changes in structural and antigenic properties.

Variation is not evenly distributed throughout the *env* gene. Two to three times more amino acid substitutions occur in the exterior gp90 compared to the transmembrane gp45. Further, within gp90 two conserved and one hypervariable region can be identified. The first conserved region within gp90 includes the N-terminal 21 amino acid leader peptide and the following 110 amino acids, while the second conserved region encompasses amino acid residues 370 to 445. In these regions, there are few substitutions, and all potential N-linked glycosylation sites and cysteine residues are absolutely conserved among the four isolates. In contrast, a variable region of gp90 spans amino acid residues 143 to 366, in

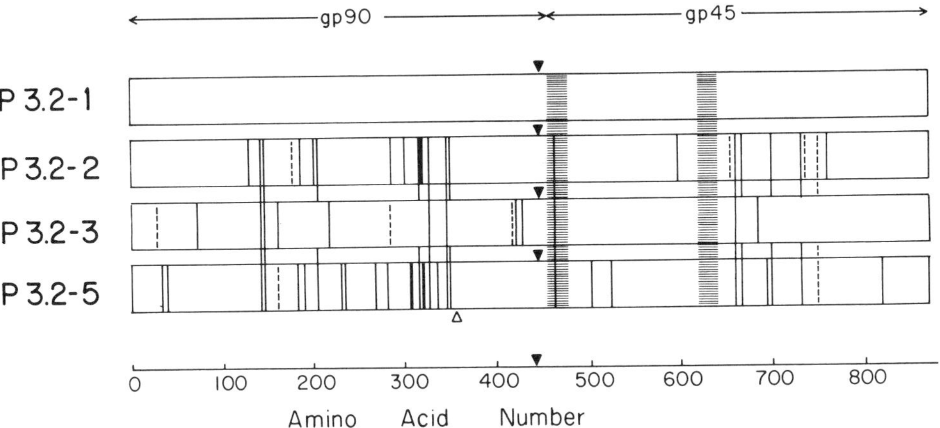

Figure 6 Schematic comparison of *env* gene sequences of four EIAV isolates, recovered during sequential febrile episodes from an experimentally infected pony (Pony 91). Nucleotide sequences for isolates P3.2-2, P3.2-3, and P3.2-5 are compared with the sequence for P3.2-1. Base substitutions not resulting in amino acid changes are indicated by dashed lines, while changes resulting in amino acid changes are represented by solid lines. Continuous lines represent nucleotide changes common to two or more virus isolates. The open triangle represents a three-base insertion in isolate P3.2-5. Th solid triangles represent the proposed precursor cleavage site. Shaded areas represent hydrophobic regions within gp45.

which pairs of virus isolates differ by 3 to 9% in amino acid sequences. A hypervariable region of 35 amino acids (residues 306-338) is located within the gp90 variable region. Within this hypervariable region, amino acid divergence between any two isolates ranges from 3 to 20%. EIAV gp90 is highly glycosylated and contains numerous potential N-linked glycosylation sites (N-X-S/T) within the variable region of the protein. Since about 40% of all amino acid substitutions in the *env* gene involve the loss or gain of an asparagine residue, it is perhaps not surprising that the number of potential glycosylation sites within the variable region of gp90 range from 6 to 10 in the different virus isolates.

In contrast to gp90, EIAV gp45 is more highly conserved among the four virus isolates, with amino acid substitutions between isolate pairs ranging from 0.7 to 2% (3-9/415 residues). Within gp45, the amino terminal half is more highly conserved than the carboxyl terminal half of the molecule, including two hydrophobic (putative transmembrane) regions (residues 448-473 and 617-636) and four N-linked glycosylation sites that are conserved among all isolates.

The sequence data also permits an estimation of the mutation rate of the EIAV *env* gene during persistent infection. This calculation uses the formula $R = D/2T$ (32), where R is the number of nucleotide substitutions per site per year, D is the divergence calculated from the proportion of nucleotide differences between pairs of isolates, and T is the divergence time represented here as the time between the isolation of the first isolate (P3.2-1) and the later isolates. Using these parameters, mutation rates of 1×10^{-1}, 2×10^{-2}, and 1×10^{-2} were obtained for isolates P3.2-2, P3.2-3, and P3.2-5, respectively. These mutation rates are about 10-fold higher than those reported for HIV (33) and 1000-fold greater than observed for other RNA viruses (34).

A final approach to both defining EIAV glycoprotein epitopes and the effect of amino acid sequence variations on antigenicity potential has been to analyze variant gp90 and gp45 sequences by computer algorithms for predicting B-cell epitopes (35). The computer analysis (36) considers hydrophilicity, flexibility, and accessibility in obtaining a final probability value for being a B-cell epitope. A representative analysis is presented in Figure 7 for the gp90 components of the four EIAV variants discussed above (see Fig. 6). The profiles indicate a number of potential B-cell epitopes (values above 50%) across the gp90 sequences. The predicted epitopes in the amino and carboxy terminal thirds of the gp90 molecule are conserved among the four EIAV variants. In contrast, predicted epitopes in the middle one-third of the gp90 molecule differ significantly in their potential values (shaded areas of Fig. 7). For example, isolates P3.2-2 and P3.2-5 contain a predicted eptiope around residue 330 that is essentially absent in the other two isolates. Similarly isolate P3.2-3 basically lacks the epitope predicted for the other three isolates around residue 200. Although the correlation of computer-predicted epitopes with those defined by monoclonal antibodies is not yet feasible, it is interesting to note that the computer-predicted "conserved and variable" regions of gp90 correspond to those deduced from gene sequence data and from the serologic reactivity of expressed segments of gp90 discussed above. Thus, it may be possible as the database is enlarged sufficiently to predict the presence or absence of particular epitopes on any variant gp90 based on deduced amino acid sequences from determined nucleotide sequences. Such an analysis would assist greatly in providing a proper perspective on the relationship between amino acid sequence variations and antigenic properties.

IMMUNE RESPONSES DURING INFECTION BY EIAV

Practical and specific diagnostic tests for EIAV-infected horses have been available since 1970, making this the first retrovirus diagnostic to be commercially available and to gain widespread usage among veterinarians (37). It was also recognized by veterinarians in the late 1960s and early 1970s that immune responses to EIAV may play a role in pathogenesis. In particular, it appears that the characteristic anemia caused by EIAV is actually the result of lysis or phagocytosis of EIAV-coated erythrocytes mediated by virus-specific antibodies produced by the horse; there does not appear to be any direct immunosuppression

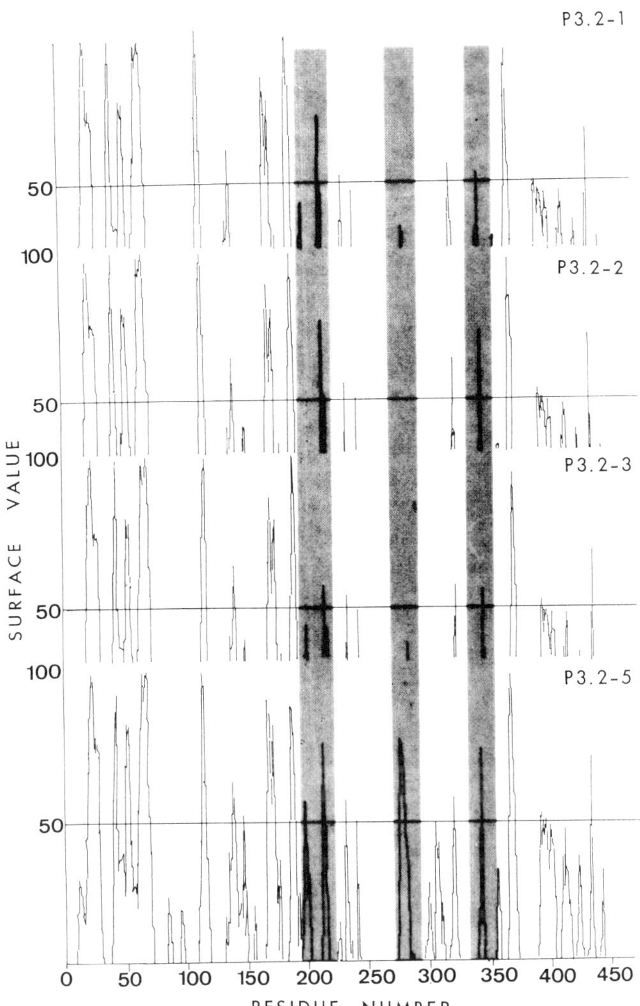

Figure 7 Comparison of computer-predicted epitopes from four EIAV variants recovered from sequential febrile episodes from pony 91. Values were derived from amino acid sequences using the programs of Parker et al. (36). These programs predict B-cell epitopes based on a combination of hydrophilicity, accessibility, and flexibility. Surface values above 50% represent potential epitopes. Shaded areas highlight changes in predicted epitopes that occur within the variable region of gp90.

by EIAV. Another early observation was that infected horses during their viremic stages frequently contain antibody-coated EIAV that remains infectious (38). Taken together, the initial deduction was that immune responses to EIAV were at best not beneficial and, most likely, actually harmful! Only recently has it been recognized that the eventual management of EIAV replication by immune responses in persistently infected horses represents a uniquely successful system in controlling retrovirus replication in general and lentivirus replication in particular.

Thus, a major focus of our current research effort is to define the kinetics and specificities of immune responses produced against the series of EIAV variants evolved during the chronic stage of disease induced by experimental infections of Shetland ponies with our standard virus inoculum. In these experimentally infected animals, the first clinical episode is typically detected 15–20 days postinfection (2), and viremia levels usually peak coincident with the first febrile episode. Analyses of humoral immune responses in experimentally infected animals (39) indicate that antibodies to the p26 antigen and to apparently group-specific determinants of gp90 are first detectable within several days following the first clinical episode. It is interesting to note that these early group-specific gp90 antibodies bind to the gp90 components of a wide variety of EIAV strains assayed in immunoblot procedures. However, these early gp90-specific antibodies typically fail to neutralize even the homologous EIAV strain, i.e., the virus predominating during the first viremia. Thus, it appears that neutralizing antibodies, at least as defined by our current in vitro assays, do not play a significant role in the cessation of the initial viremia. Instead, neutralizing antibodies to EIAV are detected later in infection, are type specific, and appear coincident with detectable levels of gp45 specific antibody. Following a second clinical episode, type-specific neutralizing antibodies are detected more rapidly than observed following the first febrile episode.

In general, the range of serum neutralization increases with each subsequent febrile episode, although the general antibody titer (as measured in ELISA) remains unchanged. Even animals that manifest only a single disease episode display more broadly neutralizing antibodies several months after infection compared to earlier time points.

Taken together, these initial studies suggest a "maturation" of EIAV-specific immune responses as the infected horse is exposed to a series of variant virus strains. In most infected horses, the sequential appearance of EIAV variants and the evolution of neutralizing antibody response are demarcated by the cyclic disease episodes characteristic of chronic EIA. In certain animals, however, the neutralizing antibody response broadens in the absence of apparent recurrent disease episodes, perhaps resulting from long-term exposure to low levels of virus replication.

Neutralizing antibodies are undoubtedly but a narrow window to view the myriad of immune responses generated in response to EIAV infection. Several nonneutralizing epitopes, recognized by mice and horses, have been identified on the EIAV gp90 and gp45 (10). In addition, lymphocytes from EIAV-infected horses can be stimulated in vitro with EIAV antigens (37). Thus, nonneutralizing humoral and cell mediated immune responses must also be examined in the immunologic management of EIAV infections.

However, with the EIAV experimental infection system, the availability of relatively large quantities of viral proteins, the elucidation of glycoprotein epitopes, and the synthesis of peptides constituting specific epitopes, it should be feasible to dissect the critical immune responses generated in response to persistent EIAV infection. For example, the kinetics of immune responses specific for particular glycoprotein epitopes can be monitored. In this manner, immunodominant and immunorecessive determinants can be assigned and, perhaps, the immune status capable of controlling virus replication identified. It is this final immune status that is clearly the beginning goal to be achieved by any candidate vaccine.

EIAV AS A VACCINE MODEL

EIAV offers a number of advantages as a model for testing different approaches to developing an effective lentivirus vaccine. Large quantities of virus and purified viral antigens and *env* gene clones for antigen expression are available from a number of well-characterized EIAV strains. The experimental infection system is highly reproducible and results in disease within 2-3 weeks, thus providing a rapid challenge to determine the efficacy of any immunization protocol. Moreover, virus challenges can be mediated using horse fly transfers of blood, thus ensuring a biologically significant level of infecting virus.

Kono and his colleagues (40) demonstrated in 1970 that immunization of horses with inactivated preparations of purified EIAV provided protection against infection by homologous, but not heterologous, strains of EIAV. However, there were no subsequent experiments to determine if a more rigorous immunization protocol, i.e., multiple inoculations, might provide protection against heterologous virus challenge. Experiments using serial immunizations with murine leukemia virus gp70 indicate the sequental appearance of type, group, and interspecies specific antibody. Thus, it may be that protective immune responses against a variety of EIAV strains can be obtained after repeated inoculations with inactivated virus preparations or subunit vaccines prepared from viral proteins or synthetic peptides. These experiments, which are currently in progress, should provide important information on approaches to producing an effective lentiviral vaccine.

REFERENCES

1. Vallee H, Carre H. Sur la natur infectieuse de l'anemie du cheval. CR Acad Sci 1904; 139:331-3.
2. Orrego A, Issel CJ, Montelaro RC, Adams WV, Jr. Virulence and in vitro gorwth of a cell-adapted strain of equine infectious anemia virus after serial passage in ponies. Am J Vet Res 1982; 43:1556-60.
3. Parekh B, Issel CJ, Montelaro RC. Equine infectious anemia virus, a putative lentivirus, contains polypeptides analogous to prototype-C oncornaviruses. Virology 1980; 107:520-5.
4. Montelaro RC, Lohrey N, Parekh B, Blakeney EW, Issel CJ. Isolation and comparative biochemical properties of the major internal polypeptides of equine infectious anemia virus. J Virol 1982; 42:1029-38.
5. Montelaro RC, Parekh B, Orrego A, Issel CJ. Antigenic variation during persistent infection by equine infectious anemia virus, a retrovirus. J Biol Chem 1984; 259:10539-44.
6. Payne S, Parekh B, Montelaro RC, Issel CJ. Genomic alterations associated with persistent infections by equine infectious anemia virus, a retrovirus. J Gen Virol 1984; 65:1395-9.
7. Salinovich O, Payne SL, Montelaro RC, Hussain KA, Issel CJ, Schnorr KL. Rapid emergence of novel antigenic and genetic variants of equine infectious anemia virus during persistent infection. J Virol 1986; 57:71-80.
8. Payne SL, Salinovich O, Montelaro RC, Issel CJ, Nauman SM. Course and extent of variation of equine infectious anemia virus during parallel persistent infections. J Virol 1987; 61:1266-70.
9. Payne SL, Fang FD, Lui CP, Dhruva B, Rwambo P, Issel CJ, Montelaro RC. Antigentic variation and lentivirus persistence: Variations in envelope gene sequences during EIAV infection resemble changes reported for sequential isolates of HIV. Virology 1987; 161:321-31.
10. Hussain KA, Issel CJ, Schnorr KL, Montelaro RC. Antigenic analysis of equine infectious anemia virus (EIAV) variants using monoclonal antibodies: Epitopes of glycoprotein 90 (gp90) of EIAV stimulate neutralizing antibodies. J Virol 1987; 61:2956-61.
11. Foil LD, Meek L, Adams WV, Issel CJ. Mechanical transmission of equine infectious anemia virus by deer flies (*Chrysops flavidus*) and stable flies (*Stomoxys calcitrans*). Am J Vet Res 1983; 44:155-6.
12. Issel CJ, Foil LD. Studies on equine infectious anemia virus transmission by insects. J Am Vet Med Assoc 1984; 184:293-7.
13. Foil LD, Adams WV, McManus JM, Issel CJ. Bloodmeal residues on mouthparts of *Tabanus fusicostatus* (Diptera: Tabanidae) and the potential for the mechanical transmission of pathogens. J Med Entomol 1987; 24:613-6.
14. Kono Y, Hirasawa K, Fukunaga Y, Taniguchi T. Recrudescence of EIA by treatment with immunosuppressive drugs. Ntl Inst Anim Health Q (Tokyo) 1976; 16:8-15.
15. Stephens RM, Casey JW, Rice NR. Equine infectious anemia virus *gag* and *pol* genes: Relatedness to visna and AIDS virus. Science 1986; 213:589-94.

16. Rushlow K, Olson K, Stiegler G, Payne SL, Montelaro RC, Issel CJ. Lentivirus genomic organization: The complete nucleotide sequence of the *env* gene region of equine infectious anemia virus. Virol 1986; 155:309-21.

17. Kawakami T, Sherman L, Dahlberg J, Gazit A, Yaniv A, Tronick S, Aaronson SA. Nucleotide sequence analysis of equine infectious anemia virus proviral DNA. Virol 1987; 158:300-12.

18. Derse D, Dorn PL, Levy L, Stephens RM, Rice NR, Casey JW. Characterization of equine infectious anemia virus long terminal repeat. J Virol 1987; 61:743-7.

19. Sherman L, Gazit A, Yaniv A, Kawakami T, Dahlberg JE, Tronick SR. Localization of sequences responsible for trans-activation of the equine infectious anemia virus long terminal repeat. J Virol 1988; 62:120-6.

20. Ball JM, Rao VSV, Robey WG, Issel CJ, Montelaro RC. Lentivirus antigen purification and characterization: Isolation of equine infectious anemia virus *gag* and *env* proteins in one step by reverse phase HPLC and application to human immunodeficiency virus glycoproteins. J Virol Meth, 1988; 19:265-77.

21. Montagnier L, Dauguet C, Axler C, Chamaret S, Gruest J, Nugeyre MT, Rey F, Barré-Sinousi F, Chermann JC. A new type of retrovirus isolated from patients presenting with lymphadenopathy and acquired immune deficiency syndrome: Structural and antigenic relatedness with EIA virus. Ann Virol (Inst Pasteur) 1984; 135E:119-34.

22. Goudsmit J, Houwers DJ, Smit L, Nauta IM. LAV/HTLV-III *gag* gene product p24 shares antigenic determinants with equine infectious anaemia virus but not with visna virus or caprine arthritis encephalitis virus. Intervirology 1986; 26:169-73.

23. Schneider J, Kaaden O, Copeland T, Oroszlan S, Hunsmann G. Shedding and interspecies type sero-reactivity of the envelope glycopeptide gp120 of human immunodeficiency virus. J Gen Virol 1986; 67:2533-8.

24. Montelaro RC, Robey WG, West MD, Issel CJ, Fischinger PJ. Characterization of the serological cross reactivity between glycoproteins of human immunodeficiency virus and equine infectious anaemia virus. J Gen Virol 1988; 69:1711-7.

25. Shane BS, Issel CJ, Montelaro RC. Enzyme linked immunosorbent assay for detection of equine infectious anemia virus p26 antigen and antibody. J Clin Micro 1984; 19:351-5.

26. Montelaro RC, West MD, Issel CJ. Antigenic reactivity of the major glycoprotein of equine infectious anemia virus, a retrovirus. Virol 1984; 136: 368-74.

27. Hussain KA, Issel CJ, Schnorr KL, West MD, Rwambo P, Montelaro RC. Epitope mapping of the envelope proteins of EIAV. Arch Virol 1988; 98: 213-24.

28. Payne SL, Rushlow K, Dhruva B, Issel CJ, Montelaro RC. Localization of conserved and variable antigenic domains of equine infectious anemia virus envelope glycoproteins using recombinant *env*-encoded protein fragments produced in *E. coli*. Virol 1989; 172:609-15.

29. Kono Y, Kobayasi K, Fukunaga Y. Antigenic drift of equine infectious anemia virus in chronically infected horses. Arch Virol 1973; 41:1-10.
30. Narayan O, Griffin DE, Chase J. Antigenic shift of visna virus in persistently infected sheep. Science 1977; 197:376-8.
31. Narayan O, Griffin DE, Clements JE. Virus mutation during "slow infection." Temporal development and characterization of mutants of visna virus recovered from sheep. J Gen Virol 1978; 41:343-52.
32. Gojobori T, Yokoyama S. Rates of evolution of the retroviral oncogene of Moloney murine sarcoma virus and of its cellular homologues. Proc Natl Acad Sci USA 1985; 82:4198-201.
33. Hahn B, Shaw G, Taylor M, Redfield R, Markham P, Salahuddin S, Wong-Staal F, Gallo R, Parks E, Parks W. Genetic variation in HTLV-III/LAV over time in patients with AIDS or risk for AIDS. Science 1986; 232: 1548-53.
34. Holland J, Spindler F, Horodyski E, Grabau E, Nichol S, Van DePol S. Rapid evolution of RNA genomes. Science 1982; 215:1577-85.
35. Ball JM, Payne SL, Zimmer EA, Issel CJ, Montelaro RC. Computer analysis of *env* variants of EIAV: Relationship to observed antigenicity and modelled lentivirus evolution. Submitted.
36. Parker J, Guo D, Hodges R. New hydrophobicity scale derived from high-performance liquid chromatography peptide retention data: Correlation of predicted surface residues with antigenicity and X-ray derived accessible sites. Biochemistry 1986; 24:5425.
37. Issel CJ, Coggins L. Equine infectious anemia: Current knowledge. J Am Vet Med Assoc 1979; 174:727-33.
38. McGuire T, Crawford T, Henson J. EIA: Detection of infectious virus-antibody complexes in the serum. Immunol Commun 1972; 1:545-51.
39. Rwambo PM, Issel CJ, Adams WV, Hussain KA, Miller M, Montelaro RC. Equine infectious anemia virus (EIAV): Humoral responses of recepient ponies and antigenic variation during persistent infection. Arch Virol, 1990; in press.
40. Kono Y, Kobayashi K, Fukunaga Y. Immunization of horses against equine infectious anemia (EIA) with an attenuated EIA virus. Natl Inst Anim Health Q (Tokyo) 1970; 10:113-22.

14

Induction of Protective Immunity Against an Immunosuppressive Mouse Retrovirus
Possible Parallels with HIV

Bruce Chesebro
Rocky Mountain Laboratory
National Institute of Allergy and Infectious Diseases
National Institutes of Health
Hamilton, Montana

Due to the recognition of human retrovirus-induced diseases such as acquired immunodeficiency syndrome (AIDS) and certain forms of leukemia, production of a vaccine for protection against retroviruses is currently of great interest. In several animal retrovirus systems protective immunity has been induced using live or killed virus or virus-infected cells, or purified viral envelope protein (1-10). However, in other models such immunizations have either been ineffective or have induced immunosuppression or enhanced disease (1,11-14). It is unclear at this time what parameters determine the success or failure of induction of protective immunity in these various retrovirus models. Failure to induce protection could be due to heterogeneity of virus populations, variability of the host in mounting an immune response due to age or genetic differences, or to variability in the regulation of expression of viral proteins or infectivity in different retroviruses perhaps resulting in a latent state not detectable by immune defenses. Similar problems and difficulties might occur during attempts to induce protective immunity against the human immunodeficiency virus (HIV); however, as yet no definitive facts are available to say whether this will be the case.

In order to avoid the problems of both virus and host genetic variability in studying mechanisms of protective immunity against retrovirus-induced diseases, it would be highly desirable to use a model involving homogeneous cloned viruses and inbred animals. The Friend murine leukemia retrovirus complex (FV) is relevant in this regard, because it induces disease in inbred strains of adult immunocompetent mice (15,16), and both components of the virus complex, the helper virus, Friend murine leukemia virus (F-MuLV), and a defective spleen focus-forming virus (SFFV), have been molecularly cloned (17-19). The disease induced by FV is a rapidly appearing erythroleukemia involving spleen, bone marrow, liver, and blood. Early cells of erythroid lineage are believed to be the primary targets of viral transformation. FV complex is also known to cause a variety immunosuppressive effects in mice including defects in B-cell, T-cell, and macrophage functions (20-25). In infected mice T cells have been shown to be unable to provide helper functions required for switching of antibody class from IgM to IgG antibody production (26). In spite of these immunosuppressive phenomena, certain mouse strains have been shown to produce a strong antiviral neutralizing antibody response during the course of progressive disease. These humoral antibodies cause a dramatic decrease in viremia and in the amount of virus released by cells in leukemic organs such as spleen (27-30). However, such antibodies alone appear to be unable to eliminate leukemic spleen cells, and mice lacking virus-specific cytolytic T cells usually die within 1 to 3 months of infection. The paradoxical occurrence of a neutralizing antiviral antibody response in the face of virus-induced immunosuppression to nonviral exogenous antigens is surprising. However, this situation appears to be quite similar to that occurring in most human AIDS patients who have serum-neutralizing antibody to HIV but are, nevertheless, severely immunosuppressed to other antigens in their environment. Thus, the Friend virus mouse model may be an interesting system in which to study problems of development of protective immunity which might have eventual relevance to HIV in humans.

PROTECTIVE IMMUNITY AGAINST CHALLENGE WITH CELL-FREE FRIEND VIRUS AND LIVE ALLOGENEIC VIRUS-INFECTED CELLS

Friend virus maintains a chronic persistent infection of many cell types in vivo. Thus, effective protective immunity should be capable of recognizing and elminating both cell-free virions and infected cells. Since viral envelope protein is expressed in external surfaces of both virions and infected cells, this protein might be an effective immunogen. However, many infected cells also express viral core polyprotein on the plasma membrane, and some studies suggest that this protein may also be good target antigen for virus-specific cytotoxic T lymphocytes (CTL) (31). Therefore, we decided to study three different immunogens, two expressing both core and envelope and one expressing envelope only (32). These were formalin-killed F-MuLV helper virus, live N-tropic Friend virus complex (FV-N), which grows as an attenuated or poorly replicating virus in the mice used, and lastly, a recombinant vaccinia virus capable of expressing the F–MuLV envelope protein (vaccinia-F–MuLV env). Control mice were either unimmunized or were immunized with vaccinia virus expressing influenza hemagglutinin (vaccinia-inf HA). Following challenge with cell-free Friend virus, mice of both H-2$^{a/b}$ and H-2$^{a/a}$ genotypes were protected by FV–N and fixed F–MuLV in complete Freund's adjuvant (CFA) (Fig. 1). In contrast, only H-2$^{a/b}$ mice were protected by vaccinia-F–MuLV env. Control mice in both strains were unprotected. Since retroviral diseases may be more efficiently transmitted by transfer of infected cells than by cell-free virus, we also tested our immunization

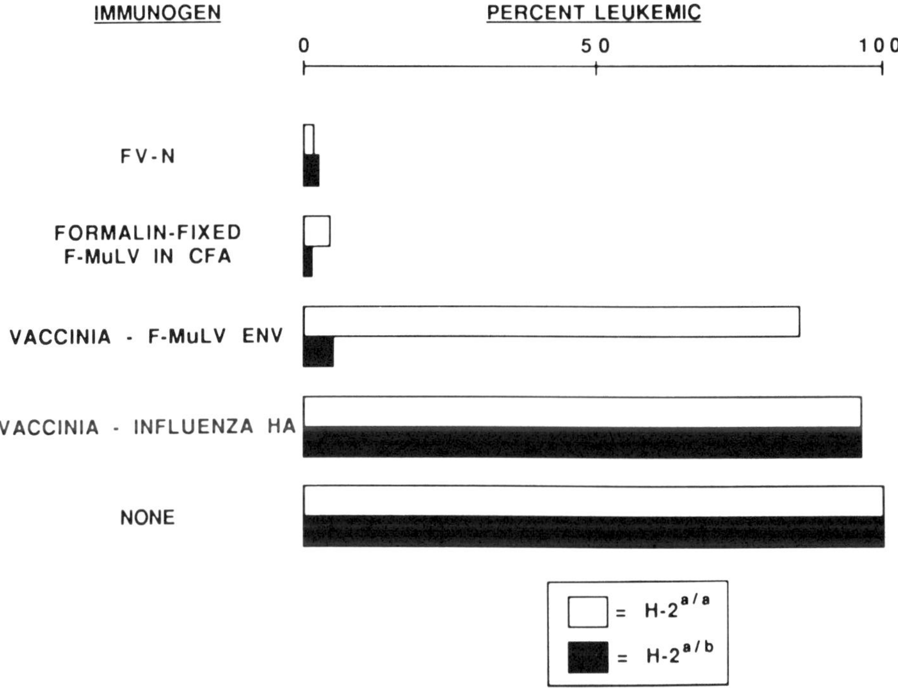

Figure 1 Protective immunization against leukemia induced by challenge with live FV. Mice: (B10.A × A/WySn)F$_1$, H-2$^{a/a}$; (B10.A × A.BY)F$_1$, H-2$^{a/b}$. Immunogens: live FV–N (N-tropic FV) 5 × 10^3 SFFU, intravenously; 44 μg formalin-fixed F–MuLV in complete Freund's adjuvant, in the foot pads; 10^7 PFU vaccinia-F–MuLV env, in a tail scratch; 10^7 PFU vaccinia-influenza HA, in a tail scratch. Twenty-six days after a single immunization, mice were challenged intravenously with B-tropic FV, 2 × 10^4 SFFU for H-2$^{a/b}$ mice and 2 × 10^3 SFFU for H-2$^{a/a}$ mice. Data are cumulative results at 14 weeks after challenge. Each group contained 18–51 mice. (Data adpated from Ref. 32.)

protocol using a challenge with live allogeneic virus-releasing leukemia cells. In these experiments protection was identical to that observed when cell-free Friend virus was used as the challenge (Fig. 2).

Mice of differing H-2 types were selected for this study because of the known strong influence of the H-2 major histocompatibility complex on Friend virus–induced leukemia in mice (33). The above results indicated that, whereas H-2 type appeared to have no influence on immunization with live attenuated FV–N or killed F–MuLV virions, H-2 played an important role in influencing induction of protective immunity by vaccinia-F–MuLV env. In order to test whether this H-2 influence was due to inability of H-2$^{a/a}$ mice to respond to all recombinant vaccinia viruses, we tested both H-2$^{a/b}$ and H-2$^{a/a}$ mice by immunization with

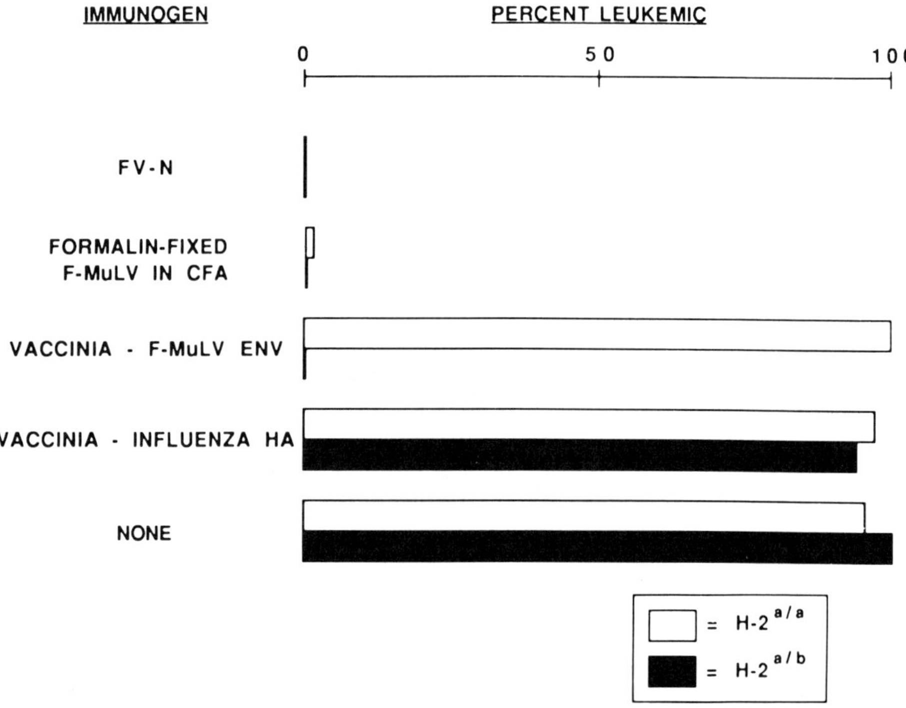

Figure 2 Protective immunization against leukemia induced by challenge with live allogeneic FV-releasing leukemia cells. Mice and immunizations were described in Figure 1. Twenty-one days after immunization mice were challenged with 2.5 X 10^7 BALB.K-fv-1, H-2^k leukemia cells. Groups had 17–20 mice each. Results shown were compiled at 20 weeks after challenge. (Data adapted from Ref. 34.)

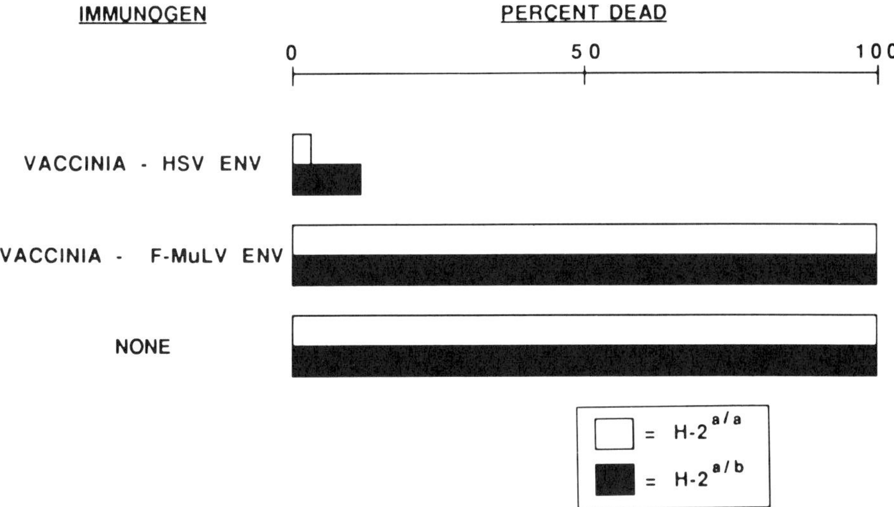

Figure 3 Protective immunization against herpes simplex virus (HSV-2). Mice and immunizations were described in Figure 1. In addition one group was immunized with vaccinia expressing HSV envelope. Twenty-four days after immunization, mice were challenged intraperitoneally with 5×10^7 PFU of HSV-2. Results shown were from 21 days after challenge. (Data adapted from Ref. 34.)

recombinant vaccinia expressing the herpes simplex virus envelope. Mice were then challenged with herpes simplex virus type 2, and it was oberved that both H-2$^{a/a}$ and H-2$^{a/b}$ mice were significantly protected (Fig. 3). These results demonstrated that H-2$^{a/a}$ mice were capable of making a good protective immune response to viral proteins expressed in recombinant vaccinia; therefore, the lack of response of H-2$^{a/a}$ mice to vaccinia-F-MuLV env was most likely due to inability of these mice to recognize the F-MuLV envelope itself rather than an inability to be immunized by recombinant vaccinia.

MECHANISMS OF PROTECTION

In order to analyze possible mechanisms of protection following immunization of mice, status of the virus-specific immune response of H-2$^{a/b}$ mice was analyzed prior to and after challenge with FV complex. Before challenge it was observed that most mice which received FV-N or killed F-MuLV had virus-specific neutralizing antibodies and cytotoxic T lymphocytes (CTL) (Table 1). In contrast, mice immunized with the vaccinia-F-MuLV env had very poor virus

Table 1 FV–Specific Immune Parameters Prior to FV Challenge in $H\text{-}2^{a/b}$ and $H\text{-}2^{a/a}$ Mice

H-2 genotype	Immunogen	FV-specific immune response before challenge		
		Neutralizing antibody	Cytotoxic T lymphocyte	T-lymphocyte proliferation
a/b	none	−	−	−
a/b	vaccinia-influenza HA	−	−	−
a/b	vaccinia-F–MuLV env	−	−	+
a/b	FV–N	+	+	+
a/b	killed F–MuLV in CFA	+	nt	+
a/a	none	−	−	−
a/a	vaccinia-influenza HA	−	−	−
a/a	vaccinia-F–MuLV env	−	−	−
a/a	FV–N	+	+	nt
a/a	killed F–MuLV in CFA	+	nt	±

FV-specific neutralizing antibodies, cytotoxic T lymphocytes, and T-lymphocyte proliferation responses were analyzed as previously described (32).

nt = not tested.

neutralizing antibody response and no detectable virus-specific CTL. In fact, these mice were positive only in a virus specific T-cell proliferation assay (Table 1 and Fig. 4), which suggested that T cells had in fact been primed by the immunization, but the antigenic stimulus was not sufficient to induce antibodies or CTL. H-2$^{a/a}$ mice were similar to H-2$^{a/b}$ mice after immunization with FV-N or killed F-MuLV, but differed from them in that there was no evidence of T-cell priming after inoculation of vaccinia-F-MuLV env (Table 1).

Immune parameters of H-2$^{a/b}$ mice were also followed *after* challenge with FV complex and were compared to the status of leukemia and frequency of Friend virus-releasing cells detected in spleen cell populations (Fig. 5). Results indicated that mice immunized with attenuated FV-N or killed F-MuLV were not infected to an extent capable of giving any detectable leukemic spleno-megaly. This was consistent with the fact that these mice had good neutralizing antibodies and CTL prior to challenge. In contrast, 40% of mice vaccinated with vaccinia-F-MuLV env developed severe splenomegaly by day 14. However, splenomegaly in these mice subsequently disappeared, resulting in a very low incidence of leukemia 40 days after challenge. After challenge, mice immunized with vaccinia-F-MuLV env developed a peak of virus-specific CTL about 15 days postchallenge which coincided with the onset of recovery from leukemic spleno-megaly. Neutralizing antibodies were also detected in these mice, and high titers were observed from 8 days onward. Thus, it appeared that mice immunized with vaccinia-F-MuLV env had only primed T lymphocytes detectable by T prolifera-tion assay prior to FV challenge, but following challenge they developed very rapid onset of a secondary IgG humoral immune (34) response and CTL re-sponse to Friend virus. Protective immunity with this vaccine did not appear to block initial infection by challenge virus, but provided protection by immuno-logically priming mice so that their secondary response to challenge virus was sufficient to mediate recovery from established infection. This interpretation was also supported by analysis of spleen virus in the various groups of mice. The results showed that spleen cells of mice which were immunized with vaccinia-F-MuLV env were successfully infected in most cases; however, the number of infected cells never rose to the high levels observed in control mice and appeared to drop as the recovery process proceeded. Nevertheless, even after complete recovery from splenomegaly, some mice still had detectable virus-releasing spleen cells 35 days after FV challenge. It is unclear whether these cells were residual, transformed leukemic cells whose growth potential was halted by continual presence of immune mechanisms or whether they were persistently infected cells with a nonleukemic phenotype which did not have uncontrolled growth poten-tial. The latter possibility seems more likely since FV is capable of infecting a variety of cell types such as capillary endothelial cells (Portis, J.L., personal communication, 1988) and megakaryocytes (35,36) without causing malignant

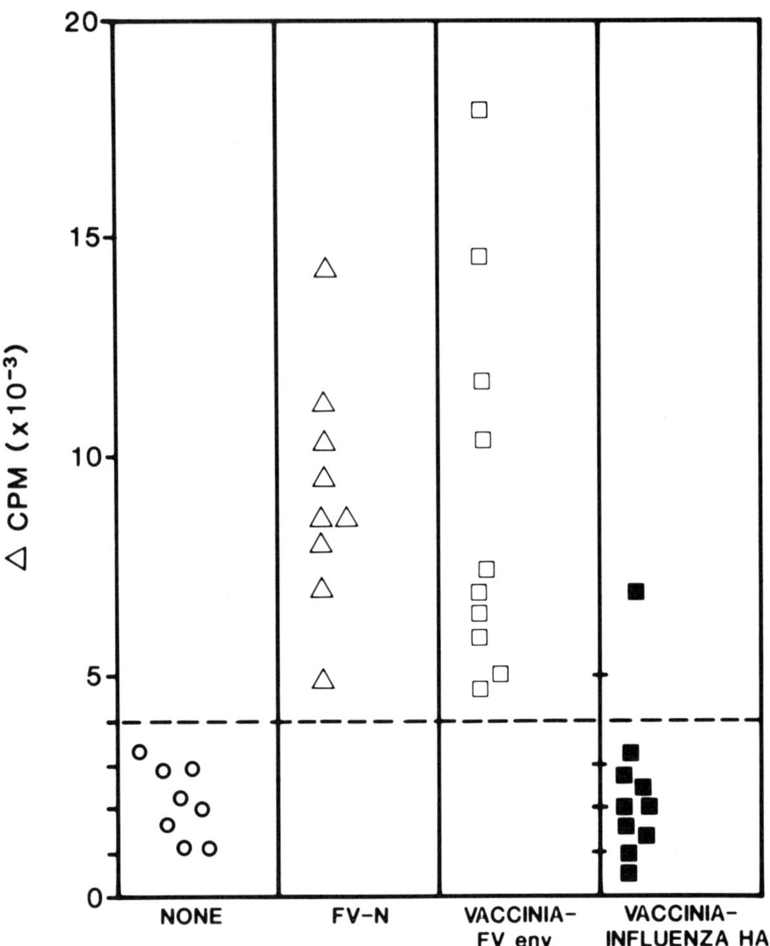

Figure 4 FV-specific T-lymphocyte proliferation before FV challenge in (B10.A X A.BY)F_1 mice (H-$2^{a/b}$) immunized 26 days previously as described in Figure 1. (Data from Ref. 49.)

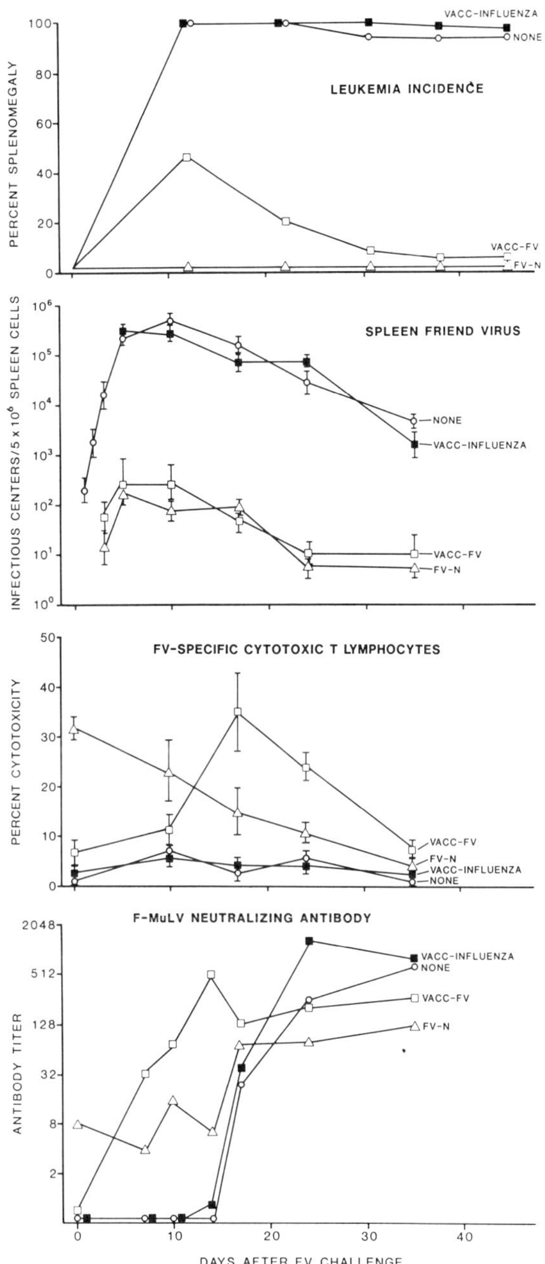

Figure 5 Leukemia incidence, spleen FV, FV-specific cytotoxic T lymphocytes, and F-MuLV neutralizing antibody in H-2$^{a/b}$ mice at various times after FV challenge. Immunizations were 26 days before challenge as described in Figure 1: Δ, FV-N; □, vaccinia-F-MuLV env; ■, vaccinia-influenza HA; ○, no immunization. (Data adapted from Ref. 32.)

transformation. In this case it would also appear likely that continued presence of virus-specific immune mechanisms might prevent virus from such nonleukemic infected cells from infecting and transforming new susceptible erythroid target cells in a second round of leukemogenesis.

POSSIBLE ROLE OF VIRUS-INDUCED IMMUNOSUPPRESSION AS A MECHANISM OF RESISTANCE TO INDUCTION OF PROTECTIVE IMMUNITY

Previous results in studies of immunized mice indicated that H-2 genotype had a strong influence on immunosuppression induced by FV complex. H-2$^{a/a}$ mice were highly immunosuppressed by Friend virus, whereas H-2$^{a/b}$ mice were not immunosuppressed in spite of the evidence for continued leukemic splenomegaly in both mouse strains (26). Typical results are shown in Table 2, where H-2$^{a/b}$ leukemic mice were capable of making strong IgG anti-SRBC antibody response, whereas leukemic H-2$^{a/a}$ mice were not. IgM anti-SRBC responses were only slightly depressed in both of these mouse strains so the primary effect of immunosuppression detected in these experiments appeared to be a reduction of T-cell help required for switching of the Ig class from the IgM to IgG anti-SRBC antibody. Since the H-2$^{a/a}$ mice were also poorly protected against FV challenge by immunization with vaccinia-MuLV env, it was hypothesized that perhaps lack of induction of protective immunity was due to the high susceptibility of these mice to FV-induced immunosuppression following challenge with infectious virus. In order to test this possibility, we used mice with recombinant H-2 genotypes in order to see whether the H-2 effect on induction of immune protection and the H-2 effect on virus-induced immunosuppression were mediated by the same H-2 subregions. The data shown in Figure 6 indicate that susceptibility to immunosuppression was mediated by the D subregion of H-2, whereas ability to mount a protective immune response to Friend challenge following immunization with vaccinia-F-MuLV env was mapped to the K or I-A subregions of H-2 (34). Subsequent experiments have mapped this effect more precisely to the I-A subregion (37). Since virus-induced immunosuppression and vaccine-F-MuLV env-induced protective immunity were mediated by different H-2 subregions, it was clear that susceptibility to immunosuppression did not by itself lead to inability to induce a protective immune respone. This was seen in both the (B10.A(5R) × A)F$_1$ and (B10.A(18R) × A)F$_1$ recombinant mice which had a high degree of virus-induced immunosuppression, but were nevertheless protected by vaccinia-F-MuLV env virus. These results are encouraging in considering the potential for immunization against human immunosuppressive retroviruses. Whereas it seems likely that the majority of humans may be susceptible to retrovirus infection and retrovirus-induced immunosuppression, this susceptibility

Table 2 Influence of H-2 Genotype on FV-Induced Immunosuppression

Strain	H-2 genotype	Rfv-3 genotype	Splenomegaly	Anti-FV antibody	IgG anti-SRBC PFC/spleen	
					Uninfected	FV-infected
(B10.A $\times$ A.BY)F$_1$	a/b	r/s	+	+	90,000	30,000
(B10.A $\times$ A)F$_1$	a/a	r/s	+	+	86,000	300

Values shown are geometric mean of indirect PFC minus direct PFC for mice 7 days after a single i.p. inoculation of 0.25 ml of a 10% suspension of washed sheep red blood cells. FV-infected mice were immunized with SRBC 25 days after i.v. inoculation with 1×10^3 SFFU of FV complex.

| | LEUKEMIA INCIDENCE | | | PLASMA ANTI-SRBC TITER | |
| STRAIN | H-2 GENOTYPE | IMMUNIZATION | | | | |

STRAIN	H-2 GENOTYPE (K, I-A, I-E, S, D)	FV-N	FIXED F-MuLV IN CFA	VACCINIA-F-MuLV env	FV INFECTED	NORMAL
(B10.A X A.BY)F₁		1/66(2%)	0/30(0%)	4/67 (6%)	1825	2632
(B10.A X A/WySn)F₁		0/56(0%)	2/30(7%)	38/46(83%)	63	3286
(B10.A(IR) X A/WySn)F₁		0/10(0%)	0/10(0%)	23/31(74%)	1855	2897
(B10.A(2R) X A/WySn)F₁		0/10(0%)	2/10(20%)	23/30(77%)	2403	3490
(B10.A(4R) X A/WySn)F₁		0/10(0%)	0/9(0%)	19/27(70%)	2048	4096
(B10.A(5R) X A/WySn)F₁		1/9(11%)	0/9(0%)	4/30 (13%)	92	4872
(B10.A(18R) X A/WySn)F₁		1/10(10%)	0/9(0%)	6/30 (20%)	63	5070

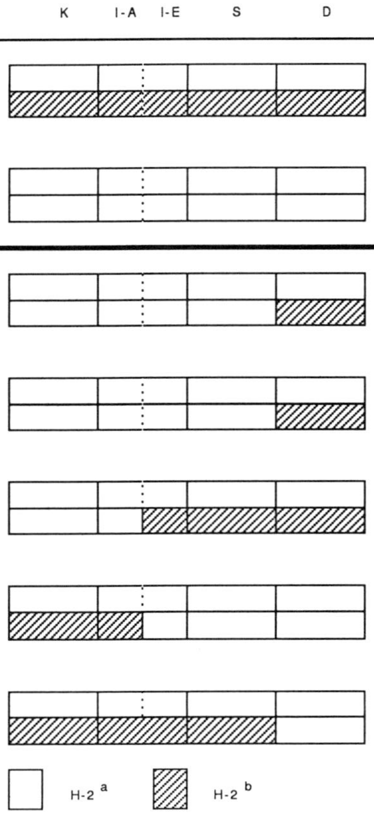

may not prevent successful induction of protective immunity if an appropriate immunogen is administered prior to virus infection.

PROTECTIVE IMMUNIZATION OF GENETIC NONRESPONDER MICE

Mice lacking the genetic potential to make a protective immune response following immunization with vaccinia-F-MuLV env required an alternative immunogen for induction of protective immunity to FV challenge. For these mouse strains both live attenuated FV-N and formalin-killed F-MuLV in adjuvant appeared to be effective in the induction of prorective immune (Fig. 6). It remains unclear why these two immunogens were successful in mice resistant to immunization by vaccinia-F-MuLV env. Since both FV-N and killed F-MuLV virions contained not only viral envelope glycoprotein, but also viral core and polymerase proteins, it was possible that these nonenvelope proteins might also play a role in induction of protective immunity. Alternatively, viral envelope protein might be the main protective immunogen in all mice; however, the different methods of immunization could be important factors distinguishing the success of these two immunogens from that of the recombinant vaccinia virus. For example, live attenuated FV-N may produce higher amounts of F-MuLV envelope protein during the immunization phase than does vaccinia-F-MuLV env, or the use of adjuvant with killed virions might have bypassed genetic resistance to immunization. Although in the present studies the adjuvant used was complete Freund's adjuvant, which has a strong local inflammatory side effects and would be unacceptable in human subjects, it seems likely that use of other less toxic adjuvant preparations might be equally successful. We are currently investigating this possibility at the present time. We are also attempting to immunize mice with purified viral core proteins or core polyproteins expressed in recombinant vaccinia viruses in order to test the induction of protective immunity by these antigens.

Regardless of the outcome in the Friend virus model, in the case of human retroviruses similar empirical studies will have to be carried out to determine which, if any, viral proteins are capable of inducing protective immune responses, and also whether there is significant variation in the humans in the ability to mount an effective protective immune response to different virion

---

Figure 6 Identification of regions of the H-2 complex involved in protective immunity and in FV-induced immunosuppression. Immunizations and FV challenge as in Figure 1. Plasma anti-sheep red blood cell titer was determined as described 7 days after immunization with SRBC (26). Infection with FV was done 18 days prior to SRBC immunization. (Data adapted from Ref. 34.)

protein antigens. Consideration of both of these factors will be important in development of a broadly effective vaccine for immunosuppressive human retrovirus disease.

VIRUS CARRIER STATUS OF PROTECTED INDIVIDUALS

One striking finding in the present studies was the observation that successful protective immunization did not usually block infection by challenge FV. Instead, immunization appeared to prime mice so that they could rapidly recover from splenomegaly induced by infection after challenge. In spite of the long-term recovery seen in protected mice, spleen cells releasing FV could still be detected at very low levels long after recovery. A similar situation might occur after immunization and subsequent exposure to HIV. Retroviruses including HIV are usually capable of infecting a variety of cell types, and levels of virus production may vary considerably even among cells derived from cloned populations. Since most immune mechanisms function best in recognition of foreign antigens expressed at high levels, it should be expected that cells expressing very little or no viral protein might escape even highly effective immune surveillance mechanisms. If so, this would not be desirable; however, if immunization were capable of preventing HIV-induced disease in a similar way to that observed with FV leukemia, then this would still be a useful preventative measure in spite of the possible persistence of rare residual cells carrying viral genomes.

CONCLUDING REMARKS

The experiments described in the preceding sections indicated that in the FV model it was possible to induce protective immunity even in the face of severe host genetic susceptibility to virus-induced immunosuppression. Furthermore, there was significant host genetic variability in ability to make a protective immune response to certain immunogens. However, even low responder individuals could be immunized if immunization was done with appropriate viral antigens and immunogenic adjuvants. It is likely that host genetic variability may also have a strong influence on the immune response of different individuals to HIV antigens. Thus, it may be necessary to consider similar ways to maximally enhance the protective immune response of humans to HIV.

The data in this report has not dealt directly with the issue of virus variability in influencing the success or failure of protective immunization. Some previous results suggest that retrovirus variability may be an important factor in allowing virus or infected cells to avoid immune defense mechanisms (38-41). Antiviral antibodies frequently appear after infection in retroviral diseases, and they may or may not play a role in restricting virus spread and selecting viral antigenic variants (42-44). Although the possibility of selection of antigenic variants has been widely discussed, the evidence from EIAV-infected horses suggests that only certain sera from early in disease show selective specificity for individual viral variants (45). Later in disease sera are highly cross-reactive and usually neutralize most virus isolates (Carpenter, S., personal communication, 1988). This latter finding is similar to what is observed in AIDS patients who usually have neutralizing antibody reactive with a wide variety of HIV isolates (46,47). Antiviral antibodies appearing after infection by EIAV, HIV, or FV are incapabe of completely eliminating established infection. However, as has been shown in certain mouse strains infected with FV, antienvelope antibodies appearing after infection may be responsible for elimination of viremia, blocking of virus spread, and decreasing of virus expression by infected cells, even in the face of persistent disease (29,30). In contrast to these findings, it seems likely that presence of cross-reactive antiviral antibodies or other immune effectors *prior* to virus infection might be much more effective at preventing disease. This is certainly the case for FV (4,48), and may also be true for HIV and other lentiviruses. This possibility should be subjected to rigorous testing in each viral system to determine the precise facts before the potential effectiveness of protective immunization can be accurately predicted.

REFERENCES

1. Kono Y, Kobayashi K, Fukunaga Y. Immunization of horses against equine infectious anemia (EIA) with an attenuated EIA virus. Natl Inst Anim Health Q 1970; 10:113-22.
2. Sachs L. Transplantability of an X-ray-induced and a virus-induced leukemia in isologous mice inoculated with a leukemia virus. J Natl Cancer Inst 1962; 29:759-64.
3. Fink MA, Rauscher FJ. Immune reactions to a murine leukemia virus. I. Induction of immunity to infection with virus in the natural host. J Natl Cancer Inst 1964; 32:1075-82.
4. Friend C. A virus-induced leukemia of adult mice. In Pollard M, ed. Perspectives in virology. New York: Wiley, 1959:231-44.
5. Mayyasi SA, Moloney JB. Induced resistance of mice to a lymphoid strain of leukemia virus (Moloney). Cancer 1967; 20:1124-30.
6. Olsen RG, Hoover EA, Mathes LE,Heding L, Schaller JP. Immunization against feline oncornavirus disease using a killed tumor cell vaccine. Cancer Res 1976; 36:3642-6.
7. Bayer H, Hunsmann G. Synthetic vaccines against Friend murine leukaemia virus-induced erythroleukaemia: *in vivo* and *in vitro* studies with synthetic oligopeptides and sequence-specific antisera. J Gen Virol 1987; 68:515-22.
8. Kleiser C, Schneider J, Bayer H, Hunsmann G. Immunoprevention of Friend leukaemia virus-induced erythroleukaemia by vaccination with aggregated gp70. J Gen Virol 1986; 67:1901-7.

9. Hunsmann G, Schneider J, Schulz A. Immunoprevention of Friend virus induced erythroleukemia by vaccination with viral envelope glycoprotein complexes. Virology 1981; 113:603-12.

10. Meyers P, Sigel MM, Holden HT. Cross protection *in vivo* against avian sarcoma virus subgroups A, B, and C induced by Rous-associated viruses. J Natl Cancer Inst 1972; 49:173-81.

11. Olsen RG, Hoover EA, Schaller JP, Mathes LE, Wolff LH. Abrogation of resistance to feline oncornavirus disease by immunization with killed feline leukemia virus. Cancer Res 1977; 37:2082-5.

12. Mathes L, Olsen R, Hebebrand L, Hoover E, Schaller J. Abrogation of lymphocyte blastogenesis by feline leukemia virus protein. Nature 1978; 274:687.

13. Mathes LE, Olsen RG, Hebebrand LC, et al. Immunosuppressive properties of a virion polypeptide, a 15,000-dalton protein, from feline leukemia virus. Cancer Res 1979; 39:950.

14. Perryman LE, Hoover EA, Yohn DS. Immunologic reactivity of the cat: immunosuppression in experimental feline leukemia. J Natl Cancer Inst 1972; 49:1357-65.

15. Friend C. Cell-free transmission in adult Swiss mice of a disease having the character of a leukemia. J Exp Med 1957; 105:307.

16. Troxler DH, Ruscetti SK, Scolnick EM. The molecular biology of Friend virus. Biochim Biophys Acta 1980; 605:305-24.

17. Linemeyer DL, Ruscetti SK, Menke JG, Scolnick EM. Recovery of biologically active spleen focus-forming virus from molecularly cloned spleen focus-forming virus-pBR322 circular DNA by cotransfection with infectious type C retroviral DNA. J Virol 1980; 35:710-21.

18. Kaminchik J, Hankins WD, Ruscetti SK, Linemeyer DL, Scolnick EM. Molecular cloning of biologically active proviral DNA of the anemia-inducing strain of spleen focus-forming virus. J Virol 1982; 44:922-31.

19. Oliff AI, Hager GL, Chang EH, Scolnick EM, Chan HW, Lowy DR. Transfection of molcularly cloned Friend murine leukemia virus DNA yields a highly leukemogenic helper-independent type C virus. J Virol 1980; 33:475-86.

20. Dent PB. Immunodepression by oncogenic viruses. Prog Med Virol 1972; 14:1-35.

21. Ceglowski WS, Friedman H. Immunosuppression by leukemia viruses. I. Effect of Friend virus disease on cellular and humoral hemolysin responses of mice to a primary immunization with sheep erythrocytes. J Immunol 1968; 101:594.

22. Kumar V, Resnick P, Eastcott JW, Bennett M. Mechanism of genetic resistance to Friend virus leukemia in mice. V. Relevance of Fv-3 gene in the regulation of in vivo immunosuppression. J Natl Cancer Inst 1978; 61:1117.

23. Mortensen RF, Ceglowski WS, Friedman H. Leukemia virus-induced immunosuppression. IX. Depression of delayed hypersensitivity and MIF

production after infection of mice with Friend leukemia virus. J Immunol 1973;111:1810.

24. Mortensen RF, Ceglowski WS, Friedman H. Leukemia virus-induced immunosuppression. X. Depression of T cell-mediated cytotoxicity after infection of mice with Friend leukemia virus. J Immunol 1974; 112: 2077.

25. Marcelletti J, Furmanski P. Infection of macrophages with Friend virus: relationship to the spontaneous regression of viral erythroleukemia. Cell 1979; 16:649–59.

26. Morrison RP, Nishio J, Chesebro B. Influence of the murine major histocompatibility complex (H-2) on Friend leukemia virus-induced immunosuppression. J Exp Med 1986; 163:301–14.

27. Doig D, Chesebro B. Antibody-induced loss of Friend virus leukemia cell surface antigens occurs during progression of erythroleukemia in F_1 mice. J Exp Med 1978; 148:1109–21.

28. Chesebro B, Wehrly K. Identification of a non-H-2 gene (Rfv-3) influencing recovery from viremia and leukemia induced by Friend virus complex. Proc Natl Acad Sci USA 1979; 76:425–9.

29. Chesebro B, Wehrly K, Doig D, Nishio J. Antibody-induced modulation of Friend virus cell surface antigens decreases virus production by persistent erythroleukemia cells: influence of the Rfv-3 gene. Proc Natl Acad Sci USA 1979; 76:5784–8.

30. Britt WJ, Chesebro B. Use of monoclonal anti-gp70 antibodies to mimic the effects of the Rfv-3 gene in mice with Friend virus-induced leukemia. J Immunol 1983; 130:2363–7.

31. Holt CA, Osorio K, Lilly F. Friend virus-specific cytotoxic T lymphocytes recognize both *gag* and *env* gene-encoded specificites. J Exp Med 1986; 164:211–26.

32. Earl PL, Moss B, Morrison RP, Wehrly K, Nishio J, Chesebro B. T-lymphocyte priming and protection against Friend leukemia by vaccinia-retrovirus *env* gene recombinant. Science 1986; 234:728–31.

33. Chesebro B, Wehrly K, Stimpfling J. Host genetic control of recovery from Friend leukemia virus induced splenomegaly: mapping of a gene within the major histocompatibility complex. J Exp Med 1974; 140:1457–67.

34. Morrison RP, Earl PL, Nishio J, Lodmell DL, Moss B, Chesebro B. Different H-2 subregions influence immunization against retrovirus and immunosuppression. Nature 1987; 329:729–32.

35. Dalton AJ, Law LW, Moloney JB, Manaker RA. An electron microscopic study of a series of murine lymphoid neoplasims. J Natl Cancer Inst 1961; 27:747–99.

36. Dennis LH, Brodsky I. Thrombocytopenia induced by the Friend leukemia virus. J Natl Cancer Inst 1965; 35:993–9.

37. Miyazawa M, Nishio J, Chesebro B. Genetic control of T cell responsiveness to the Friend murine leukemia virus envelope antigen: identification of

class II loci of the *H-2* as immune response genes. J Exp Med 1988; 168: 1587–605.

38. Kono Y. Recurrences of equine infectious anemia. In Bryans JT, Gerber H, eds. Proceedings of the 3rd international conference on equine infectious diseases. Basel: S.Karger, 1972:175–86.

39. Narayan O, Griffin DE, Chase J. Antigenic shift of visna virus in persistently infected sheep. Science 1977; 197:376–8.

40. Reitz MS Jr, Wilson C, Naugle C, Gallo RC, Robert-Guroff M. Generation of a neutralization-resistant variant of HIV-1 is due to selection for a point mutation in the envelope gene. Cell 1988; 54:57–63.

41. Hahn BH, Gonda MA, Shaw GM, et al. Genomic diversity of the acquired immune deficiency syndrome virus HTLV-III: different viruses exhibit greatest divergence in their envelope genes. Proc Natl Acad Sci USA 1985; 82:4813–7.

42. Kono Y, Kobayashi K, Fukunaga Y. Antigenic drift of equine infectious anemia virus in chronically infected horses. Arch Gesamte Virusforsch 1973; 41:1–10.

43. Montelaro RC, Parekh B, Preggo A, Issel CJ. Antigenic variation during persistent infection by equine infectious anemia virus, a retrovirus. J Biol Chem 1984; 259:10539–44.

44. Clements JE, Gdovin SL, Montelaro RC, Narayan O. Antigenic variation in lentiviral diseases. Annu Rev Immunol 1988; 6:139–59.

45. Carpenter S, Evans LH, Sevoian M, Chesebro B. Role of the host immune response in selection of equine infectious anemia virus variants. J Virol 1987; 61:3783–9.

46. Prince AM, Pascuel D, Kosolapov LB, Kurokawa D, Baker L, Rubinstein P. Prevalence, clinical significance, and strain specificity of neutralizing antibody to the human immunodeficiency virus. J Infect Dis 1987; 156:268–72.

47. Weiss RA, Clapham PR, Cheinsong-Popov R, et al. Neutralization of human T-lymphotropic virus type III by sera of AIDS and AIDS-risk patients. Nature 1985; 316:69–72.

48. Chesebro B, Wehrly K. Studies on the role of the host immune response in recovery from Friend virus leukemia. I. Antiviral and antileukemia cell antibodies. J Exp Med 1976; 143:73–84.

49. Morrison RP, Chesebro B, Earl P, Nishio J, Wehrly K, Moss B. Induction of primed T lymphocytes and protection against Friend murine leukemia by recombinant vaccinia virus expressing the Friend retrovirus envelope gene. In Chanock RM, Lerner RA, Brown F, Ginsberg H, eds. Vaccines 87: Modern approaches to new vaccines. Cold Spring Harbor, New York: Cold Spring Harbor Laboratory, 1987:268–72.

15

Epitopes Responsible for Fusion and Virus Neutralization in the Glycoprotein of Ovine and Caprine Lentiviruses
A Challenge for Vaccine Development

Susan L. Gdovin
The Johns Hopkins University School of Hygiene and Public Health
Baltimore, Maryland

Sharon E. Crane, Opendra Narayan, and Janice E. Clements
The Johns Hopkins University School of Medicine
Baltimore, Maryland

Viral infections involve complex host–parasite interactions. A wide variety of strategies employed in the replication mechanisms of viruses are pitted against a multitude of host defense mechanisms. The host immune system, for the most part, is very effective, and most infections result in elimination of the virus. Persistence of virus in an infected animal is usually the result of either virus replication in an immunologically impaired host or a replication-defective virus in a normal immune host. Lentiviruses are a unique group of viruses that not only persist indefinitely in the infected host but also replicate continuously, often in the presence of neutralizing antibodies (1–3). These viruses pose formidable problems to the host immune system as well as to those attempting vaccine development.

Lentiviruses are so named (lenti = slow) because they cause diseases characterized by long incubation periods and slowly progressive clinical courses (4). These agents are nononcogenic retroviruses that infect cells of the immune system and are transmitted horizontally through body fluids. The lentivirus group includes visna-maedi virus of sheep, caprine arthritis encephalitis virus (CAEV) of goats, equine infectious anemia virus (EIAV) of horses, human immunodeficiency (HIV) virus in man, simian immunodeficiency virus (SIV) in nonhuman primates, the bovine lentivirus (BIV) of cattle, and the feline lentivirus (FTLV) of cats (5-9). The lentiviruses are enveloped viruses that contain a positive-stranded RNA molecule which encodes the three major structural genes, 5′-*gag-pol-env*-3′ (10;11). In addition, there are small open reading frames between the *pol* and *env* genes that encode regulatory proteins required for the complex regulation of virus gene expression (10,12). Visna and CAE viruses are prototypes of the lentiviruses, and host responses to them have been the most thoroughly investigated. This review examines several viral strategies used by these agents in escaping immunologic control.

Visna-maedi virus causes chronic progressive pneumonitis and leukoencephalomyelitis in sheep (13-15). These sheep diseases were first described in Iceland as classic examples of viral diseases that have unusually long incubation periods and slowly progressive clinical courses (4). CAEV, the lentivirus most closely related to visna virus (16,17), causes chronic diseases involving the joints, brain, and lungs of goats (2). Visna and CAE viruses are transmitted horizontally through respiratory exudates and milk (18,19).

Close examination of the life cycles of visna and CAE viruses reveals several mechanisms that may contribute to the persistence of these viruses in the presence of normal host immunity. The most obvious virus strategy involves a common property of all retroviruses: invasion of the host cell genome. The target cells for visna and CAEV are cells of the monocyte-macrophage lineage (20). After the virus enters the cell, viral RNA is reverse transcribed into a DNA provirus which integrates into the host cell genome (21). The host immune system cannot recognize the unexpressed integrated viral genome and, therefore, only cell death will eliminate the viral nucleic acid. However, due to the finite life span of these target cells, this sequestration provides only temporary protection for the virus. Studies of persistently infected sheep show that monocyte precursors in the bone marrow contain viral nucleic acid (22). This may provide a reservoir of virus in stem cells in the bone marrow for lifelong persistence.

Lentiviral gene expression is very tightly regulated (23-25). In vivo there appears to be a downregulation of virus transcription and expression and, as a result, very limited virus production. Indeed, cell-free virus is only rarely recovered from visna-infected sheep, and virus antigens are seldom found by immunofluorescence. This is in contrast to the promiscuous and cytopathic virus replication in tissue culture cells. Regulation of viral gene expression is also dependent upon the stage of differentiation of the infected cell. Virus expression is barely detectable in latently infected monocytes; however, when these cells differentiate into macrophages there is a substantial increase in viral mRNA and virus production. This restricted expression and production of virus also protects the virus from exposure to the host immune system. Therefore, lifelong virus persistence can be attributed to provirus integration into the host genome in both circulating mononuclear cells and stem cells, and downregulation of virus expression mediated by viral and cellular regulatory factors.

These features undoubtedly contribute to virus persistence, however, they fail to explain the slow progression of disease illustrated by both acute and chronic lesions seen in lung and brain (26). Chronic progressive disease requires continuous virus replication and spread to other target cells. Since budding virions are potentially exposed to neutralizing antibodies, this dissemination can be accomplished only through evasion or modulation of the host immune response. Both visna virus and CAEV have developed multiple strategies to combat the humoral immunity of the immunocompetent host. First, CAEV does not induce development of neutralizing antibodies in the host (27-29). Despite the production of a multitude of nonneutralizing antibodies to all viral proteins, epitopes responsible for virus neutralization are not recognized by the host immune system. In the absence of neutralizing antibody, virus can replicate and spread in the animal. Second, lentiviruses undergo antigenic drift in infected hosts (30-33). During replication, the viral genome accumulates point mutations due to an error-prone viral reverse transcriptase which lacks editing function. Point mutations in the *env* gene which alter the neutralization epitopes give mutant viruses a selective growth advantage in an immune animal. These antigenic variants are not neutralized by antibody and can therefore replicate and spread in the host. Finally, the antibodies elicited by visna virus and CAEV are inefficient in virus neutralization (34). Neutralizing antibodies are produced in low titer and must be incubated with the virus for prolonged periods to accomplish virus neutralization. Therefore, virus spread in the animal occurs more rapidly than virus neutralization.

The targets for CAEV and visna virus neutralization are the highly glycosylated outer membrane proteins, gp135, encoded in the viral *env* gene regions (16,35). These outer membrane proteins are larger and more highly glycosylated than other retrovirus glycoproteins. The *env* gene regions of these viruses also encode a glycosylated hydrophobic transmembrane protein, which spans the membrane of the virus and probably serves as an anchor for the outer membrane protein.

Another function of the outer membrane glycoprotein is cell fusion. Replication of both visna and CAEV in cell culture causes the tissue culture cells to fuse, forming large multinucleated giant cells. In addition, visna virus can cause fusion from outside of the cell at a m.o.i. of 4 virions/cell (36). This "fusion from without" requires no viral replication, and can be blocked by antibody to the viral outer membrane protein, gp135 (37). Therefore, the outer membrane glycoprotein of visna virus and CAEV contain epitopes responsible for virus neutralization, virus-induced cell fusion, and probably virus receptor interaction.

II. IMMUNE RESPONSE TO CAEV

Goats infected naturally or experimentally with CAEV develop a lifelong persistent infection. These animals produce binding antibodies against all viral proteins, but fail to produce any detectable antibody that will neutralize virus infectivity (27-29). Previous studies demonstrated that these CAEV-infected animals, when superinfected with visna virus, did produce neutralizing antibody against visna virus. This indicates that their immune systems were not impaired (29). One interpretation of this is that epitopes responsible for CAEV neutralization are hidden or covert on the surface of virus, and therefore are masked from the host immune system.

Attempts to produce CAEV-neutralizing antibodies by using adjuvants, purified virus, disrupted virus, and hyperimmunization were unsuccessful. Recent studies using large amounts of inactivated *Mycobacterium tuberculosis* in conjunction with infectious virus have succeeded in inducing a neutralizing antibody response to CAEV (29). Activation of macrophages by *M. tuberculosis* may have altered the processing of the virus in the macrophage. The neutralizing antibody produced has extremely narrow specificity and neutralizes only the virus used for immunization. No other strains of CAEV or visna virus are recognized, including strains isolated from goats from the same herd from which the original immunizing virus had been obtained. This suggests that, in addition to being poor inducers of neutralizing antibody, various CAE virus strains contain neutralization epitopes that are distinct.

Molecular analyses of three cloned strains of CAEV reveal widely divergent restriction endonuclease maps (16,38-41). Until recently, the extent of antigenic heterogeneity of CAEV had not been determined. The inability of CAEV to induce neutralizing antibody made it impossible to detect neutralization differences between strains of viruses circulating in nature in different animals, as well as viruses isolated from the same animal. Therefore, the experimentally obtained neutralizing antisera described above was used to detect antigenically distinct viruses present in the CAEV parental stocks. This experiment demonstrated that 1 in 10^4 parental virus was not neutralized by the sera, suggesting an extremely high rate of antigenic mutation (42,43). The rate of spontaneous antigenic mutation of visna virus is at least 100 times lower (44). It must be emphasized that these mutations occurred without the selective pressure of neutralizing antibodies. This high rate of spontaneous mutation may be responsible for the heterogeneity of CAEV strains observed in nature.

ANTIGENIC VARIATION AND PERSISTENT REPLICATION
OF VISNA VIRUS

Antigenic drift, or change in the antigenicity of the surface glycoprotein, is a well-established strategy among various parasites, viruses, and bacteria for escaping immune elimination. Antigenic alteration and subsequent immune selection is a mechanism used by many organisms as a means of persistence within a population or within a single host. Viral antigenic drift is responsible for sequential epidemics of influenza virus, and has been implicated in the occasional failures of rabies and measles vaccines (45-47). The best models for viral antigenic drift in a single animal, however, come from studies of lentiviruses.

Sheep infected naturally or experimentally with visna virus become persistently infected. However, unlike infections with CAEV, visna virus does induce neutralizing antibodies 3-4 weeks postinfection (32,48). These antibodies fail to eliminate the virus and virus can be isolated throughout the life of these animals by co-cultivation of peripheral blood mononuclear cells (20,25,33,49). A recurrent inflammatory response in the CNS leads to a slowly progressive and fatal disease. Early studies were done to explain the failure of neutralizing antibodies to clear the virus and subsequent development of disease. Two sheep were inoculated with plaque-purified visna virus, strain 1514, and studied over a period of 3.5 years. At various intervals, blood was drawn as a source of peripheral blood leukocytes for virus isolation and serum for measuring neutralizing antibodies (33). Early immune sera from these animals contained neutralizing activity to the parental virus and also to subsequent viruses isolated from the animals within the first year after infection (Fig. 1). After the first year, however, viruses were isolated that were no longer neutralized by the sheep early immune sera. These mutant viruses were fully virulent in animals and stable in tissue culture. Antibody responses in these animals broadened with time, and the sheep eventually developed neutralizing antibody to the mutant viruses late in infection. Late immune sera neutralized all virus isolates but were still able to distinguish between mutant and parent viruses, further illustrating antigenic differences. It is important to note that these variant viruses did not replace the infecting strain, 1514, and parent virus could be isolated at all times from these persistently infected sheep. This is not surprising, however, since the virus does integrate into the host genome. The infecting virus could be sequestered in circulating cells as well as stem cells, providing a reservoir of parent virus that can persist for the life of the animal.

The stock of parental virus was tested to rule out the presence of preexisting variant viruses. A suspension of 1×10^7 plaque-forming units (pfu) was mixed with early immune sera and examined for nonneutralizable variants. After 6 hours of incubation at 37°C followed by overnight incubation at 4°C, all surviving viruses were of parental phenotype. Therefore, less than 1 infectious virus in 10^7 of parental virus was antigenically distinct (42,44). This is a low rate of spontaneous antigenic mutation in contrast to CAEV. The variant viruses isolated from these persistently infected sheep most likely developed under the selective pressure of neutralizing antibody.

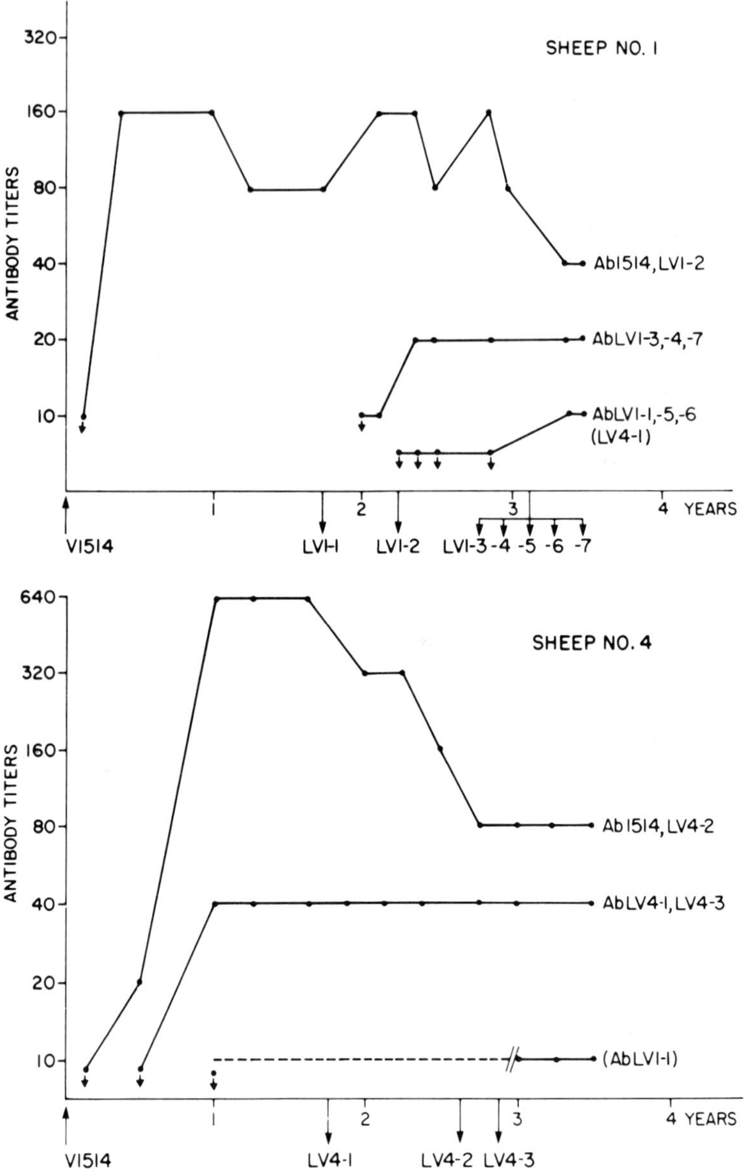

Figure 1 Sequential development of antibody to antigenic mutants of visna virus in sheep. Sheep No. 1 and No. 4 were inoculated intracerebrally with plaque-purified stock of virus 1514 (arrow pointing up). The identification and time of recovery of viruses (LV) from peripheral blood leukocytes of these animals is indicated by arrows pointing down. Line graphs indicate the temporal development and levels of neutralizing antibody (Ab) in these animals to the strain of virus inoculated and also to the viruses isolated from blood. Antibody titers are reported as the last doubling dilution of serum which neutralized 100 TCD_{50} of virus. (From Ref. 33.)

This immune selection of antigenic mutant viruses can be duplicated in a tissue culture system (50,51). Cell cultures inoculated with plaque-purified 1514 virus and maintained in medium containing neutralizing early immune sera produced stable mutant viruses within 3 weeks. These mutant viruses are no longer neutralized by the sera used to select them and are thus in vitro-derived antigenic variants.

MOLECULAR ANALYSES OF ANTIGENIC VARIANTS OF VISNA VIRUS

In order to investigate the molecular basis of antigenic variation of visna virus, the seven antigenic mutants isolated from sheep 1 were analyzed. The RNA genomes of these variants were cleaved with RNase T1, labeled with ^{32}P, and the resulting oligonucleotides were separated by two-dimensional gel electrophoresis (44,52). Comparison of the fingerprints revealed that these virus isolates were all very closely related and differed from parental virus by only a few oligonucleotide changes (Fig. 2). These altered oligonucleotides were mapped to the 3' end of the viral genome corresponding to the *env* gene region. Some variants had accumulated more mutations than others. The variants with the most changes were also the variants that were most antigenically distant from parental virus. The number of genetic changes ranged from 2 in LV1-2, which was of parental phenotype, to 6 in LV1-1, the variant most antigenically distinct from parent virus. These results are consistent with the original serologic classification of the variants (Fig. 1).

Nucleotide sequence analysis of the unique oligonucleotides revealed that: 1) the altered oligonucleotides were the result of single base changes in the viral genome, 2) many of the variants had a common subset of oligonucleotide changes, reflecting the same point mutations. This suggested that antigenic drift of visna virus is the result of a progressive accumulation of point mutations. The fact that these mutations are cumulative indicates that these variant viruses evolved sequentially, one from the ohter, during persistent infection. The conserved point mutations in the *env* gene appear to be selected for by host antibody and are probably responsible fo the lack of neutralization of the viruses by antibodies in early immune sera. Very few oligonucleotide changes were identified outside of the *env* gene, and none of these were seen in more than one variant virus. The fact that changes detected outside of the *env* gene were not conserved in other variants suggests that they were random point mutations that conferred no selective growth advantage.

Antigenic variant viruses from the second experimentally infected animal, sheep 4, were analyzed. Unexpectedly, the same oligonucleotide changes and corresponding point mutations were also detected in these mutants (Fig. 2) (44).

| VIRUS | NEUTRALIZATION | | GENETIC CHANGES |
	early	late	
1514	+ + + +	+ + + +	
L V 1-2	+ + + +	+ + + +	A B
L V 1-7	-	+ +	A B
L V 1-4	-	+ +	A B
L V 1-3	-	+ +	A B C
L V 1-6	-	+	A B C
L V 1-5	-	+	A B C
L V 1-1	-	+	A B C D E F
L V 4-2	+ + + +	+ + + +	A E F
L V 4-3	-	+ +	A E F
L V 4-1	-	+ +	A C E F
A D 1-1	-	+ +	A B E
A D 4-1	-	+ +	A B E

Figure 2 Progressive mutational changes occurring during antigenic drift of visna virus. Antigenic variants of visna virus strain 1514 were isolated from two persistently infected sheep and from tissue culture. The LV1 viruses were isolated from sheep 1 and the LV4 viruses from sheep 4. The tissue culture-derived variants AD1-1 and AD4-1 were selected with early immune sera from sheep 1 and 4, respectively. The genetic changes are those located in the 3′ region of the genome. (From Ref. 69.)

The fact that mutant viruses from two different animals contained identical genomic point mutations suggests that this immune selection requires very specific genomic alterations. During replication, mutations probably occur throughout the genome, but only a small specific subset of them confer a selective growth advantage, particularly those that alter sites on the viral glycoprotein that are responsible for virus neutralization. Analyses of mutant viruses selected in cell culture lend further support. RNase T1-resistant oligonucleotide fingerprinting revealed that antigenic variants produced in vitro in the presence of sheep early immune sera had similar oligonucleotide changes as those variants produced in an infected animal. The altered oligonucleotides detected in in vitro-derived mutants were a subset of those seen in the antigenic variants isolated from sheep.

Studies are currently in progress to determine the number, location, and biological significance of the point mutations in these antigenic variants of visna virus. The mutant viruses from sheep 1 are being cloned and the entire nucleotide sequences of the envelope gene regions determined. In LV1-1, the variant most distant from parent, 11 nucleotide changes were detected when the nucleotide sequence was compared to that of parent strain 1514 (Gdovin, unpublished). This was far fewer than expected. None of these changes affected N-glycosylation sites, and only 7 of these 11 changes resulted in amino acid changes (Fig. 3). There is a region of three clustered changes within a 27-basepair stretch at the carboxy-terminus of the outer membrane glycoprotein. Two of these amino acid changes are not only adjacent, but also represent the only charge changes detected. Both of the changes were from uncharged amino acids in the parent strain to charged amino acids in the mutant LV1-1 strain. This region of the envelope glycoprotein may play an important role in virus neutralization. These amino acids may either be an integral part of an epitope responsible for virus neutralization, or perhaps indirectly affect the neutralization epitope by changing the tertiary structure of the glycoprotein. Nevertheless, it is evident that very few amino acid changes can markedly affect the antigenicity of the viral glycoprotein.

Experiments using monoclonal antibodies directed against visna glycoprotein, gp135, further support the observation that relatively few changes are needed to drastically alter viral epitopes (53). In addition, these studies suggest that primary amino acid changes are magnified by the alteration of the three-dimensional structure of the gp135. Monoclonal antibodies prepared against purified gp135 identified five partially overlapping epitopes. These five epitopes can be divided into two domains: one overt or exposed on the native virus, and the other covert or not recognized on the virus but exposed on purified glycoprotein. Binding assays using these monoclonals against the antigenic variant viruses from sheep 1 detected alterations in all five epitopes (Fig. 4). On the contrary, monoclonal antibodies directed against the p27 core protein detected no changes in these mutant viruses.

Monoclonal antibodies that bound to exposed epitopes gp135a, gp135b, and gp135c on parent virus 1514 lost avidity subsequent to antigenic drift (Fig. 4). These three epitopes appeared lost on variant viruses. However, when these variant viruses were treated with nonionic detergents or reducing agents, avidity was restored and monoclonal antibodies were able to detect these epitopes. Conversely, the binding of monoclonal antibodies to covert epitopes gp135d and gp135e increased during antigenic drift. These epitopes appeared to be more exposed and available on the variant viruses than on parent virus. When 1514 virus was treated with reducing agents, however, avidity to epitope gp135e was increased three- to fivefold. These data suggest that antigenic drift involves the topographical rearrangement of the viral glycoprotein; and, rather than creating

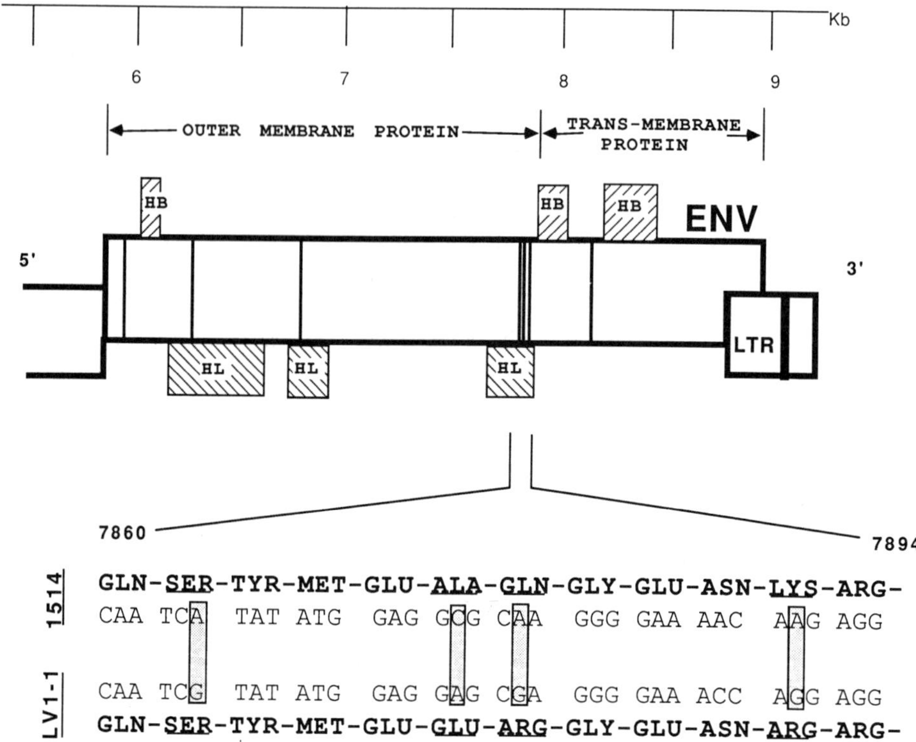

Figure 3 Amino acid changes in the viral glycoprotein of visna virus antigenic variant LV1-1. The seven single base substitutions in the *env* gene resulting in amino acid differences between 1514 and LV1-1 glycoproteins are represented by vertical lines. The hypervariable region is enlarged at the bottom. Three amino acid changes occurred within a six-amino-acid region. ALA-to-GLU and GLN-to-ARG were the only charge changes. HB = hydrophobic; HL = hydrophilic.

new epitopes, this rearrangement may hide or expose other epitopes that are not specifically recognized by neutralizing antibodies. In addition, the fact that reducing agents increase the availability of some epitopes suggests that disulfide bonds on gp135 may play a role in this conformational rearrangement.

The outer membrane glycoprotein of visna virus is a large and highly glycosylated protein. The dynamic tertiary structure of this envelope glycoprotein may allow visna virus to sequester biologically active epitopes from the immune system. It was mentioned earlier that early immune sera from sheep infected

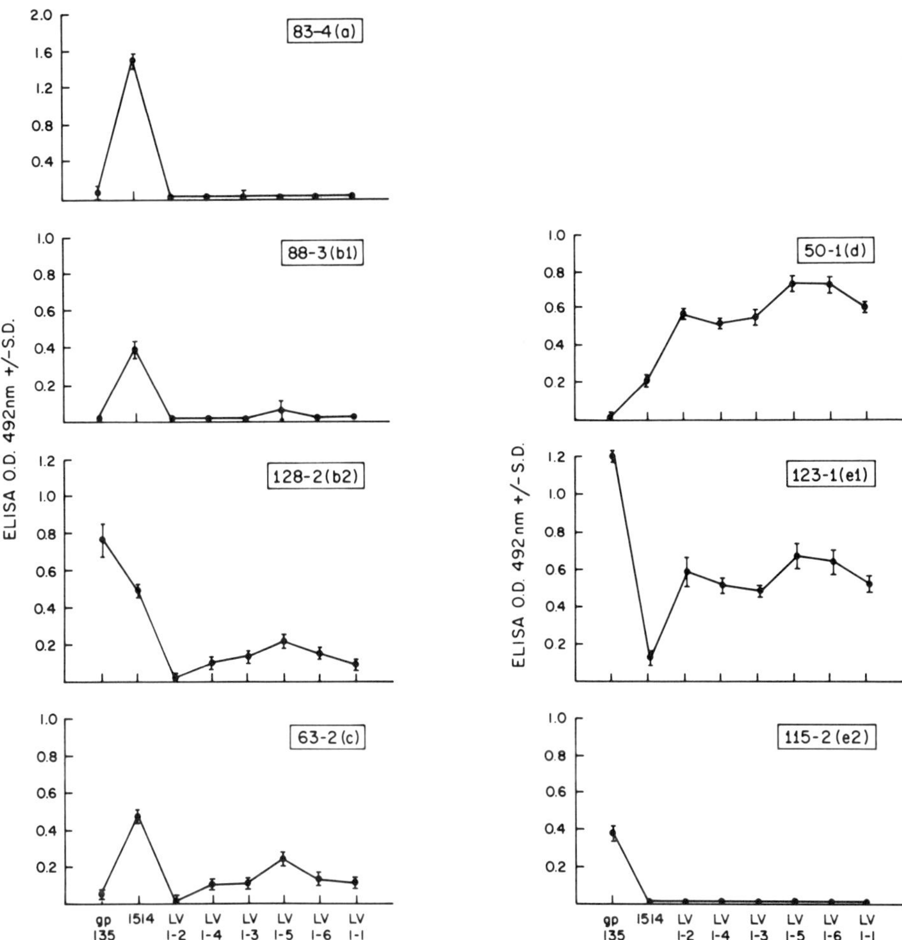

Figure 4 Topographical changes in visna gp135 during antigenic drift, shown by differential mAb binding to purified gp135 (strain 1514), virus strain 1514, or the six LV1 antigenic variants. The LV1 viruses are ordered along the abscissa from left to right by increasing genetic divergence from strain 1514. The five gp135 epitopes are marked a through e (boxes); mAb against epitopes b and e displayed two distinct ELISA patterns, which suggested that each epitope might be subdivided: (b1), (b2), (e1), (e2). Abbreviations: O.D. 492nm = optical density at 492 nm; S.D. = standard deviation. (From Ref. 53.)

with visna virus strain 1514 did not neutralize mutant virus LV1-1 (33). However, when another sheep was hyperimmunized with strain 1514 that was disrupted with nonionic detergent, the animal produced antibodies that neutralized both 1514 and mutant LV1-1 (43). This suggests that the epitopes responsible for LV1-1 neutralization are present on the surface of strain 1514, but are hidden from the immune system. Detergent disruption must conformationally expose these epitopes. This exposure of covert epitopes is strikingly similar to exposure of epitopes gp135d and gp135e on sheep 1 mutant viruses subsequent to antigenic drift.

It is important to note that none of the monoclonal antibodies produced against gp135 neutralize visna virus (53). However, LV1-2, which is indistinguishable from parent strain 1514 in neutralization tests, did demonstrate alterations in all five epitopes in the monoclonal antibody binding assays (Fig. 4). The five epitopes detected by monoclonal antibodies and the epitopes responsible for neutralization appear to be distinct, but changes in these epitopes still gave LV1-2 a selective growth advantage in vivo; therefore, the immune pressure that selected these antigenic variants may not have been neutralization alone. This suggests that both neutralizing and nonneutralizing antibodies play roles in antigenic drift and selection, and that there are global changes that confer growth advantages that are undetected by neutralization tests using polyclonal sera.

Recent studies have reported that antigenic mutation of visna virus can be detected in 25% of persistently infected sheep (54,55). This was interpreted as a rare occurrence that could neither account for virus persistence nor continued virus replication in immune animals. The fact that antigenic variants were isolated from one quarter of all infected animals suggests that this is clearly not a rare event. Indeed, the frequency of significant antigenic changes in visna virus during long-term persistent infection may have been higher had a single post-infectious serum been used to detect mutants instead of pooled sera. Our studies just described demonstrated that pooled polyclonal sera may fail to distinguish antigenic variants (53). The biological significance of antigenic variation among the lentiviruses is not fully understood. The phenomenon is not a prerequisite for virus persistence. If it is an epiphenomenon resulting from mistakes made during the unedited reverse transcription of the viral genome, then the significance will lie chiefly in its effect on a vaccine program.

VISNA VIRUS-INDUCED CELL FUSION

In contrast to their replication in vivo, both visna and CAE viruses replicate productively and cause cell fusion in certain cell cultures derived from host tissues. CAEV-infected monolayer cultures produce virus continuously for 2 to

3 weeks with development of fusion in about 50% of the cells (17). Visna virus is more virulent and kills tissue culture cells between 4 and 7 days after inoculation at a m.o.i. of 1 (36,56). During the productive phase of replication, cell fusion progresses to lysis in 1 to 2 days. This is fusion "from within," and it occurs late in the virus life cycle. Uniquely, visna virus also causes fusion "from without" when tissue culture cells are infected at a m.o.i. of greater than 3 (36). This type of fusion occurs within a few hours after inoculation and does not require virus replication. Cells degenerate by toxic fusion before completion of a single cycle of virus replication. This fusion "from without" can also be caused by UV-inactivated virus and is similar to that caused by paramyxoviruses (57).

The biological importance of cell fusion by lentiviruses is not clear. In our laboratory we have examined the mechanisms and kinetics of visna virus–induced cell fusion by using fusion "from without" as an in vitro tissue culture assay (37). Experiments have demonstrated that this fusion could be blocked by antiviral antibodies and also by antisera prepared against purified viral glycoprotein, gp135. These results suggest that, in addition to virus-neutralizing epitopes, the viral outer membrane glycoprotein contains epitopes responsible for cell fusion. The kinetics of inhibition of these two phenomena, however, appear to be quite distinct. It has been shown that visna virus neutralization requires preincubation of antibodies with virus for at least 15 min at 37°C, and that the efficiency of the neutralization increases slowly if allowed to preincubate up to 90 min. In contrast, the inhibition of virus-induced cell fusion appears to be quite rapid. Dilutions of sheep hyperimmune serum and virus were mixed and immediately inoculated onto goat synovial membrane cells. After 1 hour at 37°C, the cultures were washed with medium and reincubated at 37°C. No fusion occurred during the first 24 hours. Therefore the binding between the fusion epitope and the fusion-inhibiting antibodies must be rapid. Also, despite the inhibition of fusion in this experiment, virus replication proceeded and cells died by day 3. These results indicate that the kinetics of antibody-mediated inhibition of infection (neutralization) and inhibition of fusion are distinct. Interaction and binding between antibodies and the epitopes involved in virus neutralization are slow, and the binding between antibodies and the fusion epitopes are rapid.

Further characterization of the fusion epitope involved attempts to antigenically separate and distinguish it from the epitope involved in virus neutralization (37). Experiments were performed, using parental visna virus 1514 and its antigenic variant LV1-1. These two viruses have a similar rate of replication in cell culture and are equally efficient at inducing fusion from without. Monospecific early immune serum which neutralized visna virus 1514 but not LV1-1 was used for fusion assays. Surprisingly, this polyclonal serum completely inhibited fusion by LV1-1 despite its inability to neutralize the virus. Also, the titer and kinetics for inhibition of fusion were similar for both viruses. These data indicate that the sites on the virus surface responsible for fusion are the same in both viruses, but the sites involved in virus neutralization have been altered. Similar results were also obtained in experiments using polyclonal sera directed against the purified outer membrane glycoprotein of visna virus 1514. These studies thus established that the fusion and neutralization epitopes of visna virus are antigenically distinct.

Fusion by visna virus may be a mechanism for entry of virus into cells. Since antibodies that block cell fusion by visna virus do not completely inhibit virus infection, it is possible that the virus is capable of infecting host cells via two pathways: one via the fusion site, and the other via the neutralization site. Infected cells that produce viral glycoproteins can possibly fuse with adjacent cells and transmit viral nucleic acids. Therefore, cell-to-cell transmission can take place without the production of virions and subsequent exposure to host antibodies. This may be an important mechanism for virus spread.

CONCLUSION

Lentiviruses are nononcogenic retroviruses that share the remarkable ability to replicate continuously in immunocompetent hosts and cause slowly progressive and fatal diseases (58). The relatively recent discovery of the human lentivirus, HIV, has spurned a renewed and unprecedented interest in the lentivirus group (59,60). The AIDS epidemic has focused worldwide attention on the vast array of problems that these viruses present to both the host immune system and to those attempting to develop immunization programs. Our studies of visna virus and CAEV described in this review illustrate several of the problems that may be encountered in the search for an efficacious human virus vaccine.

One mechanism by which lentiviruses escape immune elimination, and a most formidable problem facing those involved in lentivirus vaccine development, is the ineffectiveness of the antibodies induced by the viruses. Antibody responses to ruminant lentiviruses range from total failure of antibodies to neutralize virus to the low efficiency of the antibodies that do neutralize. In addition, these viruses have a tropism for macrophages, one of the main cell types involved in virus clearance. Whether or not the infection of antigen-presenting macrophages plays a role in the induction of inefficient antibodies is not clear. However, the poor neutralizing capacity of induced antibodies, together with the tropism of these viruses for cells of the immune system, may provide enough of an advantage for these viruses to be able to replicate in immunocompetent hosts. Indeed, the problem of ineffective neutralizing antibodies has also been documented in patients infected with HIV (61,62); and, in addition to the tropism for T-helper cells, HIV may also infect and replicate in macrophages (63-66).

Although it may not be a major mechanism for virus persistence in the infected host, antigenic drift of lentiviruses poses a further complication for any potential immunization program. As exemplified by visna virus, lentiviruses undergo antigenic drift within a single infected host and neutralizing antibodies are strain specific. Envelope-specific differences have also been demonstrated in isolates of HIV (67,68). In addition, there is extreme genetic variability in HIV isolates from different sources, as seen with CAEV. It is clear that immunization with whole virus or the undenatured envelope glycoprotein of any one lentivirus will neither protect against rapidly emerging mutants during infection, nor protect against an exogenous antigenic variant. Our studies suggest that there are hypervariable regions in the envelope genes of these viruses. Further investigation of the high rate of mutation within these small genetic regions may provide information needed to genetically engineer novel immunogens that could induce a broad range of neutralizing antibodies to lentiviruses.

The antigenicity of the lentivirus glycoproteins cannot be explained simply by nucleotide sequence and genomic mutations. Antigenic phenotypes of these viruses involve complex folding of the envelope glycoproteins. Studies of the structure of these outer membrane proteins may shed light on how tertiary structure determines the recogniition of epitopes by the immune system.

It is important to mention that antibodies can only neutralize cell-free virus, and in nature lentiviruses are transmitted through infected cells; therefore, even if highly effective neutralizing antibodies could be induced through immunization, it seems doubtful that they would prevent infection. Since cell-to-cell transmission of lentiviral nucleic acids can occur through direct contact and fusion, further investigation of the fusion site on the viral glycoprotein may provide another avenue for possible prophylaxis. The potential for macrophage-to-macrophage spread through phagocytosis presents yet another possible mode of transmission that must be considered. Indeed, the lentiviruses seem to be the ultimate challenge for our traditional methods of vaccine development. Perhaps our hope for the future lies in the development of vaccines that prolong latency and prevent active disease.

ACKNOWLEDGMENTS

This work was supported by grants from the National Institute of Health NS21916, NS16145, and NS07000.

REFERENCES

1. Cheevers WP, McGuire TC. Equine infectious anemia virus. Immunopathogenesis and persistence. Rev Infect Dis 1985; 7:83–8.

2. Narayan O, Cork LC. Lentiviral diseases of sheep and goats. Chronic pneumonia, leukoencephalitis and arthritis. Rev Infect Dis 1985; 7:89–98.
3. Popovic M, Sarngadharan MG, Read E, Gallo RC. Detection, isolation and continuous production of cytopathic retroviruses (HTLV-III) from patients with AIDS and pre-AIDS. Science 1984; 224:497–500.
4. Sigurdsson B. Maedi, a slow progressive pneumonia of sheep: an epizootiological and pathological study. Br Vet J 1954; 110:255–70.
5. Gonda MA, Wong-Staal F, Gallo RC, Clements JE, Narayan O, Gilden RV. Sequence homology and morphologic similarity of HTLV-III and visna virus, a pathogenic lentivirus. Science 1985; 227:173–7.
6. Gonda MA, Braun MJ, Clements JE, Pyper JM, Casey JW, Wong-Staal F, Gallo RC, Gilden RV. HTLV-III shares sequence homology with a family of pathogenic lentiviruses. Proc Natl Acad Sci USA 1986; 83:4007–11.
7. Murphy-Corb M, Martin L, Rangan S, Baskin G, Gormus B, Wolf R, Andes A, West M, Montelaro R. Isolation of an HTLV-III-related retrovirus from macaques with simian AIDS and its possible origin in asymptomatic mangabeys. Nature 1986; 321:435–7.
8. Gonda MA, Braun MJ, Carter SG, Kost TA, Bess JW, Arthur LO, Van Der Maaten MJ. Characterization and molecular cloning of a bovine lentivirus related to human immunodeficiency virus. Nature 1987; 330:388–91.
9. Pedersen NC, Ho EW, Brown ML, Yamamoto JK. Isolation of T-lymphotropic virus from domestic cats with an immunodeficiency-like syndrome. Science 1987; 235:790–3.
10. Sonigo P, Alizon M, Staskus K, Klatzman D, Cole S, Danos O, Retzel E, Tiollais P, Haase A, Wain-Hobson S. Nucleotide sequence of the visna lentivirus: Relationship to the AIDS virus. Cell 1985; 42:369–82.
11. Wain-Hobson S, Sonigo P, Danos O, Cole S, Alizon M. Nucleotide sequence of the AIDS virus, LAV. Cell 1985; 40:7–17.
12. Davis JL, Molineaux S, Clements JE. Visna virus exhibits a complex transcriptional pattern: One aspect of gene expression shared with the acquired immunodeficiency syndrome retrovirus. J Virol 1987; 61:1325–31.
13. Sigurdsson B, Palsson PA, Grissom H. Visna, a demyelinating transmissable disease of sheep. J Neuropath Exp Neurol 1957; 16:389–403.
14. Sigurdsson B, Palsson PA. Visna of sheep, a slow demyelinating infection. Br J Exp 1958; 39:519–28.
15. Georgsson G, Palsson PA. The histopathology of maedi, a slow viral pneumonia of sheep. Vet Pathl 1971; 8:63–80.
16. Pyper JM, Clements JE, Molineaux SM, Narayan O. Genetic variation among ovine-caprine lentiviruses: Homology between visna virus and caprine arthritis-encephalitis virus is confined to the 5′ gag-pol region and a small portion of the env gene. J Virol 1984; 51:713–21.
17. Narayan O, Clements JE, Strandberg JD, Cork LC, Griffin DE. Biological characterization of the virus causing leukoencephalitis and arthritis in goats. J Gen Vir 1980; 41:343–52.
18. Adams DS, Oliver RE, Ameghino E, DeMartini JC, Verwoerd DW, Houvers DJ, Waghela S, Gorham JR, Hyllseth B, Dawson M, Trigo FJ, McGuire TC.

Global survey of serological evidence of caprine arthritis-encephalitis virus infection. Vet Rec 1984; 115:493–5.

19. Dawson M, Venables C, Jenkins CE. Experimental infection of a natural case of sheep pulmonary adenomatosis with maedi-visna virus. Vet Rec 1985; 116;588–9.

20. Narayan O, Wolinsky JA, Clements JE, Strandberg JD, Griffin DE, Cork LC. Slow virus replication: The role of macrophages in the persistence and expression of visna viruses of sheep and goats. J Gen Virol 1982; 59:345–56.

21. Haase AT, Varmus HE. Demonstration of DNA provirus in the lytic growth of visna virus. Nature New Biol 1973; 245:237–9.

22. Gendelman HE, Narayan O, Molineaux S, Clements JE, Ghotbi, Z. Slow persistent replication of lentiviruses: Role of tissue macrophages and macrophage precursors in bone marrow. Proc Natl Acad Sci USA 1985; 82:7086–90.

23. Narayan O, Sheffer D, Clements JE, Tennekoon G. Restricted replication of lentiviruses: Visna viruses induce a unique interferon during interaction between lymphocytes and infected macrophages. J Exp Med 1985; 162:1954–69.

24. Kennedy PGE, Narayan O, Ghotbi Z, Hopkins J, Gendelman HE, Clements JE. Persistent expression of Ia antigen and viral genome in visna-maedi virus-induced inflammatory cells. Possible role of lentivirus-induced interferon. J Exp Med 1985; 162:1970–82.

25. Gendelman HE, Narayan O, Kennedy-Stoskopf S, Kennedy PGE, Ghotbi Z, Clements JE, Stanley J, Pezeshkpour G. Tropism of sheep lentiviruses for monocytes: Susceptibility to infection and virus gene expression increase during maturation of monocytes to macrophages. J Virol 1986; 58:67–74.

26. Sigurdsson B, Palsson PA, Van Bogaert L. Pathology of visna. Acta Neuropath 1962; 1:343–62.

27. Crawford TB, Adams DS. Caprine arthritis-encephalitis: Clinical features and presence of antibody in selected goat populations. J Amer Vet Med Assoc 1981; 178:713–9.

28. Klevjer-Anderson P, McGuire TC. Neutralizing antibody response of rabbits and goats to caprine arthritis-encephalitis virus. Infect Immun 1982; 38:455–61.

29. Narayan O, Sheffer D, Griffin DE, Clements JE, Hess J. Lack of neutralizing antibodies to caprine arthritis-encephalitis lentivirus in persistently infected goats can be overcome by immunization with inactivated *Mycobacterium tuberculosis*. J Virol 1984; 49:349–55.

30. Kono Y, Kobayashi K, Fukunaga Y. Antigenic drift of equine infectious anemia virus in chronically infected horses. Arch Virusforschung 1973; 41:1–10.

31. Montelaro RC, Parekh B, Orrego A, Issel CJ. Antigenic variation during persistent infection by equine infectious anemia virus, a retrovirus. J Biol Chem 1984; 259:10539–44.

32. Narayan O, Griffin DE, Chase J. Antigenic shift of visna virus in persistently infected sheep. Science 1977; 197:376–8.

33. Narayan O, Griffin DE, Clements JE. Virus mutation during "slow infection." Temporal development and characterization of mutants of visna virus recovered from sheep. J Gen Virol 1978; 41:343–52.

34. Kennedy-Stoskopf S, Narayan O. Neutralizing antibodies to visna lentivirus: Mechanism of action and possible role in virus persistence. J Virol 1986; 59:37–44.

35. Vigne R, Filippi P, Querat G, Sauze N, Vitu C, Russo P, DeLori P. Precursor polypeptides to structural proteins of visna virus. J Virol 1982; 42: 1046–56.

36. Harter DH, Choppin PW. Cell fusing activity of visna virus particles. Virology 1967; 31:279.

37. Crane SE, Clements JE, Narayan O. Separate epitopes in the envelope of visna virus are responsible for fusion and neutralization: Biological implications for anti-fusion antibodies in limiting virus replication. J Virol 1988; 62:2680–5.

38. Roberson SM, McGuire TC, Klevjer-Anderson P, Gorham JR, Cheevers WP. Caprine arthritis-encephalitis virus is distinct from visna and progressive pneumonia viruses as measured by genome sequence homology. J Virol 1982; 44:755–8.

39. Chiu IM, Yaniv A, Dahlberg JE, Gazit A, Skuntz SF, Tronick SR, Aaronson SA. Nucleotide sequence evidence for relationship of AIDS retrovirus to lentiviruses. Nature 1985; 317:366–8.

40. Pyper JM, Clements JE, Gonda MA, Narayan O. Sequence homology between cloned CAEV and visna virus, two neurotropic lentiviruses. J Virol 1986; 58:665–70.

41. Yaniv A, Dahlberg JE, Tronick SR, Chiu IM, Aaronson SA. Molecular cloning of integrated caprine arthritis-encephalitis virus. Virology 1985; 145: 340–5.

42. Narayan O, Clements JE, Kennedy-Stoskopf S, Royal W. Antigenic variation in the lentiviruses that cause visna-maedi in sheep and arthritis-encephalitis in goats. In Birkbeck TH, Penn CW, eds. Antigenic variation in infectious diseases, Vol. 19. Oxford: IRL Press,1986:25–40.

43. Narayan O, Clements JE, Kennedy-Stoskopf S, Sheffer D, Royal W. Mechanisms of escape of visna lentiviruses from immunological control. In Cruse JM, Lewis RE, eds. Contributions to microbiology and immunology, Vol 8. Basel: Karger, S, 1987:60–76.

44. Clements JE, D'Antonio N, Narayan O. Genomic changes associated with antigenic variation of visna virus. II. Common nucleotide changes detected in variants from independent isolations. J Mol Biol 1982; 158:415–34.

45. Webster RG, Laver WG, Air GM, Schild GC. Molecular mechanisms of variation in influenza virus. Nature 1982; 296:115–21.

46. Wiktor TJ, Koprowski H. Antigenic variants of rabies virus. J Exp Med 1980; 152:99–112.

47. Ter Muelen V, Loffler S, Carter MJ, Stephenson JR. Antigenic characterization of measles and SSPE virus haemmaglutinin by monoclonal antibodies. J Gen Virol 1981; 57:357–64.

48. Griffin DE, Narayan O, Adams RJ. Early immune response in visna, a slow viral disease of sheep. J Infect Dis 1978; 138:340–50.

49. Gudnadottir M. Visna-maedi in sheep. Prog Med Virol 1974; 18:336–49.

50. Dubois-Dalzq M, Narayan O, Griffin DE. Cell surface changes associated with maturation of visna virus in antibody-treated cell cultures. Virology 1979; 92:353–66.

51. Narayan O, Clements JE, Griffin DE, Wolinsky JS. Neutralizing antibody spectrum determines the antigenic profiles of emerging mutants of visna virus. Infect Immun 1981; 32:1045–50.

52. Clements JE, Pederson FS, Narayan O, Haseltine WS. Genomic changes associated with antigenic variation of visna virus during persistent infection. Proc Natl Acad Sci USA 1980; 77:4454–8.

53. Stanley J, Bhaduri LM, Narayan O, Clements JE. Topographical rearrangements of visna virus envelope glycoprotein during antigenic drift. J Virol 1987; 61:1019–28.

54. Lutley R, Petursson G, Palsson PA, Georgsson G, Klein J, Nathanson N. Antigenic drift in visna. Virus variation during long term infection of Icelandic sheep. J Gen Virol 1983; 64:1433–40.

55. Thormar H, Barshatzky MR, Arnesen K, Koslowski PB. The emergence of antigenic variation is a rare event in long term visna virus infection in vivo. J Gen Virol 1983; 64:1427–32.

56. Thormar H. The growth cycle of visna virus in monolayer cultures of sheep cells. Virology 1963; 19:273–8.

57. Bratt MA, Gallaher WR. Preliminary analysis of the requirements for fusion from within and fusion from without by Newcastle disease virus. Proc Natl Acad Sci 1969; 64:536–43.

58. Clements JE, Narayan O. Two mechanisms for escape from immune surveillance by neurotropic retroviruses. Bioessays 1986; 2:259–62.

59. Barre-Sinoussi F, Chermann JC, Rey F. Isolation of a T-lymphotropic retrovirus from a patient at risk of acquired immunodeficiency syndrome (AIDS). Science 1983; 220:868–71.

60. Popovic M, Sarngadharan MG, Read E, Gallo RC. Detection, isolation and continuous production of cytopathic retroviruses (HTLV–III) from patients with AIDS and pre-AIDS. Science 1984; 224:497–500.

61. Robert-Guroff M, Brown M, Gallo RC. HTLV–III neutralizing antibodies in patients with AIDS and AIDS-related complex. Nature 1985; 316:72–4.

62. Weiss RA, Clapham PR, Cheingsong-Popov R, Dalgleish AG, Carne CA, Weller IV, Tedder RS. Neutralization of human T-lymphotropic virus type III by sera of AIDS and AIDS-risk patients. Nature 1985; 316:69–72.

63. Gartner S, Markovitz P, Markovitz DM, Kaplan MH, Gallo RC, Popovic M. The role of mononuclear phagocytes in HTLV–III/LAV infection. Science 1986; 233:215–9.

64. Salahuddin SZ, Rose RM, Groopman JE, Markham PD, Gallo RC. HTLV-III infection of human alveolar macrophages. Blood 1986;68:281-4.
65. Ho DD, Rota TR, Hirsch MS. Infection of monocyte/macrophages by human T lymphotropic virus type III. J Clin Invest 1986;77:1712-5.
66. Koyanagi Y, Miles S, Mitsuyasu RT, Merrill JE, Vinters HV, Chen ISY. Dual infection of the CNS by AIDS viruses with distinct cellular tropisms. Science 1987;236:819-22.
67. Hahn BH, Gonda MA, Shaw GM, Popovic M, Hoxie JA, Gallo RC, Wong-Staal F. Genomic diversity of the acquired immunodefiency syndrome virus HTLV-III: Different viruses exhibit greatest divergence in their envelope genes. Proc Natl Acad Sci USA 1985;82:4813-7.
68. Hahn BH, Shaw GM, Taylor ME, Redfield RR, Markham PD, Salahuddin SZ, Wong-Staal F, Gallo RC, Parks ES, Parks WP. Genetic variation in HTLV-III/LAV over time in patients with AIDS or at risk for AIDS. Science 1986;232:1548-53.
69. Clements JE. Hypothesis on the molecular basis of nononcogenic retroviral diseases. Rev Infect Dis 1985;7:68-74.

16

Infection of Nonhuman Primates with Human and Simian Immunodeficiency Viruses

Patricia N. Fultz, Harold M. McClure, and Daniel C. Anderson
Yerkes Regional Primate Research Center
Emory University
Atlanta, Georgia

INTRODUCTION

An important step in the development of any vaccine is testing that vaccine for efficacy in the prevention of infection and/or disease. Testing for efficacy, as well as for safety and immunogenicity, is facilitated by the use of animal models, especially in cases where the potential success of a vaccine is questionable. Because of the worldwide spread of the human immunodeficiency virus (HIV) epidemic and the fact that HIV is associated with a disease with essentially 100% mortality, the need for a vaccine against HIV is self-evident. Almost from the time that HIV was identified as the etiologic agent of acquired immunodeficiency syndrome (AIDS), it was apparent that the generation of a vaccine might be difficult for at least two reasons. First, no fully efficacious vaccine against a retrovirus, and none against a lentivirus, existed and, second, all HIV isolates differed from one another in nucleotide sequence, which suggested they might also differ significantly at the antigenic level. These factors emphasized the potential importance of animal models that could be used to test putative vaccines for efficacy, especially those that reproduced the natural history of and disease progression resulting from HIV infection.

The major requirements for an animal model to be useful in vaccine efficacy studies are that 1) essentially all animals become infected following inoculation of virus, 2) infection be easily detected by isolation of virus, which can be quantitated, 3) seroconversion occurs, and 4) infection elicits disease, preferably analogous to disease induced by the same virus in humans. The latter is important if the vaccine does not provide absolute protection against infection, in which case one could monitor and assess the effects of the putative vaccine on prevention or the severity of ensuing disease. This chapter summarizes some of our work on the development and characterization of animal models for AIDS that may be relevant to the generation of a vaccine against HIV. The two model systems described are HIV-1 infection of chimpanzees and simian immunodeficiency virus (isolate SIV/SMM) infection of mangabey and macaque monkeys. Work is in progress to develop a third system—HIV-2 infection of macaques—but the percentage of animals that become infected with HIV-2 following intravenous inoculation is significantly lower than that achieved in the other two systems. At the present time, therefore, this model is not suitable for vaccine studies, but it could be used in the future if a strain of HIV-2 is identified that readily establishes infection in or is adapted for infection of macaques.

HIV-1 INFECTION OF CHIMPANZEES

Although many investigators have attempted to establish infections with HIV-1 in various nonhuman primate and small animal species (1,2), they have, to date, only been able to demonstrate reproducible infections with some strains of HIV-1 in chimpanzees (3-5). Using the LAV-1 strain of HIV, we showed that infections are easily established in chimpanzees by intravenous inoculation of cell-associated or cell-free virus (5) or by application of cell-free virus to vaginal mucosa (6). Within 2 weeks of inoculation and at any time thereafter, HIV-1 was recovered from peripheral blood mononuclear cells (PBMC), irrespective of the inoculum or the route of inoculation, and seroconversion occurred by 1 month after infection, at which time antibodies to *env* and *gag* gene products were easily detected by immunoblot or radioimmunoprecipitation (RIP) assays. Moreover, infections can be established in chimpanzees with relatively low doses of HIV-1 (40 to 100 $TCID_{50}$) (7,8), which is important for vaccine challenge trials.

Aspects of the Model Relevant for Vaccine Testing

Following intravenous inoculation of chimpanzees with LAV-1, virus can be recovered from PBMC within 2 weeks, although with low dose inocula (less than 100 $TCID_{50}$), this interval may be extended by a few weeks. Quantitation of numbers of infected cells in peripheral blood have shown that during the first 2 to 3 months after virus inoculation, 10^3 to 10^4 infectious cells can be detected per 10^7 PBMC. These numbers decrease over time and plateau between 1 and 10 infectious cells per 10^7 PBMC during the first year after infection (5). Isolation of cell-free virus from plasma is more variable; only 6 of 33 samples collected from 2 weeks to 44 months after infection were positive, and all positive samples (6 of 15, 40%) were collected during the first 6 weeks (PNF, unpublished data). These data suggest that, if a vaccine against HIV does not protect absolutely against infection, then it might be possible to detect decreased numbers of infectious cells in vaccinated animals early after challenge, which would provide information on whether a vaccine limited virus replication and/or spread of virus relative to nonvaccinated animals.

Despite the fact that the majority of chimpanzees inoculated with HIV-1 seroconvert within 4 weeks after inoculation and antibody levels increase over subsequent months to titers of greater than 100,000 (as determined by enzyme immunoassay [EIA]), the development of neutralizing antibodies is more variable. Among HIV-infected chimpanzees we tested, the time after infection at which neutralizing antibodies were first detected in serum (tested at a 1:10 dilution) varied from 3 to 9 months. Since all animals developed antibodies to the envelope glycoprotein, gp120, within 4 weeks after inoculation, onset of neutralizing activity did not correlate with the development of antibodies to this protein or to total EIA titers (Table 1). Once detectable, however, neutralizing antibodies persisted and titers generally increased with time. Nara et al. (9) demonstrated that in HIV-infected chimpanzees antibodies capable of neutralizing diverse strains of HIV were generated, but the time course was delayed compared with the type-specific response.

Table 1 Lack of Correlation Between Time After Infection at Which Neutralizing Antibodies Were First Detected and Total HIV–Specific Antibody Titers

Chimpanzee	Virus	Neutralizing antibodies[a]	Antibody EIA titer[b]
C-463	LAV	3 mo	12,800
C-477	LAV	4 mo	12,800
C-550	LAV	6 mo	25,600
C-499	ARV	6 mo	3,200
C-459	LAV	6 mo	51,200
C-487	LAV	9 mo	25,600
C-560	LAV	3 mo	6,400

[a]Months after infection when neutralizing activity was first detected in a 1:10 dilution of serum.
[b]Titers are the last dilution of serum that was positive using the Abbott HTLV-III EIA kit.

The fact that the appearance of neutralizing antibodies is often delayed may present problems in vaccine challenge trials. Even though a vaccine may elicit high titers of antibodies, neutralizing antibodies may not be detected in some animals, or only at low levels, until after an extended period. Thus, challenge trials might have to be delayed and the animals boosted several times before high titers of neutralizing antibodies are generated. It may be that continued exposure to virus in infected animals is necessary to elicit high titers of neutralizing activity capable of neutralizing diverse strains of HIV, in which case it might not be possible for any vaccine to elicit high titers of neutralizing antibodies without multiple, frequent inoculations.

Although there are approximately 100 chimpanzees in the United States that are infected with HIV-1, some for more than 5 years, only two animals have developed any signs of disease (3,7), and both of these animals had persistent generalized lymphadenopathy that regressed after 6 to 8 months. No signs of acute illness have been reported. The fact that no HIV-infected chimpanzee has developed disease resembling AIDS-related complex or AIDS is the only detrimental factor to use of this model system in vaccine testing, and this factor only becomes important if it is impossible to develop a vaccine that protects absolutely from infection. In that instance it is hoped that a vaccine might be developed that could prevent or decrease the severity of disease; however, this could not be tested in the HIV-chimpanzee system.

With respect to lack of HIV-induced disease in chimpanzees, it should be mentioned that, at the present time, this observation may not be significant. Medley et al. (10) estimated that 8 years is the mean incubation time for development of AIDS among persons in the same age range as most HIV-infected chimpanzees. Since only a small number of chimpanzees (probably less than 20) have been infected for as long as 5 years and only about 15% of infected persons might be expected to develop AIDS within a comparable time, it cannot be determined from the available data whether or not HIV-infected chimpanzees will develop disease. Among six chimpanzees at our facility that have been infected with HIV for at least 4 years, two animals have lost antibodies to p24 and a third animal was lymphopenic and thrombocytopenic for more than 1 year. These observations suggest that perhaps some chimpanzees may progress to clinical disease, as has been documented for HIV-infected persons who lose antibodies to p24 (11–13).

Infection of a Chimpanzee with Two Strains of HIV-1

One possible explanation for lack of disease in HIV-infected chimpanzees, other than insufficient elapsed time, could be that multiple exposures to different strains of HIV might be necessary. In experiments that have been reported (14), and that are indirectly related to vaccine development, we addressed the question of whether a chimpanzee could be infected with two distinct isolates of HIV-1 when the second strain was injected after the first had already established infection. If an animal with an ongoing humoral and cellular immune response to one strain of HIV-1 could not be superinfected with a second strain, it would suggest that immune protection may have occurred and that development of a vaccine against HIV might be possible. However, if superinfection could be demonstrated, it would suggest either that it might not be possible to generate an effective vaccine against HIV or that a vaccine against one strain of HIV might not protect against other strains.

A chimpanzee (C-499) was inoculated with the ARV-2 strain (15) (now designated HIV-1$_{SF2}$) of HIV-1. Antibodies to the virus were first detected by EIA at 3 months and virus was first isolated from PBMC at 5 months after inoculation, indicating that ARV-2 could infect chimpanzees, but that the time course of antibody development and ability to isolate virus was slower than observed following inoculation of LAV-1. At 15 months after initial injection of ARV-2, when EIA antibody titers to HIV-1 were 64,000, the chimpanzee was given an intravenous injection of 10^4 TCID$_{50}$ of LAV-1. At the time of LAV-1 inoculation, antibodies capable of neutralizing both ARV-2 and LAV-1 were detectable in serum at titers of 1:20 and 1:10, respectively, and PBMC from the chimpanzee responded normally to mitogenic stimulation, suggesting that cellular immune responses were not defective. Within 6 weeks after injections of LAV-1, total EIA antibody titers increased 10-fold and numbers of infectious cells in PBMC increased more than 1000-fold to levels comparable to those seen early after primary infections (5).

These data suggested that either 1) inoculation of LAV-1 elicited an anamnestic antibody response, 2) LAV-1 elicited antibodies with new specificities and LAV-1 inoculation activated and enhanced replication of ARV-2, or 3) superinfection occurred. To obtain unequivocal evidence that superinfection had occurred, which was the most likely possibility, restriction enzyme analysis of virus recovered from PBMC of chimpanzee C-499 4 weeks after inoculation of LAV-1 was performed. High molecular weight genomic DNA or DNA in Hirt supernatants was obtained from co-cultures of PBMC from C-499 and human PBMC. Following enzymatic digestion with *Kpn*I, the DNA fragments were electrophoresed on an agarose gel, transferred to nitrocellulose paper, and hybridized to a 1.5-kilobase (Kb) fragment from the 3' end of the HIV-1 *env* gene (Fig. 1). After exposure of the nitrocellulose to film, a 4.9-Kb band derived from ARV-2 was detected as well as a 2.7-Kb fragment indicative of LAV-1 (lane 5).

These data provided incontrovertible evidence that LAV-1 established infection in the ARV-2-infected chimpanzee despite the presence of high titers of HIV-specific antibodies and a functional immune system. It can be inferred from this study that the generation of an effective vaccine against HIV may be difficult. It should be noted, however, that at the same time we superinfected the

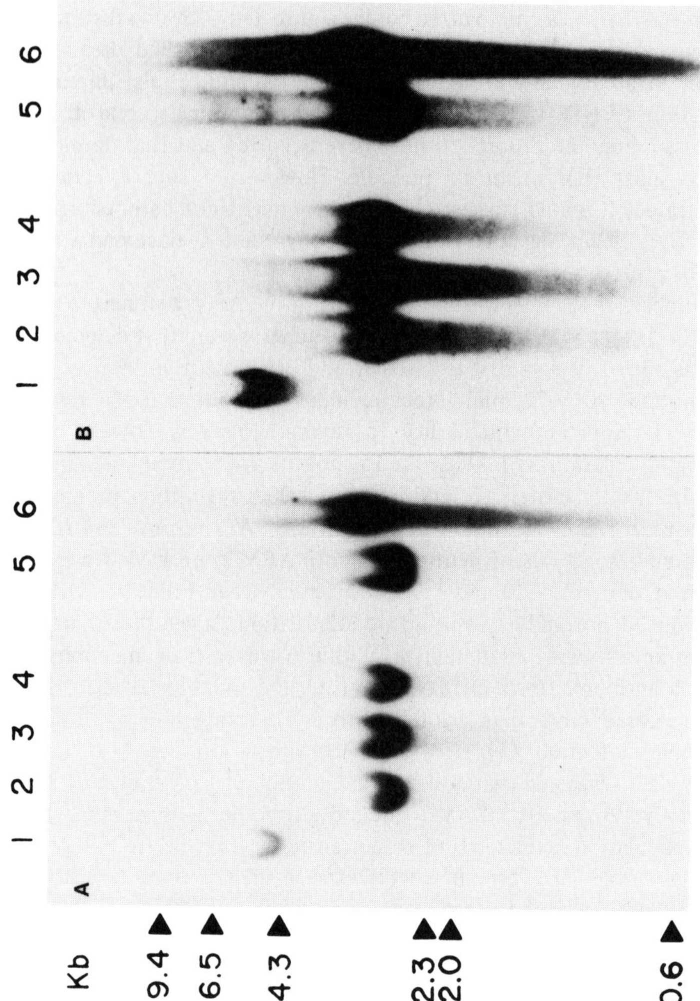

ARV-2-infected chimpanzee with LAV-1, we also reinoculated an LAV-1-infected chimpanzee with LAV-1. No significant changes in antibody titers or numbers of infectious PBMC were detected, which suggests that protection against the homologous strain may have occurred.

SIV/SMM INFECTION OF MACAQUES

SIV/SMM was isolated from naturally infected sooty mangabey monkeys (*Cercocebus atys*) in a breeding colony at the Yerkes Regional Primate Research Center (16). The infection in mangabeys is characterized as a long-term infection that persists in the presence of antibodies to the major *env*- and *gag*-encoded proteins; however, these antibodies have little or no neutralizing activity. Infected mangabeys appear to have high titers of SIV/SMM since infectious virus can be recovered not only from PBMC but also from plasma as cell-free virus (18). Although a majority of the animals tested are infected with SIV/SMM, and the virus has been present in the colony for more than 7 years, there is no apparent difference in the incidence of disease in mangabeys compared with that in other species housed at the Yerkes Center, indicating that SIV/SMM is not usually pathogenic for mangabey monkeys.

To determine whether SIV/SMM was pathogenic for another species of monkey, three groups of macaques (a total of 13 animals that included 12 rhesus and one pig-tailed macaque) were inoculated intravenously with SIV/SMM. All of the animals seroconverted, and virus was isolated on multiple occasions from PBMC of 12 of the 13 animals. The animals have now been infected up to 43 months, during which time eight (62%) animals died between 14 and 43 months after inoculation. Among the animals that died and the survivors that show clinical signs of disease, we have observed (to varying degrees) weight loss, diarrhea, lymphadenopathy, pneumonia, hepatosplenomegaly, skin rash, ataxia, anemia,

---

Figure 1 Southern blot analysis of DNA from PBMC infected with virus obtained from chimpanzees at various times after inoculation of HIV-1 isolates. Autoradiogram developed after 1 (A) or 3 (B) days of exposure. Lane 1, genomic DNA from lymphocytes infected with virus isolated from C-499 6 months after inoculation of ARV-2; lanes 2, 3, and 4, genomic DNA from lymphocytes infected with virus isolated from C-560 at 1, 2, and 6 months, respectively, after inoculation of ARV-2; lanes 5 and 6, Hirt and genomic DNA, respectively, from lymphocytes infected with virus isolated approximately 4 weeks after superinfection of C-499 with LAV-1. *Hind*III-cleaved lambda DNA was used as molecular weight markers, as indicated by arrowheads. DNA from uninfected lymphocytes did not show hybridization with the probe used in our experiments. (From Ref. 14.)

neutropenia, lymphopenia with preferential loss of CD4$^+$ cells, thrombocytopenia, intestinal cryptosporidiosis, and hypo- and hypergammaglobulinemia. Histopathologic analysis of tissue sections from animals that died showed that multinucleated giant cells were a characteristic feature of infection and were observed in large numbers in most tissues, including lymph nodes, spleen, lung, and brain in two of the five animals. These giant cells were shown to be of macrophage lineage, as demonstrated by immunoperoxidase staining for macrophage-specific enzymes (in collaboration with J. Ribas).

Following inoculation of SIV/SMM, the majority of macaques developed antibodies to *env*- and *gag*-encoded proteins between 3 and 6 weeks; however, in agreement with what was observed in mangabeys, little or no neutralizing antibodies were detected in serum from rhesus macaques up to 30 months after infection. Analysis of antibody profiles to SIV/SMM proteins in serum from animals that died of an AIDS-like disease showed that responses varied in different animals: 1) antibodies to all of the major viral proteins persisted throughout infection, 2) antibodies to either *gag* gene products or to a putative *pol* gene product, p32, were lost several months before death, or 3) antibodies to the major *gag* gene product, p28, were not observed at any time during infection. A specific antibody profile, therefore, does not appear to be predictive of severe disease or death, although a pattern may become more apparent when data are obtained on a larger group of animals. We have found, however, that infectious virus can be recovered from both PBMC and serum or plasma of those animals that have more frequent and persistent symptoms of disease but not from those animals that remain well or show only intermittent signs of disease (18).

Infection of macaques with SIV/SMM elicits a spectrum of disease states. At various times after inoculation of SIV/SMM, animals can be identified which have immunologic and clinical profiles comparable to persons classified as asymptomatic or presenting with lymphadenopathy, ARC, or with AIDS. This model, therefore, appears to be an excellent model for HIV infection of humans. It also meets the requirements necessary for vaccine studies (Table 2) in that 100% of inoculated animals became infected and seroconverted and disease analogous to that seen in HIV-infected persons developed in a majority of the animals after a variable latent period. The fact that the SIV group of viruses is diverse at the molecular level (17) also will enable testing of potential vaccines for their ability to protect against homologous and heterologous virus challenge. In addition, because macaques are more readily available, it will be possible to perform vaccine trials by using different routes of virus inoculation for challenge, e.g., via vaginal mucosa, and by challenging with virus-infected cells as well as cell-free virus. It is possible that a vaccine might not protect against intravenous cell-free virus challenge, but could protect against challenge via mucosal surface with cell-associated virus. In the event no vaccine candidate (either HIV

Table 2 Important Elements of the SIV/SMM–Macaque Model System

1. SIV/SMM is a T-lymphotropic lentivirus with regulatory genes and elements analogous to those of HIV.

2. Different SIV isolates display molecular and antigenic heterogeneity analogous to that seen with HIV isolates.

3. Essentially 100% of macaques become infected following inoculation of SIV/SMM.

4. SIV-infected macaques develop an AIDS-like disease.

5. Macaques are more abundant, easier to handle, and cheaper to work with than chimpanzees.

or SIV) can be shown to provide absolute protection against infection, then the SIV-macaque system will be useful for testing potential vaccines for their ability to interfere in disease development.

CONCLUSIONS

Excellent animal models exist for testing candidate vaccines for efficacy against HIV or the closely related simian viruses. Direct testing of vaccines for eventual use in humans is possible using the chimpanzee-HIV model; however, our experiment demonstrating superinfection of a chimpanzee with two diverse strains of HIV-1 suggested an effective universal vaccine might be difficult to produce. This is supported by data from at least three immunization and challenge studies (7,8,19) performed in chimpanzees, all of which failed to protect against infection. All of the first-generation vaccine candidates were composed of different preparations of the envelope glycoproteins in the form of either purified native or recombinant gp120 or gp120 plus gp41 expressed in recombinant vaccinia virus. These early failures underscore the fact that we do not know the identity of the HIV antigens or the types of immune responses necessary for a successful HIV vaccine and indicate that various combinations of antigens administered by different immunizing regimens should be tested. However, the limited number of chimpanzees makes their use prohibitive for such studies and increases the value of the SIV-macaque model for testing prototype vaccines.

ACKNOWLEDGMENTS

This work was supported in part by NIH grant RR-00165 and CDC contract 200-83-0626. The Yerkes Regional Primate Research Center is fully accredited by the American Association for Accreditation of Laboratory Animal Care.

REFERENCES

1. Fultz PN, Morrow WJW. Experimental models of HIV infection. In Wormser GP, ed. AIDS and other manifestations of HIV infection. New Jersey: Noyes Publications, 1987:257–69.
2. Morrow WJW, Wharton M, Lau D, Levy JA. Small animals are not susceptible to human immunodeficiency virus infection. J Gen Virol 1987; 68: 2253–7.
3. Alter HJ, Eichberg JW, Masur H, Saxinger WC, Gallo R, Macher AM, Lane HC, Fauci AS. Transmission of HTLV–III infection from human plasma to chimpanzees: An animal model for AIDS. Science 1984; 226:549–52.
4. Gajdusek DC, Gibbs CJ, Jr., Rodgers-Johnson P, Amyx HL, Asher DM, Epstein LG, Sarin PS, Gallo RC, Maluish A, Arthur LA, Montagnier L, Mildvan D. Infection of chimpanzees by human T-lymphotropic retroviruses in brain and other tissues from AIDS patients. Lancet 1985; 1:55–6.
5. Fultz PN, McClure HM, Swenson RB, McGrath CR, Brodie A, Getchell JP, Jensen FC, Anderson DC, Broderson JR, Francis DP. Persistent infection of chimpanzees with HTLV–III/LAV: A potential model for acquired immunodeficiency syndrome. J Virol 1986; 58:116–24.
6. Fultz PN, McClure HM, Daugharty H, Brodie A, McGrath CR, Swenson B, Francis DP. Vaginal transmission of human immunodeficiency virus (HIV) to a chimpanzee. J Infect Dis 1986; 154:896–900.
7. Hu S-L, Fultz PN, McClure HM, Eichberg JW, Thomas EK, Zarling J, Singhal MC, Kosowski SG, Swenson RB, Anderson DC, Todaro G. Effect of immunization with a vaccinia-HIV *env* recombinant on HIV infection of chimpanzees. Nature 1987; 328:721–3.
8. Arthur LO, Robey WG, Pyle SW, Bess JW, Nara P, Kelliher J, Gilden RV, Fischinger PJ. Preparation and evaluation of an HIV outer envelope glycoprotein prototype vaccine. Presentation at Meeting on Modern Approaches to New Vaccines including Prevention of AIDS, September, 1987, Cold Spring Harbor.
9. Nara PL, Robey WG, Arthur LO, Asher DM, Wolff AV, Gibbs CJ, Jr., Gajdusek DC, Fischinger PJ. Persistent infection of chimpanzees with human immunodeficiency virus: Serological responses and properties of reisolated viruses. J Virol 1987; 61:3173–80.
10. Medley GF, Anderson RM, Cox DR, Billard L. Incubation period of AIDS in patients infected via blood transfusion. Nature 1987; 328:719–21.
11. Allain J-P, Laurian Y, Paul DA, Verroust F, Leuther M, Gazengel C, Senn D, Larrieu M-J, Bosser C. Long-term evaluation of HIV antigen and antibodies to p24 and gp41 in patients with hemophilia. N Engl J Med 1987; 317:1114–21.
12. Lange JMA, Paul DA, Huisman HG, deWolf F, vandenBerg H, Coutinho RA, Danner SA, vanderNoordaa J, Goudsmit J. Persistent HIV antigenaemia and decline of HIV core antibodies associated with transition to AIDS. Br Med J 1986; 293:1459–62.

13. Weber JN, Weiss RA, Roberts C, Weller I, Tedder RS, Clapham PR, Parker D, Duncan J, Carne C, Pinching AJ, Cheingsong-Popov R. Human immunodeficiency virus infection in two cohorts of homosexual men: Neutralising sera and association of anti-gag antibody with prognosis. Lancet 1987; 1:119-21.

14. Fultz PN, Srinivasan A, Greene CR, Butler D, Swenson RB, McClure HM. Superinfection of a chimpanzee with a second strain of human immunodeficiency virus. J Virol 1987; 61:4026-9.

15. Levy JA, Hoffman AD, Kramer SM, Landis JA, Shimabukuro JM, Oshiro LS. Isolation of lymphocytopathic retroviruses from San Francisco patients with AIDS. Science 1984; 225:840-2.

16. Fultz PN, McClure HM, Anderson DC, Swenson RB, Anand R, Srinivasan A. Isolation of a T-lymphotropic retrovirus from naturally infected sooty mangabey monkeys (*Cercocebus atys*). Proc Natl Acad Sci 1986; 83:5286-90.

17. Kestler HW, Li Y, Naidu YM, Butler CV, Ochs MF, Jaenel G, King NW, Daniel MD, Desrosiers RC. Comparison of simian immunodeficiency virus isolates. Nature 1988; 331:619-22.

18. Fultz PN, Stricker RB, McClure HM, Anderson DC, Switzer WM, Horaist C. Humoral response to SIV/SMM infection in macaque and mangabey monkeys. J AIDS 1990; 3: in press.

19. Berman PW, Groopman JE, Gregory T, Clapham PR, Weiss RA, Ferriani R, Riddle L, Shimasaki C, Lucas C, Lasky LA, Eichberg JW. Human immunodeficiency virus type 1 challenge of chimpanzees immunized with recombinant envelope glycoprotein gp120. Proc Natl Acad Sci 1988; 85:5200-4.

17

Relevant Aspects of HIV-Related Viruses to Vaccine Development

Phyllis J. Kanki and Max Essex
Harvard AIDS Institute
Harvard University
Boston, Massachusetts

Jorg W. Eichberg
Southwest Foundation for Biomedical Research
San Antonio, Texas

For centuries, scientists have studied various animal species and their diseases as models of disease in people. The evolutionary similarities of various members of the order Primates have frequently provided unique parallels of natural and disease processes in humans. Monkeys and apes have sometimes been the only animal species other than man infected with important human viruses such as polio, hepatitis B virus, measles, yellow fever, and Marburg virus. In the cases of yellow fever, Marburg virus, and measles, it has been thought that wild monkeys harbor these infections and in some instances may be the source of human infections. In addition, these primate models have proven invaluable for the study of disease pathogenesis and ultimate vaccine and therapeutic testing. The close phylogenetic relationship of primates to man obviously increases the significance and practical applicability of these studies to human disease. It was therefore not surprising that simian (monkey) relatives to the known human retroviruses have been identified. The first of these simian viruses discovered was simian T-lymphotropic virus (STLV), the simian counterpart of human T-lymphotropic virus (HTLV) in people (1). STLV shares many properties with HTLV including virus structure, antigens, genomic organization, and in vitro immortalization capabilities. The viral antigens of STLV and HTLV are highly cross-reactive and virtually indistinguishable by most standard serologic techniques (2). Genetic studies showed that STLV viruses had a similar genomic organization and were 90-95% homologous in nucleotide sequence to the human virus, HTLV (3). Besides these virological similarities, the monkey and human viruses also showed similar in vivo properties. Asian macaques with malignant lymphoma at the New England Regional Primate Research Center showed high rates of STLV when compared to normal healthy macaques (2). Thus, it appears that STLV may be capable of inducing lymphoid neoplasm in monkeys similar to HTLV-induced ATLL in people.

The discovery of STLV prompted numerous studies to determine the distribution of this virus in various primate species worldwide. It was hoped that this data would provide some clues as to the geographic or evolutionary origin of HTLV. STLV infects both Asian and African Old World primates and apes, including the gorilla and chimpanzee; in various antibody studies, rates of infection in these species varied from 1 to 40% (4). Unfortunately, the geographic distribution of STLV—infected primates and HTLV-infected humans did not seem to overlap. However, genetic studies of STLVs from Asian and African primates showed that the human virus was more closely related to African chimpanzee or African green monkey STLV (95%) and less related to the Asian macaque STLV (90%) (3).

The distribution of STLV infection in all species of Old World primates and apes appeared to indicate that the progenitor virus of HTLV and STLV infected the anthropoid ancestor primate after the divergence of New World primates, dating back to the Eocene period 40 million years ago. One hypothesis regarding the origin of HTLV relies on the premise that the 5-10% genetic sequence difference between STLV and HTLV is significantly great enough to rule out the possibility that human infection by the monkey virus could have occurred some time after the Eocene period. Therefore, HTLV would have evolved from the virus infecting the hominoid ancestor that gave rise to the Great Apes, which include the chimpanzee, orangutan, gorilla, and man. Parallel evolution of the STLV and HTLV viruses within their respective species hosts would have to be virtually identical, resulting in viruses that are presently less than 5% different. Other scientists felt that it was unlikely that retroviruses could maintain such a high degree of similarity after millions of years of evolution in an evolving host species. This would mean that STLV-infected primates could have infected humans in more recent times, within the last 40 million years. Regardless of how STLV and HTLV entered their respective host species, it is obvious from the data available that their evolutionary origins were inextricably linked. This provided the impetus to look for related monkey viruses when the human immunodeficiency virus (HIV) was later discovered. The STLV system provides an important animal model in which T-lymphotropic virus pathogenesis may be studied either through investigations of naturally infected animals or through inoculation experiments. Relevant vaccine candidates for HTLV-1 can be readily tested in the monkey system to evaluate protection from the closely related STLV-1 virus.

By 1985, the virus responsible for human AIDS, eventually termed HIV-1, had been largely characterized. Based on our experience with the T-lymphotropic viruses of monkeys and man, STLV and HTLV, we investigated the possibility that a simian relative to HIV-1 might exist. We were successful in finding HIV-1 cross-reactive antibodies in serum samples from immunosuppressed Asian macaque monkeys (*Macaca* sp.) housed at the New England Regional Primate Research Center (NERPRC) in Southborough, Massachusetts (5). In studies done in collaboration with the NERPRC, this virus was isolated and characterized (5,6). This new simian retrovirus, simian immunodeficiency virus (SIV), previously termed STLV, was clearly related to HIV, as predicted by the antibody studies.

Subsequent genetic studies have shown that SIV is approximately 50% related to HIV-1 based on nucleotide sequence (7,8). The organization of the various structural and regulatory genes of SIV is virtually identical to that of HIV-1. Notable exceptions are the *vpx* gene of SIV and HIV-2, which is not found in HIV-1, and the lack of a *vpu* gene, which is unique to HIV-1. In experiments where SIV was injected into Asian macaques, infection caused a decrease in T4 lymphocytes with ensuing immunosuppression and antibodies to *vpx* were detected (9,10). These animals died with opportunistic infections bearing striking similarity to the clinical picture of human AIDS. The virology, host immune response, and disease induction of SIV provide striking parallels to HIV and AIDS. SIV therefore represents a system in which various AIDS drugs and vaccines can be readily tested. SIV is the closest known animal retrovirus to HIV-1, based on antigenic, genetic, and pathobiologic features. The utility of this simian lentivirus model for the study of human AIDS viruses can be summarized in the following areas: virology, host immune response, and disease pathogenesis.

VIROLOGY OF SIV

SIV (STLV-3) was first described in captive macaques in 1985 (5,6) as a primate T-lymphotropic virus related to HIV-1. Evidence of SIV has also been described in African green monkeys, African sooty mangabeys, and captive macaques (11–16). The results of seroepidemiologic studies in a variety of primate species are given in Table 1. Antibody status was determined by immunoblot and radioimmunoprecipitation analysis on SIV antigens. The similarities of this virus to HIV-1 include: T-cell tropism, ultrastructural morphology, antigenic similarities

Table 1 Antibodies to SIV in Primates

Species	Total number tested	Antibodies SIV
African		
Gorilla	5	0 (0%)
Chimpanzee	30	0 (0%)
Baboon	126	0 (0%)
Colobus monkey	5	0 (0%)
Patas monkey	95	0 (0%)
Mandrill	5	2 (40%)
Mangabey	10	2 (20%)
Talpoins	11	11 (100%)
African green monkey	772	243 (31%)
Asian		
Macaca sp.		
Captive—AIDS-like syndrome	153	35 (23%)
Macaca sp.		
Captive—healthy	206	0 (0%)
Macaca sp.		
Wild-caught—healthy	266	0 (0%)

and cross-reactivity, genomic organization, and 50–60% genetic homology. Importantly, SIV infection in macaques induces an immunodeficiency syndrome similar to that of human AIDS.

A number of virologic issues important to our understanding of HIV viruses of people may be addressed in the SIV system. The role of genetic diversity in SIVs from various primate species and within one infected primate needs to be evaluated. At present, full nucleotide sequence is available on a few SIV isolates (7,8) with approximately 10% nucleotide difference. The fact that SIV is not found in wild-caught Asian macaques (17) indicates the possibility that SIVmac resulted from infection from another primate species. Prior to evaluation of species-specific genetic diversity, the origin of the SIVmac must be determined.

SIV is similar to HIV-2 and possesses a number of accessory genes with variable homology to HIV-1 genes; these include: *tat, rev, nef, vif,* and *vpr.* Functional evidence of *tat* activity has been shown for SIV, similar and cross-reactive with HIV-1 *tat* (18). A unique gene to SIV and HIV-2, termed *vpx*, appears to be expressed in the SIV virus and is immunogenic in infected monkeys (19). Mutational studies have shown that *vpx* is dispensable for virus replication (19). Comparative analysis of the various regulatory genes' function and correlation to the biological effects of these viruses may provide important clues to the unique pathogenicity of HIV-1.

The existence of conserved epitopes in the major viral antigens of SIV and HIV was the mechanism by which these viruses were first discovered (5,11). Studies on the major envelope protein of HIV-1 have delineated a number of important functional domains that are highly conserved in SIV (7,20). Selected regions of the SIV and HIV-1 envelope genes show up to 45% amino acid homology; these are frequently regions that are also highly conserved between HIV-1 isolates. Such conserved epitopes on the envelope antigens of SIV and HIV-1 may be important as future vaccine candidates. These may be readily tested in the SIV model prior to testing in the HIV-1 system with chimpanzees or people.

HOST IMMUNITY TO SIV

The identification of protective host immune factors in HIV infection is central to the development of an effective vaccine. SIV infection in Asian macaques is linked to immunodeficiency; however, SIV infection in African green monkeys appears to be innocuous. African green monkeys, also called grivets, vervets, and guenons, are a heterogeneous group of Cercopithecine subspecies that are widely distributed throughout most of sub-Saharan Africa. Not only do Cercopithecine monkeys have the highest rates of SIV infection, but they also are among the more ecologically successful African primate species. This seems to indicate that the SIV virus infection could not be causing long-term adverse selection pressure in the species.

SIV does not appear to be immunosuppressive in other African primates such as the sooty mangabey (13,14), talopoin, or mandrill (21). SIV inoculation in baboons resulted in successful infection but no evidence of immunosuppressive disease (10). Why SIV fails to cause disease in African monkeys, in which the infection appears to be endemic, but causes severe immunosuppressive disease in captive Asian macaques, is an enigma. It seems quite possible that infection in captive Asian monkeys may have inadvertently begun when they were accidentally exposed to African monkeys in holding facilities. However, the severe disease induced in Asian monkeys by SIV suggests that the pathogenic determinants of this virus may be dependent on host factors for expression. The infected species of African monkeys would presumably then have evolved protective mechanisms to prevent a potentially lethal pathogen from causing disease. This situation might then be similar to that seen with the Epstein-Barr virus (EBV) in people. Almost all of us become latently infected with EBV for life, and some may experience mild mononucleosis, but few if any develop a lethal disease. It seems logical that retroviruses, like other infectious agents, may be most highly pathogenic when they first enter a new species. Evolutionary selection for survival on the part of both the virus and the species might then ensue. The apparent species-specific pathogenicity of SIV may provide important clues to viral-host mechanisms that results in protection from disease development. The West African HIV-2 virus that is more closely related to SIV than HIV-1 also appears to demonstrate a difference in relative pathogenicity (22–24).

The humoral immune response of SIV-infected primates appears to parallel that of people to HIV-1. The envelope antigens appear to be the most immunogenic in exposed primates and less frequently antibody response to *pol*- and/or *gag*-encoded antigens is seen (5,10,11).

Naturally infected African green monkeys show a significant anti-*env* response but less frequently mount antibodies to the *gag* or *pol* gene products (11,12). In contrast, inoculated macaques that have gone on to develop AIDS-like syndromes show antibodies to the *env, gag,* and *pol* encoded antigens of SIV (10). In some inoculation studies rapid progress to AIDS-like syndromes and death have been reported; in some of these no detectable antibody response has been found by Western blot or radioimmunoprecipitation techniques. The evidence for SIV's role in the immunosuppression and subsequent death relies solely on virus isolation results (9,21,25). The humoral response in infected primates appears to follow similar kinetics to that of HIV-1–infected people and antibodies are persistent throughout. Virus-neutralizing titers appear to be low and variable in infected primates (14,25, D. Ho and P. J. Kanki, unpublished data), similar to HIV-1 infected people. The role of cell-mediated responses in the SIV system has been less well studied to date.

DISEASE PATHOGENESIS IN SIV

One of the most significant aspects of the SIV model is the ability of this virus to induce immunodeficiency in the macaque monkey. There are many similarities in the natural history of SIV-induced immunodeficiency and human AIDS. SIV infected macaques have shown T4-cell diminution and dysfunction with death due to opportunistic infections. In addition, it is believed that SIV is also capable of crossing the blood brain barrier. Inoculated macaques develop neuropathologic disease similar to the viral encephalopathies observed in AIDS patients (9). An animal model system that demonstrates a similar disease process in a primate host has obvious utility for drug and vaccine development. However, standardization of inoculation protocols and virus titration will be necessary prior to more general use of the SIV system for HIV therapeutic testing. Acutely pathogenic strains of SIV may be useful for certain types of studies; however, the normal long latency of SIV infection is one of the most striking parallels to the HIV system.

There is no doubt that the SIV system will play an important role in the continued research on HIV viruses. As standardization of SIV inoculation protocols in macaques is established, this system will provide an excellent animal model system for AIDS drug and vaccine testing. The close relationship of this simian virus to human AIDS viruses provides an excellent animal system for comparative studies. Importance must be placed on the utility of this system to better understand the pathogenesis of HIV/SIV-induced disease. The complexities of the virus-host interactions that lead to pathology may well be worked out in such an animal system and shed new light on the pathogenesis of HIV-induced disease in people.

ACKNOWLEDGMENT

This work was supported by DAMD 17-87-C-7072.

REFERENCES

1. Miyoshi I, Yoshimoto S, Fujishita M, Taguchi H, Kubonishi I, Niiya K, Minezawa M. Natural adult T-cell leukemia virus infection in Japanese monkeys. Lancet 1982; 2:658.
2. Homma T, Kanki PJ, King NW, Hunt RD, O'Connell MJ, Letvin NL, Daniel MD, Desrosiers RC, Yang CS, Essex M. Lymphoma in macaques: Association with exposure to virus of human T lymphotropic family. Science 1984; 225:716-8.
3. Watanabe T, Seiki M, Hirayama Y, Yoshida M. Human T-cell leukemia virus type I is a member of the African subtype of simian viruses (STLV). Virology 1986; 148, 385-8.
4. Hayami M, Komuro A, Nozawa K. Prevalence of antibody to adult T-cell leukemia virus-associated antigens (ATLA) in Japanese monkeys and other non-human primates. Intl J Cancer 1984; 33:179.
5. Kanki PJ, McLane MF, King NW Jr, Letvin NL, Hunt RD, Sehgal P, Daniel MD, Desrosiers RC, Essex M. Serological identification and characterization of a macaque T-lymphotropic retrovirus closely related to HTLV–III. Science 1985; 228:1199-201.
6. Daniel MD, Letvin NL, King NW, Kannagi M, Sehgal PK, Hunt RD, Kanki PJ, Essex M, Desrosiers RD. Isolation of T-lymphotropic retrovirus related to HTLV III-like retrovirus from Macaques. Science 1985; 228:1201-4.
7. Franchini G, Gurgo C, Guo HG, Gallo RC, Collalti E, Fargnoli KA, Hall LF, Wong-Staal F, Reitz MS. Sequence of simian immunodeficiency virus and its relationship to the human immunodeficiency viruses. Nature 1987; 328: 539-43.
8. Chakrabati L, Guyader M, Alizon M, Daniel MD, Desrosiers RC, Tiollais P, Sonigo P. Sequence of simian immunodeficiency virus from macaque and

its relationship to other human and simian retroviruses. Nature 1987; 328:543-7.

9. Letvin NL, Daniel MD, Sehgal PK, Desrosers RD, Hunt RD, Waldron LM, Mackey JJ, Schmidt DK, Chalifoux LV, King NW. Induction of AIDS-like disease in macaque monkeys with T-cell tropic retrovirus STLV-III. Science 1985; 230:71-3.

10. Kanki PJ, Eichberg JW, and Essex M. Differential pathogenicity of SIV in macaques and baboons. In preparation.

11. Kanki PJ, Kurth R, Becher W, Dreesman G, Mclane MF, Essex M. Antibodies to simian T-lymphotropic virus type III in African green monkeys and recognition of STLV-III viral proteins by AIDS and related sera. Lancet 1985; 2:1330-2.

12. Kanki PJ, Alroy J, Essex M. Isolation of T-lymphotropic retrovirus related to HTLV-III/LAV from wild-caught African green monkeys. Science 2985; 230:951-4.

13. Murphey-Corb M, Martin LN, Rangan SRS, Baskin GB, Gormus BJ, Wolf RH, Andes WA, West M, Montelaro RC. Isolation of an HTLV-III related retrovirus from macaques with simian AIDS and its possible origin in asymptomatic mangabeys. Nature 1986; 321:435-7.

14. Fultz, PN, McClure HM, Anderson DC, Swenson RB, Anand R, Srinivasan A. Isolation of a T-lymphotropic retrovirus from naturally infected sooty mangabey monkeys (Cercocebus atys). PNAS 1986; 83:5286-90.

15. Benveniste RE, Arthur LO, Tsai C, Sowder R, Copeland TD, Henderson LE, Oroszlan S. Isolation of a lentivirus from a macaque with lymphoma. Comparison with HTLV-III/LAV and other lentiviruses. J Virol 1986; 60: 483-90.

16. Lowensteine LJ, Pederson NC, Higgins J, Pallis KC, Uyeda A, Marx P, Lerche NW, Munn RJ, Gardner MB. Seroepidemiologic survey of captive Old World primates for antibodies to human and simian retroviruses and isolation of a lentivirus from sooty mangabeys. Int J Cancer 1986; 38: 563-74.

17. Chou MJ, Kanki PJ, Essex M. Absence of natural SIV infection in healthy macaque monkeys, in preparation.

18. Arya SK, Beaver B, Jagodzinski L, Ensoli B, Kanki PJ, Albert J, Fenyo E-M, Biberfeld G, Zagury JF, Laure F, Essex M, Norrby E, Wong-Staal F, Gallo RC. New human and simian HIV-related retroviruses possess functional transactivator (tat) gene. Nature 1987; 328:548-50.

19. Yu XF, Ito S, Essex M, Lee TH. A naturally immunogenic virion-associated protein specific for HIV-2 and SIV. Nature 1988; 335:262-5.

20. Hirsch V, Riedel N, Mullins JI. The genome organization of STLV-3 is similar to that of the AIDS virus except for a truncated transmembrane protein. Cell 1987; 49:307-19.

21. Kanki PJ, Essex M. Unpublished data.

22. Barin F, M'Boup S, Denis F, Kanki P, Allan JS, Lee TH, Essex M. Serological evidence for virus related to simian T-lymphotropic retrovirus III in residents of West Africa. Lancet 1985; 2:1387-9.

23. Kanki PJ, M'Boup S, Ricard D, Barin F, Denis F, Boye C, Sangare L, Travers K, Albaum M, Marlink R, Romet-Lemonne J.-L, Essex M. Human T-lymphotropic virus type 4 and the human immunodeficiency virus in West Africa. Science 1987; 236:827–31.

24. Marlink R, Ricard D, M'Boup S, Kanki P, Romet-Lemonne J-L, N'Doye I, Diop K, Simpson M-A, Greco F, Chou M-J, DeGruttola V, Hseih C-C, Boye C, Barin F, Denis F, McLane M-F, Essex M. Clinical, hematological, and immunological evaluation of individuals exposed to human immunodeficiency virus type 2 (HIV-2). AIDS Research & Human Retroviruses 1988: 4:137–48.

25. Kannagi M, Kiyotaki M, Desrosiers RC, Reimann KA, King NW, Waldron LM, Letvin NL. Humoral immune responses to T-cell tropic retrovirus simian T-lymphotropic virus type III in monkeys with experimentally induced acquired immunodeficiency-like syndrome. J Clin Invest 1986; 78:1229–36.

18

Use of Simian Immunodeficiency Virus for AIDS Vaccine Research

Ronald C. Desrosiers, Yen Li, and Muthiah D. Daniel
New England Regional Primate Research Center
Harvard Medical School
Southborough, Massachusetts

The development of most viral vaccines for use in humans relied heavily on animal models for safety and efficacy testing. It has been estimated that tens of thousands of macaque monkeys were used for the development of the polio-virus vaccines (1,2), and thousands continue to be used each year for testing of production lots. It is conceivable that a vaccine against the human AIDS virus could be developed without significant involvement of animal models. In fact, two products are currently in phase I trials in humans in the United States without any demonstrated efficacy in an animal model (3). Over the long run, however, it seems likely that animal model testing will play an important role in the development of the best possible AIDS vaccines.

The viruses that cause AIDS in humans, HIV-1 and HIV-2, are members of the lentivirus subfamily of retroviruses. Several characteristics that are unique to this subfamily suggest that the best models for AIDS vaccine development will be the lentiviral ones. The lentiviruses have a more complicated life cycle than the other retroviruses. This more complicated life cycle is reflected by their increased genetic complexity and a wealth of viral and host factors which exert controlling effects on viral gene expression. HIV, for example, contains six genes that other retroviruses do not; three of these (*tat*, *rev*, and *nef*) are thought to play a role in controlling viral gene expression. Another feature that appears somewhat unique to the lentiviruses is the nature of the persistent infection and the chronic disease that is eventually induced. The lentiviruses are not oncogenic but instead induce chronic, debilitating disease following long-term persistent infection. In spite of a strong immune response, virus persists throughout the body by mechanisms that are not yet well understood. After a prolonged course, usually years, the immune defenses can be defeated and the host succumbs.

HIV is able to infect chimpanzees (see Chapters 9 and 16), rabbits (4,5), and humanized SCID mice (6,7); these systems can thus be considered for use in AIDS vaccine research. Other species might also be infectable by HIV, and continued research along these lines is warranted. Work with rabbits and SCID mice is still at a very early stage, and their eventual utility is not yet clear. Infection of chimpanzees has a number of attractive features for vaccine studies. They are readily infected with the same virus that is the primary cause of AIDS in humans, HIV-1. Furthermore, the infection is persistent, apparently similar to persistent infection of humans with HIV. Thus, HIV-1 vaccine materials can be tested in chimpanzees for their ability to protect against infection following challenge by live HIV-1. Use of chimpanzees for such research suffers from two main drawbacks. First, chimpanzees do not develop disease following HIV-1 infection. It is conceivable that a vaccine could protect against disease induction without preventing infection. In the HIV-chimpanzee system, there is no disease to measure. Second, chimpanzees are available only in very limited numbers. Well-organized national chimpanzee breeding and usage programs are in place to help enforce conservative use of chimpanzees and to guarantee their continued availability and well-being; however, their numbers remain small. Chimpanzees will undoubtedly play an important role in AIDS vaccine research and development, but it is obvious that the number of experiments that can be done with them is limited.

The simian immunodeficiency viruses (SIVs) are nonhuman primate lentiviruses related to the human AIDS viruses HIV-1 and HIV-2; they are the closest known relatives to the HIVs (for review, see Ref. 8). To date, SIV has been isolated from macaques, African green monkeys, sooty mangabeys, and mandrills (Table 1).

The importance of SIV systems for AIDS vaccine research is derived from the following:

1. *Extensive genetic similarity*: To date, the genomes of SIV from macaques (SIV$_{mac}$) and SIV from African green monkeys have been sequenced in their entirety (9,10). These SIV sequences reveal a genome organization very similar or identical to that of HIV-1 or HIV-2 with extensive homology over each of the corresponding genes. Differences have been noted in some of the open reading frames of the intergenic region, but even HIV-1 and HIV-2 differ in this regard (Table 2). Recent sequence information actually suggests that SIV from sooty mangabey monkeys may be a source of cross-species infection of humans for the origin of HIV-2 in west

Table 1 Infection of Nonhuman Primates with SIV

New World Primates
  No known examples
Asian Old World primates
  Macaques
    Captivity (SIVmac) (rare)
    Wild (no known examples)
African Old World primates
  Green monkeys
    Captivity (SIVagm)
    Wild (SIVagm) (20–50%)
  Mangabeys
    Captivity (SIVsmm or man)
    Wild (SIVsmm or man)
  Baboons
    Captivity (no known examples)
    Wild (SIVagm?) (rare 2/279)
  Mandrills
    Captivity (?)
    Wild (SIVmand) (2/16)

Africa and of macaques in captivity for the origin of SIVmac (11, 19).

2. *Ability to induce AIDS*: Natural infection of green monkeys and sooty mangabeys with their own SIV does not appear to be associated with any disease. Infection of macaque monkeys with at least some strains of SIV,

Table 2 Open Reading Frames of Intergenic Region

Gene	HIV-1	HIV-2	SIVmac	SIVagm
VPU	+	–	–	–
VPX	–	+	+	+
VPR	+	+	+	–
TAT	+	+	+	+
REV	+	+	+	+
VIP	+	+	+	+

most notably those obtained from macaques and sooty mangabeys, can cause a fatal disease remarkably similar to AIDS in humans (12-18). Some early passage stocks of SIV are able to induce AIDS and death in 3-5 months (12,13,18). One isolate of SIV kills macaques in 1-2 weeks (P. Fultz, personal communication). Even in cases where death is not so rapid, macaques remain persistently infected and eventually succumb 1-3 years or even later following initial infection. Macaques that die with SIV infection exhibit clinical signs and pathologic findings remarkably similar to AIDS in humans. These include diarrhea, wasting, thymic atrophy, immune abnormalities, decreases in T4-cell numbers, opportunistic infections, lymphomas, and a characteristic encephalitis. Opportunistic infections that have been observed include cytomegalovirus, *Pneumocystis carinii*, adenovirus, *Mycobacterium avium–M. intracelluris* complex, *Cryptosporidium*, and *Candida*. The brain lesions have been described as a multifocal, perivascular granulomatous encephalitis with multinucleated macrophages harboring SIV, very similar if not identical to the brain pathology observed in human AIDS (15). Thus, the use of SIV for AIDS vaccine research allows study not only of the ability to protect against virus infection, but also the ability to protect against disease induction in a reasonable time frame.

3. *Availability of experimental animals*: Rhesus monkeys (*Macaca mulatta*) and cynomolgus monkeys (*Macaca fascicularis*) are not endangered in the wild, and they still can be purchased at a reasonable cost ($1,000-$2,000) from importers. Furthermore, macaques breed well in captivity and with suitable planning can be made available in large numbers for vaccine studies. The seven U.S. Regional Primate Research Centers alone have over 15,000 total macaque monkeys, including approximately 9500 rhesus; this certainly must represent only a small fraction of the total U.S. captive macaque population. A single male and 10 females can be expected to yield eight viable births per year in a suitable breeding situation.

The similar genome organization, the extensive sequence homology, and the similarity in biological properties both in vitro and in vivo suggest a certain commonality between the SIVs and the HIVs. Most fundamental observations made in the SIV system are likely to be extrapolatable to HIV in humans and vice versa.

In our own vaccine studies to date, we have obtained results using purified, inactivated, whole SIV as immunogen and live SIV for challenge (20). These studies are considered to be in a preliminary stage, but a brief summary will be given here. In our first study using inactivated whole virus, vaccinated macaques were challenged intravenously with 1 ml of undiluted, cell-free, cell culture–grown SIV long after the peak of vaccine-induced antibody titer.

All four vaccinated-challenged macaques became persistently infected, and three of these four died with AIDS 258–347 days postinoculation. In subsequent experiments using a total of six vaccinated macaques and four controls, we improved the regimen of inactivated whole virus administration such that vaccinated macaques had SIV-neutralizing antibody titers of ~1:160 (sensitive MT4 cell killing assay) on the day of live virus challenge. Macaques were challenged intramuscularly with 1 ml of 10^{-3} or 2×10^{-4} dilution of the same strain of SIV that was used for vaccination; we know these amounts to represent 1000 and 200 animal infectious doses, respectively, since the challenge stock has been titered in rhesus macaques by the same IM route. Four of four control unvaccinated macaques became infected with these challenge doses, as expected. SIV recovery from peripheral blood and induction of an anamnestic antibody response were used to assess SIV infection in vaccinated-challenged macaques; two of six previously vaccinated macaques appear to have been protected against SIV infection at this time. Experiments to detect DNA in blood and in lymph nodes by PCR and by in situ hybridization are in progress.

Is there any reason to gain encouragement from apparent protection of only two of six macaques in a highly artificial, optimized laboratory setting? We think so. This represents the first apparent vaccine protection in any lentivirus system and suggests that vaccine protection against HIV is at least theoretically possible. Furthermore, inactivated SIV (or HIV) is not in general a good immunogen because the gp120 *env* protein is highly underrepresented in virus preparations. It seems likely that much better results could be obtained with better immunogens.

The road to a safe, effective AIDS vaccine is not likely to be easy. Careful, systematic comparison of a variety of vaccine approaches as well as the variables associated with each approach will be needed if we are to develop the best

Table 3 Possible Vaccine Strategies for AIDS

Inactivated whole virus

Subunit proteins

Synthetic peptides

Immune stimulatory complexes (ISCOMS)

Anti-idiotypes

Infectious recombinant viruses such as vaccinia

Recombinant microorganisms

Live attenuated virus

Table 4 Critical Variables for AIDS Vaccine Research

Adjuvants and delivery systems

Routes and schedules of delivery

Effect of dose of live challenge virus

Cell-free vs. cell-associated challenge virus

Route for live virus challenge (IM vs. IV, etc.)

Effect of strain diversity (i.e., vaccinate with one strain and challenge with
another

---

possible vaccines. Systematic testing of various vaccine strategies (Table 3) and
critical variables (Table 4) will certainly require large numbers of experimental
animals. There are lessons to be learned from Salk, Sabin, and others who accepted the challenge of developing poliovirus vaccines. "It was obvious in 1952 that
there was still much to learn about the biologic properties of polioviruses and
that the challenge to develop live poliovirus vaccines of each of the three recently identified antigenic types was no job for someone in a hurry" (2). It is
disappointing that many are still looking for the quick fix, the AIDS vaccine
that will work first try in chimpanzee or human trials, and are ready to quit
when it doesn't work. We need to realize that developing a vaccine for AIDS is
also no job for someone in a hurry and encourage more widespread use of
macaques, SIV, and other lentiviral models for this purpose.

REFERENCES

1. Salk D, Salk J. Vaccinology of poliomyelitis. Vaccine 1984; 2:59–74.
2. Sabin AB. Oral poliovirus vaccine: History of its development and use
   and current challenge to eliminate poliomyelitis from the world. J Infect
   Dis 1985; 151:420–36.
3. Koff WC, Hoth DF. Development and testing of AIDS vaccines. Science
   1988; 241:426–32.
4. Filice G, Cereda PM, Varnier OE. Infection of rabbits with human immunodeficiency virus. Nature 1988; 335:366–9.
5. Kulaga H, Folks TM, Rutledge R, Kindt T. Infection of rabbit T-cell and
   macrophage lines with human immunodeficiency virus. Proc Natl Acad Sci
   USA 1988; 85:4455–9.
6. Namikawa R, Kaneshima H, Lieberman M, Weissman IL, McCune JM. Infection of the SCID-hu mouse by HIV-1. Science 1988; 242:1684–6.
7. Mosier DE, Gulizia RJ, Baird SM, Wilson DB. Transfer of a functional human
   immune system to mice with severe combined immunodeficiency. Nature
   1988; 335:256–9.

8. Desrosiers RC. Simian immunodeficiency viruses. Ann Rev Microbiol 1988;
    42:607–25.

9. Chakrabarti L, Guyader M, Alizon M, Daniel MD, Desrosiers RC, Tiollais
    P, Sonigo P. Sequence of simian immunodeficiency virus from macaque and
    its relationship to other human and simian retroviruses. Nature 1987; 328:
    543–7.

10. Fukasawa M, Miura T, Hasegawa A, Morikawa S, Tsujimoto H, Miki K,
    Kitamura T, Hayami M. Sequence of simian immunodeficiency virus from
    African green monkey, a new member of the HIV/SIV group. Nature 1988;
    333:457–61.

11. Li Y, Naidu Y, Fultz, P, Daniel MD, Desrosiers RC. Genetic diversity of
    simian immunodeficiency viruses. J Med Primatol 1989; 18:261–9.

12. Letvin NL, Daniel MD, Sehgal PK, Desrosiers RC, Hunt RD, Waldron LM,
    MacKey JJ, Schmidt DK, Chalifoux LV, King NW. Induction of AIDS-like
    disease in macaque monkeys with T-cell tropic retrovirus STLV–III. Science
    1985; 230:71–3.

13. Daniel MD, Letvin NL, Sehgal PK, Hunsmann G, Schmidt DK, King NW,
    Desrosiers RC. Long-term persistent infection of macaque monkeys with
    the simian immunodeficiency virus. J Gen Virol 1987; 68:3183–9.

14. Ringler DJ, Hancock WW, King NW, Letvin NL, Daniel MD, Desrosiers RC,
    Murphy GF. Immunophenotypic characterization of the cutaneous exan-
    them of SIV-infected rhesus monkeys. Amer J Path 1987; 126:199–207.

15. Ringler DJ, Hunt RD, Desrosiers RC, Daniel MD, Chalifoux LV, King NW.
    Simian immunodeficiency virus-induced meningoencephalitis: Natural
    history and retrospective study. Annal Neurol 1988; 23:S101–7.

16. Ringler DJ, Wyand MS, Walsh DG, MacKey JJ, Chailfoux LV, Popovic M,
    Minassian AA, Sehgal PK, Daniel MD, Desrosiers RC, King NW. Cellular
    localization of simian immunodeficiency virus (SIV) in lymphoid tissues.
    I. Immunohistochemistry and electron microscopy. Amer J Path 1989;
    134:373–83.

17. Wyand MS, Ringler DJ, Naidu YM, Mattmuller M, Chalifoux LV, Sehgal
    PK, Daniel MD, Desrosiers RC, King NW. Cellular localization of simian
    immunodeficiency virus (SIV) in lymphoid tissues. II. *In situ* hybridization.
    Amer J Path 1989; 134:385–93.

18. Baskin GB, Murphey-Corb M, Watson EA, Martin LN. Necropsy findings in
    rhesus monkeys experimentally infected with cultured simian immuno-
    deficiency virus (SIV)/Delta. Vet Pathol 1988; 25:456–67.

19. Hirsch VM, Olmsted RA, Murphey-Corp M, Purcell RH, Johnson PR. An
    African primate lentivirus (SIV$_{sm}$) closely related to HIV-2. Nature 1989;
    339:389–91.

20. Desrosiers RC, Wyand MS, Kodama T, Ringler DJ, Arthur LO, Sehgal PK,
    Letvin NL, King NW, Daniel MD. Vaccine protection against simian im-
    munodeficiency virus infection. Proc Natl Acad Sci USA 1989; 86:6353–7.

19

A Specific Antibody Activity that Neutralizes HIV Infectivity In Vivo

Emilio A. Emini
Merck Sharp and Dohme Research Laboratories
West Point, Pennsylvania

The successful development of a vaccine that will protect against human immunodeficiency virus (HIV) infection is a formidable undertaking. The task is complicated by a lack of fundamental knowledge concerning vaccine-relevant immune responses against the virus. While much information has been obtained on the general anti-HIV responses elicted during persistent HIV infection, the significance of these immune responses in protection against the infection remains a question.

The simplest approach to the development of a successful vaccine involves the identification of a virus-specific immunogen capable of inducing circulating protective antibody. However, it is not a given fact that such an antibody exists against HIV. The ability of the virus to efficiently infect CD4-positive cells and the ubiquity of such cells in vivo present significant obstacles to an antibody-dependent immune response. Seemingly, the antibody is afforded little opportunity to interfere with the interaction between the virus and the target cell. Nonetheless, the results of recent investigations would suggest that an appropriately protective antibody species may exist.

IN VITRO HIV-NEUTRALIZING ANTIBODY

Early attempts to identify an anti-HIV protective immunogen focused on the use of the viral surface envelope protein, gp120, and its unprocessed precursor, gp160. This emphasis was appropriate since an antibody capable of preventing viral infection would most likely bind to the viral surface. Lasky et al. (1) and Robey et al. (2) first demonstrated that gp120 isolated from genetically engineered expressing mammalian cells or from persistently virus-infected lymphoid cells, respectively, elicits an in vitro virus-neutralizing antibody response in laboratory animals. It was demonstrated subsequently that this gp120-induced neutralizing activity is virus-isolate-specific and is not capable of cross-neutralizing divergent HIV isolates (3). Significantly, the immunogen used by Robey and coworkers had been denatured during the purification process. Its ability to nonetheless elicit neutralizing antibody suggests that the responsible gp120 antigenic determinant(s) is not dependent upon the glycoprotein's tertiary structure. This was confirmed when Putney et al. (4) showed that a denatured, unglycosylated, bacterially expressed carboxy-terminal fragment of gp120 (PB1) could still elicit HIV isolate-specific neutralizing activity.

Unfortunately, protective efficacy studies with the viral surface glycoprotein did not yield encouraging results. gp120 from genetically engineered mammalian cells (5) and the precursor gp160 expressed by a recombinant vaccinia virus vector (6) were found to be poor immunogens in chimpanzees with respect to the induction of neutralizing antibodies. In both studies, because of the unstable nature of the neutralizing immune response, the inoculated animals were challenged with live HIV at a time when measurable circulating neutralizing antibodies were not present. No protection was noted in either case.

These chimpanzee experiments emphasized the need for a precise identification of that portion of the gp120 protein expressing the neutralization determinant in the hope that the isolated determinant could be constructed as a reliable immunogen. Ho et al. (7) showed that synthetic peptide representations of several regions of the viral surface glycoprotein can elicit virus-neutralizing antibodies. Palker et al. (8) confirmed this observation with respect to one particular site, which was shown to induce HIV isolate-specific neutralizing activity. This same region also was found to be responsible for the isolate-specific activity elicited by the bacterially expressed carboxy-terminal PB1 fragment of gp120 (9) and was shown to be capable of binding isolate-specific neutralizing monoclonal antibodies (10,11). The determinant appears to be a closed loop bounded by two conserved Cys residues at positions 296 and 331 of gp120 (HTLV–IIIb isolate sequence). The loop is present in all sequenced HIV isolates and, with the exception of a centrally conserved portion, is generally quite variable among the different isolates. Clearly, this variability accounts for the isolate-specific nature of the neutralizing response.

The importance of the 296–331 region as a dominant antigenic site for the elicitation of virus-neutralizing antibody is underscored by the finding that the isolate-specific neutralizing activity appearing early following HIV infection of chimpanzees is directed exclusively to this determinant (12). It should be noted that a second broader neutralizing activity typically develops later in infection (13). However, this activity is poorly characterized, and attempts to map the responsible antigenic site have not succeeded.

FAVORABLE CHARACTERISTICS OF THE DOMINANT NEUTRALIZING ANTIBODY SPECIES

A strict correlation does not always exist between an antibody's in vitro neutralizing capacity and its ability to mediate protection in vivo against infection. One would expect this to be especially true for HIV-neutralizing antibodies, given the efficiency of HIV infection and the in vivo availability of appropriate target cells. Nevertheless, the antibody species directed against the dominant isolate-specific neutralization determinant does appear to exhibit certain characteristics which would favor its ability to act as a protective antibody in vivo.

Skinner et al. (13) showed that this antibody does not neutralize by inhibiting the interaction between HIV and its cellular receptor. Instead, neutralization appears to occur at a postbinding step. Given the ability of the antibody to prevent HIV-mediated cell fusion (10,13), it is suggested that the antibody may prevent virus penetration by fusion. However, the mechanism by which this may occur is not certain.

In addition, the neutralizing antibody species retains its ability to bind to virus after the virus has attached to its target cell (11). As expected, the antibody fully neutralizes HIV in vitro without the requirement for an interactive period between virus and antibody prior to target cell addition. The neutralization appears to be instantaneous.

IN VIVO PROTECTIVE EFFICACY OF THE DOMINANT NEUTRALIZING ANTIBODY SPECIES

The in vitro characteristics of the major isolate-specific neutralizing antibody are appropriate and necessary for an antibody elicited by a protective vaccine. Nevertheless, it remained to be demonstrated that in vitro antibody-mediated HIV neutralization translates into in vivo protection. HIV infects numerous cell types in vivo, and the possibility exists that, with certain target cells, antibody-mediated neutraliziation may be bypassed. One specific example might involve the uptake of virus–antibody complexes by macrophages and the establishment of infection in these susceptible target cells.

Prince et al. (14) reported a study in which HIV-specific immunoglobulin, prepared from an HIV-seropositive human plasma pool, was passively administered to susceptible chimpanzees. The immunoglobulin preparation contained a high level of HIV-neutralizing activity. The activity was present in the chimpanzee 24 hours after the immunoglobulin administration, at the time of virus challenge. No protection against virus infection was seen. The result of this study is not considered discouraging since a number of explanations are possible to explain the protection failure. The explanation may involve purely technical considerations such as the method of challenge or the dose of challenge virus. However, more significantly, it was determined that the neutralizing activity present in the human immunoglobulin pool did not contain antibody directed against the isolate-specific neutralization determinant of the HIV isolate (HTLV-IIIb) used for challenge (T. J. Matthews, personal communication). Hence, the protective efficacy of this particular antibody species remained to be established.

This was done in a study, performed by the author et al., which involved the in vitro interaction between neutralizing antibody and the challenge HIV followed by the inoculation of the virus–antibody mixture into chimpanzees. This method was chosen to guarantee the binding of virus and antibody and to avoid the uncontrollable technical elements of a passive protection experiment.

Four different purified antibody preparations were tested: (1) IgG from an infected chimpanzee which had been inoculated previously with the HTLV–IIIb challenge isolate of HIV. It was determined that the anti-HTLV–IIIb neutralizing activity present in this preparation was directed exclusively against the dominant isolate-specific neutralization determinant. (2) A specific neutralizing murine monoclonal antibody, 0.5β, directed against this site (10). (3) IgG from an HIV-seropositive human which did not neutralize the challenge HIV isolate, but which contained a high level of nonneutralizing anti-HIV activity. This preparation was included to control for any virus-specific, nonneutralizing antibody-mediated effects. (4) IgG from a normal, uninfected chimpanzee. The characteristics of each antibody preparation are summarized in Table 1.

The IgG samples were independently mixed with approximately 100 chimpanzee infectious doses of the HTLV–IIIb challenge isolate virus. Following a 90-minute incubation at room temperature, the virus–antibody mixtures were inoculated, by the intravenous route, into each of four chimpanzees. A portion of each inoculated sample was retained to confirm in vitro neutralization. As expected, the polyclonal IgG from the infected chimpanzee and the 0.5β monoclonal antibody completely neutralized the infectivity of the challenge virus in cell culture. No neutralization was noted with the anti-HIV human or control chimpanzee IgG samples.

The establishment of infection in the inoculated chimpanzees was assessed by the development of HIV-specific antibody responses. The results are presented in Table 2. Anti-HIV activity was first seen at 4-6 weeks after inoculation in the two chimpanzees which received nonneutralized virus. In contrast, the animal inoculated with virus which had been completely neutralized by the

Table 1 Characteristics of Antibody Preparations Used for In Vitro Neutralization of Chimpanzee Infectivity

Source of IgG preparation[a]	In vitro neutralizing titer[b]	Anti-HIV antibody activity[c]	Binding activity against the dominant neutralization determinant[d]
HIV-infected chimpanzee	1:640	+	+
0.5β monoclonal antibody	1:5120	ND	+
HIV-infected human	<1:10	+	-
Uninfected chimpanzee	<1:10	-	-

[a]See text for complete description.
[b]Measured as described by Robertson et al. (15). The amount of input virus (HTLV-IIIb isolate) was identical to the amount used for the chimpanzee challenge.
[c]Determined using the clinical HIV-1 Western blot assay. (+) Positive reactivity at an antibody preparation dilution of 1:100. (-) No reactivity at a 1:100 dilution. (ND) Not done.
[d]Measured by ELISA using a synthetic peptide substrate incorporating the amino acid sequence of the dominant neutralization determinant of the HTLV-IIIb isolate. (+) Positive binding. (-) No reactivity.

polyclonal chimpanzee IgG exhibited no immunologic signs of HIV infection during the course of the experiment. A delayed, apparently low-level infection developed in the chimpanzee inoculated with the monoclonal antibody-neutralized virus. The latter infection may have been due to a neutralization-escape mutant or to the inefficient in vivo clearance of circulating complexes of murine antibody and neutralized virus. Nevertheless, the results of the study suggest that antibody to the isolate-specific dominant neutralization determinant will mediate at least some degree of in vivo protection. This ability, along with the ability of the antibody to rapidly neutralize the virus, supports the view that a successful HIV vaccine should incorporate the dominant neutralization determinant.

Of course, there are many obstacles to be crossed before the hope for the successful development of an HIV vaccine becomes tangible. It remains to be demonstrated that circulating antibody against the neutralization determinant will be effective. Also appropriate immunogens which will efficiently elicit the desired antibody response need to be constructed. Finally, and probably of most importance, the variability of the neutralization determinant among HIV isolates needs to be studied carefully. A vaccine containing the determinant can be developed only if some restriction to the variability exists and if the immunologically important variability is not too great. Nevertheless, in spite of these

Table 2 Anti-HIV Antibody Development Following Chimpanzee Inoculation of Virus-Antibody Mixtures

Week, p.i.	ELISA titer[a]	Neutralization titer[b]	Western blot pattern[c]
Animal #222 (virus + control chimpanzee IgG)[d]			
0	<1:20	<1:10	—
2	<1:20	<1:10	—
4	<1:20	<1:10	—
6	1:40	<1:10	p24, p55
8	1:20	<1:10	p17, p24, p55, p66
10	1:640	<1:10	p17, p24, p55, p66, gp120, gp160
12	1:1280	1:20	p17, p24, gp41, p55, p66, gp120, gp160
14	1:2560	1:160	p17, p24, gp41, p55, p66, gp120, gp160
16	1:5120	1:160	p17, p24, gp41, p55, p66, gp120, gp160
17	1:5120	1:320	p17, p24, gp41, p55, p66 gp120, gp160
19	1:10,240	1:320	p17, p24, gp41, p55, p66, gp120, gp160
21	1:10,240	1:320	p17, p24, gp41, p55, p66, gp120, gp160
23	1:10,240	1:320	p17, p24, gp41, p55, p66, gp120, gp160
25	1:5120	1:320	p17, p24, gp41, p55, p66, gp120, gp160
27	1:5120	1:320	p17, p24, gp41, p55, p66, gp120, gp160
31	1:10,240		p17, p24, gp41, p55, p66, gp120, gp160
Animal #177 (virus + anti-HIV human IgG)[d]			
0	<1:20	<1:10	—
2	<1:20	<1:10	—
4	1:20	<1:10	—
6	1:160	<1:10	p24, p55

Table 2 (Continued)

Week, p.i.	ELISA titer[a]	Neutralization titer[b]	Western blot pattern[c]
8	1:320	<1:10	p24, p55, p66
10	1:160	1:10	p17, p24, gp41, p55, p66, gp120, gp160
12	1:320	1:10	p17, p24, gp41, p55, p66, gp120, gp160
14	1:320	1:40	p17, p24, gp41, p55, p66, gp120, gp160
16	1:160	1:40	p17, p24, gp41, p55, p66, gp120, gp160
17	1:640	1:40	p17, p24, gp41, p55, p66, gp120, gp160
19	1:640	1:40	p17, p24, gp41, p55, p66, gp120, gp160
21	1:1280	1:80	p17, p24, gp41, p55, p66, gp120, gp160
23	1:640	1:80	p17, p24, gp41, p55, p66, gp120, gp160
25	1:1280	1:80	p17, p24, gp41, p55, p66, gp120, gp160
27	1:1280	1:80	p17, p24, gp41, p55, p66, gp120, gp160
31	1:5120		p17, p24, gp41, p55, p66, gp120, gp160

Animal #81 (virus + neutralizing chimpanzee IgG)[d]

Week, p.i.	ELISA titer[a]	Neutralization titer[b]	Western blot pattern[c]
0	<1:20	<1:10	—
2			—
4			—
6			—
8			—
10			—
12			—
14			—
16			—

Table 2 (Continued)

Week, p.i.	ELISA titer[a]	Neutralization titer[b]	Western blot pattern[c]
17			−
19			−
21			−
23	<1:20	<1:10	−
25			−
27	<1:20	<1:10	−
31	<1:20		−
Animal #30 (virus + neutralizing 0.5β monoclonal antibody)[d]			
0	<1:20	<1:10	−
2	<1:20		−
4	<1:20		−
6	<1:20		−
8	<1:20		−
10	<1:20		−
12	<1:20		p24, gp160
14	1:20		p24, gp160
16	1:20		p24, gp160
17	1;20		p24, gp160
19	1:40		p17, p24, gp160
21	1:40		p17, p24, gp160
23	1:80	<1:10	p17, p24, gp160
25	1:80		p17, p24, gp160
27	1:80	<1:10	p17, p24, gp120, gp160
31	1:80		p17, p24, gp120, gp160

[a]Measured using the clinical HIV-1 ELISA.
[b]Measured against the HTLV-IIIb isolate as described by Robertson et al. (15).
[c]Determined using the clinical HIV-1 Western blot assay. Positively stained HIV-specific antigen bands are designated. (−) No viral antigen bands were visible.
[d]See text for complete description.

potential difficulties, the path toward a vaccine is becoming clearer, and specific goals are in view.

REFERENCES

1. Lasky LA, Groopman JE, Fennie CW, Benz PM, Capon DJ, Dowbenko DJ, Nakamura GR, Nunes WM, Renz ME, Berman PW. Neutralization of the AIDS retrovirus by antibodies to a recombinant envelope glycoprotein. Science 1986; 233:209-12.
2. Robey WG, Arthur LO, Matthews TJ, Langlois A, Copeland TD, Lerche NW, Oroszlan S, Bolgnesi DP, Gilden RV, Fischinger PJ. Prospect for prevention of human immunodeficiency virus infection: Purified 120-kDa envelope glycoprotein induces neutralizing antibody. Proc Natl Acad Sci USA 1986; 83:7023-7.
3. Matthews TJ, Langlois AJ, Robey WG, Chang NT, Gallo RC, Fischinger PJ, Bolognesi DP. Restricted neutralization of divergent human T-lymphotropic virus type III isolates by antibodies to the major envelope glycoprotein. Proc Natl Acad Sci USA 1986; 83:9709-13.
4. Putney SD, Matthews TJ, Robey WG, Lynn DL, Robert-Guroff M, Mueller WT, Langlois AJ, Ghrayeb J, Petteway SR, Weinhold KJ, Fischinger PJ, Wong-Staal F, Gallo RC, Bolognesi DP. HTLV-III/LAV-neutralizing antibodies to an *E. coli*-produced fragment of the virus envelope. Science 1986; 234:1392-5.
5. Berman PW, Groopman JE, Gregory T, Clapham PR, Weiss RA, Ferriani R, Riddle L, Shimaski C, Lucas C, Lasky LA, Eichberg JW. Human immunodeficiency virus type I challenge of chimpanzees immunized with recombinant envelope glycoprotein gp120. Proc Natl Acad Sci USA 1988; 85: 5200-4.
6. Hu S-L, Fultz PN, McClure HM, Eichberg JW, Thomas EK, Zarling J, Singhal MC, Kosowski SG, Swenson RB, Anderson DC, Todaro G. Effect of immunization with vaccinia-HIV *env* recombinant on HIV infection of chimpanzees. Nature 1987; 328:721-3.
7. Ho DD, Sarngardharan G, Hirsch MS, Schooley RT, Rota TR, Kennedy RC, Chanh TC, Sato VL. Human immunodeficiency virus neutralizing antibodies recognize several conserved domains on the envelope glycoproteins. J Virol 1987; 61:2024-8.
8. Palker TJ, Clark ME, Langlois AJ, Matthews TJ, Weinhold KJ, Randall RR, Bolognesi DP, Haynes BF. Type-specific neutralization of the human immunodeficiency virus with antibodies to *env*-encoded synthetic peptides. Proc Natl Acad Sci USA 1988; 85:1932-6.
9. Rusche JR, Javaherian K, McDanal C, Petro J, Lynn DL, Grimaila R, Langlois A, Gallo RC, Arthur LO, Fischinger PJ, Bolognesi DP, Putney SD, Matthews TJ. Antibodies that inhibit fusion of human immunodeficiency virus-infected cells bind a 24-amino acid sequence of the viral envelope, gp120. Proc Natl Acad Sci USA 1988; 85:3198-202.

10. Matsushita S, Robert-Guroff M, Rusche J, Koito A, Hattori T, Hoshino H, Javaherian K, Takatsuki K, Putney S. Characterization of a human immunodeficiency virus neutralizing monoclonal antibody and mapping of the neutralizing epitope. J Virol 1988;62:2107-14.

11. Skinner MA, Ting R, Langlois AJ, Weinhold KJ, Lyerly HK, Javaherian K, Matthews TJ. Characteristics of a neutralizing monoclonal antibody to HTLV-III$_B$ envelope glycoprotein. AIDS Res Hum Retroviruses 1988; 4: 187-97.

12. Goudsmit J, Debouck C, Meloen RH, Smit L, Bakker M, Asher DM, Wolff AV, Gibbs CJ, Gajdusek DC. Human immunodeficiency virus type I neutralization epitope with conserved architecture elicits early type-specific antibodies in experimentally infected chimpanzees. Proc Natl Acad Sci USA 1988;85:4478-82.

13. Skinner MA, Langlois AJ, McDanal CB, McDougal JS, Bolognesi DP, Matthews TJ. Neutralizing antibodies to an immunodominant envelope sequence do not prevent gp120 binding to CD4. J Virol 1988; 62:4195-200.

14. Prince AM, Horowitz B, Baker L, Shulman RW, Ralph H, Valinsky J, Cundell A, Brotman B, Boehle W, Rey F, Piet M, Reesink H, Lelie N, Tersmette M, Miedema F, Barbosa L, Nemo G, Nastala CL, Allan JS, Lee DR, Eichberg JW. Failure of a human immunodeficiency virus (HIV) immune globulin to protect chimpanzees against experimental challenge with HIV. Proc Natl Acad Sci USA 1988; 85:6944-8.

15. Robertson GA, Kostek BM, Schleif WA, Lewis JA, Emini EA. A microtiter cell-culture assay for the determination of anti-human immunodeficiency virus neutralizing antibody activity. S Virol Methods 1988; 20:195-202.

CLINICAL TRIALS AND REGULATORY CONSIDERATIONS

20

Recombinant-Derived Hepatitis B Vaccine
A Paradigm for Other Subunit Vaccines

Ronald W. Ellis
Merck Sharp and Dohme Research Laboratories
West Point, Pennsylvania

INTRODUCTION

The yeast-derived hepatitis B vaccine is the first recombinant-derived vaccine approved for human use. Infection with the hepatitis B virus (HBV), the major etiologic agent of infectious human liver disease, is responsible for one of the world's most widespread public health problems. Infection with this virus is endemic in many parts of the world, with the most common mode of transmission being from chronically infected mothers to their newborns; neonates exposed to the virus in this fashion most often develop chronic hepatitis B infections. In addition, many adults and adolescents exposed to the virus acquire an acute infection; while most of these individuals completely recover, a minority also develop chronic hepatitis B. The number of hepatitis B carriers worldwide has been estimated at over 25,000,000 (1). Hundreds of thousands of these carriers die annually from long-term sequelae of chronic hepatitis B, namely cirrhosis and hepatocellular carcinoma (2). Since there is no effective treatment available for chronic hepatitis B, control and prevention become paramount.

A unique first-generation hepatitis B vaccine was derived from the plasma of chronic carriers who are in the replicative phase of their disease (3). In the plasma of such carriers, a substantial quantity of hepatitis B surface antigen (HBsAg), the major viral surface protein, is not incorporated into virions in the infected liver cells. Rather, in the rough endoplasmic reticulum and secretory vesicles, this excess HBsAg is assembled with cellular lipids into noninfectious lipoprotein spheres ca. 22 nm in diameter. Following secretion from cells, these particles circulate in plasma at very high levels (up to 500 μg/ml). Following collection and during purification, chemical and physical inactivation steps are employed to kill any residual HBV or other adventitious agents present. In the vaccine licensed in the United States (Heptavax-B, Merck Sharp and Dohme), three inactivation steps are used: pepsin at pH 2, 8 M urea, and 0.01% formaldehyde (3). These steps have been demonstrated to be extremely effective at inactivating the infectivity of HBV and representative agents from all known groups of viruses (4), including HIV (5). However, despite the excellent safety profile of the plasma-derived vaccine used by millions of recipients worldwide, acceptance has been less than anticipated. Furthermore, the human source for HBsAg has been a limiting factor in the production of sufficient quantities of vaccine for worldwide use. Therefore, a need developed for a second-generation hepatitis B vaccine.

The plasma-derived hepatitis B vaccine was shown to be very effective at eliciting antibodies to HBsAg (anti-HBs). Early experiments in chimpanzees, one of the few species other than humans known to be susceptible to HBV infection, showed that anti-HBs represented the protective immune response in animals vaccinated with HBsAg prior to challenge with HBV (6). Clinical trials, culminating in a double-blind placebo-controlled study in a male homosexual population of New York City in the late 1970s, first demonstrated that the protection against clinical hepatitis B afforded by vaccination could be correlated with the levels of anti-HBs elicited in vaccinees (7). Specifically, a protective level of anti-HBs has been considered to be greater than 10 sample ratio units, i.e., S/N $\geqslant$ 10 (8,9). This level is approximately equal to 10 milli-International Units (mIU)/ml (10), which is being defined relative to an internationally accepted reference standard. Thus, 10 mIU anti-HBs/ml has become the benchmark target for immunogenicity in developing non-plasma-derived second-generation hepatitis B vaccines.

Recombinant DNA (rDNA) technology moved to the forefront as a research tool in the late 1970s. During this period, even while first-generation hepatitis B vaccines were being developed, the need for a second-generation vaccine became apparent. The relaxation of guidelines for biological and physical containment coupled with early breakthroughs in several research areas made rDNA technology attractive as a means for providing such a second-generation vaccine, in particular one which would be efficient in eliciting $\geqslant$ 10 mIU anti-HBs/ml in vaccinees.

This chapter describes the use of rDNA technology for developing a hepatitis B vaccine. Unless referenced otherwise, this chapter will describe the development of the Merck recombinant yeast-derived vaccine, known as Recombivax HB or H–B–VAX II. This was the first recombinant-derived vaccine developed and approved for human use. Other than hepatitis B, no other types of recombinant-derived vaccines have been approved for human use as of the publication of this volume. Thus, this product represents a paradigm for the development of subunit vaccines. The principles for the development of live attenuated or live recombinant vaccines are somewhat different and apply to subunit vaccines only to a limited degree (11).

There are many aspects of the development of the subunit hepatitis B vaccine which potentially relate to the development of subunit AIDS vaccines. This review describes some of these general aspects, i.e., molecular biology, fermentation, purification, formulation and testing in vitro and in vivo, and how these might be applicable to subunit AIDS vaccines. However, there is a major limitation in the degree of applicability of these general considerations to potential AIDS vaccines. Unlike the case for hepatitis B, the type of immune response that correlates with protection against HIV infection remains unknown. In lieu of such knowledge, the best candidate antigen(s) for a subunit AIDS vaccine remains to be defined. Nevertheless, all other parts of the work on the recombinant-derived hepatitis B vaccine should be applicable to some extent.

DEVELOPMENT OF THE RECOMBINANT YEAST-DERIVED HEPATITIS B VACCINE

Molecular Biology

In order to utilize rDNA technology to produce a hepatitis B vaccine, it was necessary to insert the HBsAg gene into an expression vector capable of directing the synthesis of large quantities of HBsAg in a heterologous host cell. Early studies of the molecular biology of HBV had been hampered by the inability of the virus to replicate in cell cultures, as mentioned earlier. Therefore, in the late 1970s (12–14) the HBV genome, a partially double-stranded DNA molecule within virions, was cloned. DNA sequence analysis of several genomes revealed the presence of four open reading grames (ORFs) capable of encoding large polypeptides (Fig. 1). In order to identify which of the four ORFs encoded HBsAg, the N-terminal amino acid sequence of plasma-derived HBsAg (15) was compared to the amino acid sequence imputed from the nucleotide sequence of each of the ORFs. By virtue of the identity of 14 consecutive N-terminal amino acids, the gene designated as S (Fig. 1) was identified as encoding HBsAg. The S gene actually is part of a larger ORF that is divided into three domains, each of which begins with an in-frame ATG codon that is capable of functioning as a translational initiation site. These domains are referred to as preS1, preS2, and S respective to their 5′ and 3′ order in the gene (16). Thus, these domains define three polypeptides referred to as S or HBsAg (226 amino acids), preS2 + S (281 amino acids), and preS1 + preS2 + S (389 amino acids). The 681-nucleotide S gene encodes the 24-kilodalton (kD) polypeptide, the predominant protein in 22 nm particles from human plasma. Therefore, the S gene became the gene of

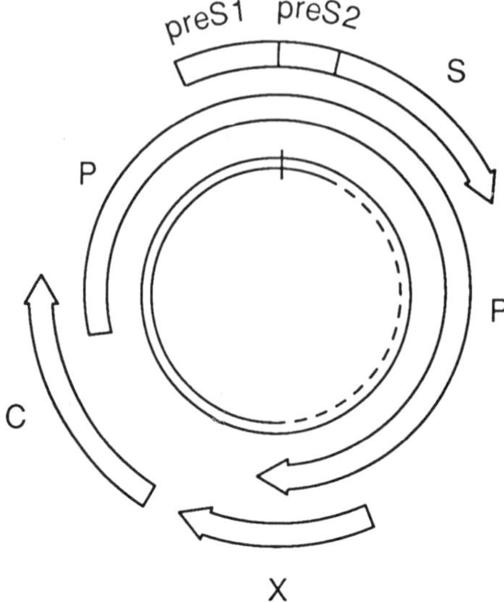

Figure 1 Diagrammatic representation of the ORFs in the HBV genome. The DNA of HBV has a nick in one strand (at the end of the X gene) and a single-stranded region (- - - -) of variable size. Nucleotide 1 of the 3.2 kilobase pair molecule is designated by convention at the top of the circle (vertical slash). The four large ORFs (P, X, C, preS1 + preS2 + S) are indicated. The arrows point in the direction in which the ORFs are translated. Each arrow begins at the ATG translational initiation codon and ends at the termination codon of the ORF. Each of the three domains of the preS1 + preS2 + S ORF is demarcated by its respective ATG initiation codon.

choice for expressing a hepatitis B vaccine in a heterologous host cell, although it is worth noting that preS-containing candidate vaccines have been prepared and are being studied (17–20).

Host System Used for Expression

Since *Escherichia coli* was the best developed heterologous expression system in the late 1970s, early attempts at expression of the S gene focused on *E. coli* as a host cell. However, all attempts were unsuccessful due to the instability of the S polypeptide and the lack of its assembly into 22 nm particles (21–23). Subsequently, satisfactory levels of expression were achieved both in bakers' yeast *Saccharomyces cerevisiae* (24–29) as well as in mammalian cells using both plasmid-based (30–32) and viral expression vectors (33,34). Both host cell systems produce HBsAg, which is assembled into 22 nm lipoprotein particles, is highly immunogenic for eliciting anti-HBs, and is highly related antigenically to plasma-derived HBsAg. All yeast-derived HBsAg is nonglycosylated; approximately 25% of mammalian-derived HBsAg is glycosylated (35), having a single asparagine-linked complex-type oligosaccharide at amino acid residue 146 (36). Nevertheless, this biochemical difference is not reflected in the antigenicity of the different particles or in their ability to elicit virus-neutralizing antibodies. In addition, the yeast-derived antigen is expressed intracellularly, while the mammalian-derived antigen is secreted from cells.

Since both *S. cerevisiae* and mammalian cells produce HBsAg, scientists had to decide which system was more desirable for producing a second-generation hepatitis B vaccine (37). There are three general considerations that are important for making a decision regarding the system of expression for most recombinant-derived biological products. These are 1) the biological activity of the expressed protein, 2) the scalability of the production process, and 3) the potential concern for safety of the final product relative to its host cell for production (38).

As discussed above, the biological activities, i.e., immunogenicity, of both the yeast-derived and mammalian-derived HBsAg are comparable. This presents no *a priori* reason for choosing one system over the other. Yeast cultures can be scaled up readily using experience gained over centuries of fermentation at an industrial scale, while attempts to scale-up mammalian cell cultures have been relatively recent. The molecular stability of recombinant yeast cells during fermentation can be controlled much more precisely than that of recombinant mammalian cells. Recombinant proteins can be produced in yeast cells at higher yields and correspondingly lower costs than in mammalian cells. While these factors should be considered in general, they apply to HBsAg in particular. Therefore, yeast is the preferred expression system for scalability of the production process.

The eventual worldwide use of a hepatitis B vaccine in hundreds of millions of healthy individuals, especially newborns, is a most important consideration in selecting a host cell for expression (37). There has been concern that mammalian cells used for expressing foreign genes generally are continuous cell lines. Such cells possess one or more properties associated with in vivo tumorigenicity or in vitro transformation and harbor endogenous protooncogenes and retroviruses, properties that can be associated with residual DNA in a product. It is essentially impossible to demonstrate the complete removal of all DNA from vaccine preparations. In contrast, yeast cells are not associated with these risk factors, such that the presence of minute quantities of yeast DNA in a vaccine is of little concern (37). Therefore, for reasons of perceived safety and production, yeast is the preferred host for the expression of recombinant-derived hepatitis B vaccines.

Intracellular HBsAg expression in yeast is directed by a high-copy number plasmid (Fig. 2). This plasmid contains the complete yeast 2μ sequences, which

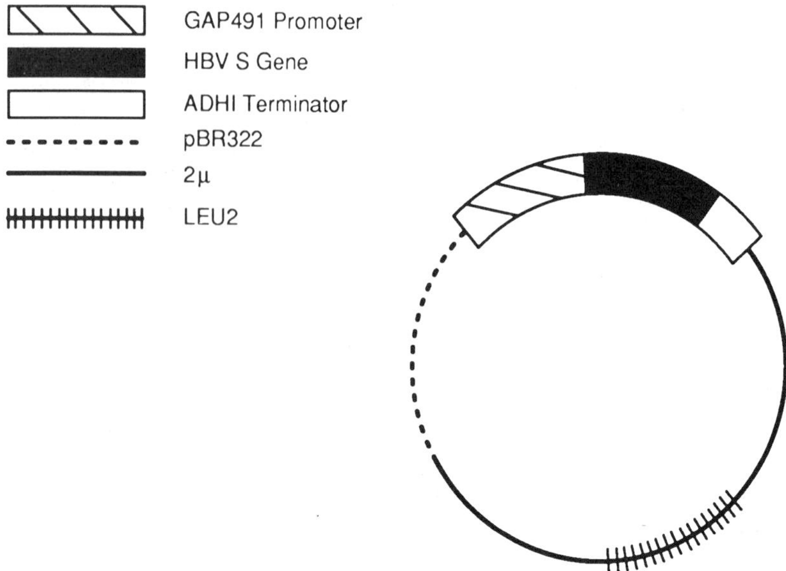

Figure 2   Structure of the plasmid that directs expression of HBsAg in yeast.

enable amplification to ca. 100 copies per cell in cir° yeast hosts (39), while the LEU2 gene enables selection for plasmid retention in leu⁻ host strains. The GAP491 gene provides one of the strongest promoters for constitutive expression of HBsAg in yeast; the GAP491 gene product, glyceraldehyde phosphate dehydrogenase, is ca. 5% of total yeast protein (40). Since expression of HBsAg is relatively nontoxic to the yeast host cell, a constitutive promoter of this type or others (24-28) can be used; HBsAg also has been expressed in yeast using repressible or inducible promoters (29,41). Besides the promoter and S gene, the other regulatory element in the expression cassette is the transcriptional termination region from the ADHI gene (42).

Scale-Up of Recombinant Yeast Fermentation

The manufacture of biological products entails the use of a seed lot system. Following transformation, a recombinant clone, obtained through the isolation of a single colony, is expanded and stored in a large number of vials as a master seed. Subsequently, one or more vials of master seed is expanded to a large number of vials as a stock seed. Each vial of stock seed is the starting material for the large-scale fermentation and manufacture of the vaccine. In this way, genetic identity of each fermentation is assured.

There is often the opportunity to improve upon the master seed for producing HBsAg. The original master seed supplied to the program for the Merck yeast-derived heptatitis B vaccine produced satisfactory levels of HBsAg. However, the productivity of the master seed over time was less stable than anticipated. Furthermore, it was highly desirable to increase the productivity of the fermentation process in terms of specific activity (HBsAg/total protein) to improve the efficiency of the entire downstream purification process. Therefore, fresh yeast were transformed at Merck with the expression plasmid (43). By careful attention to the selection conditions, propagation, and storage of the culture as well as subsequent steps in the course of scale-up, a second master seed was derived which was several-fold more productive than the original master seed. The use of this more productive master seed coupled with improvements in the purification process resulted in an improved immunogenicity of the final vaccine (see below).

The seed lot system is one of several considerations which must be applied to the manufacture by rDNA-based processes of biological products in general and hepatitis B vaccines in particular (38,44). Many of the considerations for the fermentation of the recombinant host cell relate to the plasmid used to direct the expression of HBsAg. Four of these considerations are overall structural stability, intactness of the S gene sequence, mitotic stability, and copy number (41). These parameters are considered significant, since a large number of cell divisions occur between establishing a master seed and harvesting cells from a large-scale fermentation. Thus, for each of these four considerations, plasmids within cells in the master seed are evaluated and compared to plasmids within cells at the end of the final fermentation.

Restriction endonuclease mapping provides a convenient assay for the overall structural stability of plasmids. While this assay is insensitive to small deletions or mutations in the plasmid, e.g., those within the coding sequence of the S gene, the assay readily will detect large (more than 0.05 kilobase pairs) deletions or rearrangements. With a panel of restriction endonucleases, it is possible to confirm identity in the sizes of restriction fragments of purified plasmid DNA before yeast transformation with plasmid DNA isolated from cells either in the master seed or at the end of full-scale fermentation.

In order to confirm the intactness of the coding region of the S gene, it is necessary to perform DNA sequence analysis for both the master seed as well as cells from a final time sample of a full-scale fermentation.

At the time of mitosis and DNA replication, yeast plasmids can segregate asymmetrically to their daughter cells. The segregation process is influenced by gene products encoded by the 2μ sequences on the plasmid (39). While some plasmid loss may occur during the course of a large-scale fermentation, it is desirable that a large and consistent percentage of the cells retain plasmid.

Simple replica plating assays have been developed to measure the degree of plasmid loss. The fraction of cells which retain the plasmid can be determined by testing for growth on leucine-deficient medium; cells that have lost the expression plasmid are unable to grow on such medium.

A final characterization of cells in the master seed compared to those after large-scale fermentation is a calculation of copy number of the expression plasmid. After extraction of cells and restriction endonuclease digestion of DNA followed by agarose gel electrophoresis, copy number can be quantitated relative to an appropriate internal control by densitometric scanning following staining or Southern blot hybridization. It is not critical that plasmid copy number be maintained in the final fermentation at as high a level as in the master seed. Rather, it is important from the perspective of regulatory agencies that copy number be consistent among all fermentations.

In summary, several parameters are important in characterizing the master seed and in monitoring fermentations. It is essential to demonstrate the structural stability of the plasmid, especially the DNA sequence of the S gene. Mitotic stability of the plasmid should be high, and plasmid copy number should be maintained at high levels. The consistency of the last two parameters across different fermentation batches is more important than an absolute maintenance of values relative to the master seed. All of these parameters have been demonstrated readily for fermentations of yeast expressing HBsAg (41). With the exception of DNA sequencing, all the other analyses can be performed rapidly through routine assays for several fermentation batches.

The final fermentation scale will depend on the economics of the process, anticipated productivity for HBsAg, and projected demand for the vaccine. Unfortunately, projecting the scale in advance is difficult: 1) process economics can change during the course of product development; 2) productivity can improve with experience in operating the process; 3) projected demand for the product often is only an educated guess. Nevertheless, a decision needs to be made relatively early in a development program in order to satisfy regulatory requirements as well as to gain process experience as early as possible.

In order to develop an efficient fermentation process for recombinant yeast, attention must be paid to the seed train, growth media, cell growth curves, volumes transferred during scale-up, and physical operating parameters of the fermentation vessels. The seed train refers to the method by which cells in the stock seed are propagated through initial stages of growth up to the stage of growth in the largest fermentor. The time and scale of growth is defined rigorously in a way which maximizes the final productivity of the process using different growth media in different stages of scale-up. It is desirable to use defined selective medium, e.g., leucine-deficient, which provides selective pressure for the maintenance of a high plasmid copy number duing the early stages of fermentation. Later, in the larger volumes of fermentation, it is desirable to use a more enriched medium which will favor the build-up of a high cellular density and large quantities of HBsAg. Growth curves should be derived to maintain cells for significant periods of time during exponential growth. The volume of cells transferred during each fermentation stage should be evaluated to optimize the production of HBsAg. Finally, physical parameters of the fermentation such as pH, dissolved oxygen, and agitation rate should be monitored and controlled closely to ensure high cellular viability, good productivity of HBsAg, and reproducibility of the process. In this regard, the assays for plasmid already described are very useful for monitoring and optimizing large-scale fermentations.

Isolation of Expressed Antigen

The major steps in the isolation process for the yeast-derived antigen are outlined in Figure 3. Since HBsAg accumulates intracellularly in yeast, the cells are harvested and washed at the end of a large-scale fermentation. Following disruption under high pressure, the cell lysate is clarified by filtration. As in the

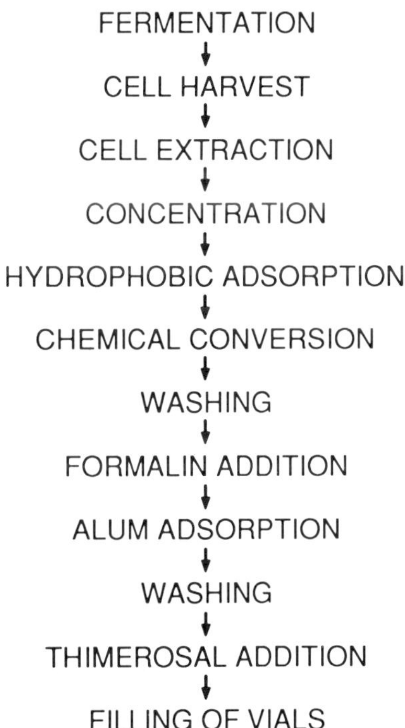

Figure 3   Outline of the isolation process for Recombivax HB.

case of all isolation processes, their design takes advantage of the particular physicochemical properties of the product. For HBsAg, both the aggregation of HBsAg polypeptides into large particles as well as the highly hydrophobic nature of the particles are exploited. The cell lysate is fractionated by hydrophobic adsorption chromatography. The purified HBsAg particles then are treated chemically to convert them into a fully disulfide-linked form similar to that of the plasma-derived particles (45). Following washing and sterilizing of the preparation by filtration, the HBsAg particle is treated with formalin, an agent commonly used for biological products other than live attenuated vaccines. The final vaccine is formulated by adsorption to aluminum hydroxide, a commonly used adjuvant. Finally, thimerosal is added as a preservative to ensure against the risk of compromising sterility by repeated needle penetrations of the same vial.

In the course of developing a purification process for the recombinant-derived hepatitis B vaccine, a prime consideration has been a very high purity level of the final product. Even though people are exposed continually to very high levels of the yeast *S. cerevisiae* without any untoward effects, the intended widespread use of the vaccine in healthy adults, children, and neonates requires that residual yeast proteins be kept to a minimum. Often, removing the last traces of yeast proteins occurs with refinements and experience in running the purification process. As previously discussed, the introduction of the second master seed provided a higher input of HBsAg into the purification process. When this improved strain was combined with a method to selectively remove residual yeast proteins, there was an increase in the minimal purity level of the product from >96% to >99% (43,46).

Immunologic studies of HBsAg have demonstrated that the aggregation of individual HBsAg polypeptides is critically important to immunogenicity. Therefore, the 22 nm particle is much more immunogenic than monomeric polypeptides in eliciting anti-HBs (47); conversely, anti-HBs binds efficiently to HBsAg particles, but not to monomeric polypeptides. While mammalian cells, either recombinant cells in vitro or infected hepatocytes in vivo, assemble and secrete 22 nm particles in their final immunogenic form, yeast cells synthesize and accumulate HBsAg polypeptides intracellularly, in which form aggregation with yeast-derived lipids occurs rather than the final assembly of the 22 nm particle. Thus, the purification process for yeast-derived HBsAg must preserve the ability of the polypeptides to aggregate with host cell lipids and enable formation of the 22 nm particle.

The ability of a process to provide yeast-derived HBsAg in a highly purified and immunogenic form (22 nm) is the most important aspect of a purification procedure. However, from the point of view of process development, several other issues must be considered. When a process is being evaluated, the prospect for scaling each step up to a manufacturing level of operation must be assured, e.g., membrane filtration may be preferred over centrifugation at different points in a process. The highest possible yield, one which assures the highest level of purity, should be attained to minimize costs incurred during production. The capital costs in setting up a production facility should be minimized; this will influence the choice of procedures during the process. There should be convenient points at which to interrupt the process and maintain HBsAg in a stable form. By testing HBsAg at various process points, stability of structure and antigenicity can be determined. Hold points (at 4°C or 20°C) are especially important for providing flexibility in the daily operation of the production facility and for establishing points in the process where individual lots of material may be pooled. Finally, the reproducibility of the process should be assured to satisfy licensure requirements for regulatory agencies. As part of this assurance, rejection criteria can be set for individual points during the process to stop the purification of poorly productive or impure batches. Examples of such rejection criteria include a contaminating microorganism being found in the fermentor, total yield of HBsAg at a particular point in the process being less than a certain predetermined level, or a yeast impurity being present at too high a level in the final level.

In Vitro Analysis of Antigen

The greatest challenge in analyzing yeast-derived HBsAg lay in selecting the most relevant assays and setting limits for acceptance of the product. The range of assays should be broad enough to ensure both a detailed physicochemical analysis as well as measurements of reproducible structure, purity, and antigenicity of the HBsAg. In practice, many assays are attempted during the development program before the most relevant ones finally are selected and validated. In terms of the point for application during the process, tests can be considered assays of the final product or in-process assays.

Several assays have been used to test the protein purity of HBsAg. These assays can be performed on samples during the process, to ensure consistent performance, and at the end of the process. Following sodium dodecyl sulfate-polyacrylamide gel electrophoresis (SDS–PAGE), gels can be stained with Coomassie Brilliant Blue or silver nitrate. By determining the sensitivity limit of an assay for the contaminating protein and for a series of control samples of known quantity, the purity level of the in-process or final product can be determined by densitometric scanning of the stained gel. For example, one might be able to determine that, at a loading level of 1 μg of final vaccine, the appearance of no polypeptides except for the HBsAg polypeptide assures a purity level of >95%. Another important piece of information from this analysis is a verification of the size of the monomeric HBsAg polypeptide. The appearance of HBsAg in stained SDS–PAGE gels as a 24-kD polypeptide establishes that full-length polypeptides are formed reproducibly and purified from each fermentation batch. Alternatively, the purity level of a sample can be determined by high performance liquid chromatography (HPLC) and spectrophotometric scanning of individual fractions. By these assays, a final product purity of >99% can be verified.

Tests for identity are performed to confirm that the 24-kD species is the HBsAg polypeptide. A sample of vaccine which has been resolved by SDS–PAGE can be subjected to immunoblot analysis with monoclonal antibodies (mAb) to HBsAg. Such analysis demonstrates identity of the 24-kD polypeptide as HBsAg. An additional such test is a demonstration of the in vitro reactivity of mAb with the vaccine. Another test for identity is amino-terminal sequence analysis of the 24-kD polypeptide, which demonstrates the presence of the same amino acid sequence as predicted from the DNA sequence and rules out comigrating contaminants.

As discussed above, the 22 nm particle isolated from plasma actually is a lipoprotein by composition. During assembly and budding from infected liver cells, the HBsAg polypeptides aggregate with host cell lipids in a proportion resembling that found in the normal cell. Similarly, the yeast-derived particle acquires lipids during the course of assembly in a proportion resembling that found in wild-type yeast (48). The purified vaccine can be assayed qualitatively and quantitatively for lipids in order to ensure consistency among batches.

Impurities in the final vaccine can be divided into two categories, extrinsic and intrinsic. Extrinsic impurities (excipients) are those which are introduced during purification and include detergents or, as used by some groups, mAb for immunoaffinity purification. It is desirable to minimize the excipient levels by the appropriate design of the purification process, as monitored by sensitive chemical assays. This is especially critical with respect to residual mAb, since there is a risk in certain individuals of immunologic sensitization to xenotypic immunoglobins.

Intrinsic impurities are those derived from the yeast host cell. As noted, lipid is *not* an impurity, since it is an integral part of the 22 nm particles. Residual yeast proteins can be detected by immunoblot or HPLC techniques, as described above. Even though there is no known biological risk associated with low levels of residual yeast DNA, the purification process should ensure the removal of as much DNA as possible. Guidelines for the preparation of recombinant-derived products require that a final dose of the product contain no more than 10 picograms of residual host cellular DNA. As assayed by quantitative DNA hybridization, this level is attainable readily in hepatitis B vaccines.

Several tests that relate to the safety of the recombinant-derived hepatitis B vaccine need to be performed. These tests are performed on all biological products and are not specific to hepatitis B vaccines per se. A general safety test is performed by inoculating a large volume, e.g., 5 ml, of the vaccine intraperitoneally into healthy young guinea pigs. These animals are observed for general health and continued weight gains relative to control animals. The vaccine is tested for pyrogenicity by following any rise in temperature of a group of inoculated rabbits; the product is considered nonpyrogenic if the temperatures rises 0.5°C or less over a 4-hour period. Finally, the vaccine is tested for sterility by standard microbiological assays.

The recombinant-derived HBsAg is formulated into a vaccine by adsorption to aluminum hydroxide, as previously described. Completeness of adsorption can be tested by assaying the supernatant of the alum-adsorbed vaccine for residual HBsAg. In addition, standard chemical tests are used for assaying pH and osmolality of the vaccine.

The assurance of stability is one of the most important determinations that needs to be made for the yeast-derived hepatitis B vaccine, as well as for any pharmaceutical product. Following the isolation and formulation process, vials are filled with doses of the vaccine. Each vial receives a label identifying the product and stating its shelf life. Typically, a period of 2–3 years at 4°C is assigned to many vaccines. A manufacturer must develop real-time stability data for the vialed product in order to be able to assign shelf life to the product. Typical assays which are performed to assure stability include SDS–PAGE analyses, in vitro reactivity with mAb, and mouse potency (see below). For 2-year dating, it is expected that assays performed 2 years postfilling will give results statistically equivalent to those performed at the time of filling.

Preclinical Evaluation of Vaccine Potency

The recombinant yeast-derived hepatitis B vaccine has undergone a wide range of tests to ensure its potency in eliciting biologically active anti-HBs. These potency tests have been performed both on the recombinant-derived vaccine per se as well as in comparison to the plasma-derived vaccine. Some of the tests are performed in vitro, while most are performed in vivo in experimental animals and humans followed by in vitro evaluation of sera by standard assays.

One of the key properties associated with the excellent immunogenicity of the recombinant-derived hepatitis B vaccine, or any other subunit vaccine for that matter, is the availability of epitopes capable of eliciting the production of specific antibodies. Among these epitopes, those considered most important to the immunogenicity of HBsAg are the *a* epitopes, present on all subtypes of HBV (*adr, adw, ayr, ayw*), which map to amino acids 124–137 in the S polypeptide (49). A mAb directed against one particular *a* epitope can neutralize the infectivity of HBV for chimpanzees (50). Furthermore, anti-*a* antibodies are the most abundant elicited by HBsAg (51,52). Therefore, an assay assuring the presence of *a* epitopes on each batch of vaccine is very useful. There is a commercial assay (AUSRIA) that employs antibodies capable of reacting in vitro with the *a* epitopes. However, these antibodies are polyclonal in origin, such that their reactivity is not exclusive with any single *a* epitope. A more specific assay is the use of mAb directed to specific *a* epitopes, including the mAb which can neutralize HBV infectivity for chimpanzees (50). An appropriate quantitative assay using such anti-*a* mAb, as well as other mAb directed to other epitopes on HBsAg, can assure the presence of key epitopes on particles in each batch of vaccine.

A commonly used immunogenicity test for hepatitis B vaccines is the mouse potency assay. In this assay, various quantities (typically 4-fold dilutions) of every vaccine lot are inoculated in a single dose into groups of 10 mice which are held for 6 weeks and bled. The sera are assayed for anti-HBs by a commercially available test (AUSAB). For each lot of vaccine, the effective dose capable of seroconverting 50% of the mice (ED_{50}) is calculated (51). The advantage of the one-dose mouse potency assay over other animal assays for immunogenicity is the availability of large numbers of mice of a single inbred strain; this assures statistical validity and reproducibility. By this assay, a consistent process can provide vaccines with ED_{50} values that fall within a reproducible range. Immunogenicity tests also have been performed in grivet monkeys in a similar multiple dose regimen as used in humans (20). These tests have been useful in demonstrating immunogenicity in a primate species. However, they suffer from the disadvantages of outbred animals, high cost, and limited supply of the animals, such that there is a lack of statistical validity (multiple doses, small groups) in calculating ED_{50}.

Efficacy in chimpanzees is the most important preclinical immunologic test. The chimpanzee is one of the few species outside of man known to be susceptible to HBV infection. A typical acute infection in this species results in the appearance of HBsAg, antibodies to hepatitis B core antigen (anti-HBc), elevations in serum liver enzyme activity, and histopathologic changes of hepatitis in liver biopsies at 6–18 weeks postinoculation with standard HBV inocula. This model offers the opportunity to test the efficacy of a candidate hepatitis B vaccine. A chimpanzee can be vaccinated, then challenged with an inoculum of HBV known to consistently cause the above-mentioned signs of infection; if the animal remains free of such signs for 24 weeks following challenge, the vaccine is deemed effective at preventing infection. This principle was demonstrated in the 1970s for the plasma-derived hepatitis B vaccine of subtype *ad*, which was shown to be able to protect chimpanzees against challenge with HBV of subtypes *ad* or *ay* (3,6,47).

In order to demonstrate that the yeast-derived hepatitis B vaccine was capable of eliciting anti-HBs of sufficient titer and specificity to protect against HBV challenge, chimpanzees received three doses of the vaccine at monthly intervals. Vaccinated animals produced anti-HBs titers of 800–3000 mIU/ml (Table 1).

Table 1 Protective Efficacy of Yeast-Derived Hepatitis B Vaccine in Chimpanzees

			Time of onset postchallenge[d]			
Chimpanzee[a]	Subtype of[b] challenge virus	Titer of anti-HBs[c] at time of challenge	HBsAg	Anti-HBc	SGOT/SGPT[e] elevation	Pathology
Vaccinated						
1	ad	1,830	—	—	—	—
2	ad	540	—	—	—	—
3	ad	3,600	—	—	—	—
4	ad	1,600	—	—	—	—
5	ay	18,300	—	—	—	—
6	ay	7,200	—	—	—	—
7	ay	3,600	—	—	—	—
8	ay	1,600	—	—	—	—
Control						
9	ad	<8	8	12	17	16
10	ad	<8	6	10	22	14
11	ad	<8	7	13	13	12
12	ad	<8	9	16	20	20
13	ay	<8	10	15	17	17
14	ay	<8	6	12	13	13
15	ay	<8	—	28	—	—
16	ay	<8	7	13	14	16

[a]Vaccinated animals were given three doses of vaccine at 40 μg/dose (#1, 2, 5, 6) or 10 μg/dose (#3, 4, 7, 8) at 0, 1, 2 months; control animals received a placebo containing the alum adjuvant at the same times of vaccination (51).
[b]All animals were challenged by intravenous inoculation of 10^3 infectious doses of HBV the indicated subtype at 1 month after the third dose of vaccine.
[c]AUSAB units/ml.
[d]Weeks after challenge for first appearance of indicated symptom of HBV infection.
[e]SGOT, serum glutamic oxalo-acetic acid transaminase (AST); SGPT, serum glutamic pyruvic transaminase (ALT).

Following challenge with HBV, none of the eight vaccinated animals showed any signs of viral infection throughout the entire observation period. In contrast, all control animals developed signs of infection. As observed with the plasma-derived vaccine, the yeast-derived vaccine (subtype *ad*) protected against HBV challenges with either subtypes *ad* or *ay*, thus highlighting the protective effect of anti-*a* antibodies (51,53).

In retrospect, the results of the efficacy tests in chimpanzees strongly suggested that the yeast-derived hepatitis B vaccine was clearly a product candidate to replace the plasma-derived vaccine.

Clinical Testing

The yeast-derived vaccine has been tested in healthy volunteers of all age groups. Before vaccination, all tested individuals were shown to be seronegative for HBsAg, anti-HBs, and anti-HBc. Following the protocol for the plasma-derived vaccine, all individuals were vaccinated at 0, 1, and 6 months. Each dose was administered intramuscularly in the deltoid muscle or, for young children, in the antero-lateral thigh; it had been shown that the plasma-derived vaccine was less immunogenic when administered in the buttock (54). Sera taken at 0, 1, 3, 6, and 7-9 months were tested for anti-HBs using the AUSAB radioimmunoassay; titers are expressed in mIU/ml.

The first stage of clinical testing for the vaccine, as well as for other pharmaceutical products, is a phase 1 clinical trial in which safety and tolerability are assured in healthy volunteers. Such a study also provides initial data on the immunogenicity of the vaccine. Subsequently, phase 2 trials are conducted. During this phase, an optimal dose is selected in all age groups and the immunogenicity of the vaccine established. Finally phase 3 trials are conducted to demonstrate that immunization with the vaccine protects against clinically apparent infection.

The yeast-derived hepatitis B vaccine has been very well tolerated. In over 8000 individuals studied to date in clinical trials, the vaccine has been generally very well tolerated (46,55,56). All clinical complaints, such as headache, fatigue, nausea, and malaise, or those related to the injection site, have been mild and transient. Despite the theoretical concern that residual yeast proteins present in the vaccine might lead to allergic reactions in vaccinees, no adverse experiences were reported during clinical trials which could be related to changes in the titers of antibodies to yeast. The lack of such a response may be related to the high titers of antiyeast antibodies in almost all individuals, owing to the widespread presence of *S. cerevisiae* in food and beverages. An initial dose-ranging study (Table 2) tested 2.5, 5, 10, and 20 µg doses of the vaccine in adults (56). While the kinetics of the immune response and the percentage of individuals seroconverting were similar for all doses, the 10 and 20 µg formulations

Table 2 Anti-HBs Responses at 8 Months Among Healthy Adults and Children Receiving Various Doses of Recombivax HB

Subject population	Dose (μg)[a]	Number of vaccinees	Percent positive anti-HBs responses[b]	GMT of responders[c]
Adults				
	2.5	57	96	295
	5	114–161	88	349
	10	509–594	97	1,286
	20	35	90	1,022
Children				
	1.25	7–21	100	2,059
	2.5	19–28	100	6,230
	5	14–21	100	15,966

[a]Three doses were administered at 0, 1, and 6 months (56).
[b]A positive anti-HBs response is defined as $S/N > 2.1$, a statistically significant immune value as compared to the background level of the assay.
[c]GMT = geometric mean titer in mIU/ml.

elicited significantly higher geometric mean titers (GMTs). Therefore, the 10-μg dose was chosen for most of the studies in adults. The GMTs of vaccine-induced anti-HBs among younger adults (20–29 years) were higher than those of older individuals ($>$50 years). By comparative testing of 1.25-, 2.5-, and 5-μg doses of vaccine in children 1–12 years of age, the 5-μg dose was chosen for all children 10 years of age or younger (Table 2). In children as compared to adults, seroconversion is more rapid (data not shown) and frequent, and GMTs are invariably much higher even at lower doses of vaccine.

The introduction of a second master seed and improvements made to the original purification process itself resulted in a more highly productive process for making the vaccine (43,46). The combination of these two developments resulted not only in an increase in product purity from 96 to 99% but also in improved immunogenicity as measured by GMTs (Table 3) (43,46).

The yeast-derived vaccine has similar antigenic properties to the plasma-derived vaccine. However, since the two vaccines have some biochemical differences, it was important to compare the properties of the antibodies elicited by each vaccine (51,52). Both vaccines 1) protect chimpanzees against challenge with HBV (subtype *ad* or *ay*); 2) elicit anti-*a* antibodies with similar kinetics and to a similar degree; 3) elicit anti-HBs of similar avidity and immunoglobulin isotype; 4) elicit antibodies which can be absorbed totally by either vaccine;

Table 3 Anti-HBs Responses at 7/8 Months Among Healthy Adults Receiving
Recombivax HB from Different Processes

Recombivax HB seed/process	No. of vaccinees[a]	Percent positive anti-HBs responses[b,c]		GMT of responders[d]
		S/N $\geqslant$ 2.1	$\geqslant$10 mIU/ml	
Original/original	739	97	95	749
Original/improved	173	98	98	1,223
Second/improved	144	99	99	1,823

[a]Three 10-μg doses were given at 0, 1, and 6 months (43,46).
[b]S/N > 2.1 is a statistically significant value as compared to the background level of the assay.
[c]GMT $\geqslant$ 10 mIU/ml is considered a level of antibodies associated with protection from HBV infection in clinical trials (7).
[d]GMT = geometric mean titer in mIU/ml.

5) elicit antibodies capable of binding to a synthetic peptide containing an *a* epitope with equivalent titers and affinities; and 6) elicit antibodies capable of binding to plasma-derived HBsAg with equivalent avidities. By these criteria, the two vaccines are immunologically comparable in vivo.

The final proof of the efficacy of the yeast-derived vaccine lay in demonstrating its effectiveness in preventing clinical infection. For the plasma-derived vaccine, efficacy was demonstrated in a double-blind placebo-controlled study with three 40-μg doses in New York City homosexual men in the late 1970s (7). In this classic study, the vaccine was shown to be 87% effective in preventing clinical hepatitis B in this high-risk group. A second study using three 20-μg doses of this vaccine showed a similar efficacy rate (8). Even though the yeast-derived vaccine is very similar immunologically to the plasma-derived vaccine, as described above, it was deemed important to demonstrate directly the protective effect of anti-HBs elicited by the yeast-derived vaccine. However, three developments had altered the proposed study design for the yeast-derived vaccine relative to the earlier study. First, since the plasma-derived vaccine had been licensed, it would have been unethical to include a placebo group, denying them access to a known effective vaccine. Therefore, the control group received the plasma-derived vaccine and the determination of efficacy was calculated relative to historical data in a high-risk group whose incidence of infection had not changed over time (57). Second, sexual habits among homosexual men had changed markedly due to the fear of AIDS, such that the incidence of HBV infection had decreased significantly in this group (58). Third, the incidence of

HBV infection had decreased in other risk groups as well, e.g., clients in institutions and staff and patients in dialysis units, such that historical data for infection rates was unreliable in these groups (9,59).

Based on these considerations, efficacy studies were carried out in newborn children born to chronic carrier mothers. In earlier studies, it had been shown that untreated infants born to viremic carrier mothers positive for HBsAg and HBeAg (an antigen marker of HBV replication) had a 70-90% rate of infection and had a high risk of becoming chronic carriers themselves (60). This perinatal mode of transmission accounts for the vast majority of hepatitis B cases worldwide (1,2). In this group of infants, passive immunization at birth with one dose of hepatitis B immune globulin (HBIG) reduced the rate of infection by ca. 50% (61). Moreover, combined passive immunization with HBIG and active immunization with the plasma-derived hepatitis B vaccine reduced the rate of infection even further (62,63). Since rates of infection were similar in untreated infants born of Asian mothers in the United States to those born in Asia, there was no suggestion that medical practices had affected the rate of perinatal transmission. Therefore, in lieu of a placebo control group, it was appropriate to calculate the efficacy of the recombinant-derived vaccine on the basis of historical data.

Among infants (born to viremic chronic carrier mothers) receiving HBIG at birth and 5-μg doses of the yeast-derived vaccine at 0, 1, and 6 months, only 5% became infected. This 94% rate of protection from infection, compared to historical controls, was comparable to a control group of infants in the same study receiving HBIG and three doses of the plasma-derived vaccine (57). Therefore, this study demonstrated that anti-HBs elicited by the yeast-derived vaccine is as effective in preventing HBV infection as that elicited by the plasma-derived vaccine. This result is consistent with the immunologic equivalence of the vaccines in terms of the qualitative properties of the anti-HBs elicited by each vaccine, as described above. Most important, this study describes the means for preventing the most common mode of transmission of HBV worldwide, one employing a vaccine which now can be produced in an essentially unlimited supply.

THE YEAST-DERIVED HEPATITIS B VACCINE AS A
MODEL FOR A POTENTIAL SUBUNIT AIDS VACCINE

The successful development of the yeast-derived hepatitis B vaccine serves as a model for future recombinant-derived subunit vaccines. A summary of some of the major issues for the development program for HBsAg (Table 4) highlights the same needs for other vaccine programs. These issues are worth considering with respect to a potential subunit AIDS vaccine, although it is impossible to apply these considerations specifically in lieu of understanding the

Table 4 Important Issues in the Development of the Yeast-Derived Hepatitis B Vaccine

---

   I. Choice of Host Cell
      A. Target population for use of the vaccine
      B. Production of biologically active antigen
      C. Concern for risk factors associated with host cell
      D. Productivity and scale-up

  II. Expression System
      A. Design of expression cassette
      B. Plasmid copy number

 III. Master Seed
      A. Stability during long-term storage
      B. Selection of an optimal yeast clone
      C. Genetic characterization

 IV. Culture Scale-Up
      A. Composition of growth medium and seed train
      B. Physical parameters of fermentation
      C. Reproducibility

  V. Purification
      A. Commercially useful yields
      B. High level of product purity
      C. Production of 22 nm particles
      D. Formulation
      E. Reproducibility

 VI. Preclinical Analysis
      A. Protein purity
      B. Identity and integrity of polypeptide
      C. Intrinsic and extrinsic impurities
      D. Potency in vitro and in vivo
      E. Safety
      F. Efficacy in chimpanzees

VII. Clinical evaluation
      A. Safety
      B. Immunogenicity
      C. Efficacy

---

immunobiology of HIV to a point where an actual candidate AIDS vaccine antigen can be identified.

The host cell must produce a biologically active antigen. This might entail the use of mammalian cells if a particular type of posttranslational modification, e.g., native glycosylation, is required for activity. If such a modification is not required, then yeast or bacterial cells would be desirable for circumventing potential safety concerns and for their advantages in scale-up and productivity. (See Fig. 4.)

All issues regarding expression, seed development and culture scale-up are similar to those for the hepatitis B vaccine. The design of the expression cassette differs somewhat among the various expression systems, although the principles for design are similar. The plasmid in the master seed would be characterized for parameters such as structural stability, intactness of the candidate gene, mitotic stability, and copy number. The master seed should be selected and grown deliberately and be well characterized genetically. Optimal growth media and seed train may differ for various expression vectors utilizing the same host cell. The reproducibility of the scaled-up process should be assured for licensure requirements as well as consistency of the downstream processing steps. The purification process should produce a sufficient quantity of antigen to meet commercial needs economically. Achieving a high level of product purity is essential, given the intended use of a vaccine in healthy individuals. As required for fermentation, reproducibility of the purification process is very important. Formulation of a subunit vaccine usually has involved adsorption to alum. However, for an HIV subunit vaccine, the use of novel adjuvants may prove worthwhile, especially if enhancement of immunogenicity is required (64,65).

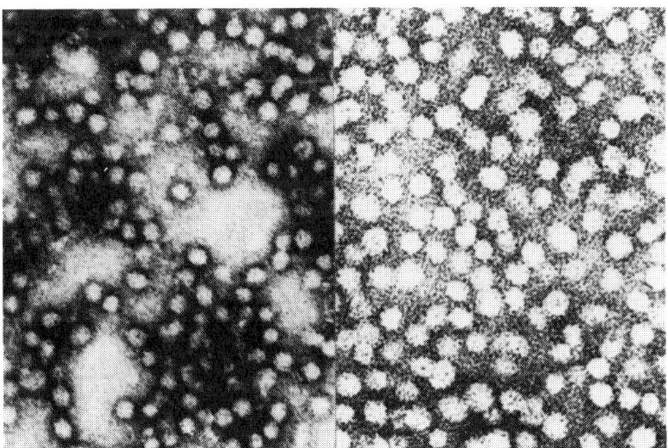

Figure 4   Electron microscopy of hepatitis B vaccine derived from (A) plasma or (B) recombinant yeast. (magnification 130,000X)

Finally, the process must be designed to maintain the antigenicity of the target antigen.

Preclinical analyses should encompass a broad range of physical, chemical, and immunologic assays. These tests should assure a detailed characterization of the target antigen, including assays for identity and integrity. Antigenic potency can be tested, both in vitro using antibodies specific for key epitopes as well as in vivo in an appropriate assay such as mouse potency. Finally, it is highly desirable to demonstrate the efficacy of a candidate vaccine in an animal model for infection, as was done for HBV in chimpanzees. For HIV, the chimpanzee may be useful. Despite debate over the validity of the use of this species as a model for AIDS in humans, it appears to be an excellent model for HIV infection.

The most difficult aspect of developing a potential subunit AIDS vaccine will be clinical testing. The basic challenge today is to identify a type of immune response that can be correlated with protection against HIV infection. Such a lead may come from studies in chimpanzees. Alternatively, a detailed immunologic characterization of long-term survivors of an HIV infection may provide a lead, as the earliest infected cohort of individuals from the late 1970s is followed for an extended period of time. However, there is currently no clue whatsoever regarding the nature of a potentially protective immune response in AIDS. In contrast, the knowledge that anti-HBs protects against HBV infection enabled scientists to focus rapidly upon HBsAg as a candidate antigen capable of eliciting this protective immune response.

As HIV subunit vaccines are tested clinically, safety should be established initially in a group of healthy volunteers. Then, in expanded clinical trials, the immune response to such vaccines will be characterized, hopefully at a time in the future when the protective immune response will have been identified. In contrast, expanded clinical trials of a subunit hepatitis B vaccine could be evaluated readily by studying the development of anti-HBs, the known protective immune response.

The final challenge to the development of an HIV subunit vaccine will be a demonstration of protective efficacy in a susceptible target population. For hepatitis B, such a study could be accomplished readily for both the plasma-derived and the recombinant-derived vaccines, given the availability of suitable target populations as well as a satisfactory understanding of the epidemiology of HBV infections. However, it is difficult to identify a suitable target population for HIV due to the rapidly changing epidemiology of the disease, one which may change even during the course of an actual clinical trial. Unlike HBV, all of whose subtypes contain *a* epitopes which elicit protective immunity, there are an undetermined number of HIV serotypes. In contrast to HBV, which is transmitted as free virus that can be neutralized by antibodies, HIV is transmitted in intact cells. Finally, there are difficult ethical issues for HIV in terms of the naure and content of material necessary to obtain informed consent in an efficacy trial, the ethics of including a placebo control group, and complex social and legal issues. Hopefully, these issues will be understood better when it is suitable to perform an efficacy trial.

Most of the technical tools are available for producing a subunit AIDS vaccine. However, it is unclear at present which polypeptide(s) should be included in such a vaccine as a candidate antigen. A much more detailed understanding of the immunobiology and protective immune response in HIV infection will be necessary before such antigens can be identified and tested clinically in a meaningful fashion. Until then, empirical approaches will be the only way to gather further information regarding candidate vaccines.

REFERENCES

1. Beasley RP, Hwang L-Y. Epidemiology of hepatocellular carcinoma. In: Vyas GN, Dienstag JL, Hoofnagle JH, eds. Viral hepatitis and liver disease. Orlando, FL: Grune & Stratton, 1984:209–24.
2. Szmuness W. Hepatocellular carcinoma and the hepatitis B virus: evidence for a causal association. Prog Med Vir 1978; 24:40–69.
3. Hilleman MR, McAleer WJ, Buynak EB, McLean AA. The preparation and safety of hepatitis B vaccine. J Inf 1983; 7:3–8.
4. Tabor E, Buynak EB, Smallwood LA, Snoy P, Hilleman MR, Gerety RJ. Inactivation of hepatitis B virus by three methods: Treatment with pepsin, urea, or formalin. J Med Virol 1983; 11:1–9.
5. Francis DP, Feorino PM, McDougal S, Warfield D, Getchell J, Cabradilla C, Tong M, Miller WJ, Schultz LD, Bailey FJ, McAleer WJ, Scolnick EM, Ellis RW. The safety of the hepatitis B vaccine. JAMA 1986; 256:869–72.
6. Hilleman MR, Bertland AV, Buynak EB, Lampson GP, McAleer WJ, Rochin RR, Tyrell AA. Clinical laboratory studies of HBsAg vaccine. In: Vyas GN, Cohen SN, Schmid R, eds. Viral hepatitis. Philadelphia: Franklin Institute Press, 1978:525–42.
7. Szmuness W, Stevens CE, Zang EA, Harley EJ, Kellner AA. Controlled clinical trial of the efficacy of the hepatitis B vaccine (Heptavax B): A final report. Hepatology 1981; 1:377–85.
8. Francis DP, Hadler SC, Thompson SE, Maynard JE, Ostrow DG, Altman N, Braff EH, O'Malley P, Hawkins D, Judson FN, Penley K, Nylund T, Christie G, Meyers F, Moore JN, Gardner A, Doto IL, Miller JH, Reynolds GH, Murphy BL, Schable CA, Clark BT, Curran JW, Redeker AG. The prevention of hepatitis B with vaccine. Ann Int Med 1982; 97:362–6.
9. Stevens CE, Alter JH, Taylor PE, Zaug EA, Harley EJ, Szmuness W. Hepatitis B vaccine in patients receiving hemodialysis: immunogenicity and efficacy. N Engl J Med 1984; 311:496–501.

10. Centers for Disease Control. Update on hepatitis B prevention. MMWR 1987; 36:353–66.

11. Ellis RW. New technologies for making vaccines. In: Plotkin S, Mortimer E., eds. Vaccines. Philadelphia: WB Saunders, 1988:568–75.

12. Galibert F, Mandart E, Fitoussi F, Tiollais P, Charnay P. Nucleotide sequence of the hepatitis B virus genome (subtype *ayw*) cloned in *E. coli*. Nature 1979; 281:646–50.

13. Pasek M, Goto T, Gilbert W, Zink B, Schaller H, MacKay P, Leadbetter G, Murray K. Hepatitis B virus genes and their expression. Nature 1979; 282: 575–9.

14. Valenzuela P, Gray P, Quiroga N, Zaldivar J, Goodman HM, Rutter WJ. Nucleotide sequence of the gene coding for the major protein of hepatitis B virus surface antigen. Nature 1979; 280:815–9.

15. Peterson DL, Roberts IM, Vyas GN. Partial amino acid sequence of two major component polypeptides of hepatitis B surface antigen. Proc Natl Acad Sci USA 1977; 74:1530–4.

16. Tiollais P, Pourcel C, Dejean A. The hepatitis B virus. Nature k1985; 317: 489–95.

17. Michael ML, Sopczak E, Malpiece Y, Tiollais P, Streek RE. Expression of amplified hepatitis B virus surface antigen genes in Chinese hamster ovary cells. Biotechnology 1985; 3:561–6.

18. Kitano K, Nakao M, Itoh Y, Fujisawa Y. Recombinant hepatitis B virus surface antigen p31 accumulates as particles in *Saccharomyces cerevisiae*. Biotechnology 1987; 5:281–3.

19. Kniskern PJ, Hagopian A, Burke P, Dunn N, Emini EA, Miller WJ, Yamazaki S, Ellis RW. A candidate vaccine for hepatitis B containing the complete viral surface protein. Hepatology 1988; 8:82–7.

20. Ellis RW, Kniskern PJ, Hagopian A, Schultz LD, Montgomery DL, Maigetter RZ, Wampler DE, Emini EA, Wolanski B, McAleer WJ, Hurni WM, Miller WJ. Preparation and testing of a recombinant-derived hepatitis B vaccine consisting of pre-S2 + S polypeptides. In: Zuckerman A, ed. Viral hepatitis and liver disease. New York: Alan R. Liss, 1988:1079–85.

21. Burrell CJ, MacKay P, Greenaway PJ, Hofschneider PH, Murray K. Expression in *Escherichia coli* of hepatitis B virus DNA sequences cloned in plasmid pBR322. Nature 1979; 279:43–7.

22. Edman JC, Hallewell RA, Valenzuela P, Goodman HM, Rutter WJ. Synthesis of hepatitis B surface and core antigens in *E. coli*. Nature 1981; 291: 503–6.

23. MacKay P, Pasek M, Magazin M, Kovacic RT, Allet B, Stahl S, Gilbert W, Schaller H, Bruce SA, Murray K. Production of immunologically active surface antigens of hepatitis B virus by *Escherichia coli*. Proc Natl Acad Sci USA 1981; 78:4510–4.

24. Valenzuela P, Medina A, Rutter WJ, Ammerer G, Hall BD. Synthesis and assembly of hepatitis B virus surface antigen particles in yeast. Nature 1982; 298:347–50.

25. Burnette WN, Samal B, Browne J, Ritter GA. Properties and relative immunogenicity of various preparations of recombinant DNA-derived hepatitis B surface antigen. Dev Biol Stand 1983; 599:113–20.

26. DeWilde M, Cabezon T, Harford N, Rutgers T, Simoen E, van Wijnendaele F. Production in yeast of hepatitis B surface antigen by R–DNA technology. Dev Biol Stand 1983; 59:99–107.

27. Hitzemann RA, Chen CY, Hagie FE, Patzer EJ, Liu C-C, Estell DA, Miller JV, Yaffe A, Kleid DG, Levinson AD, Opperman H. Expression of hepatitis B virus surface antigen in yeast. Nucl Acids Res 1983; 11:2745–62.

28. McAleer WJ, Buynak EB, Maigetter RZ, Wampler DE, Miller WJ, Hilleman MR. Human hepatitis B vaccine from recombinant yeast. Nature 1984; 307:178–80.

29. Miyanohara A, Toh-E, Nozaki C, Hamada F, Ohtomo N, Matsubara K. Expression of hepatitis B surface antigen gene in yeast. Proc Natl Acad Sci USA 1983; 80:1–5.

30. Liu C-C, Yansura D, Levinson AD. Direct expression of hepatitis B surface antigen in monkey cells from an SV40 vector. DNA 1982; 1:213–21.

31. Crowley CW, Liu C-C, Levinson AD. Plasmid-directed synthesis of hepatitis B surface antigen in monkey cells. Mol Cell Biol 1983; 3:44–55.

32. Carloni, G, Malpiece Y, Michel M-L, le Patezour A, Sobczak E, Tiollais P, Streeck RE. A transformed Vero cell line stably producing the hepatitis B virus surface antigen. Gene 1984; 31:49–57.

33. Hsiung N, Fitts R, Wilson S, Milne A, Hamer D. Efficient production of hepatitis B surface antigen using a bovine papilloma virus-metallothionein vector. J Mol Appl Genet 1984; 2:497–506.

34. Davis AR, Kostek B, Mason BB, Hsaio CL, Morin J, Dheer SK, Hung PP. Expression of hepatitis B surface antigen with a recombinant adenovirus. Proc Natl Acad Sci USA 1985; 82:7560–4.

35. Heerman KH, Goldman V, Schwartz W, Seyffarth T, Baumgarten H, Gerlich WH. Large surface proteins of hepatitis B virus containing the pre-S sequence. J Virol 1984; 52:396–402.

36. Peterson DL. Isolation and characterization of the major protein and glycoprotein of hepatitis B surface antigen. J Biol Chem 1981; 256:6975–82.

37. Hilleman MR, Ellis RW. Vaccines made from recombinant yeast cells. Vaccine 1986; 4:75–6.

38. Ellis, R.W. Vaccines, diagnostic proteins and hormones. In: Rehm HJ, Reed G, eds. Biotechnology, a comprehensive treatise (Vol 7b): Gene technology. Weinheim, West Germany: Verlag Chenne, 1988:167–94.

39. Jayaram M, Li Y-Y, Broach JR. The yeast plasmid in 2u circle encodes components required for its high copy propagation. Cell 1983; 34:95–104.

40. Holland JP, Holland MJ. Structural expression of two nontandemly repeated yeast glyceraldehyde-3-phosphate dehydrogenase genes. J Biol Chem 1980; 255:2596–605.

41. Harford N, Cabezon T, Colau B, Delisse A-M, Rutgers T, De Wilde M. Construction and characterizatin of a *Saccharomyces cerevisiae* strain

(RIT4376) expressing hepatitis B surface antigen. Postgrad Med J 1987; 63(2):65–70.

42. Bennetzen JL, Hall BD. The primary structure of the *Saccharomyces cerevisiae* gene for alcohol dehydrogenase I. J Biol Chem 1982; 257:3018–25.

43. Ellis RW, Kniskern PJ, Hagopian A, Schultz LD, Montgomery DL, Maigetter RZ, Wampler DE, Yamazaki S, Kubek DJ, Sitrin R, Lehman ED, Emini EA, Miller WJ, Zajac BA, West DJ, Gerety RJ. The yeast *Saccharomyces cerevisiae* as a host for current and potential future generation recombinant-derived hepatitis B vaccines. In: Lasky L, ed. Technological advances in vaccine development. New York: Alan R. Liss, 1988:127–36.

44. Peetermans JH. Specifications and quality control of a yeast-derived hepatitis B vaccine. Postgrad Med J 1987; 63(2):97–100.

45. Wampler DE, Lehman ED, Boger J, McAleer WJ, Scolnick EM. Multiple chemical forms of hepatitis B surface antigen produced in yeast. Proc Natl Acad Sci USA 1985; 82:6830–4.

46. West DJ, Zajac BA, Ellis RW, Gerety RJ. Improved immunogenicity of a yeast-derived hepatitis B vaccine. Infektionsklinik 1988;1:1–4.

47. Hollinger FB, Dressman GR, Sanchez Y, Cabral GA, Melnick JL. Experimental hepatitis B polypeptide vaccine in chimpanzees. In: Vyas GN, Cohen SN, Schmid R, eds. Viral hepatitis. Philadelphia: Franklin Institute Press, 1978:557–74.

48. Valenzuela P, Tekamp-Olson P, Coit D, Heberlein U, Kuo G, Masiarz FR, Medina-Selby MA, Rosenberg S, Whitney J, Burlingame A, Rutter WJ. Hepatitis-B vaccine: characterization of hepatitis-B antigen particles produced in yeast. In: Chanock RM, Lerner RA, eds. Modern approaches to vaccines. Cold Spring Harbor: Cold Spring Harbor Press, 1984:209–13.

49. Waters JA, O'Rourke SM, Richardson SC, Papaevangelou G, Thomas HC. Qualitative analysis of the humoral immune response to the "a" determinant of HBs antigen after inoculation with plasma-derived or recombinant vaccine. J Med Virol 1987; 21:155–160.

50. Iwarson S, Tabor E, Thomas HC, Godall A, Waters J, Snoy P, Shih JW-K, Gerety R. Neutralization of hepatitis B virus infectivity by a murine monoclonal antibody: an experimental study in the chimpanzee. J Med Virol 1985; 16:89–96.

51. Emini EA, Ellis RW, Miller WJ, McAleer WJ, Scolnick EM, Gerety RJ. Production and immunological analysis of recombinant hepatitis B vaccine. J Inf 1986; 13(A):3–9.

52. Hauser P, Voet P, Simoen E, Thomas HC, Petre J, DeWilde M, Stephenne J. Immunological properties of recombinant HBsAg produced in yeast. Postgrad Med J 1987; 63(2):83–91.

53. Schellekens H, de Reus A, Peetermans JH, van Eerd PACM. The protection of chimpanzees against hepatitis B viral infection using a recombinant yeast-derived hepatitis B surface antigen. Postgrad Med J 1987; 63(2): 93–96.

54. Centers for Disease Control. Suboptimal response to hepatitis B vaccination by injection into the buttock. MMWR 1985; 34:105-9.

55. Scolnick EM, McLean AA, West DJ, McAleer WJ, Miller WJ, Buynak EB. Clinical evaluation in healthy adults of a hepatitis B vaccine made by recombinant DNA. JAMA 1984; 251:2812-5.

56. Zajac BA, West DJ, McAleer WJ, Scolnick EM. Overview of clinical studies with hepatitis B vaccine made by recombinant DNA. J Inf 1986; 13:39-45.

57. Stevens CE, Taylor PE, Tong MJ, Toy PT, Vyas GN, Krugman S. Yeast-recombinant hepatitis B vaccine: Efficacy with hepatitis B immune globulin in prevention of perinatal hepatitis B virus transmission. JAMA 1987; 257: 2612-6.

58. Stevens CE, Taylor PE, Zang EA, Morrison JM, Harley EJ, DeCordoba SR, Bacino C, Ting RCY, Bodner AJ, Sarngadharam MG, Gallo RC, Rubinstein P. Human T-cell lymphotropic virus type III infection in a cohort of homosexual men in New York City. JAMA 1986; 255:2167-72.

59. Alter HJ, Favero MS, Maynard JE. Impact of infection control strategies on the incidence of dialysis-associated hepatitis in the United States. J Inf Dis 1986; 153:1149-51.

60. Okada K, Kamiyama I, Inomata M, Imai M, Miyakura Y, Mayumi M. e Antigen and anti-e in the serum of asymptomatic carrier mothers as indicators of positive and negative transmission of hepatitis B virus to their infants. N Engl J Med 1976; 294:746-9.

61. Beasley RP, Hwang L-Y, Stevens CE, Lin C-C, Hsieh F-J, Wang K-Y, Sun T-S, Szmuness W. Efficacy of hepatitis B immune globulin for prevention of perinatal transmission of the hepatitis B virus carrier state: Final report of a randomized double-blind, placebo-controlled trial. Hepatology 1983; 3:135-41.

62. Beasley RP, Hwang LY, Lee GC-Y, Lau CC, Roan CH, Huang F, Chen CL. Prevention of perinatally transmitted hepatitis B virus infections with hepatitis B immune globulin and hepatitis B vaccine. Lancet 1983; 2: 1099-102.

63. Stevens CE, Toy PT, Tong MJ, Taylor PE, Vyas GN, Nair PV, Gudavalo M, Krugman S. Perinatal hepatitis B virus transmission in the United States: Prevention by passive-active immunization. JAMA 1985; 253:1740-5.

64. Morein B, Simons K. Subunit vaccines against enveloped viruses: Virosomes, micelles and other protein complexes. Vaccine 1985; 3:83-93.

65. Allison AC, Byars NE. An adjuvant formulation that selectively elicits the formation of antibodies of protective isotypes and of cell-mediated immunity. J Imm Meth 1986; 95:157-68.

21

HIV-1 Infection in Central Africa
Some Epidemiologic and Prevention Aspects

Gérard Agius, Isabelle Desportes, Gigliola Flamminio-Zola,
and Daniel Zagury
Université P. et M. Curie
Paris, France

Z. Lurhuma
Cliniques Universitaires
Kinshasa, Zaire

J. J. Salaun
Institut National de Recherches Biomédicales
Kinshasa, Zaire

Robert C. Gallo
National Cancer Institute
National Institutes of Health
Bethesda, Maryland

Acquired immunodeficiency syndrome (AIDS) and human immunodeficiency virus (HIV) confront humanity with an unprecedented problem, which equally affects both developing and industrialized countries. Although Africa is considered the continent from which HIV emerged (35), little is known about the true origin of this retrovirus. Most existing data is compatible with its absence or, at best, presence as a low-level infection prior to 1970 (11,35,46). Since that time, pathologic manifestations were documented which have been retrospectively considered as AIDS related (2,10,15,23,47,53). Finally, it appears that the African epidemic roughly coincides in time with the American and Haitian epidemics (43).

SELECTED EPIDEMIOLOGIC ASPECTS

The sex ratio of African AIDS cases is approximately 1:1 (2,28,37,40,47,52). In Kinshasa, the mean age of AIDS cases is 34 years, with 90% of cases occurring between 20 and 49 of age. The average age is significantly higher in men (37 years) than in women (30 years) (28). The number of seropositive cases may also vary with age. Seroepidemiologic studies of healthy populations in Kinshasa have demonstrated a bimodal distribution of seropositive cases. A striking initial peak incidence was observed among children aged from 1 to 14 years with a second in young adults aged from 16 to 29 years (43).

In Rwanda and Zaire, city populations are predominantly affected by HIV infection (28,40). In Uganda, AIDS cases appear to be more frequent in rural areas or small towns (47). HIV infection rates vary also according to the socio-economic status of populations (6,29). It is difficult to accurately assess the magnitude of the epidemic in Africa in terms of the geographic scope and intensity of HIV infection. The clinical definition for AIDS cases proposed by the Center for Disease Control (CDC) and the World Health Organization (WHO) requires sophisticated laboratory support to diagnose opportunistic infections and malignancies (54). Nevertheless, central Africa and adjacent areas to the east and west as well as southern Africa appear to be more severely affected than other areas (26,31,49).

Moreover, HIV was recently detected in areas thought to be free of infection. However, it is difficult to establish a distinction between infections due to reintroduction of the virus and those in which the infection existed but has only recently been detected. Circulation of HIV-1 within African populations has been extensively studied, especially in central Africa (33,38). Some HIV-1 seroprevalence rates have been reported in selected populations in Africa (Table 1) (38).

It would appear that several million Africans may already be infected with HIV (27), even though only 8652 AIDS cases have been reported to WHO as of 9 December, 1987 (Table 2) (39). Moreover, a new human retrovirus, HIV-2, which also generates immunodeficiency, was detected in 1986 (14). HIV-2 infections have been reported in west Africa (Senegal, Ivory Coast, and Guinea Bissau). To date, this virus seems to be less widespread and perhaps less virulent than HIV-1.

TRANSMISSION OF HIV INFECTION

As in Western countries, HIV is transmitted by blood, sexual intercourse, and perinatally (5-7). Blood contamination results from transfusions or intravenous injections of medications by means of nonsterile needles or syringes (16,22). Furthermore, specific traditional practices may contribute to blood

Table 1 HIV-1 Seroprevalence Rates in Different Geographic Areas in Africa

Population group	Countries	Year	% Seroprevalence	Reference
General population	Cameroon	1985	1	18
	Central African Republic (Bangui)	1985	4	33
	Congo (Brazzaville)	1985	5	33
	Uganda (Kampala)	1985	15	11
	Uganda (West Nile)	1985	1.4	11
	Zaire (Equateur)	1986	0.8	36
Pregnant women	Ivory Coast (Abidjan)	1986	5	17
	Zaire (Kinshasa)	1986	8	40
	Zambia (Lusaka)	1985	9	32
Prostitutes	Cameroon (Meiganga)	1985	8	18
	Ivory Coast (Abidjan)	1986	20	17
	Rwanda (Butare)	1984	88	51
	Zaire (Equateur)	1986	11	36
Men with STD	Rwanda (Butare)	1984	28	52
	Zambia (Lusaka)	1985	29	32

Source: Ref. 38.

Table 2 AIDS Cases Reported to WHO as of 9 December 1987

Continent	No. of cases	No. of countries reporting	
		One or more cases	No case
Africa	8,642	37	10
Americas	55,354	42	2
Asia	224	19	9
Europe	8,775	27	1
Oceania	742	4	10
Total	73,747	129	32

Source: Ref. 39.

contamination. These include ritual tattoos, scarifications (28), as well as circumcision and infibulation, all of which are performed with shared devices. In addition, blood letting, blood exchange, or the local use of blood or blood byproducts in healing wounds, performed by traditional practitioners, can also be a cause of HIV infection (7).

The question of HIV infection via insect vectors has been raised (58). Until now, available data argues against such a mode of transmission. There is a lack of increased infection risks for household contacts living closely with AIDS cases but not sexually involved with them (30). There are also clear differences in the geographic distribution of malaria and HIV infection in a well-studied area of central Africa (J. M. Mann, unpublished observations).

Sexual transmission appears to be a major cause of HIV infection. The role of homosexuality, which has been the most important mode of transmission in Western countries, is negligible in Africa. Indeed, traditional cultures emphasize procreation rather than individual pleasure. Infection of newborns by HIV-positive mothers is also a dramatic source of infection (12,42). As in Western countries, most infected individuals are asymptomatic carriers. They are unaware of their contagious condition, and this is a major cause for widespread HIV-1, especially in the cities (28).

In an effort to summarize the distribution of HIV-1 infection in the world, Piot et al. (39) have proposed a classification with three patterns. One of these defines the main characteristics of HIV-1 transmission in Africa (Table 3), but also includes its distribution in the Caribbean and South America.

Table 3 Characteristics of HIV Transmission in Africa

Transmission	Epidemiologic characteristics
Sexual	Predominantly heterosexual
	Up to 25% of the 20- to 40-year age group
	Up to 90% of female prostitutes
Parenteral	HIV-infected blood
	Use of nonsterile needles and syringes
Perinatal	Significant problem in those areas where 5–15% of women are HIV positive

Source: Ref. 39.

CLINICAL FEATURES OF AIDS IN AFRICA

African AIDS patients present the entire spectrum of outcomes seen in American and European patients (5) as defined by the CDC, Atlanta. Numerous opportunistic infections such as candidiasis, cryptococcal meningitis, or mucocutaneous Herpes simplex, the rare encephalitis following an acute HIV seroconversion, a generalized and persistent lymphadenopathy, and the aggressive form of Kaposi's sarcoma are common in African patients (5,6). Two clinical features of AIDS in Africa stand out. First, the "slim" disease, initially reported from Uganda (47), is mainly characterized by weight loss and a recurrent diarrhea. Second, the aggressive form of Kaposi's sarcoma associated with HIV infection is rapidly progressive. This plaque-forming disease affects the trunk, the face and the internal organs. Conversely, the endemic form of Kaposi's sarcoma in Africa is not associated with HIV (9) or other forms of immunodeficiency (3).

Other clinical manifestations are commonly reported, such as tuberculosis and malaria (8,39,41). Cases of B-cell leukemia appear to be associated with AIDS in Kinshasa. It is noteworthy that the chronic activation by endemic agents may contribute to immunodeficiency and accelerate AIDS manifestations (25).

SOCIAL AND CULTURAL FACTORS

Africa's population consists of a variety of people with their own language, religion, customs, and traditions. All of these aspects must be taken into account in planning a strategy for AIDS control. The concept of group social life, strongly anchored in the African mind, has a fundamental impact on sexual behavior. Tribal customs are still important in spite of the colonial influence, and the dramatic changes inherent in the development of large cities. Bantus, the tribe most involved in the studies discussed below, live in traditional villages. Migration of entire families for economic reasons contributes to the development of urban areas, but people remain conditioned by their traditions in spite of Western influences. Sexuality is essentially linked to procreation, which assures group survival. Thus, marriage involves a relationship between two groups rather than an association of two individuals. Extraconjugal intercourse is allowed within the group, and a woman may belong as much to her husband's group as to her husband (34).

According to such concepts, having children is not only a duty towards the group but also a means of personal status and social promotion. Increasing fertility requires conditions favoring procreation such as aphrodisiacs, body care (baths, ointments, elaborate hairstyles), and erotic dances, which have an important place in traditional cultures.

These social and cultural factors have the following consequences with regard to AIDS control:

Absence or low development of homosexuality, rendering it a negligible factor of HIV-1 transmission.

Difficulties encountered in promoting use of condoms in AIDS prophylaxis.

Development of prostitution which is due not only to nonexclusive heterosexuality but also to migration of people, severe economic need, and foreign influences. Prostitution represents a major source of HIV-1 transmission in Africa, especially in large cities where the virus is endemic (24).

EDUCATION AND INFORMATION

Information provided in schools or by the media may contribute to AIDS control. Three different levels of education may be considered:

1. Informal and empiric knowledge which is communicated through influential people such as soothsayers, religious leaders, village chiefs, or government officials.
2. Formal education in school (4).
3. Graduate studies in urban centers, which are eventually completed in foreign universities.

AIDS-related communication may be transmitted by means of formal or informal education. In villages, information may pass by word of mouth. It is also diffused by means of media which have a growing influence due to the recent progress of communication facilities that even reach isolated villages.

HEALTH AND HEALTH CARE STRUCTURES

Until 1985, most public health services had not considered AIDS and HIV-1 infection as a high priority health problem. Known AIDS cases were indeed small compared to the number of preventable deaths from endemic diseases. On the other hand, classic sexually transmitted diseases (STDs), such as syphilis, gonorrhea, or chlamydiae, are fairly widespread in subsaharan Africa and are a high priority for health care (42), despite organized structures for efficient therapy and prevention. In addition, infertility is as high as 50% in some areas, and as much as 80% of infertility is attributed to STDs (42). As pertains to HIV infection, among 139 patients seen in the STD clinic in Lusaka, Zambia, 41 (29.5%) had antibodies against HIV-1 (32). Patients who had attended an STD clinic before had a higher likelihood of being seropositive (37.3%) than did first-time attenders (22.8%) (32).

Thus, existing STD centers, although not always well provisioned, are suitable platforms for screening HIV-1 carriers. Besides urologic, gynecologic, and dermatologic consultations in hospitals, there are specific venereal disease (VD) protocols in urban dispensaries. One of these is the Institut d'Hygiène Sociale at Dakar, Senegal, which treats prostitutes. These centers are coordinated through their connection with the International African Union against Venereal Diseases. This nongovernmental organization represents both French- and English-speaking countries as well as WHO. Linking HIV-1 infection and STD should trigger greater activity of VD Health Centers and lead to improvement in the control of classic STDs.

Other health care organizations may also be of interest in AIDS control. Vaccination programs and maternal health centers with follow-up care for pregnant women, mothers, and infants would be ideal for treatment of HIV-1-infected offspring. Family planning centers now have effective programs on birth control, sepsis complications, and eclampsia.

These programs are also useful for dissemination of AIDS information. Blood banks are found in many African cities, either autonomous (Abidjan, Ivory Coast) or integrated in a hospital complex (Kinshasa, Zaire), and represent pre-existing platforms for blood donor control. They are technically and operationally organized to support and coordinate regional HIV-1 testing. In fact, in some countries, such as Congo, HIV-1 tests have been conducted since 1985 and reveal a 5-6% seropositivity for blood donors. These centers must be largely expanded.

In the African health care concept, it is important to recruit and incorporate midwives and nurses, who play a major role in small cities in the fight against HIV-1 infection. The primary role of traditional practitioners should also be particularly emphasized. Such individuals contribute heavily to health care within villages and are also consulted in the cities. This is often complementary to contemporary medical treatment. While physicians deal directly with clinical symptoms, traditional practitioners have the mission to exorcise the spirits, ghosts, or genii that the patients consider to be their illness. If spiritual healers are included in AIDS control in Africa, they may facilitate the work of the physician.

FRENCH–ZAIRIAN PROPHYLACTIC AND THERAPEUTIC PROGRAM

Modern medical practices and education programs represent key elements for successful AIDS control in African countries, especially in endemic areas like subsaharan Africa. Consequently, preventive and therapeutic programs are urgently required to impact on the epidemic. These programs should aim at offering an AIDS vaccine to noninfected individuals and treatment options to AIDS patients which would halt or delay the present fatal evolution of the disease. In addition, such programs should encourage infected subjects to become identified through volunteer testing.

Prophylactic Program

The knowledge necessary for developing a vaccine preparation against HIV includes a complete understanding of the virus and of its molecular biology, the selection of appropriate antigenic targets, which take into account the extreme variability of the virus, appropriate animal models where disease is an endpoint, and the confidence that both safety and efficacy are assured (48). Only then will large clinical trials on healthy human volunteers become feasible.

A prophylactic program supervised by the University Clinic of Kinshasa (Professor Lurhuma), the Institut National de Recherche Biomedicale in Kinshasa (Professor Salaun), and the Laboratoire de Physiologie Cellulaire de l'Université P. et M. Curie in Paris (Professor Zagury) was launched in Kinshasa within the framework of a French-Zairian cooperation. This program was supported by Zairian authorities and had the consent of the Zairian Ethics Committee.

Three classical approaches exist for a vaccine development: generation of attenuated virus stocks, inactivated viral preparations, and subunit vaccines (19). We have employed two strategies to date (56,57):

1. Priming with a live vaccinia recombinant virus (VR), whose genome carries the HIV-1 gp160 *env* gene (13). Cells infected by VR express HIV-1 *env* proteins at the cell surface.
2. An immunization with VR-infected autologous blood cells subsequently fixed by paraformaldehyde (1% in PBS at 4°C for 4 minutes).

Cytopathogenic studies (55) provided the rationale for these immunization procedures. Infected T cells produce virus only after immune activation. In order to prevent extensive viral dissemination, infected cells must be destroyed before "the production of virus." Immune responses against HIV-1 infection may be triggered directly by viral gene products. In this regard, it is known that HIV-1 undergoes frequent mutations and consequently new serotypes continuously appear. Restriction enzyme analysis of HIV-1 has demonstrated considerable divergence, particularly for the *env* gene (20,50). In addition, this extensive degree of envelope variation among different HIV-1 isolates also exists with viruses isolated at different times in the same individual (21,44). Neutralizing antibodies are directed primarily to epitopes on the outer virus envelope glycoprotein. These are both conserved and variable in nature (50). Immune recognition also occurs through fragments of the viral molecules, which are expressed at the cell surface in association with products of the major histocompatibility complex (MHC) (51). The aim of our strategy was to amplify the cell surface viral signals to trigger cell-mediated immunity (CMI).

These immunization procedures were tested on different primates like Cercopithecus, baboons, and chimpanzees. No important side effects were observed in these animals; only local 0.5-1 cm pustulas appeared after VR scarifications.

A vaccine program based on these principles has been established at Kinshasa. Thirty-nine healthy volunteers (27 French and 12 Zairian) were enrolled in this preliminary vaccine program. All these subjects were HIV-1 seronegative. They were primed either by VR or purified gp160 antigen, either mixed with an oil adjuvant or water soluble. These individuals underwent a boost with different preparations:

Autologous cells infected with VR and subsequently fixed.
VR by scarification.
Purified cell membrane fractions from autologous cells infected in vitro with
   VR.

Individuals boosted with VR showed low titer of neutralizing antibodies against two strains of HIV-1 (IIIB and RF). Subjects who received purified cell membrane fractions as a booster exhibited high titers of neutralizing antibodies but only for a short time. An optimal CMI and long-lasting neutralizing antibodies at high titers (Figs. 1 and 2) were obtained with autologous cells infected with VR and subsequently fixed. Unfortunately, this protocol, using fixed infected cells as a booster, would not be appropriate for a large-scale vaccine trial. For this purpose, purified gp160 antigen, either mixed with a mineral oil or in water, is presently being studied in a new series of volunteers.

In the near future, a large prophylactic trial including two groups of subjects—one receiving control immunogens and the other the "candidate vaccine"—will be launched with healthy HIV-1–seronegative individuals. Such a trial requires the full approval of local authorities and will have to be performed in compliance with the policies of and with the assistance of the WHO.

Therapeutic Program

As a complement to the studies described above, 10 HIV-exposed individuals (2 in July 1986 and 8 in December 1986) were inoculated with candidate immunogens. All the patients presented clinical manifestations of African AIDS with biological characteristics of immune defect, i.e. a T4 cell count <300, a T4 and T8 ratio <0.5, and PHA-induced IL-2 production by blood mononuclear cells much lower than normal. These patients received injections of $2 \times 10^{7-8}$ fixed

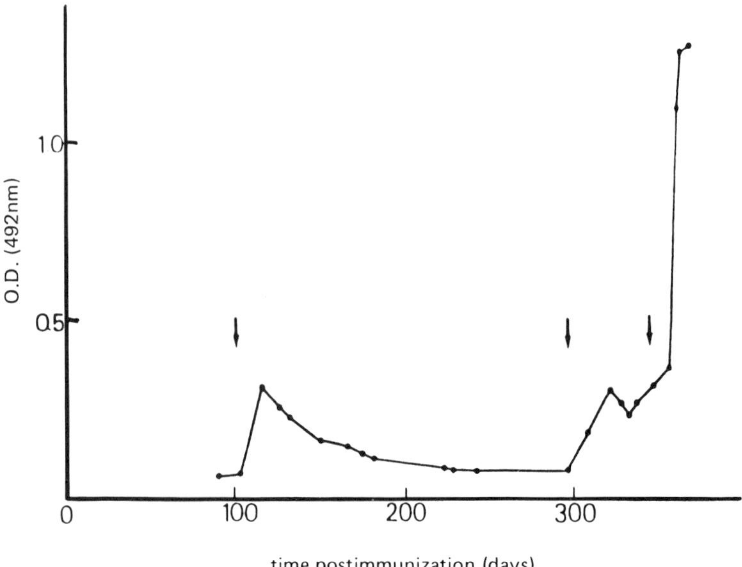

time postimmunization (days)

Figure 1 Serologic analysis of a subject (DZ) during the course of immunization for antibodies to HIV-1. Sera for antibodies to HIV envelope antigens were analyzed by an enzyme immunoassay. Arrows indicate the time of each of three immunization boosts. The control of DZ serum was collected prior to any immunization, and it did not show any evidence of antibody (not shown). (From Ref. 57.)

autologous cells infected with either HIV or the vaccinia recombinant (VR). Cells were given intravenously and subcutaneously about every 3 months.

Though clinical benefit cannot be unequivocally assessed thus far, most of the patients have gained weight (2-10 kg) and returned to their social and professional activities. Although T4 cell numbers were not restored to normal, the immune system has functionally improved, as assessed by IL-2 production. In addition, specific cell-mediated cytotoxicity against autologous infected cells was seen in two studied cases (R. Cheynier, personal communication).

These preliminary results indicate on the one hand that active immunization against HIV-1 as described above appears to be innocuous in individuals already exposed to the virus. However, more documented data are needed to draw conclusions on whether specific immunization against HIV-1 infection should be considered as an alternative or adjuvant therapy with chemical antiviral agents. A similar suggestion has been made by Salk (45) as a prophylactic postexposure vaccine.

Prevention of Infection in Neonates

The final French-Zairian project is adoptive immunotherapy to protect offspring of infected women. This program entails three steps: preparation of purified antibodies that neutralize HIV-1 virus, animal testing for safety and protection against infection, and inoculation of mothers and newborns with analysis of effective protection by follow-up. We are currently at stage one. Indeed, we have already prepared human monoclonal antibodies against HIV-1 from Epstein-Barr virus–transformed B-cells from a previously vaccinated subject (DZ).

OVERVIEW OF MEASURES FOR AIDS CONTROL IN AFRICA

AIDS control in Africa implies that various measures are to be taken focusing primarily on cities with populations of >50,000-100,000. This is where mobility

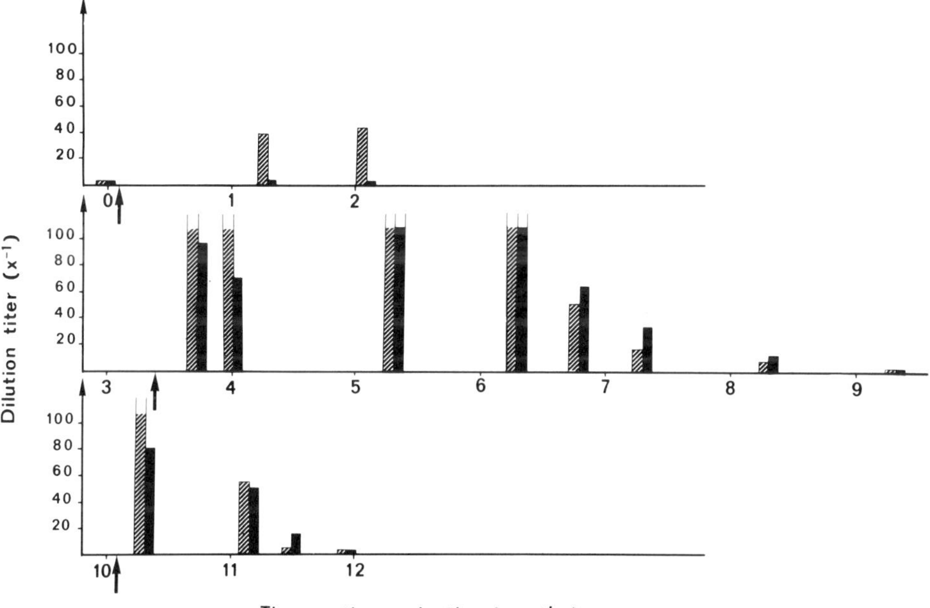

Figure 2   Serum-neutralizing antibodies to HIV, obtained from DZ at various periods before and after various stages of immunization, and tested for their capacity to inhibit infection of H9 cells by the homologous strain of HIV, HTLV–III$_B$ (hatched bars), and the divergent strain HTLV–III$_{RF}$ (solid bars). Arrows indicate times of immunization. (From Ref. 57.)

of people, promiscuity, permissive sexual exchanges, prostitution, as well as improper health care favor HIV-1 transmission.

The measures concern therapeutic and protective cures related to different categories of individuals: AIDS patients, asymptomatic carriers, high-risk sero-negatives, and offspring of infected mothers. It is most urgent to promote medical action for several reasons. First, this would tend to reduce AIDS to a common STD and would suppress both the stigmatization against infected people and the assumption that we are in the midst of a twentieth century plague. Second, epidemiologic spread may well be reduced by treatment of AIDS patients and infected individuals because of its proven ability to decrease viral load in patients. Finally, and perhaps most importantly, the availability of treatment should prompt voluntary testing and the subsequent identification of HIV-1-infected people. This could limit the epidemic spread currently due to unawareness of infection.

The second measure aims to block transmission by infected biological fluids like blood and semen. This can be accomplished by prophylaxis.

The third measure concerns the development of readily available tests and other initiatives to encourage volunteer identification of HIV-1-infected individuals. Compulsory testing for HIV-1 infection should be avoided for ethical considerations, and testing facilities need to be developed for use by high-risk populations.

The last measures concern education and information. Mass education through media has two goals: reducing AIDS to the level of any STD and prophylaxis against HIV-1 infection. A WHO program is actually established in Africa for prophylaxis, tests, and education.

ACKNOWLEDGMENT

We are grateful to Dr. Dani P. Bolognesi for helpful discussions.

REFERENCES

1. Barin F, Mc Lane MF, Allan JS, et al. Virus envelope protein of HTLV–III represents major target antigen for antibodies in AIDS patients. Science 1985;228:1094–6.
2. Bayley AC. Aggressive Kaposi's sarcoma in Zambia: 1983. Lancet 1984; 1318–20.
3. Bayley AC, Downing RG, Cheinsong-Popov R, et al. HTLV–III serology distinguishes atypical and endemic Kaposi's sarcoma in Africa. Lancet 1985;359–61.
4. Bekombo M, et al. L'institution scolaire et l'éducation traditionnelle en Afrique. UNESCO Paris: 1978.

5. Biggar RJ. The clinical features of HIV infection in Africa. B Med J 1986; 293:1453–4.

6. Biggar RJ. The AIDS problem in Africa. Lancet 1986; 79–83.

7. Biggar RJ, Agius G. AIDS in subsaharan Africa. In: AIDS and other manifestations of HIV infection. Wormser GP, Stahl RE and Bottone EJ, ed. Park Ridge, NJ: Noyes Publications, 1987: 108–23.

8. Biggar RJ, Gigase PL, Melbye M, et al. Elisa HTLV retrovirus antibody reactivity associated with malaria and immune complexes in healthy Africans. Lancet 1985; 520–3.

9. Biggar RJ, Melbye M, Kestens L, et al. Kaposi's sarcoma in Zaire is not associated with HTLV–III infection. N Engl J Med 1984; 16:1051.

10. Brunet JB, Bouvet E, Chaperon J, et al. Acquired immunodeficiency syndrome in France. Lancet 1983; 700–1.

11. Carswell JW, Sewankambo N, Lloyd G, et al. How long has the AIDS virus been in Uganda? Lancet 1986; 1217.

12. Centers for Disease Control. Recommendation for assisting the prevention of perinatal transmission of human T-lymphotropic virus type III/lymphadenopathy-associated virus and acquired immunodeficiency syndrome. MMWR 1985; 34:721–6, 731–2.

13. Chakhabarti S, Robert-Guroff M, Wong-Staal F, et al. Expression of the HTLV–III envelope gene by a recombinant vaccinia virus. Nature 1986; 320:535–7.

14. Clavel F, Guetard D, Brun-Vezinet F, et al. Isolation of a new human retrovirus from West African patients with AIDS. Science 1986; 233:343–6.

15. Clumeck N, Mascart-Lemone F, de Maulbeuge J, et al. Acquired immunodeficiency syndrome in black Africans. Lancet 1983; 642.

16. Clumeck N, Robert-Guroff M, Van de Perre P, et al. Seroepidemiological studies of HTLV–III antibody prevalence among selected group of heterosexual Africans. JAMA 1985; 254:2599–602.

17. Denis F, Barin F, Gershy-Damet G, et al. Prevalence of human T-lymphotropic retroviruses type III (HIV) and type IV in Ivory Coast. Lancet 1987; 408–11.

18. Durand JP, Garrigue GP, Bouloumie P, et al. AIDS in Cameroon. II International Conference on AIDS, Paris, 1986.

19. Ferdinand FJ, Dorner F, Kurth R. Perspectives of HIV vaccine developments. J Virol Meth 1987; 17:63–7.

20. Hahn BH, Gonda MA, Shaw GM, et al. Genomic diversity of the acquired immunodeficiency syndrome virus HTLV–III: Different viruses exhibit greatest divergence in their envelope genes. Proc Natl Acad Sci 1985; 82: 4813–7.

21. Hahn BH, Shaw GM, Taylor ME, et al. Genetic variation in HTLV-III/LAV overtime in patients with AIDS or at risk for AIDS. Science 1986; 232:1548-53.

22. Izzia KW, Lepira B, Kayembe M, et al. Syndrome d'immunodéficience acquise et drépanocytose homozygote à propos d'une observation zairoise. Ann Soc Belge Med Trop 1984; 64:391–6.

23. Katlama C, Leport C, Matheron S, et al. Acquired immunodeficiency syndrome (AIDS) in Africans. Ann Soc Belge Med Trop 1984; 64:379–89.

24. Kreiss JK, Koech D, Plummer EA, et al. AIDS virus infection in Nairobi prostitutes: Spread of the epidemic to East Africa. N Engl J Med 1986; 314:414–8.

25. Lauré F, Leonard R, Zagury D, et al. Prevalence of HIV infection in Zaire: Biological expression in relation to clinical specifities. AIDS Res Hum Retroviruses 1987; 3:343–53.

26. Lyons SF, Shoub BD, Mc Gillivray GM, et al. Lack of evidence of HTLV-III endemicity in Southern Africa. N Engl J Med 1985; 312:1257–8.

27. Mann JM. The epidemiology of LAV/HTLV–III in Africa. Ann Inst Past/Virol 1987; 138:113–8.

28. Mann JM, Francis H, Quinn TC, et al. Surveillance for AIDS in a central African city: Kinshasa, Zaire. JAMA 1986; 255:3255–9.

29. Mann JM, Francis H, Quinn TC, et al. HIV seroprevalence among hospital workers in Kinshasa, Zaire: Lack of association with occupational exposure. JAMA 1986; 256:3099–102.

30. Mann JM, Quinn TC, Francis H, et al. Prevalence of HTLV–III/LAV in household contacts of patients with AIDS and controls in Kinshasa, Zaire. JAMA 1986; 256:721–4.

31. M'boup, Prince-David M, Boye CS, et al. Serological evidence that HTLV-III is present in Senegal, West Africa. International Symposium on African AIDS, Brussels, 1985.

32. Melbye M, Njelesani EK, Bayley A, et al. Evidence for heterosexual transmission and clinical manifestations of human immunodeficiency virus infection and related conditions in Lusaka, Zambia. Lancet 1986; 1113–6.

33. Merlin M, Josse R, Gonzales JP, et al. Epidemiology of HIV-1 infection among randomized representative central African populations. Ann Inst Past/Virol 1987; 138:503–10.

34. Moyo D. Fighting AIDS in Africa. Africasia 1987; 41:54–5.

35. Newmark P. Trailing AIDS in Central Africa. Nature 1985; 315:273.

36. Nzila N, Mann JM, Francis H, et al. LAV/HTLV–III seroprevalence among tuberculosis patients in Zaire. II International Conference on AIDS, Paris, 1986.

37. Odio W, Kapita B, Bendi N, et al. Le syndrome d'immunodéficience acquise (SIDA) à Kinshasa (Zaire): observations cliniques et épidémiologiques. Ann Soc Belge Med Trop 1985; 65:357-61.

38. Piot P, Colebunders R, Laga M, et al. AIDS in Africa: A public health priority. J Virol Meth 1987; 17:1–10.

39. Piot P, Plummer FA, Mhalu FS, et al. AIDS: An international problem. Science 1988; 239:573–9.

40. Piot P, Quinn TC, Taelman H, et al. Acquired immunodeficiency syndrome in a heterosexual population in Zaire. Lancet 1984; 65–9.

41. Pitchenik AE, Cole C, Russel BW, et al. Tuberculosis, atypical mycobacteria and the acquired immunodeficiency syndrome among Haitian and non-Haitian patients in South Florida. Ann Intern Med 1985; 101:641–5.

42. Rosenbert MJ, Schulz KF, Burton N. Sexually transmitted diseases in Sub-saharan Africa. Lancet 1986; 152.
43. Quinn TC, Mann JM, Curran JW, et al. AIDS in Africa: An epidemiologic paradigm. Science 1986; 234:955–63.
44. Sakai K, Casareale D, Sonnabend J, et al. Molecular differences in the genomes of HTLV-III/LAV viruses isolated on two different occasions from a patient with lymphadenopathy. Ann Inst Pat/Virol 1986; 137E: 311–5.
45. Salk J. Prospects for the control of AIDS by immunizing seropositive individuals. Nature 1987; 327:473-6.
46. Saxinger WC, Levine PH, Dean AG. Evidence for exposure to HTLV-III in Uganda before 1973. Science 127:1036–8.
47. Serwadda D, Mugerwa RD, Servan NK, et al. Slim disease: A new disease in Uganda and its association with HTLV-III infection. Lancet 1985; 849–52.
48. Sever JL. AIDS virus. Vaccine prospects. Clin Immunol Newslett 1986; 7: 125-7.
49. Sher RS. Serological studies in Southern Africa. International Symposium on African AIDS, Brussels, 1985.
50. Starcich BR, Hahn BH, Shaw GM, et al. Identification and characterization of conserved and variable regions in the envelope gene of HTLV-III/LAV, the retrovirus of AIDS. Cell 1986; 45:637–48.
51. Unanue ER, Allen PM, Kurt-Jones EA, et al. Molecular nature of T-cell recognition of antigen in immune regulation. Feldman M and Mitchison NA, ed. Humana Press Inc, 1985, 225-30.
52. Van de Perre P, Rouvroy D, Lepage P, et al. Acquired immunodeficiency syndrome in Rwanda. Lancet 1984; 62-5.
53. Van de Pitte J, Verwilghen R, Zachee P. AIDS and cryptococcosis: Zaire, 1977. Lancet 1983; 925-6.
54. World Health Organization. Acquired immunodeficiency syndrome WHO/ CDC case definition for AIDS. Wkly Epidemiol Rec 1986; 10:69–73.
55. Zagury D, Bernard J, Leonard R, et al. Long term cultures of HTLV-III infected T-cells: a model of cytopathology of T-cell depletion in AIDS. Science 1986; 231:850–3.
56. Zagury D, Leonard R, Fouchard M, et al. Immunization against AIDS in humans. Nature 1987; 326:249-50.
57. Zagury D, Bernard J, Cheynier R, et al. A group specific anamnestic immune reaction against HIV-1 induced by a candidate vaccine against AIDS. Nature 1988; 332:728–31.
58. Zuckerman AJ. AIDS and insects. B Med J 1986; 292:1094-5.

22

Clinical Trials of AIDS Vaccines

Wayne C. Koff, Susan L. Wescott, and Daniel F. Hoth
National Institute of Allergy and Infectious Diseases
National Institutes of Health
Bethesda, Maryland

Recent advances in studying the host immune response against human immunodeficiency virus (HIV) infection have led to novel approaches in AIDS vaccine development. Utilizing molecular biological and functional analyses, epitope maps have been generated for sites on the HIV structural proteins, representing neutralization, T-cell cytolytic, and antibody-dependent cytotoxicity functional domains (1–5). Despite these elegant studies, the basic questions of whether immunization against HIV is possible and which immune functions must be stimulated to elicit protection against HIV challenge remain unanswered. This lack of understanding of the mechanisms of protective immunity against HIV has proven to be a major obstacle thus far in AIDS vaccine development and is due in large part to the lack of an ideal animal model for AIDS, i.e., an animal model in which HIV infection can be established followed by the development of AIDS-like disease. Nonetheless, several lentivirus animal models for AIDS including HIV-chimpanzee, simian immunodeficiency virus (SIV)-rhesus monkey, and others have been developed (6) and are currently being used to evaluate the pathogenesis of lentivirus infections and to define parameters for AIDS vaccine evaluation.

Concomitant with the efforts in preclinical AIDS vaccine development, preliminary clinical trials of experimental AIDS vaccines have been initiated in the absence of demonstrable protective immunity in animal models. These steps were undertaken for a number of reasons including the urgency of the AIDS pandemic, the capacity of obtaining important scientific knowledge on HIV antigenic stimulation of the human immune system, and a lack of standardized challenge criteria for examining protective immunity in animal models. These initial clinical trials have already demonstrated the complexities and challenges that clinical researchers will face as AIDS vaccine trials proceed from preliminary safety and immunogenicity studies to large-scale evaluation of vaccine efficacy.

In this review, we address the major issues associated with clinical trials of AIDS vaccines including design of phase 1, 2, and 3 trials; populations for testing AIDS vaccines; update on vaccines currently in clinical trials; social/ethical/ considerations in AIDS vaccine testing; international issues; and future directions.

DESIGN OF AIDS VACCINE TRIALS

Clinical trials of viral vaccines are carried out in a series of three phases. Table 1 lists the characteristics of phase, 1, 2, and 3 trials anticipated for AIDS vaccines. Phase 1 trials primarily address the issue of safety. In this regard, since HIV antigens may possess immunoregulatory activities (7), clinical evaluation of experimental AIDS vaccines will by necessity require a more comprehensive immunologic analysis than any other viral vaccine that has previously undergone testing. Moreover, low levels of nonneutralizing antibody against HIV have been shown to enhance infection of peripheral blood monocytes in vitro (8), suggesting that antibody-dependent enhancement may need to be monitored in vaccine recipients. Due to the extensive immunologic analysis being undertaken in phase 1 AIDS vaccine trials, the sample size and length of follow-up is greater in these trials than in previous phase 1 studies of other viral vaccines. In addition, there are difficulties in determining whether observed changes in immunologic parameters are due to the experimental AIDS vaccine being tested or are simply nonspecific responses to immunization with any protein antigen. Therefore, the first experimental AIDS vaccine product undergoing testing in the United States (recombinant gp160, MicroGeneSys, Inc.) is being compared with another

Table 1   Design of AIDS Vaccine Trials

Phase	No. of volunteers	Duration	Risk of HIV infection[a]	Evaluation
1	25–100	0.5–1.0 yr	Low	Safety and immunogenicity
2	100–400	1.0–2.0 yr	Low and high	Safety and immunogenicity
3	Currently estimated in 1000s	>2.0 yr	High	Safety and efficacy

[a]Indicates study population's risk for HIV infection as determined during the prescreening process.

Table 2 Endpoints for Phase 1 and 2 Viral Vaccine Studies

Vaccine	No. of subjects	Duration (days)	Endpoint	Reference
Adenovirus	15	28	Neutralizing ab	9
Adenovirus	47	21	Neutralizing ab	9
Influenza	24	120	HAI, ANAB	10
Influenza	111	365	HAI	11
Varicella	91	49	Fluorescent ab	12
Hepatitis B	110	210	Antibody (Anti HBs)	13
Hepatitis B	220	365	Antibody (Anti-HBs)	14
Hepatitis B	79	210	Antibody (Anti-HBs)	15
Rotavirus	20	21	EIA, Neutralizing ab	16
Rotavirus	25	28	EIA, Neutralizing ab	16
Rotavirus	43	180	Plaque reduction neutralization	17
Rift-Valley fever	52	365	Plaque reduction neutralization	18
Yellow fever	258	30	Plaque reduction neutralization, HAI	19

HAI = Hemagglutination-inhibition; ANAB = antineuraminidase antibody; Anti-HBs = Antihepatitis B surface antigen; EIA = enzyme linked immunoabsorbent assay.

vaccine (recombinant hepatitis B vaccine) in an attempt to differentiate AIDS vaccine-induced effects from nonspecific effects. Finally, phase 1 trials address preliminary immunogenicity questions with the aim of identifying safe and immunogenic doses which can be further evaluated in later phases of vaccine testing.

One of the major difficulties in evaluating experimental AIDS vaccines is the current lack of fundamental knowledge regarding parameters of HIV-induced immune responses which may be considered immunogenic endpoints for phase 1 and phase 2 vaccine trials. Table 2 lists several other virus vaccine trials in which immunogenicity endpoints have been established (9–19). For example, with hepatitis B (HB) virus vaccine, antibodies against HB surface antigen of 10 or more IU/1 (20) are indicative of protection against HB virus. No such correlate for HIV infection has been defined, thus complicating the design and testing of AIDS vaccines. As a result, immunologic analysis of humoral and cell-mediated immune responses to experimental AIDS vaccines is being carried out along with extensive natural history studies in efforts to identify mechanisms of immunity in HIV infection which may be applicable to vaccine strategies.

Given the lack of correlates for protective immunity in HIV infection, guidelines for progressing from phase 1 to phase 2 studies have not been established. Since the current state of the art in AIDS vaccine development assumes that an effective AIDS vaccine may need to induce both humoral and cell-mediated immune responses (21), candidate AIDS vaccines currently in phase 1 studies may be subjected to a more rigorous standard for progression into phase 2 studies than other viral vaccines.

Although phase 2 trials of candidate AIDS vaccines have not yet begun, it is anticipated that these trials will involve larger numbers of volunteers and will be designed to determine optimal dosage schedules based on safety and immunogenicity data. These trials may detect safety concerns or adverse reactions with low event rates, and provide the baseline for phase 3 efficacy studies. Similar to the decision point considerations for progressing from phase 1 to phase 2 (see above), the criteria for moving from phase 2 to phase 3 are currently undefined. However, due to the large scale and complex nature of the anticipated phase 3 studies (see below), it is presently hypothesized that no experimental AIDS vaccine will progress to efficacy studies unless protective immunity has been demonstrated in either chimpanzees, macaques, or another relevant animal model. Phase 3 trials will most likely be carried out as placebo-controlled, randomized, and double-blind studies, with the numbers of volunteers in each group determined by incidence of infection rates in the population being studied and statistical parameters sought for analysis of protection from infection or development of disease (21). Given the large numbers of volunteers required and the difficulties in determining the efficacy of AIDS vaccines, it is anticipated that only the most promising vaccine candidates will be evaluated in phase 3.

POPULATIONS FOR AIDS VACCINE TRIALS

Considerable debate occurred regarding the choices of study population for phase 1 AIDS vaccine trials. Ideally, individuals at no risk for HIV infection would be optimal for phase 1 trials, since safety and immunogenicity studies could be compromised by concurrent HIV infections. However, difficulties in recruitment of volunteers for these trials (see below) necessitated a pragmatic strategy. Thus, phase 1 trials are being carried out in volunteers whose risk for acquiring HIV infection is low or minimal. Healthy adult volunteers who are not engaged in high-risk behavior for acquiring HIV infection are currently the study population for phase 1 AIDS vaccine trials in the United States. In contrast, phase 2 trials will be carried out in both high- and low-risk populations, in order to determine whether the vaccine is safe and immunogenic in persons at high risk for acquiring HIV infection and to compare responses among the various population groups.

Table 3 lists the populations at high risk for HIV infection which potentially could be used in phase 3 vaccine efficacy trials of AIDS vaccines. Due to a decrease in incidence of infection rates among homosexual men in the United States, the capacity to carry out phase 3 studies in this group may be limited (22). Incidence rates of HIV infection in intravenous drug users including prostitutes continues to increase, suggesting that these populations may be amenable to vaccine studies as long as successful approaches to long-term follow-up can be demonstrated. Among other potential populations, partners and spouses of hemophiliacs may have limited utility for efficacy trials because of relatively small numbers, and ethical/legal considerations are involved in the decision-making process of using prisoners for biomedical research studies (23,24). As a result, consideration may be given to including several population groups at high risk for acquiring HIV infection in phase 3 efficacy studies.

AIDS VACCINES CURRENTLY IN CLINICAL TRIALS

Table 4 lists the experimental AIDS vaccines currently in clinical trials (25–30). These trials are all phase 1, with safety and immunogenicity of the various vaccine types being evaluated in the various populations indicated (Table 4). Clinical trials of candidate AIDS vaccines began in November 1986, with the first immunizations of HIV-seronegative healthy volunteers with recombinant vaccinia virus expressing the complete gp160 envelope protein of HIV-1 (25) (trial 1, Table 4). This Franco-Zairian study demonstrated that primary immunization with a vaccinia-HIV recombinant virus could produce low levels of

Table 3 Potential Target Populations for Phase 3 AIDS Vaccine Trials

Homosexual men

Partners/spouses of hemophiliacs

Intravenous drug users

Prostitutes

Prisoners

Military personnel in regions of high HIV incidence

Newborns of seropositive mothers

Sexually transmitted disease patients

Other high-risk groups in international locations

Table 4 Clinical Trials of Candidate AIDS Vaccines

Trial #	Candidate vaccine	Source	Location	Study population	References
1	Recombinant vaccinia-HIV env + autologous vaccinia-HIV env infected cells + recombinant gp160	D. Zagury, University Pierre et Marie Curie	Zaire	HIV-seronegative healthy individuals	25,26
2	Recombinant gp160	MicroGeneSys, Inc.	U.S.	HIV-seronegative healthy homosexual men	27
3	Recombinant gp160	MicroGeneSys, Inc.	U.S.	HIV-seronegative healthy adults	—
4	Recombinant vaccinia-HIV env	Bristol Myers, Inc.	U.S.	HIV-seronegative healthy homosexual/ bisexual men	—
5	Gamma-irradiated HIV	Immune Response Corp.	U.S.	AIDS-related complex (ARC) HIV viremia homosexual men	28
6	Monoclonal anti-CD4	Becton Dickinson	U.K.	AIDS-related complex (ARC)	29
7	Recombinant gp120	Biocine Company	Switzerland	Healthy men	30

neutralizing antibodies and could also induce cell-mediated immune responses as measured by lymphocyte proliferation. The induction of neutralizing antibodies in humans by a single immunization with a vaccinia-HIV recombinant contrasts the lack of detectable neutralizing antibodies in chimpanzees immunized by a similar procedure (31), suggesting potential difficulties in extrapolating immunogenicity studies from chimpanzees to humans. This first clinical trial was expanded to evaluate various strategies for boosting the weak primary immune response of vaccinia-HIV recombinants (26). These strategies included boosting with either a) the original vaccinia-HIV recombinant, b) intravenous infusion with paraformaldehyde fixed autologous cells infected with the vaccinia-HIV recombinant followed by two subsequent boosts with recombinant purified gp 160, c) intramuscular injections of purified autologous cell membranes infected with vaccinia-HIV recombinant, or d) scarification with a fragment of the gp120 envelope protein which reacted with an anti-gp120 monoclonal antibody. The multiple boosting protocol (b, above) induced an anamnestic humoral and cell-mediated immune response which persisted for more than one year following the primary immunization, and these responses were group specific, suggesting that combination of various strategies in AIDS vaccine development may potentially be necessary to produce the optimal anti-HIV immunologic responses.

The first FDA-approved AIDS vaccine for study in the United States involves a recombinant envelope glycoprotein, gp160, derived from HIV and expressed in a baculovirus vector-insect cell system (27) (trials 2, 3, Table 4). Trial 2 is a dose escalation phase 1 study in seronegative and HIV culture-negative healthy homosexual men with primary immunization at day 0, followed by booster at day 30. Trial 3 involves seronegative, HIV culture-negative healthy heterosexual and homosexual adults at low risk for HIV infection. This study includes booster immunization with gp160 at 1 month and 6 months post-primary immunization. Preliminary data from trial 2 indicates that the gp160 elicited minimal adverse reactions, and appears safe at low doses over the short term (27). Completion of both of these studies will include a detailed immunologic analysis and aims to determine the immunogenicity of the candidate vaccine. Recently, the FDA approved a second candidate AIDS vaccine for study, a recombinant vaccinia expressing the envelope glycoproteins of HIV strain LAV-1 (trial 4, Table 4). This study should greatly add to the preliminary information regarding vaccinia recombinants obtained from the Franco-Zairian study discussed above.

In a different strategy, gamma-irradiated HIV was inoculated into nine homosexual men with ARC and active HIV viremia (28) (trial 5, Table 4). This safety and immunogenicity study demonstrated an absence of adverse reaction to the inactive HIV and preliminary evidence of restoration of delayed type hypersensitivity reactions in all nine volunteers. This postinfection immunization strategy is based on the hypothesis that immunization of seropositive individuals with HIV antigens may boost immunologic responses necessary to reduce the viral burden and prevent further development of disease (32). This preliminary study, demonstrating lack of toxicity of inactivated HIV administered to ARC patients, paves the way for expanded studies in a more immunocompetent group of HIV-positive asymptomatic subjects (28).

In another preliminary study, monoclonal anti-CD4 is being administered to ARC patients in an attempt to evaluate the safety of this product, and to study whether anti-idiotypic antibodies which mimic CD4 and exhibit anti-HIV effects can be elicited (29) (trial 6, Table 4), as has previously been shown in animal model systems (33,34). Finally, another AIDS vaccine trial has recently been initiated (30) (trial 7, Table 4). Trial 7 is a phase 1 study of recombinant gp120 produced in yeast and aims to test the safety and immunogenicity of this glycoprotein using different adjuvant formulations.

Thus, several candidate AIDS vaccines have already reached the clinic for phase 1 analysis, and it is anticipated that several others will be nearing completion of preclinical evaluation in the near future, thereby increasing the potential number of experimental AIDS vaccines in clinical trials. As more vaccine candidates become available for testing, the numbers of volunteers required for these trials will increase, thereby exacerbating the logistical, social, and ethical challenges unique to AIDS vaccine testing. These are discussed briefly below.

SOCIAL/ETHICAL ISSUES SURROUNDING AIDS VACCINE TESTING

Recruitment of volunteers at low risk for HIV infection is proving to be a formidable task, as evidenced by the preliminary phase 1 trials (35). This is due in part to the issue of confidentiality, and concern that inappropriate release of information regarding a volunteer's participation in an AIDS vaccine trial may carry social risks. Already, a study subject in an experimental AIDS vaccine testing program has filed a complaint that alleges discrimination because of his participation in the vaccine trial (36). The confidentiality issue becomes more complex when prescreening of sexual partners of potential vaccine trial volunteers is included in the study protocol when recruiting persons at low risk for HIV infection. Trial design should address the issue of partner notification, especially if potential volunteers are found to be HIV-infected during the prescreening process. In addition, in trials of recombinant viruses where transmission of the recombinant virus to an unsuspecting contact is theoretically possible, both institutional review boards (IRBs) which review trial design and potential volunteers need to be apprised of these risks and of mechanisms to minimize potential transmission.

AIDS vaccine trial study subjects may also face the social risks of vaccine-induced seroconversion (21), which may affect any situation where HIV antibody testing occurs, including hospitalizations, applications for insurance, military service, traveling or living in foreign nations, and donating blood. Thus, altruistic healthy volunteers participating in AIDS vaccine trials may suddenly find themselves in compromising situations due to positive ELISA and Western blot tests resulting from a successful immunogenic response to a candidate AIDS vaccine. Efforts have been established to decrease the social consequences of vaccine-induced seroconversion through identification cards and registries of vaccine trial subjects, yet these concerns certainly impact on the difficulties in recruiting sufficient numbers of volunteers for AIDS vaccine trials.

While the recruiting concerns discussed above primarily affect phase 1 and 2 vaccine trials in the near future, phase 3 trials may also face these concerns as well as the difficult dilemma of trying to obtain statistically significant efficacy data while at the same time maintaining efficient counseling of volunteers from high-risk behavior for HIV infection. Resolution of this dilemma may rest on the development of placebo-controlled, randomized, double-blind studies using extremely large sample sizes, the presumption being that even with highly effective counseling, a percentage of volunteers will still not abstain from high-risk behavior for HIV infection.

INTERNATIONAL ISSUES

The AIDS pandemic has rapidly expanded to global distribution, and three infection patterns worldwide have been described (37). Extremely high infection rates have been described for urban populations in Zambia, Zaire, Uganda, Rwanda, Tanzania, the Congo, and in other developing nations, suggesting that these areas should be included when considering potential sites for phase 3 efficacy trials of AIDS vaccines (38). However, undertaking large-scale vaccine trials in these areas may be confounded by social, political, and logistical concerns.

Although currently there is no AIDS vaccine candidate on the horizon which appears ready for consideration for phase 3 efficacy trials, the complex logistics which will be required indicates that planning for such trials should begin immediately. The planning can best be coordinated through a collaborative process involving all countries involved, including participation by the World Health Organization. This process would include international clinical epidemiology studies, establishment of cohorts for potential vaccine trials, laboratory training and support, resource allocation, and cultural studies to understand ethical considerations of vaccine testing in different cultural milieu. A long-term planning process for phase 3 AIDS vaccine trials could thereby significantly decrease the start-up time required for these large-scale studies when a suitable vaccine candidate is identified for testing.

FUTURE DIRECTIONS

Clinical trials of AIDS vaccines continue to advance our knowledge of the human immune response to HIV antigens. The immunogenicity of HIV antigens appears to be low, particularly when neutralizing antibody titers during infection are used in comparative analyses with other retroviruses (39). These findings suggest that potentiation of the immune response against HIV antigens might be a necessary component of HIV vaccine strategies in order to induce levels of humoral and/or cell-mediated immunity necessary to protect against HIV disease. In this regard, since alum is the only adjuvant licensed for use in the United States, future directions in AIDS vaccine development should address the development of more effective adjuvants. Table 5 lists several new adjuvant approaches currently being explored as immune potentiators of candidate AIDS vaccines (40-52).

Finally, despite the difficult challenges posed by the testing of AIDS vaccines, the preliminary trials of experimental AIDS vaccines when taken together have demonstrated a lack of adverse reactions to the varied immunogens, and in the case of the Franco-Zairian studies (26) have initially demonstrated that a group-specific human immune response to HIV immunogens can be obtained by combining different vaccine approaches. The demonstration that immunity to HIV can be achieved in human beings by vaccination is the first step on the road to demonstration of protective immunity. While the road is long and contains many

Table 5 Adjuvants to Potentiate the Immune
Response to Candidate AIDS Vaccines

Adjuvant	References
Liposomes	40,41
ISCOMs	42
Synthetic polymers	43,44
Lipid A analogs	45
Muramyl dipeptide derivatives	46-48
Antigen modification	49
Monokines and lymphokines	50-52

obstacles, the continued collaborative efforts of the international scientific community in AIDS vaccine development combined with the triumphant history of vaccine development against other formidable pathogens (53), raises hope that the clinical testing of AIDS vaccines will eventually lead to the successful distribution of a safe and effective vaccine to prevent AIDS.

REFERENCES

1. Cease KB, Margalit H, Cornette JL, Putney SD, Robey WG, Ouyang C, Streicher HZ, Fischinger PJ, Gallo DeLisi C, Berzofsky JA. Helper T-cell antigenic site identification in the acquired immunodeficiency syndrome virus gp120 envelope protein and induction of immunity in mice to the native protein using a 16-residue synthetic peptide. Proc Natl Acad Sci USA 1987;84:4249.
2. Palker TJ, Clark ME, Langois AJ, Matthews TJ, Weinhold KJ, Randall RR, Bolognesi DP, Haynes BF. Type-specific neutralization of the human immunodeficiency virus with antibodies to env-encoded synthetic peptides. Proc Natl Acad Sci USA 1988; 85:1932.
3. Takahashi H, Cohen J, Hosmalin A, Cease KB, Houghten R, Cornette JL, DeLisi C, Moss B, Germain RN, Berzofsky JA. An immunodominant epitope of the human immunodeficiency virus envelope glycoprotein gp160 recognized by class I major histocompatibility complex molecule-restricted murine cytotoxic T lymphocytes. Proc Natl Acad Sci USA 1988; 85:3105.
4. Langlade-Demoyen P, Michel F, Hoffenbach A, Vilmer E, Dadaglio G, Garcia-Pons F, Mayaud C, Autran B, Wain-Hobson S, Plata F. Immune recognition of AIDS virus antigens by human and murine cytotoxic T lymphocytes. J Immunol 1988; 141:1949.
5. Rusche JR, Javaherian K, McDanal C, Petro J, Lynn DL, Grimaila R, Langlois A, Gallo RC, Arthur LO, Fischinger PJ, Bolognesi DP, Putney SD, Matthews TJ. Antibodies that inhibit fusion of human immunodeficiency virus-infected cells bind a 24-amino acid sequence of the viral envelope, gp120. Proc Natl Acad Sci USA 1988; 85:3198.
6. Desrosiers RC, Letvin NL. Animal models for acquired immunodeficiency syndrome. Rev Infec Dis 1987; 9:438.
7. Siliciano RF, Lawton T, Knall C, Karr RW, Berman P, Gregory T, Reinherz EL. Analysis of host-virus interactions in AIDS with Anti-gp120 T cell clones: Effect of HIV sequence variation and a mechanism for CD4+ cell depletion. Cell 1988; 54:561.
8. Takeda A, Tuazon CU, Ennis FA. Antibody-enhanced infection by HIV-1 via Fc receptor-mediated entry. Science 1988; 242:580.
9. Dudding BA, Bartelloni PJ, Scott RM, Top Jr FH, Russell PK, Buescher EL. Enteric immunization with live adenovirus type 21 vaccine, I. Tests for safety, infectivity, immunogenicity, and potency in volunteers. Inf and Imm 1972; 5(3):295.

10. Wright PF, Sell SH, Shinozaki T, Thompson J, Karzon DT. Safety and antigenicity of influenza A/Hong Kong/68-ts-I [E] (H$_3$N$_2$) vaccine in young seronegative children, J Pediatrics 1975; 87(6):1109.

11. Feldman S, Wright PF, Webster RG, Roberson PK, Mahoney J, Thompson J, Doolittle M, Lott L, Johnson P, Cristoph RC. Use of influenza A virus vaccines in seronegative children: Live cold-adapted versus inactivated whole virus. J Inf Dis 1985; 152(6):1212.

12. Arbeter AM, Starr SE, Weibel RE, Plotkin SA. Live attenuated varicella vaccine: Immunization of healthy children with the OKA strain. J Pediatrics 1982; 100(6):886.

13. Papaevangelou GJ, Vissoulis CG, Roumeliotou-Karayannis AJ, Kolaitis N, Krugman S. Comparison of safety and immunogenicity of adw and ayw hepatitis B vaccines. J Virology 1982; 9:231.

14. Scheiermann N, Gesemann KM, Kreuzfelder E, Paar D. Effects of a recombinant yeast-derived hepatitis B vaccine in healthy adults. Postgraduate Medical Journal 1987; 63(suppl.2):115.

15. Crovari P, Crovari PC, Petrilli RC, Icardi GC, Bonanni P. Immunogenicity of a yeast-derived hepatitis B vaccine (Engerix-B) in healthy young adults. Postgraduate Medical Journal 1987; 63(suppl.2):161.

16. Vesikari T, Isolauri E, Delem A, D'Hondt E, Andre FE, Zissis G. Immunogenicity and safety of live oral attenuated bovine rotavirus vaccine strain RIT 4237 in adults and young children. Lancet 1983; 807.

17. Maldonado Y, Hestvik L, Wilson M, Townsend T, O'Hare J, Wee S, Yolken R. Safety and immunogenicity of bovine rotavirus vaccine RIT 4237 in 3-month-old infants. J Pediatrics 1986; 109(6):931.

18. Meadors III, Gilcin F, Gibbs Paul H, Peters CJ. Evaluation of a new rift valley fever vaccine: safety and immunogenicity trials. Vaccine 1986; 4: 179.

19. Roche JC, Jouan A, Brisou B, Rodhain R, Fritzell B, Hannoun C. Comparative clinical study of a new 17D thermostable yellow fever vaccine. Vaccine 1986; 4(3):163.

20. Jilg W, Schmidt M, Deinhardt F, Zachoval R. Hepatitis B vaccination: How long does protection last? Lancet 1984; 2:458.

21. Koff WC, Hoth DF. Development and testing of AIDS vaccines. Science 1988; 241:426.

22. Curran JW, Jaffe HW, Hardy AM, Morgan WM, Selik RM, Dondero TJ. Epidemiology of HIV infection and AIDS in the United States. Science 1988; 239:610.

23. Walters L. Ethical issues in the prevention and treatment of HIV infection and AIDS. Science 1988; 239:597.

24. Code of Federal Regulations: Title 45, Part 46.

25. Zagury D, Leonard R, Fouchard M, Reveil B, Bernard J, Ittele D, Cattan A, Zirimwabagabo L, Kalumbu M, Justin W, Salaun J, Goussard B. Immunization against AIDS in humans. Nature 1987; 326:249.

26. Zagury D, Bernard J, Cheynier R, Desportes I, Leonard R, Fouchard M, Reveil B, Ittele D, Zirimwabagangabo L, Mbayo K, Wane J, Salaun J, Goussard B, Dechazal L, Burny A, Nara P, Gallo R. A group specific anamnestic immune reaction against HIV-1 induced by a candidate vccine against AIDS. Nature 1988; 332:728.

27. Kovacs JA, Megil ME, Deyton L,Metcalf JA, Salzman N, Vasudevachari M, Baseler M, Martin M, Fauci AS, Lane HC. Phase 1 trial of a recombinant gp 160 candidate AIDS vaccine. Abst. 6569, IV International Conference on AIDS, Stockholm, Sweden, 1988.

28. Levine, AM, Henderson BE, Dworsky R, Ascher MS, Sheppard HW, Cullman LC, Hicks DR, Munson C, Carlo DJ, Abrahamson J, Salk J. Response of HIV infected individuals with ARC to inoculation of gamma-irradiated HIV. Abst. 6567, IV International Conference on AIDS, Stockholm, Sweden, 1988.

29. Dalgleish AG, Kennedy RC, Chanh TC, Habeshaw J, Maddon P, Malkovsky M, Thomson B, Clapham P, Axel R, Webster ADB, Weiss R. Therapeutic strategies against HIV based on the CD4 molecule: Monoclonal antibody therapy, soluble CD4 and anti-idiotype vaccines. Abst., 3061, IV International Congress on AIDS, Stockholm, Sweden, 19xx.

30. Coles P. AIDS vaccine trials to begin in Geneva. Nature 1988; 333:792.

31. Hu S, Fultz PN, McClure HM, Eichborg JW, Thomas EK, Zarling J, Singhal MC, Kosowski SG, Swenson RB, Anderson DC, Todaro G. Effect of immunization with a vaccinia-HIV env recombinant on HIV infection of chimpanzees. Nature 1987; 328:721.

32. Salk J. Prospects for the control of AIDS by immunizing seropositive individuals. Nature 1987; 327:473.

33. Kennedy RC, Maino VC, Warner NL, Chanh TC, Koff W. CD4-gp 120 interaction: Idiotype mimicry as putative vaccines and therapeutics against HIV infection. In: AIDS vaccine: Basic research and clinical trials, Putney SD, Bolignesi DP, eds). Marcel Dekker Inc., in press.

34. Dalgleish AG, Thompson BJ, Chanh TC, Malkovsky M, Kennedy, RC. Neutralization of HIV isolates by anti-idiotypic antibodies which mimic the T4 (CD4) epitope: A potential AIDS vaccine. Lancet 1987; 1: 1047.

35. Ogata-Arakari D, Davey V, Lee, Dianne. Human immunodefieincy virus vaccine: Recruitment of healthy volunteers. Abst. 6574, IV international Conference on AIDS, Stockholm Sweden, 1988.

36. Ex-executive files MCAD complaint. Boston Globe, August 2, 1988. "A Massachusetts man who says he was fired for participating in an experimental AIDS vaccine test program filed a complaint yesterday against his employer with the Massachusetts Commission Against Discrimination in Boston.

37. Piot P, Plummer FA, Mhalu FS, Lamboray J, Chin J, Mann JM. AIDS: An international perpsective. Science 1988; 239:573.

38. Mann JM, Chin J, Piot P, Quinn T. The international epidemiology of AIDS. Scientific American 1988; 259:82.

39. Weiss RW, Clapham PR, Cheinsong-Popov Dalgleish AG, Carne CA, Weller IVD, Tedder RS. Neutralization of human T-lymphotropic virus type III by sera of AIDS and AIDS-risk patients. Nature 1985; 316:69.

40. Allison AC, Gregoriadis G. Liposomes as immunologic adjuvants. Nature 1974; 252:252.

41. Van Roijen N, Van Nieuwmegen R. Use of liposomes as biodegradable and harmless adjuvants. Methods Enzymol 1983; 93:83.

42. Morein B, Jundquist B, Hoglond S, Dalsgaard K, Osterhaus A. Iscom, a novel structure for antigenic presentation of membrane proteins from enveloped viruses. Nature 1984; 308:457.

43. Hunter R, Strickland F, Kezdy F. The adjuvant activity of non-ionic block polymer surfactants. I. The role of hydrophile-lipophile balance. J Immunol 1981; 127:1233.

44. Hunter RL, Bennett B. The adjuvant activity of nonionic block polymer surfactants. II. Antibody formation and inflammation related to the structure of triblock and octablock copolymers. J Immunol 1984; 133:3167.

45. Kotani S, Takada H, Tsujimoto M, Ogawa T, Harada K, Mori Y, Kawasaki A, Tanaka A, Nagao S, Tanaka S, Shiba T, Kosumoto S, Imoto M, Yoshimura H, Yamamoto M, Shimamoto T. Immunologically active lipid A analogs synthesized according to a revised structural model of natural lipid A. Infect Immun 1984; 45:293.

46. Chedid L, Audibert F, Lefrancier P, Choay J, Lederer E. Modulation of the immune response by a synthetic adjuvant and analogs. Proc Nat Acad Sci USA 1976; 73:2472.

47. Azuma I, Sugimura K, Taniyama T, Yamawaki M, Yamamura Y, Kusumoto S, Ikada S, Shiba T. Adjuvant activity of mycobacterial fractions: Immunological properties of synthetic N-acetylmuramyl dipeptide and related compounds. Infec Immun 1976; 14:18.

48. Allison AC, Byars NE. Vaccine technology: Adjuvants for increased efficiacy. Biotechnology 1987; 5:1041.

49. Warren HS, Vogel FR, Chedid LA. Current status of immunological adjuvants. Ann Rev Immunol 1986; 4:369.

50. Weinberg A, Mesigan TC. Recombinant interleukin-2 as an adjuvant for vaccine-induced protection. J Immunol 1988; 140:294.

51. Dinnarello CA. Interleukin-1. Rev Inf Dis 1984; 6:51.

52. Merluzzi UJ, Last-Barney K. Potential use of human interleukin 2 as an adjuvant for the therapy of neoplasia, immunodeficiency, and infectious disease. Int J Immunopharmacol 1985; 7:31.

53. Hilleman MR. Newer directions in vaccine development and utilization. J Inf Dis 1985; 151:407–19.

23

AIDS Vaccines
Regulatory, Scientific, and Ethical Issues

Alec E. Wittek and Gerald V. Quinnan, Jr.
Center for Biologics Evaluation and Research
Food and Drug Administration
Bethesda, Maryland

INTRODUCTION

Since its recognition in 1981, the acquired immunodeficiency syndrome (AIDS) has evolved into a health concern of global proportions. While counseling and education have reduced the risk of HIV infection in some high-risk populations, and sensitive antibody screening tests have significantly reduced the risk of HIV transmission by blood transfusion, HIV infection continues to spread in many populations and in most regions of the world. The development of safe and effective vaccines for the prevention of HIV infection would provide a major weapon in the global effort towards the control and eradication of AIDS. This chapter will summarize regulatory, scientific, and ethical considerations pertinent to the development of vaccines for the prevention of HIV infections and AIDS.

SOURCES OF INFORMATION FOR VACCINE DEVELOPERS

Formal regulatory requirements for specific vaccines are normally developed by the Food and Drug Administration (FDA) at the time of licensure when necessary data to assure safety and efficacy have been developed. Accordingly, the FDA does not have formal requirements for AIDS vaccine manufacture and testing at present. However, a variety of documents exist which can provide vaccine developers with many of the scientific principles applicable to AIDS vaccine development. These documents are listed in Table 1.

Table 1 Existing Regulatory Documents Relevant to Experimental AIDS Vaccines

Type	Subject	Reference
Regulations	Good laboratory practices	21 CFR 58
	Good manufacturing practices General	21 CFR 200–299
	Additional standards for biological products	21CFR 600–699
Guidelines	Numerous topics concerning manufacture, study considerations, and documentation	Director CBER[a]
Points to consider	Production and testing of new drugs and biologicals produced by recombinant DNA technology	Director, CBER[a]
	Characterization of cell lines used to produce biological products	Director, CBER[a]
	Manufacture and testing of monoclonal antibody products for human use	Director, CBER[a]
Summary basis for approval	Recombinant hepatitis B vaccine	Director, CBER[a]
	Recombinant alpha-interferon	Director, CBER[a]

[a]Available from the Director, Center for Biologics Evaluation and Research, 8800 Rockville Pike, Bethesda, MD 20892.

The regulations enforced by FDA are included in Title 21 of the Code of Federal Regulations (CFR). There are general requirements for good manufacturing and laboratory practices that apply to all products. In addition, more specific requirements exist for biological products and establishments that manufacture biological products. When feasible, experimental products should be produced in accord with Good Manufacturing Practice regulations (1,2), and preclinical evaluation of the product should be performed in conformity with Good Laboratory Practice standards (3). The FDA recognizes that full compliance with these regulations may be difficult and unnecessary for adequate assurance of safety at early stages of product development.

The Additional Standards for Biological Products (4) describe the general requirements for all biological products. Among these regulations are requirements for the prerelease testing of representative samples from each lot of product. This testing includes, among other things, in vitro and/or in vivo evaluation of product potency; general safety tests for the detection of toxic contaminants in a product, sterility, identification, and qualification of all product components, and purity and identity of the biological product. Some regulations in these sections pertain to the manufacture of specific vaccine products, including influenza, live and inactivated poliovirus, measles, mumps, rubella, and smallpox vaccines. The World Health Organization has issued international requirements for the manufacture of a number of other viral vaccines including plasma-derived hepatitis B, yeast-derived recombinant hepatitis B, yellow fever, influenza, and duck embryo and continuous cell line-derived rabies virus vaccines. If a regulation that applies to an already licensed vaccine can be applied to an investigational product to provide increased assurance of safety and efficacy, normally it should be applied. An example of such a regulatory concept would be the requirements for the qualification of cell banks and virus stocks. Certain portions of the Additional Standards for Human Blood and Blood Products (5) would be relevant to the manufacture of HIV immune globulin for passive immunization.

The FDA often publishes guidelines, a less formal type of requirement than a regulation. These guidelines deal with concerns that are common to many products. Examples of guidelines are documents that describe methods for equipment validation, for control and monitoring of sterile filling operations, and other critical routine functions. Guidelines contain details of methods consistent with good manufacturing practice regulations.

Another type of document that FDA makes available to provide guidance to product developers is referred to as "Points to Consider." These draft documents do not carry the weight of regulatory requirement. They represent a spectrum of opinions provided by scientists within and outside the agency and are developed in situations where many individuals or groups are attempting to develop a certain type or range of products using a specific technology. These documents serve to convey to these interested parties the concepts relating to the product or technology in question that FDA believes are relevant to consider early in the course of product development. Points to Consider are always in draft form and are updated from time to time to reflect revised or additional concepts.

With respect to AIDS vaccine development, there exist several Points which are likely to be of relevance. The "Points to Consider in the Characterization of Cell Lines Used to Produce Biological Products" was recently revised. This document describes the information that should be provided by manufacturers on cell lines used for the production of biological products, including cell seed systems and characterization of working cell banks. In addition, the document provides guidelines on testing for the presence of adventitious agents, tumorigenicity, and karyology.

The "Points to Consider in the Manufacture of Monoclonal Antibody Products for Human Use" addresses concerns about freedom from contamination, especially from adventitious murine viruses and those potentially introduced by interspecies hybridoma fusions. Other issues discussed in this document include product characterization and preclinical evaluation of potency and specificity. Some of the safety-related concepts expressed in this document may also be applicable to processes that use monoclonal antibodies as a step in the production of another biological product, as in antibody affinity columns for protein purification.

Suggestions for the characterization of products made by recombinant DNA technology are contained in the "Points to Consider in the Production and Testing of New Drugs and Biologics Produced by Recombinant DNA Technology." This document also provides guidelines pertaining to technical aspects of recombinant manufacturing processes, and recommendations for the preclinical evaluation of potency, purity, and safety of recombinant biological products. In addition, the production of new biologicals by recombinant DNA technology should generally follow the NIH Guidelines for Research Involving Recombinant DNA Molecules.

Another type of document which vaccine developers may find useful is known as a Summary Basis for Approval (SBA). These documents are issued by the FDA upon the licensure of a specific product and contain points related to the development, manufacture and testing of that product which FDA considered relevant to licensure. The SBA for recombinant hepatitis B vaccine and the SBA for recombinant alpha-interferon may provide useful information for vaccine developers using recombinant DNA techniques.

AN OVERVIEW OF THE INVESTIGATIONAL NEW DRUG
REVIEW PROCESS

The Center for Biologics Evaluation and Research (CBER), formerly the Office of Biologics Research and Review, of the U.S. Food and Drug Administration (FDA) has the responsibility for the regulation and licensure of new biological products including vaccines (6).

For any new biologic product subject to FDA regulation to enter clinical trials, the sponsor of that product must file a "Notice of Claimed Investigational Exemption for a New Drug," also known as an Investigational New Drug application (IND). Such an exemption is required because the Food, Drug, and Cosmetics Act ordinarily prohibits the administration of unlicensed biologic products to humans. An original IND submission is comprised of several sections, which are summarized in the application form (Form 1571) (7). The submission includes a detailed product description, details of its manufacture, a summary of preclinical data, a summary of any clinical data that may exist (for example, a product developed and tested in other countries), a listing of the proposed clinical investigators and their qualifications, details of the proposed clinical trials including institutional review board approval, and a description of the environmental effect of manufacture and testing.

Prior to the submission of the IND application, CBER encourages vaccine developers to meet with FDA staff. These pre-IND meetings provide the product developer with an opportunity to receive feedback from the FDA regarding various aspects of biological product development and manufacture. The meetings allow the FDA to identify early on issues for which new data or additional advice are needed for regulatory decision making. Experience has shown that a series of such meetings are likely to be useful, even if a manufacturer is experienced in vaccine development. Pre-IND meetings are most valuable when a well-characterized product has been developed and has been evaluated by appropriate preclinical methods. In some cases, however, it may be determined in fairly early stages of product development that major revisions in the developmental plans are appropriate. Early resolution of scientific or regulatory issues can occur through this mechanism, permitting a more expeditious review of the completed IND submission and enabling a more rapid implementation of clinical trials. The occurrence of such pre-IND meetings and any proprietary information communicated to the FDA before the filing of an IND is protected by the same confidentiality rules that apply to formal submissions to the agency.

The most recently revised IND regulations (March, 1987) emphasize safety as the prime determinant of the appropriateness of early clinical trials (8). Thus, initial review of an IND is oriented toward establishing whether there exists sufficient data to reasonably conclude that it is safe to begin clinical trials of a product in humans. If the results of this review indicate that there exist important outstanding safety concerns, FDA may require that the sponsor not initiate clinical trials. Elements that would lead FDA to conclude that the safety of a product is in question would include inadequate description of the manufacturing process, insufficient product characterizaion, or inadequacy in the extent or quality of preclinical studies upon which FDA would rely for safety evaluation. In addition, if the planned clinical investigations are unlikely to provide adequate protection for human subjects, then such investigations would not be permitted.

CANDIDATE VACCINE ANTIGENS

Enormous strides have been made in defining the molecular biology and genomic organization of HIV. The nature of the immune response to infection with HIV, while studied with equal vigor, has not been as well characterized.

In other viral infections, including retroviral infections in lower mammals, protective immune responses, or immune responses associated with resistance to or recovery from disease, are effected by both the humoral and cell-mediated immune systems (9,10). Specific antiviral immune responses include the production of neutralizing antibodies, those that are functional in antibody dependent cellular cytotoxicity, and cytotoxic T lymphocytes. While all these responses have been observed in HIV-infected individuals, the presence or absence of these responses, to date, has not been clearly shown to influence the natural history of HIV infection. Any or all of these responses may be protective if immunity is established prior to primary infection. In the absence of firm data to indicate which responses must be elicited in order to establish protective immunity to HIV, vaccine antigen selection must be based on the expectation that the antigen can elicit responses associated with protection in other viral systems.

To date, several approaches to the development of AIDS vaccines have been pursued. A number of such strategies are listed in Table 2, and many are described in detail elsewhere in this text.

HIV Envelope-Based Vaccines

Most vaccine development efforts have to date focused on the surface antigens of HIV as the potential immunogens. The envelope of HIV is composed to two viral glycoproteins, gp120, which projects from the envelope surface, and the

Table 2 Candidate AIDS Vaccines

Type	Antigen	Source
Subunit	Envelope	Virus
Recombinant DNA-derived	Envelope	*E. coli* Yeast Insect cells Mammalian cells
Live virus vectors	Envelope	Vaccinia Adenovirus Herpes simplex virus
	Core	Vaccinia
Synthetic peptides	Core	Solid-phase synthesis
Anti-idiotype antibodies	Envelope	Mouse monoclonal antibodies
HIV hyperimmune globulin	Whole virus	Human plasma
Inactivated	Whole virus	Whole virus

transmembrane anchor, gp41 (11). Both of these products are produced from a gp160 envelope precursor, which is cleaved before viral assembly (12,13). Antibodies to both these molecules and the gp160 precursor are found in the sera of most patients infected with HIV (11-14). Binding of HIV to T-helper cells is mediated through interactions between regions of the viral envelope and CD4, the T-helper cell surface marker. Syncytium formation is also effected through interactions between the HIV envelope glycoproteins and cell membranes. Given their immunogenic nature, their involvement in entry of HIV into susceptible cell types, their localization on the surface of virions, and their expression on the surface of HIV infected cells (12,13), the envelope glycoproteins of HIV would seem to be important targets for effective immune responses.

The genes that code for the complete gp160 and for the cleaved products gp120 and gp41 have been cloned and expressed in several prokaryotic and eukaryotic systems. The gene products expressed in yeast (15) and bacteria (16-18) are nonglycosylated, whereas those expressed in invertebrate (19,20) and vertebrate (21) cells are in glycosylated form. Both forms are recognized by sera from patients infected with HIV (16-18,20). Envelope sequences critical to T-cell binding and others important for virus neutralization have been defined and expressed in a variety of systems (22,23).

Native envelope glycoprotein gp120 has also been produced by purification of fluids of bulk cultures of HIV in permissive cell lines (18,24-26). In addition to the expression of HIV proteins and glycoproteins in cell culture, for the purpose of producing purified viral antigens, recombinant vaccinia viruses have been produced which contain genetic material coding for components of HIV for potential use as live AIDS vaccine preparations (27,28).

A theoretical safety concern pertinent to HIV envelope-based vaccines is the potential for the HIV envelope glycoprotein to be immunosuppressive. It is unclear whether the binding of the virus to the CD4 determinant on T-helper cells in and of itself affects T-cell function (29-31). Synthetic peptide fragments of gp41 were recently shown to be immunosuppressive in vitro (32). The CD4 receptor of man has significant homology only to the CD4 molecule of other primate species, so that animal models using nonprimate mammals cannot test for this potentially adverse interaction. Thus, primates closely related to man are the most relevant animal model system for assessment of CD4-envelope protein interactions. Another means for evaluating deleterious CD4-envelope protein interactions would involve the in vitro analysis of T-helper cell functions in the presence of envelope glycoprotein products. Such in vitro and primate testing should be essential elements of the evaluation of all vaccines based on HIV envelope constituents.

A potentially serious shortcoming of HIV envelope-based vaccines relates to the genetic variation among individual isolates of HIV. This variability is most extensive in the *env* gene, and differences in envelope amino acid sequences in excess of 20% have been shown between HIV isolates from diverse geographic regions (33,34). Studies of neutralizing antibody have shown marked differences in the capacity of sera from infected individuals to neutralize even a limited number of laboratory strains of HIV (25,35–37). In preclinical evaluations of candidate envelope glycoprotein vaccines, the antibody responses of immunized animals are often type specific, recognizing only the envelope of the immunizing virus strain (25,26).

The isolation and identification of newer human retroviruses complicates the issue even more. The recently described HIV-2 shows only 50–60% genetic homology with HIV-1, and its envelope glycoprotein is antigenically distinct (38,39). It would not be surprising if more members of the HIV family are identified in the future. Thus, successful vaccination against one virus would not necessarily confer immunity against other AIDS viruses. Multivalent vaccines containing different envelope glycoproteins from strains of both HIV-1 and HIV-2 may be required to confer immunity against the divergent strains present in nature. This strategy has been firmly established in the development of influenza vaccines (40).

HIV *gag*-Based Vaccines

The role of HIV core antigens as potential vaccine candidates is unclear. Antibodies or other immune rsponses directed against viral antigens present on the surface of virions or infected cells would seem to be the most likely functions to mediate protective immunity. However, it is possible that internal viral structural proteins could also be important antigens (41–43). Recently, human anti-p24 antibodies were implicated in the lysis of HIV-infected cells by ADCC (44). Clinical data seems to indicate that the level of antibody to p24, the major core protein of HIV, correlates with the clinical status of patients with HIV infection (45–47). A progressive loss of antibody to p24, with a concurrent increase in the level of circulating p24 antigen is observed as disease progresses (46). The clinical significance of this association is unknown. Thus, antibodies directed against the major internal structural protein of the virus may be involved in protective immune responses.

The *gag* gene of HIV has been successfully cloned into yeast cells (48), and recombinant vaccinia viruses expressing p24 have been produced (49).

The p17 *gag* gene product has been reported to be localized just internal to the envelope of HIV (50), although this interpretation is not universally accepted. No function has yet been ascribed to this protein. A 30-amino-acid synthetic peptide with partial homology to p17 and thymosin alpha$_1$ has been proposed as an HIV vaccine candidate (51). The rationale forwarded for this vaccine strategy is that antibodies to thymosin alpha$_1$ cross-react with HIV-1 p17 and can neutralize viral infectivity (52). These observations have not been verified by other investigators (53,54).

Vaccines Based on Other HIV Proteins

Evidence for the role of other HIV structural, functional, and regulatory gene products in eliciting potentially protective immune responses is less clear. High levels of serum antibodies to the reverse transcriptase of HIV has been associated with difficulty in virus isolation from peripheral blood cells (55). This observation may represent a virus neutralization phenomenon and is worthy of further investigation. In addition, reverse transcriptase has been shown to be a target of cytotoxic lymphocytes in HIV-infected individuals (56). The reverse transcriptase gene of HIV has been cloned and an enzymatically active molecule synthesized. However, this product has not been evaluated as an immunogen (57).

PRECLINICAL EVALUATION OF CANDIDATE AIDS VACCINES

The initiation of human AIDS vaccine trials is incumbent upon the satisfactory demonstration that a particular product is reasonably safe and would not constitute an unacceptable risk if administered to human subjects. The preclinical evaluation of candidate AIDS vaccines must address a variety of issues.

Rationale

There should be an experimental basis for the incorporation of any specific viral antigen in a candidate vaccine. For full-length viral proteins and glycoproteins, as well as recombinant subunit and recombinant and synthetic peptide vaccines, the immunogen should be thoroughly characterized and its immunogenicity, biological function, and immunologic importance elucidated to as great an extent as possible.

Biological Activity

If an HIV vaccine antigen is expected to be biologically active in its own right, the consequences of such activity should be defined. The example of HIV envelope vaccines and the theoretical risk of binding to CD4 was discussed earlier. Another example of a biologically active immunogen would be anti-idiotypic monoclonal antibodies that mimic the CD4 cell surface marker (58). Normal immunologic interactions requiring CD4 recognition may be influenced by the presence of the anti-idiotype. Experiments should evaluate the potentially deleterious effects of such biological activity.

Generally Applicable Principles of Production Control Management and Cell Banking

Cell Substrate

One concern relevant to products developed by most strategies is the cell substrate used in vaccine antigen production. The cell line used in vaccine production is selected because it has characteristics that make it particularly suitable for the given application. Experience has shown that the best approach to the management of such cell cultures to assure consistent quality is through a cell banking system.

The production of cell substrates should be based on the use of cell bank systems starting with master cell banks, which are the sources of cells used for the production of working cell banks, the pools of cells which are stored and propagated for use in the actual production of biologic products. Such a system helps ensure homogeneity of the cell substrate throughout manufacturing and aids in the production of a standard and reproducible final product. The history and genealogy of cell lines used in the manufacturing process are important parts of this characterization. Quality assurance testing for cell banks includes testing of the cell line for growth potential, tumorigenicity, karyology, and adventitious agents. The cell line is characterized as having either a limited potential for growth as a stable line or as having an indefinite or continuous potential for stable growth. Positive tumorigenicity tests will not necessarily disqualify a cell line for use in manufacturing. However, the tumorigenic potential is a biological characteristic that should be defined. If a cell line is continuous or tumorigenic, special attention is paid to testing for transforming viruses and activated oncogenes, and the removal of cell DNA during the manufacturing process. Karyology testing is done to document the species of origin of the cell line and whether it is diploid or aneuploid. Extensive testing for adventitious agents is done taking into account the passage history of the cell line.

Virus Seed Lot System

Just as a cell banking system is an important element for cell substrate consistency, a virus seed lot system helps assure the homogeneity of virus strains used in vaccine production. Strains of virus used for vaccine development should be adequately characterized with respect to origin and passage history. For attenuated or recombinant viruses, a complete record of procedures used to develop the vaccine strain is essential. Methods for the identification of vaccine strains, and their differentiation from wild strains are important elements of product qualification. The vaccine strain is expanded to produce a master virus seed, which is the source of working virus seeds, which are stored and propagated for use in actual vaccine production. The relationship between cell banks and virus seed stock as applied to live virus vaccine production is shown in Figure 1.

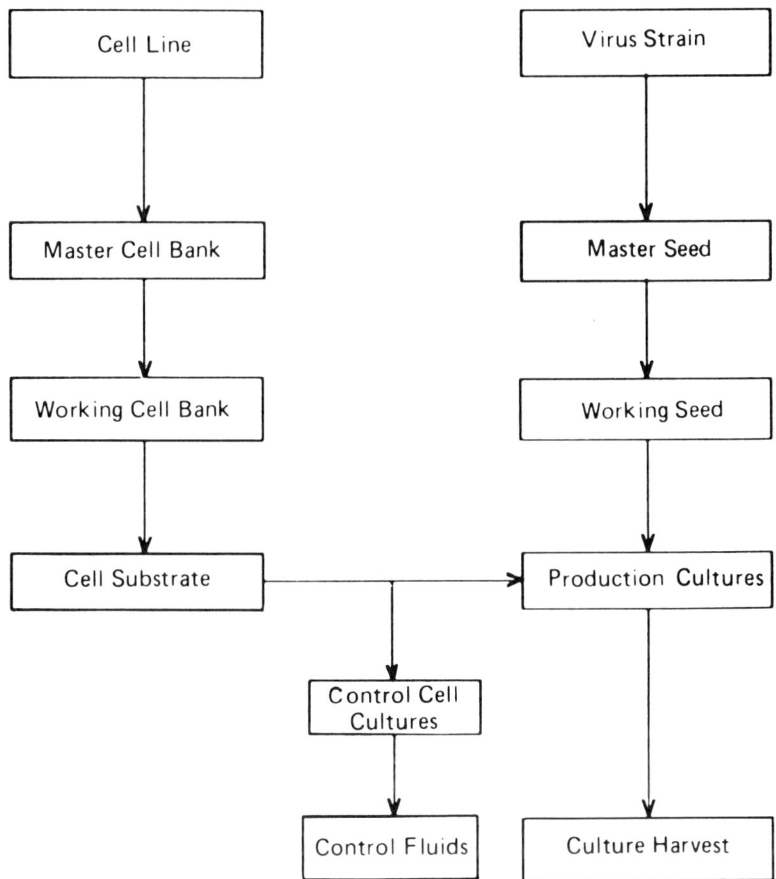

Figure 1 Diagrammatic representation of vaccine antigen production using a master cell bank and master virus seed system.

In the actual production process, an aliquot of the working cell bank is thawed and expanded to produce the cell substrate. Similarly, the vaccine virus is propagated from an aliquot of the working seed until a predetermined passage level which provides a yield adequate for vaccine production. Following inoculation of the cell substrate with the vaccine strain virus, and an appropriate incubation period, the cultures are harvested and further processed to yield the final product.

The virus seed system is also applicable to recombinant vaccines such as those produced in baculovirus expression vectors and live viral vector vaccines such as recombinant vaccinia viruses containing genes for HIV envelope glycoproteins. For subunit vaccines produced in recombinant bacteria, yeast, or mammalian cells, there is no virus used in production, and, consequently, no virus seed; the cell substrate itself produces the vaccine antigen. For such vaccines, the production involves propagation of the cell substrate to a predetermined passage level, harvesting of the cells or supernatant, and processing of the culture harvest.

Using this system, each lot of vaccine is produced from cells and viruses at approximately the same passage level beyond the master cell bank and master virus seed, respectively. This consistency in production should help minimize lot to lot variability in terms of product yield, composition, and purity.

Product-Specific Control Issues

Just as each candidate vaccine antigen raises specific concerns, issues relating to several or individual manufacturing processes merit specific attention.

Purified Subunit Vaccines Produced by Recombinant DNA Methodology

For vaccines produced by recombinant DNA technology, the basis for evaluation of potential risks and benefits in clinical trials includes assessment of the methods used for gene cloning, biochemical characterization of the vector and the expressed gene and gene product, characterization of the transformed cell line if one is involved, and lot-by-lot testing to assure that the product has appropriate biochemical and biological characteristics. Stability of the specific expression system is a critical issue evaluated by DNA sequencing and restriction enzyme analysis at a cell passage level at or beyond that used routinely for vaccine antigen production. Characterization of the recombinant product includes a detailed description of the purification methods employed, extensive chemical characterization, such as by complete amino acid analysis, carboxy- and amino-terminal amino acid sequencing, peptide mapping and polyacrylamide gel electrophoresis, as well as biological demonstration of identity and potency. The final product should be largely free from host cell and vector DNA, and free of contaminating host cell and vector-coded proteins.

The specific strategy used for recombinant vaccine antigen production can greatly influence the characteristics and scope of preclinical evaluations. Some specific examples are discussed below.

Insect protein allergy is a potential safety concern with vaccine antigens produced in insect cells. Cell lines derived from insects whose bite or sting cause allergic reactions in man would be inappropriate for vaccine production. Animal toxicity testing should include tests for potential allergic reactions to trace insect cellular proteins which may be present in the final product. Recombinant insect viruses used as vectors for vaccine antigen expression in insect cells should also be evaluated for potential allergenicity. Baculoviruses currently used or proposed as vectors for vaccine production in insect cells have been extensively tested and three Baculovirus species are approved by the United States Environmental Protection Agency for insect pest control on food crops. While proteins synthesized in insect cells can be glycosylated, the pattern of glycosylation may influence the immunogenicity of recombinant glycoproteins produced in this expression system.

Most mammalian cell lines used for production of recombinant proteins are transformed, continuous cell lines, and some contain endogenous retrovirus particles. The quality assurance procedures for such cell substrates and the recombinant product produced in these cells is a reflection of the potential presence of contaminating retroviruses and the inherent risks of human transmission of intact retrovirus particles or retroviral genomic material through an inadequately purified product. The presence of retrovirus-like transposons or transposable DNA elements in yeast cells and mammalian cells is another cause of concern. The requirements for elimination of contaminating nucleic acid in a final product reduces the risk of inadvertent transmission of protentially harmful genetic elements to man.

For yeast-derived recombinant products, quality control issues would include testing for the presence of contaminating yeast proteins. The use of protease inhibitors such as phenylmethylsulfonyl fluoride to prevent degradation of the recombinant product in culture harvests may modify protein structure, changing its immunogenicity. This problem may also be encountered in the purification of recombinant products made in bacteria.

Specific issues relevant to vaccine production strategies utilizing recombinant bacteria include differences in the N-terminal processing of proteins synthesized in bacteria as compared to eukaryotes. Bacterially coded proteins contain a formyl-methionine residue at the N-terminal. The presence of this amino acid rather than the appropriate N-terminal residue may alter protein structure and immunogenicity. Other modifications of the vaccine antigen may occur during purification, where disulfide reagents such as *n*-ethyl maleimide, used to increase solubility of the recombinant protein, may degrade intermolecular disulfide bonds and lead to changes in tertiary structure of the product.

Live Recombinant Viral Vector Vaccines

Live recombinant viral vaccines raise substantial safety issues in addition to those relevant to other recombinant DNA-derived products. The genetic stability of the recombinant virus must be clearly demonstrated. Freedom from adventitious agents may be difficult to demonstrate. For example, vaccinia virus is highly lytic in tissue culture and can mask the cytopathic effects of other contaminating viruses in tissue culture. Vaccinia virus tends to aggregate in suspension so that not all particles are accessible to neutralizing antibodies. Thus, neutralizing antisera to vaccinia are insufficient to fully neutralize vaccinia virus in an undiluted preparation, and dilution of vaccine preparations to the point where all vaccinia could be neutralized would in all likelihood prevent the detection of low levels of contaminating viruses. For this reason, control cells uninfected with vaccinia, but otherwise processed in an identical manner, are maintained during vaccine production and tested for the absence of adventitious viral agents. Appropriate animal models to test for virulence, infectivity, and immunogenicity of the recombinant viral vector must also be developed.

HIV-Derived Vaccines

The administration of inactivated whole HIV has been proposed as a mechanism for the augmentation of specific immune responses in individuals already infected with HIV (60). This strategy would be aimed at the prevention of clinical progression to AIDS, not at preventing HIV infection. Regarding this approach, there are a number of relevant safety issues. There is a need for complete assurance of the efficacy of the viral inactivation procedure. In addition, the role of immunologic stimulation in the pathogenesis of AIDS remains unclear. Generation of activated T cells could theoretically accelerate HIV replication, leading to further depletion in helper T cells and progression of the immunodeficiency state. Principles generally relevant to inactivated viral vaccines produced in cell cultures are pertinent.

Antigen preparations have been produced for animals studies by the extraction and purification of viral components from bulk cultures of infectious HIV. It is not likely that this method would be used to produce vaccines for humans because of safety concerns. It would be extremely difficult to demonstrate the complete absence of infectious virus and viral nucleic acid in such a product. It is also likely that a candidate vaccine containing an antigen of similar quality could be produced more efficiently by other techniques.

Several currently available viral vaccines are produced by attenuation of wild viruses. The prospect for the development of similar vaccines for AIDS is bleak. It is unlikely that a virus unable to become incorporated into the cellular DNA as a provirus could be developed with current technology. Concerns would exist about the potential for recombination with, or activation of, cellular proto-oncogenes. The absence of an appropriate animal model to assess attenuation would also hinder development of such a vaccine.

Synthetic Peptide Vaccines

Production of vaccines by the solid-phase synthesis of immunogenic peptides is a strategy that eliminates a number of safety concerns, namely freedom from contaminating viruses, DNA, and proteins. Synthetic peptide antigens can be designed to include neutralizing or otherwise biologically active epitopes, making the use of synthetic peptides a potentially powerful approach to selective immunization. However, there are a number of potential difficulties associated with this approach. Many apparently important peptide sequences may be functionally active only as a result of the secondary or tertiary structure involved in the intact protein. Some epitopes are comprised of parts of proteins that are not in linear sequence but are juxtaposed spatially. Purity of synthetic peptides is difficult to assure. Synthetic reactions occur with incomplete fidelity resulting in mixtures of synthetic peptides of many types which may be very difficult to separate. Even a pure synthetic peptide might be considered a mixture in the sense that the molecule may be capable of existing in a wider range of conformations than would be possible for the sequence as part of the intact protein. There is the paradoxical situation, therefore, that the highly selected epitope may induce unpredictable aberrant immune responses. Synthetic peptides tend to be poorly immunogenic, and there are novel concerns about safety and process control that relate to the needs for linkage to carriers and use with adjuvants.

Anti-Idiotype Monoclonal Antibodies

The use of anti-idiotype monoclonal antibodies rather than native, recombinant, or synthetic peptide antigens offers several theoretical advantages. The anti-idiotype approach could overcome limitations of antigen source and would eliminate potential problems with aberrant antigenic configurations that might occur with recombinant or synthetic antigens. Depending on the nature of the epitope represented by the tertiary structure of the antibody, concerns relevant to that epitope must be addressed. For anti-idiotype monoclonal antibodies, product-specific manufacturing and control issues would include the rationale for and characterization of the specific immunogen used and the description of production and purification methods. Of importance for monoclonal antibody products is the demonstration of freedom from adventitious agents. Since many murine myeloma cell lines are contaminated with murine retroviruses, manufacturing processes include steps which inactivate these adventitious agents, and their removal is documented by appropriate assays of in-process and final materials. For human hybridomas, absence of human pathogens, especially Epstein-Barr virus, is demonstrated. Specificity of the final product and the absence of cross-reactivity with normal human cell proteins is a critical issue.

HIV Immune Globulin

Passive immunization with high titered naturally occurring antibodies to HIV may be clinically useful. Hepatitis B immune globulin administered in the immediate postpartum period accompanied by active immunization with hepatitis

B vaccine is effective in the prevention of vertical transmission of hepatitis B virus infection at the time of delivery (61). While the mode of transmission of HIV infection in the newborn has not been clearly defined, natal acquisition of infection is considered a possible mechanism. Were this the case, an analagous passive or passive/active immunization regimen may be effective in the prevention of perinatal transmission of HIV infections. The demonstration of freedom from infectious HIV would be a major safety requirement for such a product, since the product would be produced from plasma derived from individuals with HIV infection. The current safety record for immune globulin products suggests that the risk of transmission of infectious viruses through immune globulin preparations is negligible or absent. Immune globulins produced between 1980 and 1985, especially hepatitis B immune globulin, were derived from plasma pools that included HIV-infected donations but did not transmit HIV infection (62,63).

Newer Vaccine Adjuvants and Conjugates

There is relatively little experience in humans with adjuvants other than alum, or with conjugates other than polysaccharides linked to diphtheria toxin. New vaccine adjuvants will undoubtedly be evaluated in parallel with AIDS vaccine development efforts. Among these newer adjuvants are immune stimulating complexes or ISCOMS, which are produced when a matrix of the glycoside Quill A, at a critical concentration, assumes a micellar form permitting interactions with membrane protein antigens (64). Muramyl dipeptide and tripeptide are synthetic analogues of a Mycobacterial cell wall component, which is the active immunologic component of Freund's complete adjuvant. They are active even when administered in aqueous solution rather than oil suspension (65,66). As with other investigational products, these compounds will require extensive preclinical evaluation both individually and as components of candidate vaccines.

Animal Models of Safety and Immunogenicity

Animal models of infection and immunization have played an integral role in the development of vaccines effective against a wide range of human pathogens. Lower mammals play an important role in some aspects of AIDS vaccine development, such as their use in potency assays for vaccine standardization. In mouse potency assays, groups of mice are immunized with a dilution series of vaccine antigen, and subsequent seroconversions are detected by an appropriate antibody assay. The dose required to cause seroconversion in a defined percentage of test animals (usually 50% is the chosen endpoint) is calculated. Potency assays are important in standardization of vaccine lots. Small animals are regularly used for acute and chronic toxicity testing. For products intended for only occasional administration, such as vaccines, chronic toxicity studies are not

needed ordinarily. Acute toxicity studies are a component of preclinical evaluation. One purpose of preclinical testing is to determine if induction of an immune response is associated with an adverse effect. This principle is especially
important when a theoretical risk of vaccine administration is immunosuppression or interference with normal immune responses. Administration of candidate
vaccines to a range of animal species is of value to assess differences in potential
toxic effects and immunogenicity. Extensive evaluations of a number of candidate vaccines in a broad range of animal species have verified that HIV vaccine
antigens can be immunogenic, as manifested by antibody production or development of cellular immune responses without induction of adverse effects (17,18,
21,24-28,49,67,68).

Animal Models for Efficacy

When available, animal models are very valuable for assessing possible vaccine
efficacy. Ideally, immunization with a candidate AIDS vaccine would protect
a susceptible animal species from infection if subsequently challenged with HIV.
Chimpanzees (*Pan troglodytes*) and gibbons (*Hylobates* spp.) are the only
species which become infected consistently when inoculated with HIV-1 (69-
73). Baboons (*Papio* spp.) are reportedly susceptible to infection with HIV-2
(73). None of these infected animals, to date, have developed signs or symptoms
of immunodeficiency clearly attributable to HIV infection, although several
animals have developed lymphadenopathy following infection (68,69). Thus,
the relevance of the chimpanzee as a model for human infection may be limited.
On the other hand, given their close relationship with man, chimpanzees may
represent the best model system for the evaluation of immunogenicity and
potentially deleterious effects of vaccination, and may also provide useful preclinical data with respect to dosage range and immunization schedules. Chimpanzees vaccinated with either recombinant gp120 or recombinant vaccinia virus
expressing HIV envelope glycoprotein were able to mount both cellular and
humoral immune responses but became infected following live virus challenge
(68,74). This vaccine failure may be attributable to many causes including inadequate vaccine potency, a suboptimal vaccination regimen, or an excessive challenge dose. Resistance to large viral inocula administered by the intravenous
route may have little or no relevance to the prevention of HIV infection in man.
The failure of large volumes of human anti-HIV immune globulins to protect a
chimpanzee from HIV infection may also be due to one or several of the reasons
cited above (75).

An alternative approach to a model for HIV vaccine evaluation involves the
use of a parallel model of AIDS in another animal species. Macaque monkeys
infected with the simian immunodeficiency virus (SIV) develop a clinical disease
characterized by wasting and immunodeficiency, not unlike AIDS in man

(8,10,76). The development of vaccines against SIV may provide important information concerning vaccine antigens that stimulate protective immunity, vaccination strategies, and the feasability of vaccines for AIDS in general. Similar animal models which may parallel HIV infection in humans and provide practical information for vaccine development may include feline immunodeficiency virus, bovine immunodeficiency virus, and other animal lentiviruses (10).

CLINICAL TRIALS

The Sequence of Clinical Trials

Clinical trials of vaccines are normally conducted in three phases (77). The three phases are summarized in Table 3. Each successive phase of clinical trials exposes an increasing number of subjects to the risks of exposure to the experimental product. While the public health benefits of an effective vaccine for the prevention of HIV infection would be substantial, every effort must be taken to assure that study volunteers are exposed to minimal risks.

Phase I trials stress safety. For this purpose, studies are deisgned to assess clinical pharmacology, pharmacokinetics, metabolism, and toxicity. They should, as a result, provide some information about vaccine immunogenicity. Depending on the product, phase 1 testing may be conducted in either healthy or ill volunteers. Initial trials are sometimes conducted in subjects who may benefit personally from the product in question. For AIDS vaccines, phase 1 study volunteers have been at low risk of natural infection to assure sensitivity to vaccine effects and to minimize immunologic variability. Phase 1 trials are not routinely conducted in a placebo-controlled fashion. It has been argued that given the theoretical risk of immunologic derangement as a consequences of some candidate AIDS vaccines, and in light of the variability of available assays to measure such immunologic parameters, inclusion of a placebo or other

Table 3 Phases of Clinical Trials of a Candidate AIDS Vaccine

Phase	Type of subjects	Duration	Purpose
1	Low risk	Up to 1 yr	Mainly safety, some immunogenicity
2	Low and high risk	Up to 2 yr	Safety, immunogenicity
3	All target populations	Up to 4 yr	Efficacy, safety, dosage

control group would control for assay variability and permit the detection of subtle immunotoxic effects. Some phase 1 trials of candidate AIDS vaccines in progress are designed as placebo-controlled trials. Phase 1 trials generally involve a relatively small number of subjects. Their duration depends on the immunization regimen being studied. Phase 1 trial results are critical to the design of later clinical trials. The results reveal essential information about dose range and vaccination schedules and could alert investigators to potential side effects that would influence the conduct of larger clinical studies.

Phase 2 studies are designed to further evaluate safety and immunogenicity. Among study participants in phase 2 would be volunteers considered to be at high risk for AIDS. Since high-risk populations would constitute initial target groups for vaccination programs, it is essential to accumulate data concerning vaccine immunogenicity and safety in such high-risk individuals.

Phase 3 trials provide the opportunity for further evaluation of vaccine safety, as well as the first large-scale evaluation of efficacy. Phase 3 trials of AIDS vaccines will involve large numbers of individuals at risk of HIV infection and may require years to complete. Vaccine efficacy may need to be determined in specific risk groups. Geographic location may influence vaccine efficacy, due to regional strain variability or other environmental factors.

As with phase 2 studies, appropriate control groups will be essential to the thorough evaluation of vaccine efficacy. Double-blind trials may be useful for the elimination of investigator bias and for the discouragement of high-risk behavior by vaccinees who perceive that vaccination may be protective. A common objection to placebo-controlled trials is that the experimental treatment may be effective, so that vaccine recipients may be protected from HIV infection, while placebo recipients are not. there are also concerns that vaccination may not be effective, may potentiate infection, and accelerate the onset of clinical disease. One mechanism to enhance the attractiveness of placebo-controlled trials is to offer vaccination with another product with proven benefit, such as hepatitis B vaccine, to the control group.

Target Groups for AIDS Vaccine Trials

Recognized risk groups for AIDS in the United States include homosexual men, intravenous drug abusers, patients with hemophilia, prostitutes, heterosexual partners of persons with HIV infection or at recognized risk for infection and children born to mothers infected with HIV. Members of all these populations would be potential vaccine candidates (Table 4). Because vaccine efficacy may differ between risk groups, it is probable that multiple populations will have to be studied to assess vaccine efficacy.

Homosexual and bisexual men remain the major group at high risk for disease due to the human immunodeficiency virus (HIV), with prevalence estimates

Table 4 Target Populations for AIDS Vaccine Clinical Trials

Group	Availability	Infection incidence
Homosexual men	Good	$<$1–3%
Drug abusers	Fair	Variable
Heterosexual partners		
Partners of hemophilia patients	Limited	High
Female prostitutes	Limited	Variable
Wives of infected men	Variable	High
Infants born to infected mothers	Good	40%
STD clinic patients	Fair	High
Prisoners	Poor	Variable
Repeated blood donors	Good	0.003%
Civilian applicants to U.S. military	Good	0.05%
Active duty, U.S. military	Good	0.007%

ranging from 10 to 70% in studies performed in various geographic regions (78). The prevalence of seropositivity for members of some of these risk groups varies with geographic region. In some cities on the east coast of the United States, prevalence of HIV infection in drug abusers ranges from 50 to 60% (78). In other regions of the country, the prevalence is generally below 5% (78). Approximately 70% of patients with hemophilia A and 35% of those with hemophilia B are seropositive for HIV (78). The prevalence of infection in these patients is consistent throughout the United States, reflecting the production of clotting factor concentrates from plasma pools representing thousands of donors. Seroprevalence data on female prostitutes vary from 0 to 45%, with the highest rates observed in large inner-city areas where the frequency of intravenous drug use among prostitutes is high (78). For heterosexual partners of individuals with or at high risk of HIV infection, the prevalence varies from 10 to 60% (78). In screening studies of filter paper blotted blood specimens from newborns in Massachusetts, 0.21% of neonates had antibodies to HIV, with the prevalence increasing to 0.80% in babies born at inner-city hospitals (79).

The widespread prevalence of HIV infection and AIDS in several nations in central Africa make these regions potentially important sites for large-scale efficacy studies of AIDS vaccines (80–82). HIV infection and AIDS severely drain the social and economic resources of these nations, so that the evaluation and identification of safe and effective vaccines would be entirely consistent with national priorities. The incidence of HIV infection in these countries may be high enough to yield information about vaccine efficacy more rapidly than could trials in any identified risk group in the United States. In recognition of these facts, the World Health Organization (WHO) is working to establish "a mechanism to ensure the open exchange of scientific, social, and ethical information necessary for advanced planning and international collaboration in the clinical testing of candidate AIDS vaccines, with particular attention to Phase III trials" (83).

Study Size Considerations

The number of participants required for an AIDS vaccine efficacy trial is dependent upon the incidence of HIV infection in the study population. While there is extensive prevalence data available for the United States, incidence data in the diverse groups at risk is, at best, incomplete (83,84). Additional studies of incidence of HIV infections in target groups is essential.

It is estimated that the current annual incidence rate for HIV infection among homosexual men in large American cities is one the order of 1–2%. (84). For intravenous drug abusers, incidence is believed to be less than 5%, even in areas of high prevalence of HIV infection (84). In risk groups where the incidence of HIV infection might be higher, such as in spouses and sexual partners of patients with hemophilia, the available population is so limited that vaccine evaluation may be impossible. A one-year placebo controlled efficacy trial, in a study group in which the annual incidence of HIV infection is 1%, would require 2004 subjects per arm (assuming 100% vaccine efficacy and a 20% type 2 error) to detect vaccine-induced protection. For a study population with a 10% incidence rate, roughly 400 subjects would be required in the treatment and control groups. Extending trial duration over a number of years would delay vaccine availability, but would also reduce the number of study participants required in order to measure real differences related to vaccination. If several vaccines need testing in parallel, there will be added strain on available subject resources.

The Design and Implementation of Clinical Trials

In the design and implementation of clinical trials of AIDS vaccines, a number of obstacles can be envisioned, of both a technical and an ethical nature.

The recruitment of volunteers from some risk groups may be difficult, given the illegal nature of some high-risk activity, and prospects for long-term follow-up may be poor. Enlistment of members of high-risk groups through existing community or medical support programs may not provide a study population representative of the risk group as a whole. For example, the incidence of HIV infection in seronegative drug abusers enrolled in methadone maintenance treatment programs may be different than the incidence of infection in untreated drug abusers (85).

The participation of high-risk subjects in clinical trials is essential to the determination of vaccine efficacy. It is unethical, however, to permit participation of high-risk subjects in trials without providing AIDS prevention education. These education efforts, if successful, should minimize risk of infection in both treatment and placebo groups and might mask the ability of an otherwise well-designed trial to detect a treatment effect.

In the course of clinical trials, it is likely that some study participants will become infected with HIV. At present, there has been no resolution of the conflicting issues of the physician's obligation to preserve patient confidentiality and the physician's responsibility to intervene when his or her patient becomes a danger to a third party. Moreover, the sexual partners of HIV-seropositive persons may be suitable candidates for efficacy studies themselves. The state of California recently enacted legislation which relieves a physician of liability for reporting a patient's seropositive status to a regular sexual partner (86). Some investigators may feel a need to include third-party notification as a component of study design and as an element of informed consent.

Trials of vaccinia-based vaccines face a number of potential problems. Vaccinia immunizations have not been carried out in general populations of most countries since the late 1960s, although selected categories of individuals such as military recruits and laboratory workers have been immunized subsequently. Thus, there exist three distinct populations with respect to vaccinia immune status: those never immunized, those with remote immunization, and those vaccinated more recently. The performance of vaccinia-based vaccines may vary widely depending upon the preexisting immune status of the vaccinee. The degree of attenuation of the recombinant virus relative to the parent strain is unknown, although it is generally believed that deletion of the thymidine kinase gene in the process of cloning the recombinant strains may further attenuate the virus (87,88). The potential for dissemination of the recombinant vaccinia virus from experimental subjects to close contacts was the reason for isolation of vaccinees in the early stages of phase 1 clinical evaluation.

Vaccine recipients will probably develop antibodies to HIV. The repercussions of seropositivity may be great. A seropositive individual cannot donate blood, is ineligible for enlistment into the United States armed services, and may be denied privileges such as life or health insurance. Immigration to some countries can be restricted, and United States residency status can be denied to seropositive foreign nationals. It is impossible to predict completely the future consequences of seropositivity. These issues should be presented to volunteers before they participate in clinical trials.

Antibody screening programs may not distinguish between natural and vaccine-induced seropositivity, although some tests such as the Western blot should be able to distinguish the serologic profiles which would be induced by some AIDS vaccines from those commonly induced by infection. Adequate clinical trial designs would provide some means to identify vaccine recipients in a way that would allow them to avoid some or all of the stigma of seropositivity. One proposed mechanism for dealing with this issue is an identity card with descriptive data and a toll-free telephone number to call for further information. A possible enhancement to such an identity card system would be the inclusion of a photograph of the volunteer's Western blot pattern somewhere on the document.

It will be necessary to monitor vaccinees in phase 3 studies for evidence of HIV infection. For most currently proposed vaccines, screening could include testing for antibody responses to viral antigens not present in the vaccine. It is possible that previous immunization might in some way influence immune response to later natural infection with HIV, and it may be necessary to monitor phase 3 study participants for infection by additional techniques such as HIV antigen detection, detection of viral nucleic acids, or virus isolation in tissue culture.

STANDARDIZATION

The diversity of candidate AIDS vaccines and the expectation that clinical trials will be conducted on a variety of products and in a variety of locations accentuate the need to develop standardized measures of vaccine-induced immunity and efficacy. Ongoing efforts include the establishment of repositories for standardized reagents, both viral isolates and immune sera, for the purpose of distribution to research laboratories throughout the world. Current international collaborative efforts are directed at establishing the comparative performance of different HIV-neutralizing antibody assays. The development and international recognition of other standardized methods would help to further simplify AIDS vaccine evaluation.

CONCLUSION

The past 7 years has seen the mobilization of a global scientific effort, which has led to the identification and extensive characterization of the AIDS virus. The first clinical trials of experimental AIDS vaccines are now in progress. It is important to recognize, however, that much remains to be learned about what immune mechanisms constitute a protective immune response. In conjunction with these vaccine development efforts, it is incumbent upon scientists to explore and implement other programs for the control of the AIDS pandemic.

REFERENCES

1. Code of Federal Regulations, Title 21, Part 211, U.S. Government Printing Office, Washington, D.C., 1987.
2. Code of Federal Regulations, Title 21, Part 606, U.S. Government Printing Office, Washington, D.C., 1987.
3. Code of Federal Regulations, Title 21, Part 58, U.S. Government Printing Office, Washington, D.C., 1987.
4. Code of Federal Regulations, Title 21, Part 610, U.S. Government Printing Office, Washington, D.C., 1987.
5. Code of Federal Regulations, Title 21, Part 640, U.S. Government Printing Office, Washington, D.C., 1987.
6. Burlington, DB, Gubish, ER. Review of investigational biological products by the United States Food and Drug Administration. J Clin Res Drug Rev 1987; 1:143–52.
7. New drug, antibiotic, and biologic drug product regulations; final rule. Federal Register 1987; 52:8798–847.
8. Code of Federal Regulations, Title 21, Part 312, U.S. Government Printing Office, Washington, D.C., 1987.
9. Daniel MD, Letvin NL, Seghal PK, Hunsmann G, Schmidt DK, King NW, Desrosiers RC. Long term persistent infection of macaque monkeys with the simian immunodeficiency virus. J Gen Virol 1987; 68:3183–9.
10. Desrosiers RC, Letvin NL. Animal models for acquired immunodeficiency syndrome. Rev Infect Dis 1987; 9:438–46.
11. Veronese, FD, DeVico AL, Copeland TD, Oroszlan S, Gallo RC, Sarangadharan MG. Characterization of gp41 as the transmembrane protein coded by the HTLV–III/LAV envelope gene. Science 1985; 229:1402–5.
12. Allan JS, Coligan JE, Barin F, McLane MF, Sodroski JG, Rosen CA, Haseltine WA, Lee TH, Essex M. Major glycoprotein antigens that induce antibodies in AIDS patients are encoded by HTLV–III. Science 1985; 228:1091–4.
13. Barin F, McLane, MF, Allan JS, Lee TH. Virus envelope proteins of HTLV–III represent the major targets for antibodies in AIDS patients. Science 1985; 228:1094–6.
14. Saah AJ, Farzadegan H, Fox R, Nishanian P, Rinaldo Jr CR, Phair JP, Fahey JL, Lee T-H, Polk BF, the Multicenter AIDS Cohort Study. Detection of early antibodies in human immunodeficiency virus infection by enzyme-linked immunosorbent assay, Western blot, and radioimmuniprecipitation. J Clin Microbiol 1987; 25:1605–10.
15. Barr PJ, Steimer KS, Sabin EA, Parkes D, George-Nascimento C, Stephans JC, Powers MA, Gyenes A, Van Nest GA, Miller ET, Higgins KW, Luciw PA. Antigenicity and immunogenicity of domains of the human immunodeficiency virus (HIV) envelope polypeptide expressed in the yeast *Saccharomyces cerevisiae*. Vaccine 1987; 5:90–101.
16. Crowl R, Ganguly K, Gordon M, Conroy R, Schaber M, Kramer R, Shaw G, Wong-Staal F, Reddy EP. HTLV–III env gene products synthesized in *E.*

coli are recognized by antibodies present in the sera of AIDS patients. Cell 1985; 41:979–86.

17. Putney SD, Matthews TJ, Robey WG, Lynn DL, Robert-Guroff M, Mueller WT, Langlois AJ, Ghrayeb J, Petteway Jr SR, Weinhold KJ, Fischinger PJ, Wong-Staal F, Gallo RC, Bolognesi DP. HTLV–III/LAV neutralizing antibodies to an *E. coli* produced fragment of virus envelope. Science 1986; 234:1392–5.

18. Krohn K, Robey WG, Putney SD, Arthur L, Nara P, Fischinger P, Gallo RC, Wong-Staal F, Ranki A. Specific cellular immune response and neutralizing antibodies in goats immunized with native or recombinant envelope proteins derived from human T-lymphotropic virus type III$_B$ and in human immunodeficiency virus-infected men. Proc Nat Acad Sci USA 1987; 84: 4994–8.

19. Cochran MA, Ericson BL, Knell JD, Smith GE. Use of baculovirus recombinants as a general method for the production of subunit vaccines. In Vaccines 87, R.A. Lerner, R.M. Channock, and F. Brown, eds. Cold Spring Harbor Laboratory, 1987: 384–8.

20. Rusche JR, Lynn DL, Robert-Guroff M, Langlois AJ, Lyerly HK, Carson H, Krohn K, Ranki A, Gallo RC, Bolognesi DP, Putney SD, Matthews TJ. Humoral immune response to the entire human immunodeficiency virus envelope glycoprotein made in insect cells. Proc Nat Acad Sci USA 1987; 84:6924–8.

21. Lasky LA, Groopman JE, Fennie CW, Benz PM, Capon DJ, Dowbenko DJ, Nakamura GR, Nunes WM, Renz ME, Berman PW. Neutralization of the AIDS retrovirus by antibodies to a recombinant envelope glycoprotein. Science 1986; 233:209–12.

22. Palker TJ, Clark ME, Langlois AJ, Matthews TJ, Weinhold KJ, Randall RR, Bologenese DP, Haynes BF. Type specific neutralization of the human immunodeficiency virus with antibodies to env-encoded synthetic peptides. Proc Nat Acad Sci USA 1988; 85:1932–6.

23. Rusche JR, Javaherian K, McDanal C, Petro J, Lynn DL, Grimaila R, Langlois A, Gallo RC, Arthur LO, Fischinger PJ, Bolognesi DP, Putney SD, Matthews TJ. Antibodies that inhibit the fusion of human immunodeficiency virus-infected cells bind a 24-amino acid sequence of the viral envelope, gp120. Proc Nat Acad Sci USA 1988; 85:3198–202.

24. Robey WG, Arthur LO, Matthews TJ, Langlois A, Copeland TD, Lerche NW, Oroszlan S, Bolognesi DP, Gilden RV, Fischinger PJ. Prospect for prevention of human immunodeficiency virus infection: Purified 120kDa envelope glycoprotein induces neutralizing antibody. Proc Nat Acad Sci USA 1986; 83:7023–7.

25. Matthews TJ, Langlois AJ, Robey WG, Chang NT, Gallo RC, Fischinger PJ, Bolognese DP. Restricted neutralization of divergent human T-lymphotropic virus type III isolates by antibodies to the major glycoprotein. Proc Nat Acad Sci USA 1986; 83:9709–13.

26. Nara PL, Robey WG, Gonda MA, Carter SG, Fischinger PJ. Absence of cytotoxic antibody to human immunodeficiency virus-infected cells in

humans and its induction in animals after infection or immunization with purified envelope glycoprotein gp120. Proc Nat Acad Sci USA 1987; 84: 3797–801.

27. Chakrabarti S, Robert-Guroff M, Wong-Staal F, Gallo RC, Moss B. Expression of the HTLV–III envelope gene by a recombinant vaccinia virus. Nature 1986; 320:535-7.

28. Hu SL, Kowalski SG, Dalrymple JM. Expression of AIDS virus envelope gene in recombinant vaccinia viruses. Nature 1986; 320:537-40.

29. Dalgleish AG, Beverley PC, Clapham PR, Crawford DH, Greaves MF, Weiss RA. The CD4 (T4) antigen is an essential component of the receptor for the AIDS retrovirus. Nature 1984; 312:763-7.

30. Klatzmann D, Champagne E, Chamaret S, Gruest J, Guetard D, Hercend T, Gluckman JC, Montagnier L. T-lymphocyte T4 molecule behaves as the receptor for human retrovirus LAV. Nature 1984; 312:767-8.

31. McDougal J, Kennedy M, Sligh J, Cort S, Mawle A, Nicholson J. The binding of HTLV–III/LAV to T4^{+} T cells by a complex of the 110 kD viral protein (gp110) and the T4 molecule. Science 1986; 231:382-5.

32. Chanh TC, Kennedy RC, Kanda P. Synthetic peptides homologous to HIV transmembrane glycoprotein suppress normal human lymphocyte blastogenic response. Cell Immunol 1988; 111:77-86.

33. Wong-Staal F, Shaw GM, Hahn BH, Salahuddin SZ, Popovic M, Markham P, Redfield R, Gallo RC. Genomic diversity of human T-lymphotropic virus type III (HTLV–III). Science 1985; 229:759-62.

34. Alizon M, Wain-Hobson S, Montagnier L, Sonigo P. Genetic variability of the AIDS virus: Nucleotide sequence analysis of two isolates from African patients. Cell 1986; 46:63-74.

35. Coffin JM. Genetic variation in AIDS viruses. Cell 1986; 46:1-4.

36. Prince AM, Pascual D, Kosolapov LB, Kurosawa D, Baker L, Rubenstein P. Prevalence, clinical significance, and strain specificity of neutralizing antibody to the human immunodeficiency virus. J Infect Dis 1987; 156:268-72.

37. Vujcic LK, Shepp DH, Klutch M, Wells MA, Hendry RM, Wittek AE, Krilov LR, Quinnan Jr GV. Prevalence and specificity of antibodies to human immunodeficiency virus (HIV) measured using a sensitive neutralization assay. J Infect Dis 1988; 157:1047-50.

38. Clavel F, Guetard D, Brun-Vezinet F, Chamaret S, Rey M-A, Santos-Ferreria MO, Laurent AG, Dauguet C, Katlama C, Rozioux C, Klatzmann D, Champalimaud JL, Montagnier L. Isolation of a new human retrovirus from West African patients with AIDS. Science 1986; 233:343-6.

39. Clavel F, Mansinho K, Chamaret S, Guetard D, Faurer V, Nina J, Santos-Ferreira MO, Champalimaud J-L, Montagnier L. Human immunodeficiency virus type 2 infection associated with AIDS in West Arica. N Engl J Med 1987; 316:1180-5.

40. Quinnan GV, Schooley R, Dolin R, Ennis FA, Gross P, Gwaltney JM. Serologic responses and systemic reactions in adults after vaccination with

monovalent A/USSR/77 and trivalent A/USSR/77, A/Texas/77, B/Hong Kong/72 influenza vaccines. Rev Infect Dis 1983; 5:723–36.

41. Townsend ARM, McMichael AJ, Carter NP, Huddleston JA, Brownlee GG. Cytotoxic T cell recognition of the influenza nucleoprotein and hemagglutinin expressed in transfected mouse L cells. Cell 1984; 39:13–25.

42. Yewdell JW, Bennick JR, Smith GL, Moss B. Influenza A virus nucleoprotein is a major target antigen for cross-reactive anti-influenza A virus cytotoxic T lymphocytes. Proc Nat Acad Sci USA 1985; 82:1785–9.

43. Holt CA, Osorio K, Lilly F. Friend virus-specific cytotoxic T lymphocytes recognize both gag and env gene-encoded specificities. J Exp Med 1986; 164:211–26.

44. Rook AH, Lane HC, Folks T, McCoy S, Alter H, Fauci AS. Sera from HTLV–III/LAV antibody positive individuals mediate andibody-dependent cellular cytotoxicity against HTLV–III/LAV infected T-cells. J Immunol 1987; 138:1064–7.

45. Kalyanaraman VS, Cabradilla CD, Getchell JP, Narayanan R, Braff EH, Chermann J-C, Barre-Sinoussi F, Montagnier L, Spira TJ, Kaplan J, Fishbein D, Jaffe HW, Curran JW, Francis DP. Antibodies to the core of lymphadenopathy-associated virus (LAV) in patients with AIDS. Science 1984; 225:321–3.

46. Lange JMA, Paul DA, Huisman HG, de Wolf F, Van der Berg H, Coutinho RA, Danner SA, Van der Noorda J, Goudsmit J. Persistent HIV antigenemia and decline of HIV core antibodies associated with transition to AIDS. Br Med J 1986; 293:1459–62.

47. Wittek AE, Phelan MA, Wells MA, Vujcic LK, Epstein JS, Lane HC, Quinnan Jr GV. Detection of human immunodeficiency virus core protein in plasma by enzyme immunoassay. Association of antigenemia with symptomatic disease and T-helper cell depletion. Ann Intern Med 1987; 107:286–92.

48. Kramer RA, Schaber MD, Skalka AM, Ganguly K, Wong-Staal F, Reddy EP. HTLV–III gag protein is processed in yeast cells by the virus pol-protease. Science 1986; 231:1580–5.

49. Zarling JM, Eichberg JW, Moran PA, McClure J, Sridhar P, Hu S-L. Proliferative and cytotoxic T cells to AIDS virus glycoproteins in chimpanzees immunized with a recombinant vaccinia virus expressing AIDS virus envelope glycoproteins. J Immunol 1987; 139:988–90.

50. Gelderblom HR, Hausmann EHS, Ozel M, Pauli G, Koch MA. Fine structure of human immunodeficiency virus (HIV) and immunolocalization of structural proteins. Virology 1987; 156:171–6.

51. Naylor PH, Naylor CW, Badamchian M, Wada S, Goldstein AL, Wang S-S, Sun DK, Thornton AH, Sarin PS. Human immunodeficiency virus contains an epitope immunoreactive with thymosin alpha$_1$ and the 30-amino acid synthetic p17 group-specific antigen peptide HGP-30. Proc Nat Acad Sci USA 1987; 84:2951–5.

52. Sarin PS, Sun DK, Thornton AH, Naylor PH, Goldstein AL. Neutrlization of HTLV–III/LAV replication by antiserum to thymosin alpha 1. Science 1986; 232:1135–7.

53. Ritter J, Septejan M, Monier JC. Lack of reactivity of anti-human immunodeficiency virus (HIV) P17/18 antibodies against al thymosin and of anti-al thymosin monoclonal antibody against P17/18 protein. Immunol Lett 16: 97–100.

54. Chen SJ, Ko HS. Serum thymosin-alpha$_1$: Lack of association between elevated levels and HIV infection. Clin Exp Immunol 1987; 70:263–7.

55. Sano K, Lee MH, Morales F, Nishanian P, Fahey J, Detels R, Imagawa DT. Antibody that inhibits human immunodeficiency virus reverse transciptase and association with inability to isolate virus. J Clin Microbiol 1987; 25:2415–7.

56. Walker BD, Flexner C, Paradis TJ, Fuller TC, Hirsch MS, Schooley RT, Moss B. HIV-1 reverse transcriptase is a target for cytotoxic T lymphocytes in infected individuals. Science 1988; 240:64–6.

57. Hizi A, McGill C, Hughes SH. Expression of soluble, enzymatically active human immunodeficiency virus reverse transcriptase in *Escherichia coli* and analysis of mutants. Proc Nat Acad Sci USA 1988; 85:1218–22.

58. Dalgleish AG, Thompson BJ, Chanh TC, Malkovsky M, Kennedy RC. Neutralisation of HIV isolates by anti-idiotypic antibodies which mimic the T4 (CD4) epitope: A potential AIDS vaccine. Lancet 1987; 2:1047–50.

59. Hsieh P, Robbins PW. Regulation of asparagine-linked oligosaccharide processing: Oligosaccharide processing in *Aedes albopictus* mosquito cells. J Biol Chem 1984; 259:2375–82.

60. Salk J. Prospects for the control of AIDS by immunizing seropositive individuals. Nature 1987; 327:473–6.

61. Hepatitis B. In *Report of the Committee on Infectious Diseases,* 20th ed. American Academy of Pediatrics, Elk Grove Village, IL, 1986, pp. 181–190.

62. Centers for Disease Control, Safety of therapeutic immune globulin preparations with respect to transmission of human T-lymphotropic virus type III/lymphadenopathy-associated virus infection, MMWR 1986; 35:231–3.

63. Centers for Disease Control, Lack of transmission of human immunodeficiency virus through Rh$_O$(D) immune globulin (human). MMWR 1987; 36:728–9.

64. Morein B, Sundquist B, Hoglund S, Dalsgaard K, Osterhaus A. Iscom, a novel structure for antigenic presentation of membrane proteins from enveloped viruses. Nature 1984; 308:457–62.

65. Audibert F, Chedid L, Lefrancier P, Choay J. Distinctive adjuvanticity of synthetic analogs of mycobacterial water soluble components. Cell Immunol 1976; 21:243–9.

66. Chedid L, Parent MA, Audibert FM, Riveau GJ, Parant FJ, Lederer E, Choay JP, Lefrancier PL. Biological activity of a new synthetic muramyl peptide adjuvant devoid of pyrogenicity. Infect Immun 1982; 35:417–24.

67. Zarling JM, Morton W, Moran PA, McClure J, Kosowski SG, Hu S-L. T-cell responses to human AIDS virus in macaques immunized with recombinant vaccinia viruses. Nature 1986; 323:344–6.

68. Hu S-L, Fultz PN, McClure HM, Eichberg JW, Thomas EK, Zarling J, Singhal MC, Kosowski SG, Swenson RB, Anderson DC, Todaro G. Effect of immunization with a vaccinia-HIV env recombinant on HIV infection in chimpanzees. Nature 1987; 328:721–3.

69. Alter HJ, Eichenberg JW, Masur H, Saxinger WC, Gallo R, Macher AM, Lane HC, Fauci AS. Transmission of HTLV–III infection from human plasma to chimpanzees: An animal model for AIDS. Science 1984; 226: 549–52.

70. Francis DP, Feorino PM, Broderson JR, McClure HM, Getchell JP, McGrath CR, Swenson B, McDougal JS, Palmer EL, Harrison AK, Barre-Sinoussi F, Chermann J-C, Montagnier L, Curran JW, Cabradilla CD, Kalyanaraman VS. Infection of chimpanzees with lymphadenopathy-associated virus. Lancet 1984; 2:1276–7.

71. Gajdusek DC, Amyx HL, Gibbs Jr CJ, Asher DM, Rodgers-Johnson P, Epstein LG, Sarin PS, Gallo RC, Maluish A, Arthur LO, Montagnier L, Mildvan D. Infection of chimpanzees by human T-lymphotropic retroviruses in brain and other tissues from AIDS patients. Lancet 1985; 1:55–6.

72. Fultz PN, McClure HM, Swenson RB, McGrath CR, Brodie A, Getchell JP, Jensen FC, Anderson DC, Broderson JR, Francis DP. Persistent infection of chimpanzees with human T-lymphotropic virus type III/lymphadenopathy-associated virus: A potential model for acquired immunodeficiency syndrome. J Virol 1986; 58:116–24.

73. Letvin NL, Daniel MD, Seghal PK, Letz JM, Solomon KR, Kannagi M, Schmidt DK, Silva DP, Montagnier L, Desrosiers RC. Infection of baboons with human immunodeficiency virus-2 (HIV-2). J Infect Dis 1987; 156: 406–7.

74. Berman PW, Groopman JE, Gregory T, Clapham PR, Weiss RA, Ferriani R, Riddle L, Shimasaki C, Lucas C, Lasky LA, Eichberg JW. Human immunodeficiency virus type 1 challenge of chimpanzees immunized with recombinant envelope glycoprotein gp120. Proc Natl Acad Sci USA 1988; 85: 5200–4.

75. Prince AM, Horowitz B, Baker L, Shulman RW, Ralph H, Valinsky J, Cundell A, Brotman B, Boehle W, Rey F, Piet M, Reesink H, Lelie N, Tersmette M, Miedema F, Barbosa L, Nemo G, Nastala CL, Langlois AJ, Allen JS, Lee DR, Eichberg JW. Failure of an HIV immune globulin to protect chimpanzees against experimental challenge with HIV. Proc Nat Acad Sci USA, 1988; 85:6944–8.

76. Letvin NL, Daniel MD, Seghal PK, Desrosiers RC, Hunt RD, Waldron LM, Mackey JJ, Schmidt DK, Chalifoux LV, King NW. Induction of AIDS-like disease in macaque monkeys with T-cell tropic retrovirus STLV–III. Science 1985; 230:71–3.

77. Code of Federal Regulation, Title 21, Part 312, section 100, U.S. Government Printing Office, Washington, D.C. 1987.
78. Centers for Disease Control, Human immunodeficiency virus infection in the United States: A review of current knowledge. MMWR 1987; 36(suppl. S-6):1–8.
79. Marwick C. HIV antibody prevalence data derived from study of Massachusetts infants. JAMA 1987; 258:171–2.
80. Clumeck N, Robert-Guroff M, Van De Perre P, Jennings A, Sibomana J, Demol P, Cran S, Gallo RC. Seroepidemiological studies of HTLV–III antibody prevalence among selected groups of heterosexual Africans. JAMA 1985; 254:2599–602.
81. Quinn TC, Mann JM, Curran JW, Piot P. AIDS in Africa: An epidemiological paradigm. Science 1986; 234:955–63.
82. Melbye M, Njelesani EK, Bayley A, Mukelabai K, Manuwele JK, Bowa FJ, Clayden SA, Levin A, Blattner WA, Weiss RA, Tedder R, Biggar RJ. Evidence for heterosexual transmission and clinical manifestations of human immunodeficiency virus infection and related conditions in Lusaka, Zambia. Lancet 1986; 2:1113–5.
83. World Health Organization, Report on informal discussions on AIDS vaccine efficacy trials in human populations, Geneva, 15–16 December, 1986, WHO Document 87.1.
84. Centers for Disease Control, Quarterly report to the Domestic Policy Council on the prevalence and rate of spread of HIV in the United States, July 26,1988.
85. Brown LS Jr, Burkett W, Primm BJ. Drug treatment and HIV seropositivity, NY State J Med 1988; 88:156–9.
86. State AIDS Reports, Number 2, State AIDS Policy Center, Washington, D.C., 1988, p. 7.
87. Mark R, Buller L, Moss B. Genetic basis for vaccinia virus virulence. In *Vaccinia viruses as vectors for vaccine antigens*, G.V. Quinnan, Jr. (Ed.). Elsevier Science Publishing Co., New York, 1985, pp. 69–75.

RECENT PROGRESS IN HIV VACCINE DEVELOPMENT

Although unsuccessful chimpanzee protection experiments (1–5) and the extensive variability of HIV (6-9) put a damper on early optimism for the possibility of vaccine development, recent progress during 1989 has shown that a vaccine may be not only possible but perhaps probable. This optimism comes from three research fronts: 1) advances in understanding HIV variability and how to design T- and B-cell memory to important determinants of the virus, 2) the first demonstration of efficacy of vaccine prototypes in lentiviral animal models, and 3) the demonstration that humans respond to certain HIV immunogens. Each of these recent advances is described in this chapter.

ANALYSIS OF DETERMINANTS RESPONSIBLE FOR PROTECTIVE IMMUNITY

An important step in HIV vaccine development has been the definition and extensive analysis of epitopes on the viral envelope protein that are likely to confer protective immunity. This type of analysis has been made possible by the advent of genetic engineering and molecular immunology and virology, and more of this type of work has been done with HIV than with any other virus. It is likely, therefore, that an HIV vaccine will be designed and constructed differently than vaccines for other viruses. Advances have been made in several directions, including an array of neutralization epitopes, T-cell epitopes that are targets for cytotoxic lymphocytes, and regions of the virus envelope that bind antibodies that mediate antibody-dependent cell cytotoxicity (ADCC). In total, nearly 20 such linear determinants have been mapped on the envelope (see Chapter 1).

The principal neutralizing determinant (PND) of HIV is situated in the third hypervariable region of the envelope, the V3 loop of the external envelope glycoprotein (gp120) (10-13). The usefulness of the PND as a vaccine candidate has been questioned because of the amino acid variability. However, recent studies in which the sequence of the PND from several hundred HIV isolates has been determined show that the sequence is less variable than originally thought (G. LaRosa et al., in preparation). In addition, there appears to be considerable pressure to conserve critical peptide sequences in the PND, and the PND may adopt particular polypeptide conformations. This could make many isolates a target for an antibody directed to a particular peptide or a polypeptide secondary structure in the PND. In addition, certain serotype classes may exist in the population (G. LaRosa et al., in preparation; J. Goudsmit, personal communication), and this may pave the way for a cocktail approach to deal with the diversity of HIV isolates in the population. It has also been found that the PND is the target for cytotoxic T lymphocytes (14,15).

Most encouraging is the finding that antibodies to the PND may protect against HIV infection in vivo. Emini and colleagues have shown that antibodies to the PND, when mixed with HIV, protect chimpanzees from HIV infection (Chapter 19). More recently, when this segment of the envelope was used to boost chimpanzees that were primed with inactivated HIV and other subunit immunogens, high titers of virus neutralizing antibodies were elicited and these appear to be responsible for protection against HIV challenge (16). Further evidence that PND antibodies may be protective is that antibodies to the PND correlate with lack of HIV transmission from infected mother to infant (17). There is still more to learn about this region of the virus before one can design an appropriate vaccine prototype. For example, other studies (18,19; G. Gray, M. White, M. Robert-Guroff, S. Putney, unpublished data) indicate that viruses can escape PND-directed neutralizing antibodies, not by altering the amino acid sequence of the PND but by harboring a mutation(s) elsewhere in the envelope. It still remains to be determined whether there are particular variants of HIV that are more infectious or that are more apt to be transmitted from donor to recipient. Such variants would be the primary focus for vaccine development.

Other neutralization targets also appear to exist on the virus envelope and one of these, situated in the transmembrane envelope (gp41), is conserved (20). This determinant has been reported to be a more potent immunogen when inserted in the VP1 neutralization determinant of poliovirus (21). Combinations of this epitope and the PND, neither of which is involved in the binding of the virus to its receptor (22,23) (so such antibodies do not have to compete against the high-affinity interaction between gp120 and CD4), are attractive as components of a vaccine prototype.

A number of determinants conferring T-cell immunity have been located on the virus envelope, core proteins, reverse transcriptase, and regulatory proteins.

T-cell helper epitopes appear to be the most plentiful, and one such site (T-1) has been linked to the PND (24). The combination of a T-cell and neutralizing B-cell determinants may allow one to avoid nonviral carrier proteins to induce high-titer neutralizing antibodies. Other T-cell determinants serve as targets for cytotoxic lymphocytes that are present in HIV-seropositive individuals (see Chapter 1). Along with a number of sites on the envelope that are targets for ADCC, a substantial arsenal is thus available with which to attack virus-infected cells. It is important to induce an immune response that acts on infected cells because: 1) natural transmission of HIV occurs with both free virus-infected cells and 2) some degree of infection of host cells may not be able to be avoided even with a vaccine that induces high neutralizing antibody titers. Thus, to be effective against these two modes of HIV transmission, a mechanism to clear the infection should be established by the vaccination regimen.

Just as determinants conferring protective immunity are being defined, epitopes of the virus that may produce such undesirable responses as immunosuppressive effects or antibodies that enhance infection are being investigated. Observations of enhancement of HIV infection have thus far been limited to in vitro experiments. It has not been documented in animal model studies of HIV or SIV vaccine testing and has been looked for and not found in humans immunized with HIV antigens (25). Nevertheless, in order to guarantee safety and maximal efficacy it will be important to eliminate any potentially harmful epitopes from vaccine prototypes.

SUCCESSFUL VIRUS CHALLENGE EXPERIMENTS WITH RELATED LENTIVIRUSES

Encouraging results have been obtained in animal model studies with simian immunodeficiency virus (SIV) (26-28), as well as with equine infectious anemia virus (EIAV) (29). In each of these experiments whole killed virus vaccines either prevented infection in some animals or delayed (or perhaps prevented as may eventually be demonstrated) the onset of disease. Notably, protection against the respective diseases caused by experimental challenge with SIV and EIAV could be achieved even in cases where actual infection by the virus was not prevented. The importance of this development is underscored with regard to HIV vaccine development because it suggests that the same general rules may apply to HIV as exist for other viruses; it may not be necessary to completely block infection in order to have a successful vaccine. If some degree of virus infection can in fact be tolerated, a vaccine against HIV will be easier to develop. It also suggests that some of the earlier studies already performed with HIV in chimpanzees (which were considered failures because infection was not prevented) might have had a more favorable outcome had a disease endpoint been available for study.

That is not to say that one should not strive to develop mechanisms to clear the virus. In this regard, studies showed evidence of protection in chimps against HIV challenge using an inactivated whole virus vaccine (30). In related studies a surprising result was seen when whole killed virus was administered to two animals previously infected with HIV, with the result that the virus was apparently cleared. Postexposure immunization in man with the same preparation has also been studied, although the results are still equivocal (31). However, long-term studies initiated in 1986 and still in progress using autologous cells expressing HIV envelope have shown positive therapeutic effects in patients with AIDS and include elevation of CD4 lymphocyte levels (D. Zagury et al., personal communication). Taken together, these results suggest that the immune system can be harnessed to protect humans from HIV infection and perhaps to affect the course of disease. From the animal model studies it should now be possible to define more precisely the nature and elements responsible for the protective immunity achieved.

Although such animal studies are important for providing concepts and strategies for vaccine development, none of these models precisely mimics the host-virus relationship of HIV and humans. In this regard, there are also other retrovirus models from which vaccine concepts have emerged and where there has also been recent success, notably with feline leukemia virus (E. Hoover, personal communication; D. Marciani, personal communication) and bovine leukemia virus (32). However, to bridge the gap between HIV and these animal models, one might look toward developments with animal models using HIV instead of related lentiviruses [such as the SCID-Hu mice (33,34)]. If such mice, which contain parts of the human immune system and can be infected with HIV, can be shown to generate human immune responses to the virus, their value for vaccine development would be considerable.

SUMMARY

These encouraging steps notwithstanding, there remain challenges standing before the development of an HIV vaccine. Ways to present HIV antigens to the immune system that will evoke protective humoral and cellular immunity are still being perfected. Much more has to be done to develop safe and effective adjuvants or constructions of innocuous replicating vectors into which protective HIV target determinants can be incorporated. It may also be necessary to induce secretory immunity to protect against transmission of HIV across mucosal surfaces. Even though such studies are in their infancy, considerable promise exists, particularly in approaches in which priming is achieved with a replicating vector followed by boosting with a subunit immunogen. As reported recently (35), this gives rise to elevated levels of T-cell immunity and increased antibody production. This partly parallels the studies by Girard and colleagues mentioned above which achieved protective immunity in chimpanzees (16).

Nevertheless, the most formidable barrier will be the evaluation of efficacy of a vaccine candidate in humans. This is due to such potential problems as the low attack rate of HIV infection and the long and variable interval between infection and disease (36). Safety and efficacy testing will thus be difficult to assess critically, particularly if the primary effect of the vaccine will be to delay or reduce disease symptoms rather than prevent infection. Finally, one must be concerned about the availability of an acceptable number of volunteers for vaccine trials. It is thus likely that restrictions will have to be placed on the number of vaccine candidates that can be tested in humans, and these may be limited to those showing efficacy and acceptable safety in chimpanzee studies or other animal models or for which there are other compelling reasons for testing in humans to occur (37). As research into the immunology of HIV progresses, such candidates will hopefully be forthcoming.

Scott D. Putney
Dani P. Bolognesi

REFERENCES

1. Berman PW, Groopman JE, Gregory T, Clapham PR, Weiss RA, Ferriani R, Riddle L, Shimasaski C, Lucas C, Lasky LA, Eichberg JW. Human immunodeficiency virus type 1 challenge of chimpanzees immunized with recombinant envelope glycoprotein gp120. Proc Natl Acad Sci USA 1988; 85:5200–4.

2. Kennedy RC, Kanda P, Dressman GR, Eichberg JW, Chanh TC. Properties of synthetic peptides that identify neutralizing epitopes on the HIV envelope glycoprotein. In: Chanock, Lerner, Brown, Ginsberg, eds. Vaccines '87. 1987 Cold Spring Harbor Laboratory, Cold Spring Harbor.

3. Hu SL, Fultz PN, McClure HM, Eichberg JW, Thomas EK, Zarling J, Singhal MC, Kosowski SG, Swenson RB, Anderson DC, Todaro G. Effect of immunization with a vaccinia-HIV *env* recombinant on HIV infection of chimpanzees. Nature 1987; 328:721–3.

4. Arthur LO, Bess JW, Waters DJ, Pyle SW, Kelliher JC, Nara PL, Krohn K, Robey WG, Langlois AJ, Gallo RC, Fischinger PJ. Challenge of chimpanzees (*Pan troglodytes*) immunized with human immunodeficiency virus envelope glycoprotein gp120. J Virol 1989; 63:5046–53.

5. Prince AM, Horowitz B, Baker L, Shulman RW, Ralph H, Valinsky J, Cundell A, Brotman B, Boehle W, Rey F, Piet M, Reesink H, Lelie N, Tersmette M, Miedema F, Barbosa L, Nemo G, Nastala CL, Allan JS, Lee DR, Eichberg JW. Failure of a human immunodeficiency virus (HIV) immune globulin to

protect chimpanzees against experimental challenge with HIV. Proc Natl Acad Sci USA 1988; 85:6944–8.

6. Starcich DH, Hahn BH, Shaw GM, McNeely PD, Modrow S, Wolf H, Parks ES, Parks WP, Josephs SF, Gallo RC, Wong-Staal F. Identification and characterization of conserved and variable regions in the envelope gene of HTLV–III/LAV, the retrovirus of AIDS. Cell 1986; 45:637–48.

7. Fisher AG, Ensoli B, Looney D, Rose A, Gallo RC, Saag MS, Shaw GM, Hahn BH, Wong-Staal F. Biologically diverse molecular variants within a single HIV-1 isolate. Nature 1988;334:444-7.

8. Hahn BH, Shaw GM, Taylor ME, Redfield RR, Markham PD, Salahuddin SZ, Wong-Staal F, Gallo RC, Park ES, Parks WP. Genetic variation in HTLV-III/LAV over time in patients with AIDS or at risk for AIDS. Science 1986; 232:1548–53.

9. Saag MS, Hahn BH, Gibbons J, Li Y, Parks ES, Parks WP, Shaw GM. Extensive variation of human immunodeficiency virus type-1 *in vivo*. Nature 1988; 334:440–4.

10. Putney SD, Matthews TJ, Robey WG, Lynn DL, Robert-Guroff M, Mueller WT, Langlois AJ, Ghrayeb J, Petteway, Jr. SR, Weinhold KJ, Fischinger PJ, Wong-Staal F, Gallo RC, Bolognesi DP. HTLV–III/LAV-neutralizing antibodies to an *E. coli*-produced fragment of the virus envelope. Science 1986; 234:1392–5.

11. Rusche JR, Javaherian K, McDanal C, Petro J, Lynn DL, Grimaila R, Langlois AJ, Gallo RC, Arthur LO, Fischinger PJ, Bolognesi DP, Putney SD, Matthews TJ. Antibodies that inhibit fusion of human immunodeficiency virus-infected cells bind a 24-amino acid sequence of the viral envelope, gp120. Proc Natl Acad Sci USA 1988; 85:3198–202.

12. Palker TJ, Clark ME, Langlois AJ, Matthews TJ, Weinhold KJ, Randall RR, Bolognesi DP, Haynes BF. Type-specific neutralization of the human immunodeficiency virus with antibodies to env-encoded synthetic peptides. Proc Natl Acad Sci USA 1988; 85:1–5.

13. Goudsmit J, Debouck C, Meloen RH, Smit L, Bakker M, Asher DM, Wolff AV, Gibbs CJ, Gajdusek DC. Human immunodeficiency virus type 1 neutralization epitope with conserved architecture elicits early type-specific antibodies in experimentally infected chimpanzees. Proc Natl Acad Sci USA 1988; 85:4478–82.

14. Takahashi H, Cohen J, Hosmalin A, Cease KB, Houghton R, Cornette JL, DeLisi C, Moss B, Germain RN, Berzofsky JA. An immunodeficiency epitope of the human immunodeficiency virus envelope glycoprotein gp160 recognized by class I major histocompatibility complex molecule-restricted murine cytotoxic T lymphocytes. Proc Natl Acad Sci USA 1988; 85: 3105–9.

15. Takahashi H, Merli S, Putney SD, Houghten R, Moss B, Germain RN, Berzofsky JA. A single amino acid interchange yields reciprocal CTL specificities for HIV-1 gp160. Science 1989; 246:118–21.

16. Girard M, Fultz P, Kleny MP, Yagello M, Desiandres A, Muchmore E, Pinter A, Nara P, Ronco J, Barre-Sinoussi F, Lecocq JP, Gluckman JC. Presented in Quatrième Colloque Des Cent Gardes, Paris, Oct. 26–28, 1989.

17. Rossi P, Moschese V, Broliden PA, Fundaro C, Quinti I, Plebani A, Giaquinto C, Tovo PA, Ljunggren K, Rosen J, Wigzell H, Jondal M, Wahren B. Presence of maternal antibodies to human immunodeficiency virus 1 envelope glycoprotein gp120 epitopes correlates with the uninfected status of children born to seropositive mothers. Proc Natl Acad Sci USA 1989; 86: 8055–8.

18. McKeating JA, Gow J, Goudsmit J, Mulder C, McClure J, Weiss R. Monoclonal antibody selection of HIV neutralization resistant mutants. In: Retro Human AIDS and Related Animal Diseases. 1988:159–64.

19. Nara P, Dunlop N, Waters D, Smit L, Goudsmit J, Gallo RC. Vth International Conference on AIDS, Montreal, Canada, June 1989 (abstr. T.C.O. 22).

20. Chahn TL, Dreesman GR, Kanda P. Induction of anti-HIV neutralizing antibodies by synthetic peptides. EMBO J 1986; 5:3065.

21. Evans DJ, McKeating J, Meredith JM, Burke KL, Katrak K, John A, Ferguson M, Minor PD, Weiss RA, Almond JW. An engineered poliovirus chimaera elicits broadly reactive HIV-1 neutralizing antibodies. Nature 1989; 339:385.

22. Skinner MA, Langlois AJ, McDanal CB, McDougal JS, Bolognesi DP, Matthews TJ. Serum from HIV infected humans prevents gp120 binding to CD4 and this activity is not elicited in animals immunized with envelope protein components. J Virol 1988; 62:4195–200.

23. Linsley PS, Ledbetter JA, Kinney-Thomas E, Hu SL. Effects of anti-gp120 monoclonal antibodies on CD4 receptor binding by the *env* protein of human immunodeficiency virus type 1. J Virol 1988; 62:3695–702.

24. Palker TJ, Matthews TJ, Langlois A, Tanner ME, Martin ME, Scearce RM, Kim JE, Berzofsky JA, Bolognesi DP, Haynes BF. Polyvalent human immunodeficiency virus synthetic immunogen comprised of envelope gp120 T helper cell sites and B cell neutralization epitopes. J Immunology 1989; 142:3612–9.

25. Bernard J, Reveil B, Najman I, Liautaud-Roger F, Fouchard M, Picard O, Cattan A, Mabondzo A, Laverne S, Gallo RC, Zagury D. Discrimination between protective and enhancing HIV antibodies. AIDS Res Human Retro 1990, in press.

26. Desrosiers RC, Wyand MS, Kodama T, Ringler DJ, Arthur LO, Sehgal PK, Letvin NL, King NW, Daniel MD. Vaccine protection against simian immunodeficiency virus infection. Proc Natl Acad Sci USA 1989; 83:6353–7.

27. Murphy-Corb M, Martin LN, Davison-Fairburn B, Montelaro RC, Miller M, West M, Ohkawa S, Baskin GB, Zhang J, Putney SD, Allison AC, Eppstein DA. A formalin-inactivated whole SIV vaccine confers protection in macaques. Science 1989; 246:1293–7.

28. Sutjipto S, Pedersen N, Gardner MB, Hanson CV, Miller C, Gettie A. J. Vth International Conference on AIDS, Montreal, Canada, June 1989 (abstr. C.Th.C.O. 45).
29. Montelaro R, Issel CJ. Immunologic management of EIAV: Evaluation of protective immune responses in ponies after experimental infection or after vaccination with inactivated virus. Meeting of the Laboratory of Tumor Cell Biology, Bethesda, Maryland, Aug. 21–26, 1989.
30. Gibbs CJ, Mora C, Peters R, Jensen FC, Carlo DJ, Salk J. Vth International Conference on AIDS, Montreal, Canada, June 1989 (abstr. C.Th.C.O. 46).
31. Levine A, Henderson BE, Groshen S, Peters R, Shepard HW, Salk J. Vth International Conference on AIDS, Montreal, Canada, June 1989 (abstr. B.Th.B.O. 44).
32. Portetelle D, Burny A, Desmettre P, Mammerickx M, Paoletti E. Development of a specific serological test and an efficient subunit vaccine to control bovine leukemia virus infection. The International Association of Biological Standardization, in press.
33. McCune JM, Namikawa R, Kaneshima H, Shultz LD, Lieberman M, Weissman IL. The SCID-Hu mouse: Murine model for the analysis of human hematolymphoid differentiation and function. Science 1988;241:1632-9.
34. Mosier DE, Gulizia RJ, Baird SM, Wilson DB. Transfer of a functional human immune system to mice with severe combined immunodeficiency. Nature 1988;335:256-9.
35. Corey L. Immunization with subunit protein enhances immune response elicited by live virus immunization. 2d Annual Meeting of the National Cooperative Vaccine Development Group for AIDS, Fort Lauderdale, Florida, Oct. 15–18, 1989.
36. Koff WC, Hoth DF. Development and testing of AIDS vaccines. Science 1988;241:426.
37. Guidelines for Phase I Evaluations: Guidelines for the Selection of Immunogens Proposed as Candidate AIDS/HIV Vaccine for Evaluation by the AIDS Vaccine Clinical Trials Network, 1989.

INDEX

ABOUT THE EDITORS

Scott D. Putney is Vice President and Director of Molecular Biology at Repligen Corporation in Cambridge, Massachusetts. He has directed Repligen's AIDS vaccine project since its inception in 1984. The author or coauthor of more than 8 publications, he collaborates with many leading international experts on HIV research. Dr. Putney received dual B.S. (biology) and B.A. (chemistry) degrees in 1976 from the University of California, Irvine, and the Ph.D. degree (1981) in chemistry from the Massachusetts Institute of Technology, where he also served as a postdoctoral fellow from 1981 to 1983.

Dani P. Bolognesi is the James B. Duke Professor of Surgery and Professor of Microbiology and Immunology at the Duke University Medical Center in Durham, North Carolina, where he has taught since 1971. The author or coauthor of some 240 articles, book chapters, and proceedings papers, he has edited one book, *Human Retroviruses, Cancer, and AIDS*. He is editor-in-chief of the journal *AIDS Research and Human Retroviruses* and serves on many professional committees, including the NIH AIDS Policy Advisory Committee, the National Cancer Institute's AIDS Task Force, and the National Institute of Allergy and Infectious Diseases' AIDS Drug Selection and AIDS Vaccine Selection Committees. He is a member of the American Society for Virology, Sigma Xi, the American Society for Microbiology, and the American Association for the Advancement of Science. Professor Bolognesi received the B.S. (biology, 1963) and M.S. (virology, 1965) degrees from Rensselaer Polytechnic Institute, and the Ph.D. degree (virology, 1967) from Duke University.